HEALTH AND HUMAN DEVELOPMENT

ALTERNATIVE MEDICINE RESEARCH YEARBOOK 2017

HEALTH AND HUMAN DEVELOPMENT
JOAV MERRICK - SERIES EDITOR
NATIONAL INSTITUTE OF CHILD HEALTH
AND HUMAN DEVELOPMENT,
MINISTRY OF SOCIAL AFFAIRS, JERUSALEM

Alternative Medicine Research Yearbook 2017
Joav Merrick (Editor)
2018. ISBN: 978-1-53613-726-2 (Hardcover)
2018. ISBN: 978-1-53613-727-9 (eBook)

Clinical Art Psychotherapy with War Veterans
Alexander Kopytin and Alexey Lebedev
2018. ISBN. 978-1-53612-975-5 (Softcover)

Cancer and Exercise
Leila Malek, Fiona Lim, Bo Angela Wan, Patrick L Diaz, Edward Chow, Joav Merrick (Editors)
2018. ISBN: 978-1-53612-747-8

Brennan Healing Science: An Integrative Approach to Therapeutic Intervention
Nina Koren, Muriel Moreno and Joav Merrick (Editors)
2018. ISBN: 978-1-53612-825-3

Palliative Care: Oncology Experience from Hong Kong
Louisa Cheuk-Yu Lui, Kam-Hung Wong, Rebecca Yeung, Joav Merrick (Editors)
2017. ISBN: 978-1-53612-397-5

Psychosocial Needs: Success in Life and Career Planning
Daniel TL Shek, Janet TY Leung, Tak Y Lee and Joav Merrick (Editors)
2017. ISBN: 978-1-53611-951-0 (Hardcover)
2017. ISBN: 978-1-53611-971-8 (eBook)

Cannabis: Medical Aspects
Blair Henry, Arnav Agarwal, Edward Chow, Hatim A Omar, and Joav Merrick (Editors)
2017. ISBN: 978-1-53610-510-0 (Hardcover)
2017. ISBN: 978-1-53610-522-3 (eBook)

Palliative Care: Psychosocial and Ethical Considerations
Blair Henry, Arnav Agarwal, Edward Chow, and Joav Merrick (Editors)
2017. ISBN: 978-1-53610-607-7 (Hardcover)
2017. ISBN: 978-1-53610-611-4 (eBook)

Oncology: The Promising Future of Biomarkers
Anthony Furfari, George S Charames, Rachel McDonald, Leigha Rowbottom, Azar Azad, Stephanie Chan, Bo Angela Wan, Ronald Chow, Carlo DeAngelis, Pearl Zaki, Edward Chow and Joav Merrick (Editors)
2017. ISBN: 978-1-53610-608-4 (Hardcover)
2017. ISBN: 978-1-53610-610-7 (eBook)

Public Health Yearbook 2016
Joav Merrick (Editor)
2017. ISBN: 978-1-53610-947-4 (Hardcover)
2017. ISBN: 978-1-53610-956-6 (eBook)

Alternative Medicine Research Yearbook 2016
Joav Merrick (Editor)
2017. ISBN: 978-1-53610-972-6 (Hardcover)
2017. ISBN: 978-1-53611-000-5 (eBook)

Pain Management Yearbook 2016
Joav Merrick (Editor)
2017. ISBN: 978-1-53610-949-8 (Hardcover)
2017. ISBN: 978-1-53610-959-7 (eBook)

Medical Cannabis: Clinical Practice
Shannon O'Hearn, Alexia Blake,
Bo Angela Wan, Stephanie Chan,
Edward Chow and Joav Merrick (Editors)
2017. ISBN: 978-1-53611-907-7 (Softcover)
2017. ISBN: 978-1-53611-927-5 (eBook)

Cancer: Treatment, Decision Making and Quality of Life
Breanne Lechner, Ronald Chow,
Natalie Pulenzas, Marko Popovic, Na Zhang,
Xiaojing Zhang, Edward Chow,
and Joav Merrick (Editors)
2016. ISBN: 978-1-63483-863-4 (Hardcover)
2015. ISBN: 978-1-63483-882-5 (eBook)

Cancer: Bone Metastases, CNS Metastases and Pathological Fractures
Breanne Lechner, Ronald Chow,
Natalie Pulenzas, Marko Popovic, Na Zhang,
Xiaojing Zhang, Edward Chow,
and Joav Merrick (Editors)
2016. ISBN: 978-1-63483-949-5 (Hardcover)
2015. ISBN: 978-1-63483-960-0 (eBook)

Cancer: Spinal Cord, Lung, Breast, Cervical, Prostate, Head and Neck Cancer
Breanne Lechner, Ronald Chow,
Natalie Pulenzas, Marko Popovic, Na Zhang,
Xiaojing Zhang, Edward Chow
and Joav Merrick (Editors)
2016. ISBN: 978-1-63483-904-4 (Hardcover)
2015. ISBN: 978-1-63483-911-2 (eBook)

Cancer: Survival, Quality of Life and Ethical Implications
Breanne Lechner, Ronald Chow,
Natalie Pulenzas, Marko Popovic, Na Zhang,
Xiaojing Zhang, Edward Chow
and Joav Merrick (Editors)
2016. ISBN: 978-1-63483-905-1 (Hardcover)
2015. ISBN: 978-1-63483-912-9 (eBook)

Cancer: Pain and Symptom Management
Breanne Lechner, Ronald Chow,
Natalie Pulenzas, Marko Popovic, Na Zhang,
Xiaojing Zhang, Edward Chow,
and Joav Merrick (Editors)
2016. ISBN: 978-1-63483-905-1 (Hardcover)
2015. ISBN: 978-1-63483-881-8 (eBook)

Alternative Medicine Research Yearbook 2015
Joav Merrick (Editor)
2016. ISBN: 978-1-63484-511-3 (Hardcover)
2016. ISBN: 978-1-63484-542-7 (eBook)

Public Health Yearbook 2015
Joav Merrick (Editor)
2016. ISBN: 978-1-63484-511-3 (Hardcover)
2016. ISBN: 978-1-63484-546-5 (eBook)

Quality, Mobility and Globalization in the Higher Education System: A Comparative Look at the Challenges of Academic Teaching
Nitza Davidovitch, Zehavit Gross,
Yuri Ribakov, and Anna Slobodianiuk
(Editors)
2016. ISBN: 978-1-63484-986-9 (Hardcover)
2016. ISBN: 978-1-63485-012-4 (eBook)

**Alternative Medicine Research
Yearbook 2014**
Joav Merrick (Editor)
2015. ISBN: 978-1-63482-161-2 (Hardcover)
2015. ISBN: 978-1-63482-205-3 (eBook)

Pain Management Yearbook 2014
Joav Merrick (Editor)
2015. ISBN: 978-1-63482-164-3 (Hardcover)
2015. ISBN: 978-1-63482-208-4 (eBook)

Public Health Yearbook 2014
Joav Merrick (Editor)
2015. ISBN: 978-1-63482-165-0 (Hardcover)
2015. ISBN: 978-1-63482-209-1 (eBook)

**Forensic Psychiatry:
A Public Health Perspective**
Leo Sher and Joav Merrick (Editors)
2015. ISBN: 978-1-63483-339-4 (Hardcover)
2015. ISBN: 978-1-63483-346-2 (eBook)

**Leadership and Service Learning
Education: Holistic Development
for Chinese University Students**
*Daniel TL Shek, Florence KY Wu
and Joav Merrick (Editors)*
2015. ISBN: 978-1-63483-340-0 (Hardcover)
2015. ISBN: 978-1-63483-347-9 (eBook)

**Mental and Holistic Health:
Some International Perspectives**
*Joseph L Calles Jr, Donald E Greydanus,
and Joav Merrick (Editors)*
2015. ISBN: 978-1-63483-589-3 (Hardcover)
2015. ISBN: 978-1-63483-608-1 (eBook)

**India: Health and Human
Development Aspects**
Joav Merrick (Editor)
2014. ISBN: 978-1-62948-784-7 (Hardcover)
2014. ISBN: 978-1-62948-794-6 (eBook)

**Alternative Medicine Research
Yearbook 2013**
Joav Merrick (Editor)
2014. ISBN: 978-1-63321-094-3 (Hardcover)
2014. ISBN: 978-1-63321-144-5 (eBook)

**Health Consequences of Human
Central Obesity**
*Kaushik Bose and Raja Chakraborty
(Editors)*
2014. ISBN: 978-1-63321-152-0 (Hardcover)
2014. ISBN: 978-1-63321-181-0 (eBook)

Public Health Yearbook 2013
Joav Merrick (Editor)
2014. ISBN: 978-1-63321-095-0 (Hardcover)
2014. ISBN: 978-1-63321-097-4 (eBook)

**Public Health: Improving Health via
Inter-Professional Collaborations**
*Rosemary M Caron and Joav Merrick
(Editors)*
2014. ISBN: 978-1-63321-569-6 (Hardcover)
2014. ISBN: 978-1-63321-594-8 (eBook)

**Textbook on Evidence-Based Holistic
Mind-Body Medicine: Holistic Practice
of Traditional Hippocratic Medicine**
Søren Ventegodt and Joav Merrick
2013. ISBN: 978-1-62257-105-5 (Hardcover)
2012. ISBN: 978-1-62257-174-1 (eBook)

**Textbook on Evidence-Based Holistic
Mind-Body Medicine: Healing the Mind
in Traditional Hippocratic Medicine**
Søren Ventegodt and Joav Merrick
2013. ISBN: 978-1-62257-112-3 (Hardcover)
2012. ISBN: 978-1-62257-175-8 (eBook)

**Textbook on Evidence-Based Holistic
Mind-Body Medicine: Sexology and
Traditional Hippocratic Medicine**
Søren Ventegodt and Joav Merrick
2013. ISBN: 978-1-62257-130-7 (Hardcover)
2012. ISBN: 978-1-62257-176-5 (eBook)

**Health and Happiness
from Meaningful Work:
Research in Quality of Working Life**
Søren Ventegodt and Joav Merrick (Editors)
2013. ISBN: 978-1-60692-820-2 (Hardcover)
2009. ISBN: 978-1-61324-981-9 (eBook)

**Conceptualizing Behavior in Health
and Social Research:
A Practical Guide to Data Analysis**
Said Shahtahmasebi and Damon Berridge
2013. ISBN: 978-1-60876-383-2 (Hardcover)
2013. ISBN: 978-1-53611-212-2 (eBook)

Adolescence and Sports
*Dilip R Patel, Donald E Greydanus,
Hatim Omar and Joav Merrick (Editors)*
2013. ISBN: 978-1-60876-702-1 (Hardcover)
2010. ISBN: 978-1-61761-483-5 (eBook)

**Pediatric and Adolescent Sexuality
and Gynecology: Principles for the
Primary Care Clinician**
*Hatim A Omar, Donald E Greydanus,
Artemis K. Tsitsika, Dilip R. Patel
and Joav Merrick (Editors)*
2013. ISBN: 978-1-60876-735-9 (Softcover)

**Human Development: Biology
from a Holistic Point of View**
*Søren Ventegodt, Tyge Dahl Hermansen
and Joav Merrick*
2013. ISBN: 978-1-61470-441-6 (Hardcover)
2011. ISBN: 978-1-61470-541-3 (eBook)

**Building Community Capacity: Case
Examples from Around the World**
*Rosemary M Caron and Joav Merrick
(Editors)*
2013. ISBN: 978-1-62417-175-8 (Hardcover)
2013. ISBN: 978-1-62417-176-5 (eBook)

Managed Care in a Public Setting
Richard Evan Steele
2013. ISBN: 978-1-62417-970-9 (Softcover)
2013. ISBN: 978-1-62417-863-4 (eBook)

Bullying: A Public Health Concern
*Jorge C Srabstein and Joav Merrick
(Editors)*
2013. ISBN: 978-1-62618-564-7 (Hardcover)
2013. ISBN: 978-1-62618-588-3 (eBook)

**Bedouin Health: Perspectives
from Israel**
*Joav Merrick, Alean Al-Krenami
and Salman Elbedour (Editors)*
2013. ISBN: 978-1-62948-271-2 (Hardcover)
2013: ISBN: 978-1-62948-274-3 (eBook)

**Health Promotion: Community Singing
as a Vehicle to Promote Health**
*Jing Sun, Nicholas Buys and Joav Merrick
(Editors)*
2013. ISBN: 978-1-62618-908-9 (Hardcover)
2013: ISBN: 978-1-62808-006-3 (eBook)

Public Health Yearbook 2012
Joav Merrick (Editor)
2013. ISBN: 978-1-62808-078-0 (Hardcover)
2013: ISBN: 978-1-62808-079-7 (eBook)

**Alternative Medicine Research
Yearbook 2012**
Joav Merrick (Editor)
2013. ISBN: 978-1-62808-080-3 (Hardcover)
2013: ISBN: 978-1-62808-079-7 (eBook)

**Advanced Cancer: Managing Symptoms
and Quality of Life**
*Natalie Pulenzas, Breanne Lechner,
Nemica Thavarajah, Edward Chow,
and Joav Merrick (Editors)*
2013. ISBN: 978-1-62808-239-5 (Hardcover)
2013: ISBN: 978-1-62808-267-8 (eBook)

**Treatment and Recovery
of Eating Disorders**
Daniel Stein and Yael Latzer (Editors)
2013. ISBN: 978-1-62808-248-7 (Softcover)

**Health Promotion: Strengthening
Positive Health and Preventing Disease**
*Jing Sun, Nicholas Buys and Joav Merrick
(Editors)*
2013. ISBN: 978-1-62257-870-2 (Hardcover)
2013: ISBN: 978-1-62808-621-8 (eBook)

Pain Management Yearbook 2011
Joav Merrick (Editor)
2013. ISBN: 978-1-62808-970-7 (Hardcover)
2013: ISBN: 978-1-62808-971-4 (eBook)

Pain Management Yearbook 2012
Joav Merrick (Editor)
2013. ISBN: 978-1-62808-973-8 (Hardcover)
2013: ISBN: 978-1-62808-974-5 (eBook)

Suicide from a Public Health Perspective
Said Shahtahmasebi and Joav Merrick
2013. ISBN: 978-1-62948-536-2 (Hardcover)
2014: ISBN: 978-1-62948-537-9 (eBook)

Food, Nutrition and Eating Behavior
Joav Merrick and Sigal Israeli (Editors)
2013. ISBN: 978-1-62948-233-0 (Hardcover)
2013: ISBN: 978-1-62948-234-7 (eBook)

**Public Health Concern:
Smoking, Alcohol and Substance Use**
Joav Merrick and Ariel Tenenbaum (Editors)
2013. ISBN: 978-1-62948-424-2 (Hardcover)
2013. ISBN: 978-1-62948-430-3 (eBook)

**Mental Health from an International
Perspective**
*Joav Merrick, Shoshana Aspler
and Mohammed Morad (Editors)*
2013. ISBN: 978-1-62948-519-5 (Hardcover)
2013. ISBN: 978-1-62948-520-1 (eBook)

**Adolescence and Chronic Illness.
A Public Health Concern**
*Hatim Omar, Donald E Greydanus,
Dilip R Patel
and Joav Merrick (Editors)*
2012. ISBN: 978-1-60876-628-4 (Hardcover)
2010. ISBN: 978-1-61761-482-8 (eBook)

**Child and Adolescent Health
Yearbook 2009**
Joav Merrick (Editor)
2012. ISBN: 978-1-61668-913-1 (Hardcover)
2012. ISBN: 978-1-62257-095-9 (eBook)

**Child and Adolescent Health
Yearbook 2010**
Joav Merrick (Editor)
2012. ISBN: 978-1-61209-788-6 (Hardcover)
2012. ISBN: 978-1-62417-046-1 (eBook)

**Child Health and Human Development
Yearbook 2010**
Joav Merrick (Editor)
2012. ISBN: 978-1-61209-789-3 (Hardcover)
2012. ISBN: 978-1-62081-721-6 (eBook)

Public Health Yearbook 2010
Joav Merrick (Editor)
2012. ISBN: 978-1-61209-971-2 (Hardcover)
2012. ISBN: 978-1-62417-863-4 (eBook)

Alternative Medicine Yearbook 2010
Joav Merrick (Editor)
2012. ISBN: 978-1-62100-132-4 (Hardcover)
2011. ISBN: 978-1-62100-210-9 (eBook)

**The Astonishing Brain and Holistic
Consciousness: Neuroscience and
Vedanta Perspectives**
Vinod D Deshmukh
2012. ISBN: 978-1-61324-295-7

Health Risk Communication
Marijke Lemal and Joav Merrick (Editors)
2012. ISBN: 978-1-62257-544-2 (Hardcover)
2012. ISBN: 978-1-62257-552-7 (eBook)

**Translational Research
for Primary Healthcare**
*Erica Bell, Gert P Westert
and Joav Merrick (Editors)*
2012. ISBN: 978-1-61324-647-4 (Hardcover)
2012. ISBN: 978-1-62417-409-4 (eBook)

**Our Search for Meaning in Life:
Quality of Life Philosophy**
Søren Ventegodt and Joav Merrick
2012. ISBN: 978-1-61470-494-2 (Hardcover)
2011. ISBN: 978-1-61470-519-2 (eBook)

**Randomized Clinical Trials
and Placebo: Can You Trust
the Drugs are Working and Safe?**
Søren Ventegodt and Joav Merrick
2012. ISBN: 978-1-61470-067-8 (Hardcover)
2011. ISBN: 978-1-61470-151-4 (eBook)

**Building Community Capacity:
Minority and Immigrant Populations**
*Rosemary M Caron and Joav Merrick
(Editors)*
2012. ISBN: 978-1-62081-022-4 (Hardcover)
2012. ISBN: 978-1-62081-032-3 (eBook)

**Applied Public Health: Examining
Multifaceted Social or Ecological
Problems and Child Maltreatment**
John R Lutzker and Joav Merrick (Editors)
2012. ISBN: 978-1-62081-356-0 (Hardcover)
2012. ISBN: 978-1-62081-388-1 (eBook)

**Treatment and Recovery
of Eating Disorders**
Daniel Stein and Yael Latzer (Editors)
2012. ISBN: 978-1-61470-259-7 (Hardcover)
2012. ISBN: 978-1-61470-418-8 (eBook)

**Human Immunodeficiency Virus (HIV)
Research: Social Science Aspects**
Hugh Klein and Joav Merrick (Editors)
2012. ISBN: 978-1-62081-293-8 (Hardcover)
2012. ISBN: 978-1-62081-346-1 (eBook)

**AIDS and Tuberculosis: Public
Health Aspects**
Daniel Chemtob and Joav Merrick (Editors)
2012. ISBN: 978-1-62081-382-9 (Softcover)
2012. ISBN: 978-1-62081-406-2 (eBook)

Public Health Yearbook 2011
Joav Merrick (Editor)
2012. ISBN: 978-1-62081-433-8 (Hardcover)
2012. ISBN: 978-1-62081-434-5 (eBook)

**Alternative Medicine Research
Yearbook 2011**
Joav Merrick (Editor)
2012. ISBN: 978-1-62081-476-5 (Hardcover)
2012. ISBN: 978-1-62081-477-2 (eBook)

**Building Community Capacity: Skills
and Principles**
*Rosemary M Caron and Joav Merrick
(Editors)*
2012. ISBN: 978-1-61209-331-4 (Hardcover)
2012. ISBN: 978-1-62257-238-0 (eBook)

**Textbook on Evidence-Based Holistic
Mind-Body Medicine: Basic Principles
of Healing in Traditional Hippocratic
Medicine**
Søren Ventegodt and Joav Merrick
2012. ISBN: 978-1-62257-094-2 (Hardcover)
2012. ISBN: 978-1-62257-172-7 (eBook)

**Textbook on Evidence-Based Holistic
Mind-Body Medicine: Basic Philosophy
and Ethics of Traditional Hippocratic
Medicine**
Søren Ventegodt and Joav Merrick
2012. ISBN: 978-1-62257-052-2 (Hardcover)
2013. ISBN: 978-1-62257-707-1 (eBook)

Textbook on Evidence-Based Holistic Mind-Body Medicine: Research, Philosophy, Economy and Politics of Traditional Hippocratic Medicine
Søren Ventegodt and Joav Merrick
2012. ISBN: 978-1-62257-140-6 (Hardcover)
2012. ISBN: 978-1-62257-171-0 (eBook)

Behavioral Pediatrics, 3rd Edition
Donald E Greydanus, Dilip R Patel, Helen D Pratt and Joseph L Calles, Jr (Editors)
2011. ISBN: 978-1-60692-702-1 (Hardcover)
2009. ISBN: 978-1-60876-630-7 (eBook)

Rural Child Health: International Aspects
Erica Bell and Joav Merrick (Editors)
2011. ISBN: 978-1-60876-357-3 (Hardcover)
2011. ISBN: 978-1-61324-005-2 (eBook)

International Aspects of Child Abuse and Neglect
Howard Dubowitz and Joav Merrick (Editors)
2011. ISBN: 978-1-60876-703-8 (Hardcover)
2010. ISBN: 978-1-61122-049-0 (Softcover)
2010. ISBN: 978-1-61122-403-0 (eBook)

Environment, Mood Disorders and Suicide
Teodor T Postolache and Joav Merrick (Editors)
2011. ISBN: 978-1-61668-505-8 (Hardcover)
2011. ISBN: 978-1-62618-340-7 (eBook)

Positive Youth Development: Evaluation and Future Directions in a Chinese Context
Daniel TL Shek, Hing Keung Ma and Joav Merrick (Editors)
2011. ISBN: 978-1-60876-830-1 (Hardcover)
2011. ISBN: 978-1-62100-175-1 (Softcover)
2010. ISBN: 978-1-61209-091-7 (eBook)

Understanding Eating Disorders: Integrating Culture, Psychology and Biology
Yael Latzer, Joav Merrick and Daniel Stein (Editors)
2011. ISBN: 978-1-61728-298-0 (Hardcover)
2011. ISBN: 978-1-61470-976-3 (Softcover)
2011. ISBN: 978-1-61942-054-0 (eBook)

Advanced Cancer Pain and Quality of Life
Edward Chow and Joav Merrick (Editors)
2011. ISBN: 978-1-61668-207-1 (Hardcover)
2010. ISBN: 978-1-61668-400-6 (eBook)

Positive Youth Development: Implementation of a Youth Program in a Chinese Context
Daniel TL Shek, Hing Keung Ma and Joav Merrick (Editors)
2011. ISBN: 978-1-61668-230-9

Social and Cultural Psychiatry Experience from the Caribbean Region
Hari D Maharajh and Joav Merrick (Editors)
2011. ISBN: 978-1-61668-506-5 (Hardcover)
2010. ISBN: 978-1-61728-088-7 (eBook)

Narratives and Meanings of Migration
Julia Mirsky
2011. ISBN: 978-1-61761-103-2 (Hardcover)
2010. ISBN: 978-1-61761-519-1 (eBook)

Self-Management and the Health Care Consumer
Peter William Harvey
2011. ISBN: 978-1-61761-796-6 (Hardcover)
2011. ISBN: 978-1-61122-214-2 (eBook)

Sexology from a Holistic Point of View
Soren Ventegodt and Joav Merrick
2011. ISBN: 978-1-61761-859-8 (Hardcover)
2011. ISBN: 978-1-61122-262-3 (eBook)

**Principles of Holistic Psychiatry:
A Textbook on Holistic Medicine
for Mental Disorders**
Soren Ventegodt and Joav Merrick
2011. ISBN: 978-1-61761-940-3 (Hardcover)
2011. ISBN: 978-1-61122-263-0 (eBook)

**Clinical Aspects of Psychopharmacology
in Childhood and Adolescence**
*Donald E Greydanus, Joseph L Calles, Jr,
Dilip P Patel, Ahsan Nazeer
and Joav Merrick (Editors)*
2011. ISBN: 978-1-61122-135-0 (Hardcover)
2011. ISBN: 978-1-61122-715-4 (eBook)

Climate Change and Rural Child Health
*Erica Bell, Bastian M Seidel
and Joav Merrick (Editors)*
2011. ISBN: 978-1-61122-640-9 (Hardcover)
2011. ISBN: 978-1-61209-014-6 (eBook)

**Rural Medical Education:
Practical Strategies**
*Erica Bell, Craig Zimitat and Joav Merrick
(Editors)*
2011. ISBN: 978-1-61122-649-2 (Hardcover)
2011. ISBN: 978-1-61209-476-2 (eBook)

**Advances in Environmental Health
Effects of Toxigenic Mold
and Mycotoxins**
Ebere Cyril Anyanwu
2011. ISBN: 978-1-60741-953-2
2011. ISBN: 978-1-53611-209-2

Public Health Yearbook 2009
Joav Merrick (Editor)
2011. ISBN: 978-1-61668-911-7 (Hardcover)
2011. ISBN: 978-1-62417-365-3 (eBook)

**Child Health and Human Development
Yearbook 2009**
Joav Merrick (Editor)
2011. ISBN: 978-1-61668-912-4

Alternative Medicine Yearbook 2009
Joav Merrick (Editor)
2011. ISBN: 978-1-61668-910-0 (Hardcover)
2011. ISBN: 978-1-62081-710-0 (eBook)

**The Dance of Sleeping and Eating
among Adolescents:
Normal and Pathological Perspectives**
Yael Latzer and Orna Tzischinsky (Editors)
2011. ISBN: 978-1-61209-710-7 (Hardcover)
2011. ISBN: 978-1-62417-366-0 (eBook)

**Drug Abuse in Hong Kong:
Development and Evaluation
of a Prevention Program**
*Daniel TL Shek, Rachel CF Sun
and Joav Merrick (Editors)*
2011. ISBN: 978-1-61324-491-3 (Hardcover)
2011. ISBN: 978-1-62257-232-8 (eBook)

**Chance Action and Therapy:
The Playful Way of Changing**
Uri Wernik
2010. ISBN: 978-1-60876-393-1 (Hardcover)
2011. ISBN: 978-1-61122-987-5 (Softcover)
2011. ISBN: 978-1-61209-874-6 (eBook)

**Bone and Brain Metastases:
Advances in Research and Treatment**
*Arjun Sahgal, Edward Chow
and Joav Merrick (Editors)*
2010. ISBN: 978-1-61668-365-8 (Hardcover)
2010. ISBN: 978-1-61728-085-6 (eBook)

**Challenges in Adolescent Health:
An Australian Perspective**
*David Bennett, Susan Towns,
Elizabeth Elliott
and Joav Merrick (Editors)*
2009. ISBN: 978-1-60741-616-6 (Hardcover)
2009. ISBN: 978-1-61668-240-8 (eBook)

**Obesity and Adolescence:
A Public Health Concern**
*Hatim A Omar, Donald E Greydanus,
Dilip R Patel and Joav Merrick (Editors)*
2009. ISBN: 978-1-60692-821-9 (Hardcover)
2009. ISBN: 978-1-61470-465-2 (eBook)

**Poverty and Children:
A Public Health Concern**
Alexis Lieberman and Joav Merrick (Editors)
2009. ISBN: 978-1-60741-140-6 (Hardcover)
2009. ISBN: 978-1-61470-601-4 (eBook)

**Living on the Edge: The Mythical,
Spiritual, and Philosophical
Roots of Social Marginality**
Joseph Goodbread
2009. ISBN: 978-1-60741-162-8 (Hardcover)
2013. ISBN: 978-1-61122-986-8 (Softcover)
2011. ISBN: 978-1-61470-192-7 (eBook)

**Alcohol-Related Cognitive Disorders:
Research and Clinical Perspectives**
*Leo Sher, Isack Kandel and Joav Merrick
(Editors)*
2009. ISBN: 978-1-60741-730-9 (Hardcover)
2009. ISBN: 978-1-60876-623-9 (eBook)

Children and Pain
*Patricia Schofield and Joav Merrick
(Editors)*
2009. ISBN: 978-1-60876-020-6 (Hardcover)
2009. ISBN: 978-1-61728-183-9 (eBook)

**Complementary Medicine Systems:
Comparison and Integration**
Karl W Kratky
2008. ISBN: 978-1-60456-475-4 (Hardcover)
2008. ISBN: 978-1-61122-433-7 (eBook)

Pain in Children and Youth
*Patricia Schofield and Joav Merrick
(Editors)*
2008. ISBN: 978-1-60456-951-3 (Hardcover)
2008. ISBN: 978-1-61470-496-6 (eBook)

**Adolescent Behavior Research:
International Perspective**s
Joav Merrick and Hatim A Omar (Editors)
2007. ISBN: 1-60021-649-8

HEALTH AND HUMAN DEVELOPMENT

ALTERNATIVE MEDICINE RESEARCH YEARBOOK 2017

JOAV MERRICK
EDITOR

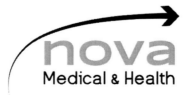

Copyright © 2018 by Nova Science Publishers, Inc.

All rights reserved. No part of this book may be reproduced, stored in a retrieval system or transmitted in any form or by any means: electronic, electrostatic, magnetic, tape, mechanical photocopying, recording or otherwise without the written permission of the Publisher.

We have partnered with Copyright Clearance Center to make it easy for you to obtain permissions to reuse content from this publication. Simply navigate to this publication's page on Nova's website and locate the "Get Permission" button below the title description. This button is linked directly to the title's permission page on copyright.com. Alternatively, you can visit copyright.com and search by title, ISBN, or ISSN.

For further questions about using the service on copyright.com, please contact:
Copyright Clearance Center
Phone: +1-(978) 750-8400   Fax: +1-(978) 750-4470   E-mail: info@copyright.com.

NOTICE TO THE READER

The Publisher has taken reasonable care in the preparation of this book, but makes no expressed or implied warranty of any kind and assumes no responsibility for any errors or omissions. No liability is assumed for incidental or consequential damages in connection with or arising out of information contained in this book. The Publisher shall not be liable for any special, consequential, or exemplary damages resulting, in whole or in part, from the readers' use of, or reliance upon, this material. Any parts of this book based on government reports are so indicated and copyright is claimed for those parts to the extent applicable to compilations of such works.

Independent verification should be sought for any data, advice or recommendations contained in this book. In addition, no responsibility is assumed by the publisher for any injury and/or damage to persons or property arising from any methods, products, instructions, ideas or otherwise contained in this publication.

This publication is designed to provide accurate and authoritative information with regard to the subject matter covered herein. It is sold with the clear understanding that the Publisher is not engaged in rendering legal or any other professional services. If legal or any other expert assistance is required, the services of a competent person should be sought. FROM A DECLARATION OF PARTICIPANTS JOINTLY ADOPTED BY A COMMITTEE OF THE AMERICAN BAR ASSOCIATION AND A COMMITTEE OF PUBLISHERS.

Additional color graphics may be available in the e-book version of this book.

Library of Congress Cataloging-in-Publication Data

ISBN: 978-1-53613-726-2
ISSN: 2162-3759

Published by Nova Science Publishers, Inc. † New York

CONTENTS

Introduction   1

Chapter 1   Introduction: Maltreatment in Children with Disabilities   3
Vincent J Palusci, Dena Nazer, Donald E Greydanus and Joav Merrick

Section one – Alternative medicine   9

Chapter 2   A review on psychotherapeutic interventions with children and adolescents   11
Roberto Flachier and Kathleen A Gross

Chapter 3   A review on behavioral and cognitive behavioral psychotherapeutic interventions with children and adolescents   23
Roberto Flachier

Chapter 4   Family therapy as an integrated care model for pediatricians   41
Galen Alessi and Colleen C Cullinan

Chapter 5   A review on psychopharmacology in children and adolescents   55
Ahsan Nazeer

Chapter 6   Long-term music-listening's effects on blood pressure, heart rate, anxiety, and depression   71
Taunjah P Bell and David O Akombo

Chapter 7   Antibacterial and antioxidant potential of organic solvents extract of mangrove endophytic fungus *Eupenicillium senticosum* Scott   81
Ambarish Cheviry Nair, Santhosh Goveas, Laveena D'Souza, Flavia D'Cunha and Viana D'Souza

Chapter 8   Exclusive role of potentized *Thuja occidentalis* on myoma recovery: Case report   93
Supriyo Ghosh, Riya Dutta, Aswini K Sasmal, Animesh Das, Subhabrata Sinha, Rathin Chakravarty and Sandhimita Mondal

Chapter 9   Grief in primary care practice: Loss of house   97
Mohammed Morad and Adam Morad

Section two - Virtual reality technologies for rehabilitation 107

Chapter 10   A participatory design framework for the gamification of rehabilitation systems   109
Darryl Charles and Suzanne McDonough

Chapter 11   Evidence-based facial design of an interactive virtual advocate   117
Wendy Powell, Tom A Garner, Daniel Tonks and Thomas Lee

Chapter 12   Reflections and early evidence of the importance of presence for three types of feedback in virtual motor rehabilitation   123
Thomas Schüler, Luara Ferreira dos Santos and Simon Hoermann

Chapter 13   Challenges in developing new technologies for special needs education: A force-field analysis   131
Patrice L (Tamar) Weiss, Susan VG Cobb, Massimo Zancanaro, Nirit Bauminger-Zviely, Sigal Eden, Eynat Gal and Sarah J Parsons

Chapter 14   Grid-pattern indicating interface for ambient assisted living   139
Zeeshan Asghar, Goshiro Yamamoto, Yuki Uranishi, Christian Sandor, Tomohiro Kuroda and Hirokazu Kato

Chapter 15   Realistic and adaptive cognitive training using virtual characters   147
Daniel Sjölie

Chapter 16   Conducting focus groups in Second Life® on health-related topics   153
Alice B Krueger, Patrice Colletti, Hillary R Bogner, Frances K Barg and Margaret Grace Stineman

Chapter 17   Self-management intervention for amputees in a virtual world environment   161
Sandra L Winkler, Robin Cooper, Kurt Kraiger, Ann Ludwig, Alice Krueger, Ignacio Gaunaurd, Ashley Fisher, John Kairalla, Scott Elliott, Sarah Wilson and Alberto Esquenazi

Chapter 18   Video-based quantification of patient's compliance during post-stroke virtual reality rehabilitation   169
Matjaž Divjak, Simon Zelič and Aleš Holobar

Chapter 19   Putting immersive therapies into PRAXIS: Towards holistic wellbeing multisensory meditation environments   177
Henry J Moller, Lee Saynor, Harjot Bal, Kunal Sudan and Lee Jones

Chapter 20   Assessment of motor function in hemiplegic patients using a virtual cycling wheelchair   185
Remi Ishikawa, Norihiro Sugita, Makoto Abe, Makoto Yoshizawa, Kazunori Seki and Yasunobu Handa

Chapter 21	Low-cost active video game console development for dynamic postural control training *Annie Pouliot-Laforte, Édouard Auvinet, Martin Lemay and Laurent Ballaz*	193
Chapter 22	Improved mobility and reduced fall risk in older adults after five weeks of virtual reality training *Shirley R Shema, Pablo Bezalel, Ziv Sberlo, Orly Wachsler Yannai, Nir Giladi, Jeffrey M Hausdorff and Anat Mirelman*	199
Chapter 23	The potentiality of virtual reality for the evaluation of spatial abilities: The mental spatial reference frame test *Silvia Serino, Francesca Morganti, Pietro Cipresso, Erika Emma Ruth Magni and Giuseppe Riva*	205
Chapter 24	Virtual spatial navigation tests based on animal research: Spatial cognition deficit in first episodes of schizophrenia *Iveta Fajnerová, Kamil Vlček, Cyril Brom, Karolína Dvorská, David Levčík, Lucie Konrádová, Pavol Mikoláš, Martina Ungrmanová, Michal Bída, Karel Blahna, Filip Španiel, Aleš Stuchlík, Jiří Horáček and Mabel Rodriguez*	213
Chapter 25	Enhancing brain activity by controlling virtual objects with the eye *Cristián Modroño, Julio Plata, Estefanía Hernández, Iván Galván, Sofía García, Fernando Zelaya, Francisco Marcano, Óscar Casanova, Gorka Navarrete, Manuel Mas and José Luis González-Mora*	223
Chapter 26	Colour-check in stroke-rehabilitation games *Veronika Szücs, Cecília Sik Lanyi, Ferenc Szabo and Peter Csuti*	229
Chapter 27	Perception of multi-varied sound patterns of sonified representations of complex systems by people who are blind *Orly Lahav, Jihad Kittany, Sharona Tal Levy and Miriam Furst*	237
Chapter 28	Outdoor navigation system for visually impaired persons *Babar Chaudary, Petri Pulli and Iikka Paajala*	245
Chapter 29	Exploring haptic feedback for robot-to-human communication *Ayan Ghosh, Jacques Penders, Peter Jones, Heath Reed and Alessandro Sorranzo*	255
Chapter 30	Raised-dot slippage perception on a fingerpad using an active wheel device *Yoshihiko Nomura and Hirotsugu Kato*	263
Section three - Children, disability and abuse		**271**
Chapter 31	Physical abuse and neglect in children with disabilities: Medical evaluation *Dena Nazer*	273

Chapter 32	Medical evaluation and management of sexual abuse in children with disabilities *Dena Nazer*	289
Chapter 33	Sexual behaviors in children with developmental disabilities *Alyse Mandel and Ellen Datner*	299
Chapter 34	Children with medical complexity: Neglect, abuse, and challenges *Alex Okun*	333
Chapter 35	Children with disabilities: Legal issues in child welfare cases *Frank E Vandervort and Joshua B Kay*	347
Chapter 36	Children with disabilities: Prevention of maltreatment *Vincent J Palusci*	365
Section four - Virtual rehabilitation system design		393
Chapter 37	Choosing virtual and augmented reality hardware for virtual rehabilitation: Process and considerations *Sebastian T Koenig and Belinda S Lange*	395
Chapter 38	Bayesian modelling for inclusive design under health and situational-induced impairments: An overview *Bashar I Ahmad, Patrick M Langdon and Simon J Godsill*	405
Chapter 39	The impact of the visual representation of the input device on driving performance in a power wheelchair simulator *Abdulaziz Alshaer, David O'Hare, Simon Hoermann and Holger Regenbrecht*	419
Chapter 40	Influence of navigation interaction technique on perception and behaviour in mobile virtual reality *Wendy A Powell, Vaughan Powell, Phillip Brown, Marc Cook and Jahangir Uddin*	431
Chapter 41	Evaluation of Leap Motion controller and Oculus Rift for virtual-reality-based upper limb stroke rehabilitation *Dominic E Holmes, Darryl K Charles, Philip J Morrow, Sally McClean and Suzanne M McDonough*	445
Chapter 42	Study of stressful gestural interactions: An approach for assessing their negative physical impacts *Sobhi Ahmed, Laure Leroy and Ari Bouaniche*	459
Chapter 43	Bringing the client and therapist together in virtual reality telepresence exposure therapy *David J Roberts, Allen J Fairchild, Simon Campion and Arturo S Garcia*	473

Chapter 44	Remote communication, examination, and training in stroke, Parkinson's, and COPD care: Work in progress testing 3D camera and movement recognition technologies together with new patient-centered ICT services *Martin Rydmark, Jurgen Broeren, Jonas Jalminger, Lars-Åke Johansson, Mathias Johanson and Anna Ridderstolpe*	**483**
Chapter 45	Visual impairment simulator for auditing and design *George W Stewart and Rachel J McCrindle*	**491**
Chapter 46	Authenticating the subjective: A naturalistic case study of a high-usability electronic health record for virtual reality therapeutics *Henry J Moller and Lee Saynor*	**509** |//

Section five – Acknowledgments   **517**

Chapter 47	About the editor	**519**
Chapter 48	About the National Institute of Child Health and Human Development in Israel	**521**
Chapter 49	About the book series "Health and human development"	**525**

Section six – Index   **531**

Index   **533**

INTRODUCTION

Chapter 1

INTRODUCTION: MALTREATMENT IN CHILDREN WITH DISABILITIES

Vincent J Palusci[1],*, MD, MS, FAAP, Dena Nazer[2], MD, FAAP, Donald E Greydanus[3], MD, DrHC(Athens), FAAP and Joav Merrick[4-8], MD, MMedSc, DMSc

[1]New York University School of Medicine, New York, New York, US
[2]Wayne State University School of Medicine, Detroit, Michigan, US
[3]Western Michigan University Homer Stryker MD School of Medicine, Kalamazoo, Michigan, US
[4]National Institute of Child Health and Human Development, Jerusalem
[5]Office of the Medical Director, Health Services, Division for Intellectual and Developmental Disabilities, Ministry of Social Affairs and Social Services, Jerusalem
[6]Division of Pediatrics, Hadassah Hebrew University Medical Center, Mt Scopus Campus, Jerusalem, Israel
[7]Kentucky Children's Hospital, University of Kentucky School of Medicine, Lexington, Kentucky, US
[8]Center for Healthy Development, School of Public Health, Georgia State University, Atlanta, Georgia, US

ABSTRACT

Professional responses today are at odds with planning a public health response to child maltreatment prevention. The absence of a public policy framework and related infrastructure for disabled children precludes common ownership of the problem while recognizing the vast differences in parenting behaviors. A universal system of assessment

---

* Correspondence: Vincent J Palusci, Professor of Pediatrics, New York University School of Medicine, Bellevue Hospital Center, 462 First Avenue, New York, NY 10016, United States. E-mail: Vincent.palusci@nyumc.org.

and support would touch all children and all families at multiple points in the developmental process and would not simply identify those at highest risk. It would be built on the premise that all parents have concerns which differ only in the extent to which they have the capacity to address these issues. We would like to highlight the importance of identifying abuse and neglect among children with disability, because of their increased risk and the harmful effects which can result from a complex interaction of disability, special needs, and our professional responses. Developmental considerations must be included in any professional response to maltreatment in children with disability, and additional research is needed to improve our understanding of how to best improve professional practice for this vulnerable population to maximize their developmental and intellectual potentials.

INTRODUCTION

Concurrent with the legal recognition of abuse and neglect and our increasing knowledge about its epidemiology among children with developmental and intellectual disabilities (IDD), professionals have developed the assessment and treatment of children with abuse and neglect and disabilities. Often this professional response addresses maltreatment or disability, but not both. It is only relatively recently that we have come to understand the profound effects of abuse and neglect on persons with disability and how to respond when children with disability are maltreated. At the time of the classic description of the battered child by C Henry Kempe (1922-1984) in 1962, physical abuse and neglect were not a stranger to children with disabilities (1). In 1989, the United Nations Convention on the Rights of the Child set out the rights that must be realized for children to develop their full potential, free from hunger and want, neglect and abuse (2). In the United States, there are a number of agencies have been put in place at different levels (e.g., local, state, federal) to improve our response. More recently, the Convention on the Rights of Persons with Disabilities codified rules and regulations which provided special protections and accommodations for people with physical and other impairments (3).

While these changes have dramatically improved our responses to child maltreatment and disabilities, children with disabilities continue to be victimized, the evaluation for which is made all the more difficult because their developmental delays affect their behavior and communication. Child protective systems strive to protect all children, but they are especially challenged to help children with disabilities and those who are medically fragile (4). Legal systems designed to intervene and to reduce potential harm from maltreatment may be unable to integratively approach both maltreatment and disability to maximize children's growth and development. Maltreatment prevention strategies, many of which have limited evidence supporting their efficacy in non-disabled populations, generally have much less information available surrounding their use among populations of children with disabilities.

ASSESSMENT AND TREATMENT

Children with disability often have contact with healthcare and other service providers whose role it is to support their safety and well-being. However, the presentation of certain disabilities may disguise potential indicators of child abuse. Beliefs and attitudes can affect how professionals view, assess and attend to children with intellectual and developmental disabilities. For example, beliefs such as that children with IDD cannot provide accurate information regarding their personal experiences; children with IDD are not affected by abuse and/or cannot benefit from interventions after a traumatic experience; and children with IDD are stressful or undesirable to work with, can negatively impact service providers and investigators interactions with this population and lead to unsupportive and less effective interventions (4).

Children develop across many domains: emotional, social and physical, and at different rates and developmental stages. Parents of children with IDDs generally take a protective stance when it comes to shielding their vulnerable children from physical injury and abuse, but sexual development is often overlooked as an expected area of development. This could be due to societal beliefs and/or parental, cultural or religious differences. The normative progression of sexual development may not apply within a clear framework if a child has a developmental disability or delay. Unfortunately, children with IDD experience maltreatment at higher rates than peers who are not developmentally delayed (5). These children are especially at risk due to cognitive, social and emotional deficits. As with typically developing peers, problematic sexual behavior can occur in children with IDD as a result of sexual abuse, but there may also be other factors at play. Those with sexualized behaviors in youth require even more specialized assessment and treatment to tease out the developmental and intellectual issues from elements of their victimization. The presence of a disability may not in and of itself change some of the basic findings of maltreatment on physical examination. Key concepts in assessing the potentially abusive nature of injuries in all age groups include the mobility and developmental abilities of the victim, the severity of the injury, the contribution of underlying medical conditions, and the ability of the victim to disclose what, if anything happened. As infants, patients are relatively immobile and passive in ways similar to frail adults. It is only with successful rehabilitation and mobilization that a child or adult may later become more vocal and more demanding of care, prompting an alleged event of abuse or neglect. When there is an unclear or inconsistent mechanism of injury reported, the caretaker-patient dyad should be observed closely and a full psychosocial assessment by a multidisciplinary team should be obtained (6).

Once concern has arisen, the medical evaluation for potential physical and sexual abuse and neglect in children with IDD requires special training, assistance, and resources to best identify their needs while reducing further trauma from the evaluation. It is important to differentiate the medical evaluations for physical abuse and neglect from sexual abuse given the different objectives during assessment, classes of findings expected, and potential for additional traumatic stress from the process. It is also important to recognize suspected medical neglect among children with medical complexity/disability, how medical complexity is defined, what distinguishes it from medical fragility, and the issues that arise for mandated reporters in the domains of ethics and professionalism (7).

The perception that all children with IDD are unreliable witnesses and lack the ability to provide accurate information can lead investigators to discount their disclosures and/or behaviors and fail to conduct forensic interviews that consider children's individual capabilities and needs (8). As with any child, children with IDD should receive individualized treatment when being interviewed about child abuse. Investigators and courts should avoid making assumptions about their functioning, should take into account the individual abilities of each child, and should obtain information about a particular child before conducting an interview. Many children with IDD have the capacity to provide accurate accounts of their personal experiences, but more research is needed on these abilities in order to inform investigators and improve the effectiveness of child abuse evaluations.

The assessment of medical neglect is often made much more complex when children have physical disabilities and special medical needs. The failure to comply with treatments and diagnostic testing is a marker of parental/caretaker noncompliance and potential neglect (9). Children in need of diagnostic testing, therapy for progressive limb contractures, or provision of orthotics and varied treatments will not perform as well when not provided with these services. These lapses may extend to the lack of provision of general medical care and failure to properly immunize children which would not only place them at jeopardy but also, in the absence of medical contraindications, limit their participation in center-based and rehabilitative programs. Intentionally not permitting a physically-challenged adult or child to access their augmentative communication and other technological devices or intentional breakage of such devices upon which they are dependent is also a form of maltreatment. Children with medical care neglect have been underidentified and underreported, partly because of the difficulties in assessing the contribution of the child's altered abilities to the failure to meet the reasonable expectations our society has for their care (10).

REPORTING AND LEGAL RESPONSE

If there are concerning examination findings or a child discloses information or behaves in such a way that leads to a suspicion of abuse or neglect, a variety of professionals and agency staff members can be legally mandated (each state/country according to their laws) to make a report to the governmental entity designed to receive such reports. This entity determines if there is enough evidence to prompt an investigation and/or begins an investigation which includes assessing the safety of the home, interviewing family members and others known to the patient, and obtaining medical and other records. This investigation can involve law enforcement and child protective services, or both. If abuse occurs in an institution or in foster care, the agencies involved may also conduct their own investigation. Given the variety of agencies that can become involved, collaboration and awareness of the needs of the patient and his/her family are essential. Efforts should be made to decrease the number of evaluations conducted by different agencies to reduce further trauma. Multiple interviews have the potential to create stress, confusion, and frustration for patients and families and lead victims to think they are not believed or are in trouble, to avoid disclosing information, accurate or not, to cope with the repetitive process. Repeated examinations can inappropriately focus a child's attention on injuries or embarrassing body parts and can also lead the child to identify medical care as painful and traumatic. For victims with IDD, these potential negative effects can be exacerbated by their difficulties coping with and understanding the evaluation process. Difficulties conducting a sound and informed evaluation can ultimately fail to protect a victim, halt an abuse investigation, and negatively impact subsequent civil and/or criminal legal proceedings (4).

Despite the multiple potential risks for child abuse in populations with IDD, few reported cases end up in the court system or result in disciplinary action against the perpetrator of abuse. In addition, criminal cases have been dismissed because of uninformed interviewers who do not ask sound questions. Investigators of child abuse should take into account the individual abilities of each child before and during a forensic interview (11). The legal framework in the US tries to respect individual rights when child maltreatment and disability intersect. Federal child welfare laws shape each state's child protection system and govern work with children and families when a child has a disability. The Child Abuse Prevention and Treatment Act, the Americans with Disabilities Act, the Individuals with Disabilities Education Act, Section 504 of the Rehabilitation Act, and the Social Security Act are the legal frameworks that provide support for determining when maltreatment has occurred while providing safety for the child and recognizing rights that parents have to raise their children. Much remains to be done in creating systems which integrate child maltreatment and disability within a unified child welfare system.

PREVENTION

Those caring for children with disabilities want to prevent child abuse and neglect to reduce their pain and suffering and future health problems. First and foremost for prevention are good professional practice and reporting. Professionals need to be able to identify and report patterns of maltreatment while excluding mimics and other confounders. Children and adults with disabilities are seen by many subspecialists, and it is important that there is one individual or group of professionals who follow them on a consistent basis, preferably in a defined 'medical home' integrated with community services to reduce the risk of abuse or neglect and permit proactive, preventative services to be put into place. Some have offered concrete ideas about how professionals in the health system can integrate prevention into the day-to-day care of children with disabilities. These strategies can be justified based on their financial savings as well as their human benefits (12).

However, the details of why, how, when, and where health care professionals can promote prevention are murky or ill-defined, especially for maltreatment of children with disability. Contemporary approaches to child protection are dominated by individualized forensically focused interventions that provide limited scope for more holistic preventative responses for children at risk and the provision of support to struggling families and communities. Investigatory and removal approaches fail in critically important ways, particularly regarding reducing the inequities that underpin neglect and abuse. There have been increasing calls for a health systems-based model for the protection of children, and it is precisely the population of children with disabilities who would most benefit from this approach (13).

CONCLUSION

Daro (14) has noted that today's professional responses are at odds with planning a public health response to child maltreatment prevention. The absence of a public policy framework and related infrastructure for disabled children precludes common ownership of the problem while recognizing the vast differences in parenting behaviors. A universal system of assessment and support would touch all children and all families at multiple points in the developmental process and would not simply identify those at highest risk. It would be built on the premise that all parents have concerns which differ only in the extent to which they have the capacity to address these issues.

We would like to highlight the importance of identifying abuse and neglect among children with disability because of their increased risk and the harmful effects which can result from a complex interaction of disability, special needs, and our professional responses. Developmental considerations must be included in any professional response to maltreatment in children with disability, and additional research is needed to improve our understanding of how to best improve professional practice for this vulnerable population to maximize their developmental and intellectual potentials.

REFERENCES

[1] Kempe CH, Silverman FN, Steele BF, Droegemueller W, Silver HK. The battered-child syndrome. JAMA 1962;181:17-24.
[2] United Nations General Assembly. Convention on the Rights of the Child A/RES/44/25. Adopted 20 November 1989.
[3] United Nations General Assembly. Convention on the Rights of Persons with Disabilities A/RES/61/106. Adopted 24 January 2007.
[4] Palusci VJ, Datner E, Wilkins C. Abuse and neglect. In: Rubin IL, Merrick J, Greydanus DE, Patel DR, eds. Rubin and Crocker, 3rd edition: Health care for people with intellectual and developmental disabilities across the lifespan. Cham, Switzerland: Springer International Publishing 2016;2011-32.
[5] Turner HA, Vanderminden J, Finkelhor D, Hamby S, Shattuck A. Disability and victimization in a national sample of children and youth. Child Maltreat 2001;16:275-86.
[6] Hershokowitz D, Lamb ME, Horowitz D. Victimization of children with disabilities. Am J Orthopsychiatr 2013;77(4):629-35.
[7] Palusci VJ. Some thoughts on counting medical neglect. Maltreat Sci 2015 Jan 16. URL: http://www.maltreat.info/index.php/contribution-articles?download=9:some-thoughts-on-counting-medical-neglect-reports.
[8] Ballard MB, Austin S. Forensic interviewing: Special considerations for children and adolescents with mental retardation and developmental disabilities. Educ Train Ment Retard Dev Disabil 1999;34(4):521-5.
[9] Jenny C, American Academy of Pediatrics. Recognizing and responding to medical neglect. Pediatrics 2007;120:1385-9.
[10] Spencer N, Devereux E, Wallace A, Sundrum R, Shenoy M, Bacchus C, Logan S. Disabling conditions and registration for child abuse and neglect: A population-based study. Pediatrics 2005;116:609-13.
[11] Poole DA, Lamb ME. Investigative Interviews of Children: A guide for helping professionals. Washington, DC: American Psychological Association, 1998.
[12] American Professional Society on the Abuse of Children. Practice Guidelines: Integrating prevention into the work of child maltreatment professionals. Columbus, OH: Author, 2010.
[13] Scott D, Lonne B, Higgins D. Public health models for preventing child maltreatment: Applications from the field of injury prevention. Trauma Violence Abuse 2016;17(4):408-19.
[14] Daro D. A public health approach to prevention: What will it take? Trauma Violence Abuse 2016;17(4):420-1.

Section one – Alternative medicine

In: Alternative Medicine Research Yearbook 2017
Editor: Joav Merrick
ISBN: 978-1-53613-726-2
© 2018 Nova Science Publishers, Inc.

Chapter 2

A REVIEW ON PSYCHOTHERAPEUTIC INTERVENTIONS WITH CHILDREN AND ADOLESCENTS

Roberto Flachier[*], PhD and Kathleen A Gross, MD

Department of Psychiatry, Western Michigan University
Homer Stryker MD School of Medicine, Kalamazoo, Michigan, US

ABSTRACT

Management of mental health disorders in children and adolescents have benefited from the significant increase in the numbers and types of interventions that have become available over the past several decades; these include psychosocial, psychotherapeutic and psycho-pharmacological treatments. Principles of psycho-therapeutic interventions for the pediatric population are considered in this discussion. It is important that primary care clinicians are able to identify mental health problems and disorders in their pediatric patients. It is also critical to the health of these patients that their clinicians are able to utilize integrated health and behavioral health care models to address them, and also have ready access to referral resources for assessment and treatment needs that require more specialized expertise.

Keywords: mental health, children, adolescents, psychotherapy

INTRODUCTION

In their roles as providers of medical care for children and adolescents, primary care physicians (PCP's), especially pediatricians, are often the first to be consulted by parents about a child's behavioral, emotional, psychological, and developmental difficulties. They

---

[*] Correspondence: Roberto Flachier, PhD, Department of Psychiatry, Western Michigan University Homer Stryker MD School of Medicine, 1717 Shaffer Street, Suite 010, Kalamazoo, MI 49048, United States. E-mail: roberto.flachier@med.wmich.edu.

frequently are asked for advice on managing a child's medical problems, such as diabetes, obesity and medical treatment non-adherence. In fact, young people often have both medical conditions and psychoemotional issues. The use of psychological applications is often indicated in these settings.

An integrated primary care system is the most effective and efficient model for delivering health care related to prevention, early intervention, and treatment of acute and chronic developmental, behavioral and mental health, and medical conditions (1). In this type of system, the PCP coordinates a primary care team that includes psychologists, social workers, nurses, behavior analysts, physician assistants, occupational therapists, and other professionals who assist with assessment, service delivery, and referral to more specialized providers (e.g., psychiatrists). Collaborative relationships among the various disciplines represented are of outmost importance in providing high quality healthcare within this model.

Beginning in the 1950s and, especially, in the last thirty years, new psychotherapeutic approaches with children and adolescents have proliferated, mostly due to the awareness of their efficacy and the significant advancement in the field. The range of available options is now broader in depth and more diverse in range, simultaneously offering greater flexibility and more precisely targeted applicability. As a consequence of this expansion, clinical use of these approaches has become more widespread. Not only has the field embraced evidence-supported psychotherapeutic treatments, but medical practitioners and society as a whole also have increasingly accepted the importance of early intervention. Research clearly shows that many youth, one in five, suffer from developmental, emotional, or behavioral problems that may be related to mood, anxiety, eating, substances of abuse, suicide proneness and autism (2, 3). Some of these problems (e.g., eating, mood, anxiety, and psychotic disorders) become even more poignant in adolescence. Interventions have evolved beyond a focus on the individual to include members of the system(s) that support the child (e.g., family and school). Family therapies, systemic and integrated approaches are now offered. In addition, the number and type of available psychopharmacological interventions has expanded.

Even with the increasing use of medication, the importance of including psychotherapeutic and psychosocial interventions as integral parts of the treatment plan has become more widely recognized. Because, children and adolescents often do not receive mental health services when needed, however, it is very important for PCPs to be skilled in assessing mental health needs, and in making appropriate referrals for more specialized mental health services. Furthermore, the use of certain therapeutic techniques in the PCP's office (e.g., Motivational Interviewing, family consultation and counseling) often is necessary to motivate the patient and the family to follow through on medical and behavioral recommendations. In this way, integrated models of primary healthcare delivery can be effective in providing comprehensive assessment and treatment of behavioral health and medical issues, including treatment adherence problems, and in enhancing follow through with referrals (2, 4).

In the following sections of this review, the general principles and categories of psychotherapeutic and psychosocial interventions for children and adolescents will be delineated and described, and a guide to the recommended interventions for specific diagnoses and problem areas will be presented.

General principles of assessment, treatment planning and referral for mental health and behavioral problems in children and adolescents

As stated before, the PCP may be the first professional to be consulted by a parent about a child's behavioral, emotional, psychological or developmental issues. The school, day care provider, relative, or other concerned adult may have suggested such a consultation. In some cases, there is an agenda, (e.g., "this child needs medication"). Therefore, the initial task is to determine what constitutes the "problem." This may entail identification of a specific disorder, behavioral problem, disability/developmental problem, and response to traumatic or stressful event, or abuse, or psychoemotional expression of a medical or neurological condition. In addition, it is vital to assess environmental factors, including stress in the family, lack of or problematic parenting skills, and difficult living conditions (e.g., housing, neighborhood, socioeconomic factors). Nutritional factors also may play a role. Consequently, PCPs and their multidisciplinary teams are greatly challenged in this complex assessment process.

Behavioral difficulties may not necessarily indicate the presence of a disorder, but the assessment of such as common problems as non-compliance, disruptive behavior (e.g., fighting and aggression, tantrum behavior, stealing, fire setting), toilet training difficulties, and school avoidance is very important. Behavioral problems may at any stage of development and, if they persist, may evolve into more enduring and persistent disorders. Thus, early intervention is recommended. Often, these behaviors indicate difficulties in parenting or are expressions of other environmental factors. Alternatively, they may symptomatic of an underlying disorder; e.g., school avoidance may be associated with social anxiety or obsessive-compulsive disorder (OCD).

It is especially important to assess for disorders that may already be evident in childhood or adolescence, including depression and bipolar disorder (the latter being more evident in adolescence); anxiety disorders, such as selective mutism, separation anxiety, panic disorder and OCD; adjustment disorders; psychosis; eating disorders; somatization disorders; body dysmorphic disorder; substance use disorders; suicide attempts (usually associated with a disorder); autism spectrum disorders; learning disabilities; developmental disabilities; and others. Assessing for these disorders can be a complex process, and may involve professionals from several disciplines.

Other assessments

A very important part of assessment includes identifying what types of assessment(s) and treatment(s) are necessary, or alternatively, determining who is qualified to assess and treat a particular condition, or to determine whether specific identified areas of difficulty exist in isolation or are expressions of an underlying disorder. For this reason, psychological evaluation can be a very important and integral part of the assessment process. For further detail on the assessment process, please consult other chapters in this book such as chapters 3 and 38 to 40.

TREATMENT PLANNING AND REFERRAL

Because the assessment of behavioral problems and disorders can be complex, PCPs and their clinics need to either have other appropriate professionals on staff; or have reliable resources for referral. It is important to survey local professionals regarding their specialized training and interests (e.g., neuropsychological assessment, learning disability assessment, OCD treatment). Assessment needs must be must be considered in the initial treatment plan, and the assessment results should be incorporated into the long-term treatment plan. Parents must be educated about this process from the outset as their cooperation is indispensable. With children and adolescents, other members of the family and of other social and support systems (e.g., school) also may need to be part of the treatment plan and process.

Addressing the psychotherapeutic needs associated with behavioral problems and disorders may be the primary form of intervention. When medication is needed as part of the treatment plan, a concurrent referral to child psychiatrist often is recommended. Specific syndromes require practitioners with specific training and experience (5, 6). OCD for instance requires specific treatment modalities (i.e., cognitive behavioral treatment involving exposure and response prevention) with a psychotherapist who is qualified to treat OCD.

Individual psychotherapy approaches

Even though there are immensely helpful individual therapy approaches for children and adolescents, it is necessary to coordinate treatment with the parent(s). PCPs and their teams can be extremely helpful in conveying the need for psychotherapy as a part of the treatment plan and process. Without the full cooperation of parents or primary caregivers (e.g., foster parents) the likelihood of attaining treatment goals diminishes. In addition, the school must often participate in the therapeutic efforts. In social anxiety, the school is often critical in the psychotherapeutic plan of action, as this type of anxiety is often associated with school avoidance. Suicide prevention and intervention, as well as treatment of depression, substance abuse, oppositional defiant disorder and ADHD often require that a treatment approach be integrated with the school program. Examples of individual therapy approaches now will be delineated and described:

Play therapy

Play therapy was first utilized in the 1930's as a psychoanalytical approach to therapy with children and adolescents. Thereafter, it became an integral part of the client-centered therapies. Currently, there are numerous applications of play in therapy, and play therapy has become part of the empirically supported therapy movement. Play may be utilized throughout the process of assessment, case conceptualization and intervention, and applications of play therapy fall under various theoretical conceptualizations; i.e., psychodynamic, cognitive, behavioral, interpersonal, client-centered, or integrationist (7, 8). Overall, it is recognized that play is one of the most important modes of interaction, and it is important to note that play and other interactive modes (drawing, storytelling) are very often integrated with other therapies described below.

Psychodynamic

Play, storytelling and development, drawing, dream recall, and other communication modes of communication are utilized in therapy with children and adolescents. In applying each, consideration is given to developmental stage and capacity, and a non-judgmental, non-punitive and non-directive approach is used. The content and meaning of what is expressed in play are considered to be metaphorical expressions of the child's internal world, and the goal is to discover the emotional world of the child or adolescent, and to understand how she gives meaning to her internal and external worlds. Impulses, internal conflicts and struggles are expressed, discussed and reintegrated. Themes and internal conflicts (i.e., forbidden internal impulses, attachment and identity struggles) are discovered and used in interpretation. Parental guidance is given intermittently in separate sessions to support the change process (8).

Interpersonal psychotherapy (IPT)

Interpersonal psychotherapy is a time-limited, psychodynamic approach, which has received significant empirical support for the treatment of mild to severe depression in adults, and also has been applied to the treatment of adolescents (9). Interventions are designed to modify problematic expectations modify about interpersonal relationships. It does not directly address transference factors in the therapeutic relationship, although is considered to be a very important part the therapeutic process. Several factors that favor this treatment approach include adequate motivation, ability to develop a therapeutic alliance, capacity to withstand internal and external stress (ego strength), relatively secure attachment, and good social support.

Cognitive behavioral therapy approaches (CBT)

A variety of therapeutic approaches have now been integrated under the rubric of CBT, including Cognitive Therapy (CT), Behavioral Therapy (BT), Cognitive Behavioral Therapy (CBT), Behavior Modification (BM), and Applied Behavioral Analysis (ABA). These approaches have the most empirically support as psychotherapies for children and adolescents and have been applied in many areas including autism spectrum disorders, anxiety disorders, mood disorders, obsessive compulsive spectrum disorders (i.e., OCD, trichotillomania, body dysmorphic disorder), Tourette's syndrome, attention deficit disorders, externalizing disorders, trauma and traumatic stress related disorders, substance abuse, eating disorders, behavioral problems, chronic medical problems (e.g., diabetes and asthma), parenting issues and other areas (10). CBT represents an integrated approach focused on emotional, behavioral and cognitive pattern change. For a thorough review of CBT, please refer to chapter 38 in this book.

Supportive psychotherapy

This is a broadly defined therapeutic approach that also can be effectively applied in the PCP office. Its theoretical support emanates from psychodynamic, cognitive behavioral and learning theory. Through a directive approach, it aims to reduce symptomatology and restore or improve self-esteem (e.g.; efficacy, confidence, hope, and self-concept), ego function (e.g., reality contact, affect, cognitive and impulse regulation), adaptive skills, and daily functioning, including socialization and problem solving. The basic process involves thorough examination and analysis of symptoms, interactions and relationships, adaptive functioning, patterns of thinking, emotional reactions, and actions or behavior.

One of the guiding concepts in psychotherapy is that a supportive approach should be applied when there is high degree of impairment, and it therefore can be useful in acute expressions of dysfunction. Supportive psychotherapy approaches also can be very useful in treating chronic medical conditions. It is imperative that the clinician be supportive, accepting, emphatic, and able to maintain a positive patient-clinician alliance. Clearly, these skills can be attained and practiced by all clinicians employed in the PCP's office. If every interaction is supportive, then treatment adherence and outcome is likely to improve.

Problem solving

This can be integrated with suicide prevention and with the treatment of medical conditions, anxiety disorders, and depression, externalizing disorders, as well as to promote healthy related behavior. Health-care providers can easily apply this method.

Social skills training

Another individual treatment modality involves social skills training, which encompasses communication, assertiveness, conflict resolution and other skills. It is widely applied in the treatment of social anxiety, externalizing disorders, ADHD, autism, developmental disorders, depression and other disorders.

Others

Other individual psychotherapy approaches are routinely applied in work with children and adolescents, either alone or integrated within the above-described approaches. *Motivational Interviewing* (MI) is an effective counseling application for use with children and adolescents who have difficulty entering into the treatment process, which is a common occurrence, for example, in cases involving substance abuse. Concomitantly, MI is utilized with parents to encourage them to make behavioral changes that promote infant, child and adolescent health and mental health. It has been applied to the treatment of diabetes, smoking, obesity, substance abuse, and to promote physical activity, healthy eating habits, medical adherence, and effective parenting. MI can easily be implemented within the primary care settings and can be utilized by physicians, nurses, physician assistants, and other health care providers. In the clinic, MI can greatly facilitate the physician's medical care and treatment plan (11). It can be said that every health-care provider would benefit from being trained in MI.

INTERVENTION WITH THE FAMILY AND FAMILY PSYCHOTHERAPY

Because children and adolescents are part of a family system, various forms of intervention with the family have been developed. One of the principal modalities is family therapy. Family therapy is often integrated with individual psychotherapy, but it is sometimes applied as the sole intervention. Since the 1960's, the family's inter-and-intra-system dynamics have been recognized as a very important focus of intervention in the process of change. Consequently, family therapy is directed at improving interfamilial relationships as well as interactional patterns within the family system and among family sub-systems. There are various theoretical conceptualizations in family therapy with specific emphasis and processes, but all approaches focus on family system or subsystems interactional patterns. The effectiveness of family therapy is well documented in literally hundreds of studies. This research has typically focused on specific areas of difficulty, such as substance abuse, depression, eating disorders and delinquency (12, 13). Family therapy usually occurs in the therapist's office, but it also may be done in the family's home (home based family therapy). Short term, focused family therapy can be practiced and integrated in the PCP clinic as discussed in the chapter "Family Therapy-An Integrated Care Model for Pediatricians." Family therapy is an integral form of intervention in substance abuse treatment programs, inpatient and partial hospitalization programs, and other acute treatment programs. It is also a very important component of treatment in juvenile delinquency and in trauma and abuse centered treatment. Family therapy is best delivered by trained family therapists, and this should be kept in mind when making referrals. Family therapists are often certified through the American Association for Marriage and Family Therapy as Licensed Marriage and Family Therapy (LMFT) therapists.

There are several other forms of intervention with families, including parenting skills training, consultation, case management, mediation between parents and the school or legal system, family crisis therapy, and others. (For a discussion of family therapy, please refer to the "Family Therapy" chapter). Oppositional Defiant Disorder (ODD) is one of the major complaints presented to PCPs. Problematic behavioral characteristics of ODD include excessive and long lasting tantrums, defiance or lack of compliance, aggression and argumentativeness. These issues negatively affect relationship satisfaction and quality for both child and parent. For ODD treatment, Parent-Child Interaction Therapy (PCIT) is a current form of family intervention that has received much empirical support (14). Its goals include developing a high degree of warmth in the parent-child interaction as well as reducing ODD behaviors.

GROUP PSYCHOTHERAPY APPROACHES

Group psychotherapy is a very effective form of intervention that has been applied to work with children and adolescents in outpatient, inpatient and acute treatment settings (15). It has been applied to the treatment of depression, substance abuse, social anxiety, bipolar disorders, psychosis, eating disorders, children of alcoholics, and others. Group therapy can be problem or syndrome specific (e.g., social anxiety, children of divorce, grief). In acute mental health treatment settings and substance abuse treatment programs, multisystemic treatment approaches and group therapy are consistently integrated into the treatment process.

In group therapy approaches with children, play therapy, role-play and other interactional processes are utilized. With adolescents, action-oriented and role-play techniques are customarily used. Various situations can be role-played, such as conflicts between parent and adolescent, issues between friends, difficulties with the expression of feelings or wishes (assertiveness), and appropriate use of social skills, among others. The focus of group therapy is often on the various developmental issues of adolescence, such as individuation, independence and autonomy, issues of control or conflict with authority figures, uncertainty about the future, dealing with peer pressure, social effectiveness and self-concept, sexuality and coping with societal demands.

Another form of group intervention with children and adolescents involves *psychoeducational groups*. These groups tend to be issue, theme or skill focused. Examples of such groups include emotional regulation, aggression and anger control, self-esteem/self-concept, social skills, conflict resolution, coping skills, stress management, or coping with a specific problem (depression, bipolar disorder, anxiety). Often, they are an integral component in acute treatment settings, such as inpatient and partial hospitalization programs, substance abuse inpatient or intensive outpatient treatment programs, and residential programs for the severely behaviorally disturbed. Participation in psychoeducational groups is also an important component of many standard outpatient treatment plans.

MULTISYSTEMIC TREATMENT APPROACHES

There are several areas of difficulty, which necessitate a multisystemic approach to intervention, such as severe and complex disorders that may require integration of the individual, family, school and, possibly, the legal system. These disorders also may integrate individual, family and group therapy (including psychoeducational groups). Multisystemic approaches have a long history, and some of the best known empirically based programs include Dialectical Behavior Therapy for suicidal patients and borderline personality disorder (16), Multisystemic Therapy for Antisocial Children and Adolescents (17), Trauma-Focused Cognitive-Behavioral Therapy for children and adolescents that have experienced trauma and traumatic grief (18), and Aggression Replacement Training for antisocial youth (19).

Table 1. Therapeutic approaches recommended for specific behavioral health disorders and problems, and clinician's type of training

Therapeutic Approach	Behavioral Health Problems and Disorders	Need for Certification, Specialized or General Training
Play Therapy	Most disorders and behavioral problems	General training in this modality
Psychodynamic Therapy	Depression, anxiety, Substance Abuse and personality issues	General training in this modality
Interpersonal Therapy	Depression, anxiety and interpersonal issues	General training in this modality
Cognitive Therapy CT)	Depression, anxiety, OCD, externalizing and internalizing disorders	Specialized training, certification is available
Cognitive Behavioral Therapy (CBT) (Behavioral Therapy)	Depression, anxiety disorders, OCD spectrum disorders, eating disorders internalizing and externalizing disorders, substance abuse and most other disorders	Specialized training, certification is available: some disorders (e.g., OCD, PTSD, trichotillomania, Tourette's require syndrome specific training)
Behavior Modification (BM) (Applied Behavioral Analysis)	Behavioral problems, autistic spectrum disorders, encopresis and enuresis, parenting issues, substance abuse, impulse control disorders, skill deficits or behavioral excesses, delinquency, aggression and other issues	Specialized training, certification is available
Motivational Interviewing (MI)	Non-adherence to treatment (behavioral or medical), increase motivation to take action	General training in this modality
Supportive Therapy	Chronic disorders, such as psychosis, personality disorders, mood disorders, bipolar disorder, other medical conditions and health issues. For depression, anxiety, and substance abuse add CBT and MI	General training in this modality and in added modalities
Problem Solving	All conditions, especially generalized anxiety disorder and complex health issues. Adjunct to other therapies	General training
Social Skills Training	Autism spectrum disorders, developmental disabilities, social anxiety, psychosis and other	Specialized training
Family Therapy	All complicated medical problems and behavioral disorders and issues	Specialized training, certification is available
Group Therapy	Medical and behavioral disorders (depression, anxiety, trauma history, social anxiety and others)	Specialized training
Dialectical Behavior Therapy (DBT)	Borderline personality disorder, high risk suicidal adolescents, significant disruptive patterns of behavior and personality, including substance abuse	Specialized training, certification is available and desired
Multisystemic Therapy for Antisocial Children and Adolescents	Antisocial children and adolescents	Specialized training
Trauma-Focused Cognitive-Behavioral Therapy	Trauma and traumatic grief	Specialized training
Aggression Replacement Training	Antisocial and aggressive youth	Specialized training

Conclusion

In the last 30 to 50 years, there has been significant growth in the number and type of mental health interventions (psychosocial, psychotherapeutic and psychopharmacological that are available for use) with children and adolescents. Nonetheless, identification and treatment of mental health problems have lagged behind. Given the large array of potential treatments, many of which are empirically supported, it behooves the primary care physician to understand their role in the overall treatment plan. Therefore, it is critical that primary care physicians be able to identify mental health issues and utilize integrated health and behavioral health care models to address them, and also have ready access to referral resources for assessment and treatment needs that require more specialized expertise.

References

[1] Stancin T, Perrin CL. Psychologists and pediatricians: Opportunities for collaboration in primary care. Am Psychol 2014;69:332-43.
[2] Irwin CE, Burg SJ, Cort CU. America's Adolescents: Where have we been? J Adolesc Health 2002;31:91-121.
[3] Evans DL, Foa EB, Gur RE, Hendin H, O'Brien CP, Seligman MEP, et al. Treating and preventing adolescent mental health disorders: What we know and what we don't know. New York: Oxford University Press, 1979.
[4] Romer D, McIntosh M. The role of primary care physicians in detection and treatment of adolescent mental health problems. In Evans DL, et al. editors. Treating and preventing adolescent mental health disorders: What we know and what we don't know. New York: Oxford University Press, 2005:579-95.
[5] American Psychological Association Task Force on Psychological Intervention Guidelines. Template for developing guidelines: Interventions for mental disorders and psychological aspects of physical disorders. Washington DC: American Psychological Association, 1995.
[6] Chorpita BF, Daleiden EL, Ebesutani C, Starace N. Evidence-based treatments for children and adolescents: An updated review of indicators of efficacy and effectiveness. Clin Psychol Sci Pract 2011;18:153-71.
[7] Russ SW, Niec LN. Play in clinical: evidence-based approaches. New York: Guilford, 2011.
[8] Chethik M. Techniques of child therapy: Psycho-dynamic strategies, 2nd ed. New York: Guilford, 2000.
[9] Mufson L, Weissman MM, Moreau RG. Efficacy of interpersonal psychotherapy for depressed adolescents. JAMA Psychiatry 1999;33:695-705.
[10] Berman SK, Weisz JR. Cognitive behavior therapy: An introduction. In: Szigethy E, Weisz JR, Findling RL, eds. Cognitive-behavior therapy for children and adolescents. Washington DC: American Psychiatric Publishing, 2012:1-28.
[11] Gayes LA, Steele RG. A meta-analysis of motivational interviewing interventions for pediatric health behavior change. J Consult Clin Psychol 2014 Feb 17. [Epub ahead of print].
[12] Couturier J, Kimber M, Szatmari P. Efficacy of family-based treatment for adolescents with eating disorders: A systemic review and meta-analysis. Int J Eat Disord 2013;46 (1):3-11.
[13] Austin AM, Macgowant MJ, Wagner EF. Effective family-based interventions for adolescents with substance abuse problems: A systemic review. Res Soc Work Pract 2005;15(2):67-83.
[14] Couturier J, Kimber M, Szatmari P. Efficacy of family-based treatment for adolescents with eating disorders: A systemic review and meta-analysis. Int J Eat Disord 2013;46 (1):3-11.
[15] Bodiford-McNeil C, Hembree-Kigin TL. Parent child interaction therapy, 2nd ed. New York: Springer, 2010.

[16] Shechtman Z. Group counseling with children and adolescents: Current practice and research. In: Delucia-Wassck JL. Gerrity D, Kalonder CR, Riva MT, eds. Handbook of group counseling and psychotherapy. Thousand Oaks, CA: Sage, 2004:429-44.
[17] Curtis N, Ronan K, Borduin CM. Multisystemic treatment: A meta-analysis of outcome studies. J Fam Psychol 2004;18(3):411-9.
[18] Cohn AC, Mannerig AP, Dubliner E. Treating trauma and traumatic grief in children and adolescents. New York: Guilford, 2007.
[19] Glik B, Gibbs JC. Aggression replacement training: A comprehensive intervention for aggressive youth, 3rd ed. Champaign, IL: Research Press, 2013.

Submitted: June 05, 2015. *Revised:* July 03, 2015. *Accepted:* July 10, 2015.

In: Alternative Medicine Research Yearbook 2017
Editor: Joav Merrick
ISBN: 978-1-53613-726-2
© 2018 Nova Science Publishers, Inc.

Chapter 3

A REVIEW ON BEHAVIORAL AND COGNITIVE BEHAVIORAL PSYCHOTHERAPEUTIC INTERVENTIONS WITH CHILDREN AND ADOLESCENTS

Roberto Flachier[*], *PhD*
Department of Psychiatry, Western Michigan University
Homer Stryker MD School of Medicine, Kalamazoo, Michigan, US

ABSTRACT

A group of psychotherapies have evolved that are referred to as behavior modification, behavior therapy, and cognitive behavioral therapy. This discussion considers these therapies now mostly commonly called cognitive behavior therapy. The range of application has reached most psychiatric diagnoses and is applied to the management of psychological factors associated with various medical conditions (i.e., asthma, diabetes mellitus, others). This discussion reviews these psychotherapeutic interventions used now in the 21st century to help children and adolescents.

Keywords: mental health, children, adolescents, behavior, psychotherapy

INTRODUCTION

In medical practice with children and adolescents, primary care physicians are often the first to be consulted by parents about a child's behavioral difficulties, emotional problems, psychological conditions, and developmental disabilities. In addition, these physicians are presented with the difficulties parents have while managing their child medical problems, such as diabetes, obesity and non-compliance. Furthermore, because psychological issues often accompany chronic and other medical conditions, the use of behavioral interventions is

---

[*] Correspondence: Roberto Flachier, PhD, Department of Psychiatry, Western Michigan University Homer Stryker MD School of Medicine, 1717 Shaffer Street, Suite 010, Kalamazoo, MI 49048, United States. E-mail: roberto.flachier@med.wmich.edu.

often necessary. Since the 1950's, a group of psychotherapies called behavior modification, behavior therapy, and cognitive behavioral therapy have been developing, evolving and integrating.

Currently, in its most general conceptualization, "Cognitive behavioral therapy (CBT)" is most commonly used to refer to this group of therapies. Their range of application has now reached most psychiatric diagnosis, and they have been applied to the management of psychological factors associated with medical conditions, such as diabetes, asthma and other chronic illnesses. Therefore, it is very important for pediatricians, family physicians, internists and medical professionals to be cognizant of the far-reaching and empirically supported applications of behavioral therapy (BT) and CBT.

In this review on BT and CBT, theoretical models and specific therapeutic approaches will be described and delineated. Currently these two approaches (BT and CBT) have become so integrated that, in practice, they are difficult to separate from each other. It is more practical to view them as integrated models and applications that fall under the rubric, "cognitive behavioral therapy". In the literature, one finds slightly different forms of the terminology, such as "cognitive therapy," "behavior therapy" and "cognitive-behavioral therapy" (1, 2). Some of these differences represent variations in treatment philosophy and either emphasizes cognition as primary in influencing behavior or view cognition, emotion, and action (operant or instrumental) as joint determinants of behavior. Currently, as an integrated model, CBT emphasizes the learning process, social environmental factors, cognitive factors (the meditational influence of cognitive processes, including information processing), emotional/affective factors, and instrumental behavioral factors (actions).

General concepts

Under the general term "CBT," there are over 46 separate treatment protocols with various names, such as prolonged exposure therapy for posttraumatic stress disorder (PE-CBT), trauma focused CBT (TF-CBT), aggression replacement therapy, cognitive behavioral treatment of insomnia (CBT-I), and others. All these treatments are "… unified by the guiding belief that an individual's thoughts (cognitions), behaviors (actions), and emotions are inextricably linked, and that maladaptive cognitions, emotional responses and behaviors can produce psychological dysfunction and impairment" (3). Thus, in the broader sense, CBT represents an integrated approach focused on emotional, behavioral (actions) and cognitive pattern change (1-3).

The concept that human experience is largely influenced by behaviors and thoughts has been formulated over two millennia within different schools of thought such as in Buddhism, Taoism, the teaching of stoicism (e.g., Epictetus), existential philosophy, and others. As indicated above, CBT integrates behavioral and cognitive models and principles. The *behavioral model* emphasizes learning principles, which are classified under operant and classical (respondent) conditioning. As expressed by Ellis (5) and Beck (6), the *cognitive model* emphasizes the mediational/information processing effect on emotional and instrumental behavior. Thus, in the cognitive model, how we attribute meaning to events, affects how we feel and react both emotionally and behaviorally (1-6).

The integration of the behavioral and cognitive models was clearly evident in the work of Meichenbaum in the 1960s and 1970s (7). Thereafter, and throughout the 1980's and 1990's, cognitive and behavioral techniques were further integrated in developing treatments for depression, anxiety, disruptive and externalizing behaviors, aggression and others. CBT also owes much in its development to the social learning theorists, of whom Albert Bandura was the most influential (8). Social learning theory places significant importance on the social environments in which behavior is acquired. Concomitantly, Bandura also emphasizes observational learning (modeling and vicarious learning, described below) and cognitive mediational processes in behavior. Lastly, the term self-efficacy was used to refer to one's own belief that one can perform well in a particular situation. These concepts were influential in the CBT movement (1-7).

Table 1. Applications of behavioral and cognitive behavioral therapy

DSM-5 Disorder Classification	Typical Specific Disorders
Neurodevelopmental Disorders	Autism, Intellectual and Developmental Delay, Language and Communication Deficits, Tic Disorders, Attention Deficit/Hyperactivity Disorders
Schizophrenia and Other Psychotic Disorders	Schizophrenia (mostly focused on negative symptoms), Delusional Psychotic Disorders
Bipolar and Related Disorders	Type I, II, and unspecified
Depressive Disorders	Major Depression, Dysthymia, Disruptive Mood Dysregulation Disorder
Anxiety Disorders	Separation Anxiety Disorder, Selective Mutism, Specific Phobia, Social Anxiety, Panic Disorder, Agoraphobia, Generalized Anxiety Disorder, Unspecified
Obsessive-Compulsive and Related disorders	Obsessive-Compulsive Disorder, Body Dysmorphic Disorder, Hoarding Disorder, Trichotillomania (hair pulling), Excoriation (skin picking), and other body focused behavior (nail biting)
Trauma and Stressor Related Disorders	Post-Traumatic Stress Disorder, Acute Stress Disorder, Adjustment Disorders
Somatic Symptom and Related Disorders	Conversion Disorder, Somatic Symptom Disorder, Illness Anxiety Disorder
Feeding and Eating Disorders	Anorexia Nervosa, Bulimia Nervosa, Binge Eating Disorder, Avoidant/Restrictive Food Intake Disorder, Pica, Rumination
Elimination Disorders	Enuresis and Encopresis
Sleep-Wake Disorders	Insomnia Disorder (psychogenic origin)
Sexual Disorders	Psychogenic origin (Mostly applied to late adolescence)
Disruptive. Impulsive-Control and Conduct Disorders	Oppositional Defiant Disorder, Intermittent Explosive Disorder, Conduct Disorder, Pyromania, Kleptomania
Substance-Related and Addictive Disorders	All Substance Use and Abuse Disorders (i.e., alcohol, opioid, stimulant, sedative, etc.)
Personality Disorders	Borderline, Avoidant, Dependent, Histrionic, Obsessive-Compulsive, Unspecified

There are hundreds of empirical trials demonstrating the efficacy of CBT and have addressed a large number of behavioral/psychological conditions affecting the pediatric population. It is important to note that in several conditions, such as ADHD, Tourette's, Obsessive Compulsive Disorder (OCD), psychosis, mood and anxiety disorders, a pharmaceutical and psycho-social intervention combined approach is indicated. While in others, a purely psychotherapeutic approach is sufficient.

Table 2. Other applications of behavioral and cognitive behavioral therapy

Family Issues: conflict, communication
Parenting and Child Behavior Management
Stress Management
Assertiveness Training
Social Skills Training
Toilet Training
Behavioral Problems (i.e., aggression, compliance, etc.)
Excessive Tantrum Behavior
Obesity
Classroom Management
Juvenile Programs
Education and Achievement Problems
Medical and Health Care Compliance and Management (e.g., Diabetes, Asthma)

Behavior therapy principles and techniques

Even though the roots of BT extend to the work of Pavlov and Watson in the early 1900's, it was around the middle of the 20th century that BT was established as a separate school of psychotherapy. BT encompasses a large array of techniques, integrating learning principles from operant (instrumental) and classical (respondent) conditioning. It also integrates psychological principles from developmental, social, and other specialized fields of psychology, as well as from allied fields of study, such as neurology, biology, sociology and anthropology. BT utilizes these principles to systematically and constructively modify or eliminate maladaptive behavioral patterns, and develop or strengthen adaptive behavior when it is absent or insufficient. Therefore, one of the central aims of BT is to eliminate or reduce consistently recurring behavioral patterns that are self-defeating and/or interfere with the welfare of others; and to replace them with more effective, flexible and adaptive patterns.

In learning theory and therefore BT, *behavior* constitutes anything a human (or organism) does. Thus, behavior includes *cognition* (thoughts, images, memories, interpretations, etc.), *affective/emotion* components (moods, feelings, emotions, interoceptive sensations or psychophysiological responses, etc.), and *actions* (operant or instrumental behavior, what we do to get or get-away-from something), which involve the musculoskeletal system. Therefore, any behavior, be it cognitive, affective, or instrumental action, is under the influence of operant and classical conditioning paradigms or operations.

Thus any of these are conditionable, and therefore can be altered or modified. Even reflexive components of affective responses or physiological responses, such as heart rate, blood pressure, galvanic skin response, and digestive responses are conditionable, modifiable or altered. When we consider the human organism as a whole, the cognitive, affective and action components of responding are all intricately integrated. Furthermore, this intricately connected behavioral system is intricately connected to environmental variables, the contexts in which behavior occurs.

In BT, case conceptualization involves developing hypotheses about *what* the patient is like and *why* he is like that. It utilizes behavioral principles in this process, and relies on empirical observation. Thus, by careful assessment of the context within which target behaviors occur, it develops testable hypothesis about causative and maintaining factors and treatment interventions (9).

It is also important to assess background socio-cultural and religious factors, historical, and developmental factors. It is important to emphasize that ongoing assessment is utilized to evaluate the effectiveness of treatment interventions and the validity of the case conceptualization upon which treatment strategies were developed.

Behavior modification

Behavior modification (9) is a term that mainly refers to applications of operant (or instrumental) learning principles to change, modify and shape overt (visible) or covert (private, internal, within our skin; i.e., thinking, imagining, remembering, physiological sensations) behavior. Operant behavior principles address behaviors that are affected by consequences or contingencies (i.e., if a child is praised for asking by saying "please," she is more likely to say "please" in the future). Behavior modification has been applied in a variety of settings such as the office, home, school, prison, juvenile home, hospitals, day treatment, other community settings, or in specialized population –specific settings; i.e., autism or developmentally disabled treatment centers. In current literature, behavioral modification is often subsumed under behavior therapy, though some subsume behavior therapy under behavior modification. Thus the two terms have become synonymous. Nonetheless, for the purpose of this chapter, "Behavior modification (BM)" will be subsumed under "behavior therapy (BT)."

Central to behavior modification (and behavior therapy) is the emphasis in defining problems in terms of behavior that can be observed and measured. Measures are attained in terms of *frequency, duration and intensity*. Secondly, treatment procedures and techniques are seen as altering the individual's *environment* to affect change. Environment involves people, objects, and events in a specific setting or set of circumstances. Stimuli or cues refer to these people, objects, contexts (stimulus complexes; such as the classroom, under one specific teacher; the dining room table; etc.) and events. In operant learning, stimuli or cues are referred to as discriminative stimuli. Specific behavior emission or inhibition become associated with specific cues where behavior is reinforced punished or put on extinction. This is called stimulus control. When stimulus control is established, there is a high probability that under a particular stimulus, a specific behavior will or will not occur.

Thirdly, in behavior modification, methods, rationales, strategies and techniques are precisely described. Furthermore, patients themselves, in real settings, often can apply the techniques. As such, a parent may be clearly instructed on how to use specific approaches to modify the child's behavior (e.g., tantrum behavior) and successfully implement these techniques at home. Lastly, in behavior modification, the scientific demonstration that a particular technique or procedure is directly connected to the attained result is emphasized.

Table 3. Behavior modification principles and procedures to increase behavior

Principles for Increasing Behavior	Procedures
Positive Reinforcement	A consequence follows after a behavior occurs, it increases the probability of that behavior to occur again
Negative Reinforcement	An aversive situation/event is immediately removed after a behavior occurs, it increases the probability of that behavior to occur again
Shaping	Positive reinforcement of successive approximations to desired behavior
Schedules of Reinforcement	Refers to how frequent reinforcement occurs, whether it is continuous or intermittent, or if it is based on a ratio, etc. This affects behavior frequency, pattern, and resistance to extinction.
Premack Principle	A high probability behavior can be used as a positive reinforcer for a less probability behavior.
Generalization	Behavior that has been learned in one situation is likely to occur in a similar situation.
Social Reinforcement (attention, praise, approval)	Social reinforcement is a form of positive reinforcement if it increases the likelihood of that behavior to occur again.
Modeling (vicarious learning, imitation)	A behavior becomes more likely to occur through observation of another individual being positively reinforced for the same type of behavior.

Table 4. Behavior modification procedures to decrease behavior

Principles for Decreasing Behavior	Procedures
Punishment	An aversive consequence follows after a behavior occurs; it decreases the probability of that behavior to occur: spanking, frowning, touching a hot stove (a naturally occurring punisher). A reward is removed (response cost, removing privileges) or the individual is removed from a rewarding situation or activity (time out).
Extinction	Behavior is no longer reinforced, no longer attended to, totally ignored.
Counterconditioning	Differential reinforcement of incompatible behavior or other (appropriate) behavior (DRI or DRO).
Negative Practice	Repeatedly practicing an undesirable behavior (nail biting) over and over again in an established schedule.
Overcorrection	Engaging in a tedious behavior after inappropriate behavior occurs (e.g., a 5 y o boy is guided to undress, wash his cloths and take a bath after he urinates on his cloths).
Vicarious Learning	Observing someone experiencing punishment or any of the above procedures, reducing probability of behavior to occur.

In behavior modification, target behaviors refer to the behaviors to be improved, developed or modified. Behavioral assessment is indispensable in developing a behavior modification plan. The behavioral assessment involves collecting and analyzing information and data to identify and describe target behaviors; it also involves identifying causes of the behavior (consequences, or what is happening in the environment that is maintaining the behavior). This process helps in deciding which interventions will be appropriate and how treatment effectiveness will be evaluated. This process is called *functional analysis*. As stated above, what occurs after a behavior is emitted (*consequences*) will affect whether the probability of the behavior occurring in the future increases or decreases. As such positive reinforcement refers to an event (reinforcer) which when presented after the occurrence of a behavior increases the likelihood of that behavior to occur again. Negative reinforcement refers to the removal of a condition, event or stimulus aversive to the organism (pain, anxiety, distress), which also has the effect of increasing the likelihood of that behavior to occur again. Punishment refers to a consequence or event that reduces the likelihood of that behavior to occur. Extinction refers to the process by which a positive or negative reinforcer is withdrawn, with the result that the previously reinforced behavior is eventually reduced or eliminated. From these operant learning principles, various procedures have been developed to shape, modify, increase or decrease behaviors. In terms of increasing behavior, there are several schedules of reinforcement (rules that specify which occurrences of a behavior, if any, will be reinforced), which differ in terms of the "strength" or resistance to extinction of the attained behavior.

The *Premack Principle (Grandma's Rule)* is an important principle in behavior modification applications. It refers to the well-researched finding that high frequency or high-probability behavior can be utilized as a positive reinforcer for a low frequency or low-probability behavior. For example if mowing the lawn is a high-frequency behavior, it can be used to reinforce a low-frequency behavior, such as picking up dirty clothes in the bedroom. Thus a person's behavior can be utilized as a reinforcer in a behavior modification program or in modifying one's own behavior, "after you clean your room, you can go out and mow the lawn (or play)."

Another important finding is that behavior can be learned by observation. This type of learning is called *vicarious learning*. Maintenance of the behavior, however, is dependent upon the basic reinforcement principles and operations described above. The utilization of modeling techniques is based on this principle (8).

In BM applications, positive reinforcement is emphasized over punishment and extinction. Although punishment and extinction are sometimes used, simply punishing or putting an undesired behavior on extinction does not guarantee that the desired behavior will occur. The desired behavior needs to be strengthened through positive reinforcement; otherwise, undesired behaviors such as escape, avoidance, anger and other negative emotions are likely to be inadvertently reinforced. Thus, to achieve the elimination of an undesired behavior, the desired or incompatible behavior needs to be reinforced. This is referred to as *differential reinforcement of incompatible behavior (DRI)* or *differential reinforcement of other behavior (DRO)*, "other behavior" being the desired behaviors.

Lastly, most parenting approaches in use today are significantly tied to the use of BM techniques. Being a parent requires an enormous amount of responsibility and effort. Teachers and other significant adults share in that responsibility from early childhood until young adulthood. BM has developed numerous applications that are consistently taught to parents to help children attain adaptive patterns during their development. It begins with such steps as helping children to walk, to be toilet trained, to talk, to comply, to do chores, etc. Other techniques address decreasing behavior that is maladaptive, such as decreasing temper tantrums, nail biting, defiance, lying, stealing, aggressive behavior, etc. The commonly used techniques of using "time out" procedures, implementing reward or chart programs (point/token systems), developing a structured home environment, promoting effective communication skills, and many others are also direct applications of BM techniques.

Behavior therapy (BT)

In the 1950s, as behavior therapists in England (Lazarus) and South Africa (Wolpe) were using Pavlovian/Classical conditioning methodology, in the United States, operant principles were popular (BM or applied behavioral analysis). Eventually, these two methodologies integrated to become what is now known as BT (10).

Classical conditioning (also known as respondent conditioning) is based on the fact that humans and other organisms learn to associate events or stimuli that frequently occur together in time. In classical conditioning there are various principles and operations. These include the *unconditioned stimulus (US)*, a stimulus that evoke an *unconditioned response (UR)*, a reflexive non-learned response, such as salivation in the presence of food, increased heart rate (and other physiological responses) in the presence of a threat, shivering when exposed to cold, sucking when nipple touches the lips of an infant, etc. The basic types of respondents or reflexes include the digestive, circulatory and respiratory systems. Respondents are also a basic component of emotions or feelings, the sensations we experience. *Conditioned stimulus (CS)* refers to a previously *neutral stimulus (NS)* (a stimulus that has no specific reflex or respondent already associated with it) that has been paired with a respondent (either an aversive or appetitive response). After several pairings this NS becomes associated with the response and when presented evokes the previously paired respondent/reflex (e.g., salivation, increased heart rate). This associated response becomes a *conditioned response*.

Table 5. Classical (respondent) conditioning principles and operations

Principle	Operation
Unconditioned Stimulus	Evokes a reflexive, non-learned response.
Unconditioned Response	Innate non--learned reflexes.
Neutral Stimulus	A stimulus that does not result in a reflexive or learned response.
Conditioned stimulus	When a neutral stimulus is repeatedly presented with an unconditioned stimulus, it eventually evokes a similar reflexive response.
Conditioned Response	The learned response evoked by a conditioned stimulus.
Extinction	When the unconditioned stimulus is repeatedly withheld during presentations of the previously associated conditioned stimulus, the conditioned response eventually stops occurring.

Generalization refers to the likelihood that a CR would be evoked in situations similar to the one in which the CR was conditioned. For example if a child has been attacked by another child wearing a red shirt (CS), a child wearing an orange shirt (generalized CS) will likely evoke the CR (fear response). The concept of *extinction* refers to the operation by which a conditioned stimulus is no longer temporally presented with the unconditioned stimulus. Eventually, the conditioned stimulus will stop evoking the conditioned response. In contemporary learning theory, extinction is considered a misnomer because associations are not actually unlearned (11). Alternatively, new associations are learned, thus the CS evoke competing conditioned responses (inhibitory learning). When a CS is presented in situations different from those present during the extinction operation, the CR is likely to be evoked again (spontaneous recovery).

It is very important to understand that classically conditioned responses, such as conditioned anxiety responses, are inseparable from operant response conditioning. For example, when the CS-CR response set for anxiety is established, escape/avoidance behaviors are almost immediately established as well. Escape/avoidance behavioral patterns are established through negative reinforcement, (i.e., the organism does something to avoid or escape the aversive response and other associated CS's). In humans, these patterns are made into association rules (e.g., "I get panic attacks when I go to the mall"), such that in the future, someone asking a particular adolescent to go to the mall will immediately result in an anxiety response (albeit small in intensity) which then will result in an avoidance response (negatively reinforced), such as an excuse; e.g., "not today, I do not feel well."

Before specific techniques and applications are discussed, it is important to note that in developing a behavioral case conceptualization, the assessment requires specification of cognitive, psychophysiological and behavioral components of the problem behavior and the stimuli (triggers) associated with those responses. For example, cognitive experiences such as worries, "what if...?" questions, associational rules and self-defeating thoughts and beliefs about effectiveness or self-worth are identified, as well as physical sensations, such as suffocation, tight chest, muscle tension, increased heart rate, etc. In addition, behavioral manifestations that are associated with a particular situation or trigger are characterized, including social withdrawal, inactivity, lack of goal directed activity, and escape and avoidance behaviors, such as making excuses and safety-seeking behavior (seeking reassurance, rituals, etc.). Contributing conditions also are identified, such as being tired, stressed, hungry, tired, and hung over, etc.

Behavioral techniques and applications

Various behavioral techniques have been developed primarily based on classical conditioning paradigms. Nevertheless, in theory and in practice, both operant and classical conditioning paradigms are always concurrently operating. For example, an adolescent suffering with panic disorder is asked by her friend to go to the movies, but because she previously had a panic attack in a crowded situation, she immediately feels anxious (a classically conditioned response). She appraises the situation as potentially dangerous with a cognitive response, such as: "What if I have a panic attack and can't get away, lose control, I'll look crazy and everyone will think I'm a total loser!" She then makes an excuse (an operant verbal behavior) that allows her to avoid going to the theater (a feared and anxiety producing situation) and, thus, her anxiety and the excuse-behavior (avoidance/escape) is negatively reinforced. In addition, this adolescent's parents feel sorry for her and indulge her with affection and extra attention (positive reinforcement, which in this case is also called "secondary gain"). In behavioral treatment, the cognitive components are targeted also, as it will be explained later.

Exposure techniques are among the most widely known BT techniques. It is confrontation with situations that evoke the anxiety/fear response in order to achieve the eventual reduction of the intensity of the response to tolerable levels, and, very importantly, to reduce escape and avoidance behaviors. This exposure has to be done repeatedly over an extended period of time until the associated anxiety response is tolerated. During this exposure, escape behavior is not allowed. This is called *response prevention*. In fact, exposure without response prevention does not result in the desired lowered anxiety/fear response or the corresponding lowered avoidance and escape behavior for that specific situation or evoking stimulus (sensations, thoughts, having to take an exam) or stimulus set (a crowded theater). If there is no response prevention, the escape/avoidance behavior continues to be negatively reinforced, and therefore the anxiety response continues to be maintained. Exposure and response prevention often involves development of *hierarchies*.

Developing hierarchies involves creating a graded list of situations in which anxiety is evoked at increasing degrees or intensity, such that the situations range from mild to moderate (30-40 in a scale of 0-100, 100 being the highest) levels of anxiety to very high levels (80-100). Various scales may be used, depending on the age or sophistication of the child or adolescent. The scales can range from 1- 5, 1- 10, or 1- 8, with the numbers representing *subjective units of distress* or *SUD's*. Exposure and response prevention gradually proceed from mild to moderate levels of distress to increasingly higher levels, but only if after the lower level is consistently tolerated; e.g., 20 to 30 or 2 to 3 SUD's.

There are two types of exposures, in-vivo and imaginal. *In-vivo exposure* refers to situations in real life in which the individual experiences much anxiety and therefore escapes or avoids; examples of in-vivo situations include crowded places, school and social situations. In-vivo exposure is often applied with specific phobias, social anxiety, post-traumatic stress disorder (PTSD), obsessive compulsive disorder (OCD), and with any condition in which the conditioned response is associated with an external situation or stimulus (trigger). There is a special form of in-vivo exposure referred to as *interoceptive exposure* (12). Basically, fear responses can be conditioned to internal physiological stimuli, and *interoceptive stimuli*, a term first used by Russian investigators, is the term that is currently utilized universally. These researchers found that interoceptive stimuli-associated learned fear was particularly resistant to extinction. In panic disorder, for example, patients often indicate the absence of external triggers, as if the attacks come "out of the blue." In reality, they are responding to an internal physiological stimulus outside their conscious awareness (12).

Interoceptive exposure involves repeatedly exposing the individual to the same physiological responses/sensations that evoke the fear response (panic). Through repeated exposures to purposely evoked sensations, these fear-associated sensations eventually result in a lowered intensity of the fear response. For example, an adolescent with panic disorder would be asked to hyperventilate until he or she experiences shallow breathing, breathlessness, or dizziness in order to elicit the fear/anxiety response. As with other exposure methods, graduated hierarchical exposure is often used, starting with a lower level anxiety producing sensation (40 SUD) and gradually progressing to higher level anxiety producing sensations. There are several manuals describing these procedures, most include cognitive restructuring procedures (13).

Imaginal exposure refers to engaging the individual in exposure to imagined stimuli, such as memories, images, impulses, thoughts (such as in generalized anxiety disorder, PTSD and OCD) and other cognitive material. The process of developing hierarchies is used in imaginal exposure, also. The individual is asked to imagine the feared situation as vividly as possible, describing the feared stimuli as clearly as possible and involving all senses (sensations) and outcomes. This process is repeated over extended periods of time and can be done verbally or in writing. It is important to note, virtual-reality scenarios currently are being utilized in this process of exposure and response prevention.

It is important to understand that exposure techniques have replaced *systematic desensitization*, which was espoused by Wolpe in the early 1950s (14, 5). Desensitization was thought to result in reduction of anxiety by pairing an anxiety evoking situation with the relaxation response. It was believed that the anxiety evoking situation eventually would be neutralized or counteracted by the relaxation response. It was later found that the relaxation response was not needed, but the graduated exposure to the anxiety provoking stimuli coupled with response prevention (preventing the avoidance or escape behavior) was necessary and also sufficient. The use of hierarchical exposure was maintained and came to be seen as key elements. Relaxation training also has been maintained as important in the treatment of anxiety disorders and other problems, such as pain management.

Relaxation training

This can take several forms, such as progressive muscle relaxation training, breathing retraining (focused or mindful breathing), autogenic relaxation training, and others, but these techniques must be applied judiciously and systematically. Relaxation training is not universally productive if used by itself in the treatment of anxiety disorders and OCD. Also, in a minority of individuals aspects of the relaxation response may actually provoke anxiety and panic. It is hypothesized that the internal sensations (interoceptive stimuli) produced by relaxation may evoke the anxiety response. This apparent paradoxical response has been extensively documented (12). Thus it is important to assess whether producing the relaxation response actually may be counterproductive. If it is tolerated, then it can be effectively utilized in conjunction with other methods (e.g., exposure methods). It is important to emphasize that just simply introducing patients to a relaxation method in session and then asking them to practice is not effective and is a misapplication of relaxation techniques as a treatment method (10).

Applied relaxation involves extensive relaxation exercises and training to develop the patient's ability to relax and, thus, achieve relaxation more quickly. It also involves training in early detection of anxiety cues. Lastly, it involves applying relaxation techniques in the presence of these cues. This process needs to be well guided and systematically applied. Self-calming techniques, including mindfulness breathing, distraction, and focused attention are often taught along with progressive relaxation techniques. Self-calming techniques and relaxation are widely utilized in helping children and adolescents cope with specific anxiety producing situations. They are also widely used as components in the treatment of anger and aggressive behavior (16); yet, these procedures are often not effective as stand-alone applications.

Biofeedback training

This is another behavioral technique that has been useful in managing tension headaches, migraines, and specific muscle tension-associated pains. In biofeedback training the patient is given feedback on his/her electrophysiological activity, most commonly via auditory or visual sensory modes. The individual is trained to reduce the intensity of the sensory input. In children, a visual cue is often used, such that an image of a train would move faster as the intensity of the electrophysiological activity is lowered.

Emotion regulation

Emotional regulation skills training is central to Dialectical Behavioral Therapy (DBT, a therapeutic program directed at the treatment of borderline personality disorder) and other applications, such as those for individuals traumatized by abuse (17, 18). Even though DBT was developed to address difficult to treat adults (especially those prone to self-destructive behavior, such as suicidal behavior), various applications have been developed for adolescents and their families (19). In general, emotion regulation skills training emphasize teaching the individual to identify the specific triggers associated with a particular emotional response, and the consequences attached to that emotion. Individuals learn to identify their emotions as they occur and to differentiate among different emotions (e.g., anger versus fear).

Patients also are taught to differentiate between those emotions directly evoked by an external trigger and those evoked by an internal trigger, such as a thought or the initially externally evoked emotion. Lastly, individuals are taught strategies that allow them to respond more calmly and adaptively. In general, emotion regulation is seen as an integral part of psychotherapy for children and adolescents, and it is applied in the treatment of various diagnoses, including anxiety disorders, depression, and externalizing and internalizing disorders (20).

Stress management

This has been an area of study and clinical development for several decades (21-23). Most approaches are integrative in nature, and they borrow from behavioral, cognitive, and other clinical approaches, such as mindfulness and yoga. These approaches involve managing distress in the moment and as it happens, daily stress/distress lowering procedures, time management and scheduling, problem solving, prioritizing, conflict management, balancing between demands and recuperative activities (socialization, leisure, exercising), cognitive techniques (how one assesses and reacts to a stressful situation), etc. Stress management is considered not only a psychological intervention, but also a medical one. It lowers the stress response in the short and long term, which when, cumulative, it can result in significant psycho-immunological effects.

Behavioral activation (BA)

BA is becoming widely used in the treatment of depression, and there are several treatment guides (24). "Activity scheduling" is an integral part of cognitive therapy, as presented by Beck (4). In 2001, based on their research, Neil Jacobson and colleagues introduced behavioral activation as a stand-alone treatment for depression. In 2006, Dimidjian (25) demonstrated that an expanded form of behavioral activation was as effective as medication and cognitive therapy, and superior to either one for severe depression. Beck originally indicated that with more severely depressed individuals, behavioral activation (activity scheduling) was the component of choice at the beginning of treatment. The stated goal is to restore functioning to premorbid levels. This approach has been applied to severely depressed adolescents, where it has been formulated as a preferred treatment approach (25). From a behavioral perspective, the characteristic inactivity of depressed adolescents precludes their exposure to the potential reinforcement which one finds either through contact with others or directly associated with certain activities. This inactivity also serves as an avoidant behavior and thus it is negatively reinforced.

The individual may feel relief from not doing something (e.g., making the effort to call a friend or doing home-work), but this negative reinforcement is short lived and reduces the potential opportunity for positive reinforcement. As these patterns increase in range and frequency, there is usually a disruption of healthy patterns of behavior, such as school attendance, participation in recreational and social activities, etc. Consequently, after a therapeutic relationship is developed and a thorough understanding of this model of depression is established, BA then directly focuses on specific areas of avoidant behavior and routine disruption. If an adolescent is socially withdrawn and isolated, but actually holds socialization as important and meaningful to her life (i.e., it is valued), that area would be targeted. Usually, through a collaborative process, the person engages in specifically planned actions regardless of how he feels (depressed, unmotivated, experiencing lack of energy, etc.).

Modeling

Modeling is a powerful procedure that has been used from both operant and classical conditioning perspective and based on the principle of vicarious conditioning. In the operant approach, certain behaviors are modeled in a specific situation and observed by another individual. Later, the individual reproduces that behavior in the same or similar situation. The behavior that is attained by modeling is maintained by the consequences that follow, resulting in both positive and negative reinforcement. This approach is often used in the attainment of skills, such as social skills. In the classical conditioning paradigm, modeling is used to facilitate exposure to feared situations (10).

For instance, if a child is afraid of the dark, the therapist first models the behavior of staying in a dark room with the door closed. Then the therapist and the child both go into the dark room together. Through graduated exposure (e.g., the door being gradually closed, and the therapist gradually exiting), the child will eventually go alone into the dark room. Much praise is used in this process. Often, modeling is integrated with guided behavioral rehearsal, and is integral to the acquisition and facilitation of new behavioral patterns. Lastly, modeling is utilized in conjunction with exposure and other cognitive and behavioral techniques.

Psychoeducation

Another aspect of behavior therapy, behavior modification and cognitive therapy is the utilization of *psychoeducation*. Because of the collaborative process and the transparency of the methodology, patients (along with parents, siblings, teachers, and others) may become cognizant of all the techniques, rationale, models, and concepts being utilized in treatment. Psychoeducation helps the patient be an active participant in treatment, with the ultimate goal being to help the individual become his/her own therapist; doing this requires psychoeducation throughout treatment, especially at the beginning. Psychoeducation usually includes in-session discussion, instruction, and assigned readings. It is an integral part of treatment for all problems addressed through a behavioral or cognitive therapy model.

Problem solving

Difficulties with *problem solving*, whether due to lack of skills or the utilization of ineffective strategies, can result in psychological problems. These types of difficulties also can be a significant factor in certain syndromes, such as in generalized anxiety disorder, social anxiety, unipolar depression, psychosis and others. The goal of problem solving skills training is to teach rational problem solving, develop a positive problem solving orientation, and eliminate impulsive and ineffective problem solving or habitual avoidance. This is very important in assertiveness training, relationship therapy, and conflict resolution. Problem solving skills training is often an integral component in parent training, stress management and in the treatment of depression, anxiety disorders, and bipolar disorder in adolescents, as well treatment of chronic illness and obesity.

Stimulus control

Currently, there are various applications of the concept of *stimulus control.* Behavioral patterns or reactions (the interaction of cognitions, operant responses/behaviors, and emotions/physiological responses) are learned in association with specific situations or stimulus complexes or contexts. In these situations, specific behavioral patterns are emitted or inhibited. Stimulus control procedures have been used in the treatment of various conditions, such as obesity, substance abuse, insomnia and others. It is also an integral part of DBT. For example, in the treatment of adult insomnia (26), the individual is instructed to utilize the bedroom solely for sleeping and sex. At the beginning of treatment, the latter is also eliminated in some cases. Together with other procedures (e.g., going to bed only when feeling sleepy and only at a specific time, getting up if unable to fall sleep within a certain amount of time, etc.), the bedroom becomes solely associated with the sleep response and not with other behaviors like watching TV, reading, eating, problem solving, worrying, etc. Given the multipurpose use of the bedroom by adolescents and children, stimulus control procedures for improving sleep require creative and thoughtful modifications of standard treatment.

Furthermore, with children and adolescents, stimulus control is utilized in establishing structured activities, such as home-work and daily routines (e.g., play-time, dinner time, bed time), in compliance training, etc. It is also utilized in the establishment of social skills. In establishing an alternative pattern of behavior to one that is not desired (faulty stimulus control), such as coming into the house and spreading one's belongings everywhere, a very common problem faced by parents. Establishing stimulus control for a specific desired pattern can effectively be attained by taking the child back to the very beginning of the desired pattern (corrective procedure).

For instance if a child is not putting her jacket and boots in the desired place when she comes into the house, the parent would ask the child to go outside with the coat and boots on, have her come back in, prompt her to put the coat and boots in the proper place and praise/reinforce her for doing so. Also, stimulus control is a very important component of behavioral procedures used in the treatment of ADHD, Oppositional Defiant Disorder (ODD) and other externalizing disorders.

Others

Token economies, point systems, and behavior management programs are operant behavioral applications often used in institutional care, such as Inpatient and Partial Hospitalization Programs, specialized population programs, such as the juvenile delinquent population, and schools. But they can also be used at home. Tokens or points can be earned for several desired behaviors, can be accumulated, and can be exchanged later for a variety of back up reinforcers, such as privileges, activities, objects or items, or even edibles. Usually, tokens are given immediately after a desired behavior occurs, to be cashed in later. As such, tokens act as an immediate reinforcer in situations where a delay exists between the target desired behavior and the backup reinforcer.

This is very important as it may be impractical or impossible to deliver a backup reinforcer immediately after the target desired behavior occurs. This is often true in schools and treatment programs, such as addiction and psychiatric treatment programs. Token economies have been very successful in the treatment and management of behavior and have been applied for use in several populations, such as in regular and special education, juvenile and pre-juvenile homes, mental health treatment programs, drug addiction programs, residential programs, etc.

Various other procedures have been developed for specific problems. These include, but are not limited to compliance training, parent training, anger management and aggression reduction, habit reversal training (e.g., trichotillomania, skin picking), behavioral intervention for tics (Tourette's syndrome), reducing tantrum behavior, toilet training, eliminating or reducing fear and phobias, school avoidance, scholastic problems, eating problems and obesity, compliance with medical management, and many others. Also, behavioral procedures, including procedures based on operant learning have been applied in numerous settings, such as school, home, institutional care, health care institutions, psychiatric institutions, and others.

Cognitive conceptualization focused treatment: Cognitive therapy and cognitive-behavior therapy

Even though there have been several cognitive models of therapy, Aaron T Beck's, Ellis' and Meichenbaum's models are the most widely known (4-7). Beck's therapy approach share commonalities with the other cognitive and behavioral approaches; from learning, psychodynamic, and social learning theory; and with the work of Piaget, Ellis, Horney, Adler, Lazarus, Meichenbaum and others. Paraphrasing Judy S. Beck, in the cognitive model, dysfunctional thinking and cognitive processes affect the patient's mood and behavior (actions), and are common to all psychological disturbances (1). Even though this view predominated during the early years of cognitive therapy (CT), current approaches based on this basic cognitive principle increasingly integrate behavioral procedures, and thus they are currently referred to as cognitive-behavior therapy (1-3). Even so, Beck, Ellis, and Meichenbaum utilized behavioral techniques in their treatment approach from the very beginning.

Thus, while focusing on current behavior, clinical formulations emphasize maladaptive thinking and behavior (actions), which maintain and are associated with psychoemotional distress and impairment (1, 3). Furthermore, this cognitive-behavior model is based on the principle that cognitions/thoughts and behavior are inextricably linked to emotional responding (3). With this in mind, treatment goals are focused both on cognitive and behavioral (action) change, with consequent changes in emotional response. Some treatment sessions and goals may be focused more on one of these integral components than on the other. Within this framework, techniques specifically directed at emotional control and change is currently utilized. Some of these include relaxation training, breathing retraining, and emotional regulation skills.

CBT techniques continue to evolve and become integrated with other identified treatments. Utilizing the cognitive formulation, Judy S Beck (1), and Berman and Weisz (3) summarize the basic principles of CBT as follows:

1) From the cognitive perspective, therapy is guided by "…ever-evolving formulation of patient's problems and an individual conceptualization of each patient in cognitive terms (1)."
2) A strongly developed therapeutic alliance is indispensable.
3) Therapy is a collaborative (team) process.
4) Therapy is "…goal oriented and problem focused (1)," and goals are defined in specific, objective, and measureable terms.
5) Therapy is focused on the here and now, but utilizes information regarding symptom origin (current and past, socio-cultural and biological factors) in formulation and treatment.
6) Therapy involves psychoeducation, "…teaches the patient to be his/her own therapist, and emphasizes relapse prevention (1, 3)."
7) From an integrated perspective, "…maladaptive behaviors and cognitions are presumed to be learned and maintained based on behavioral learning principles (3)."
8) Therapy is structured in such ways that it strives to be time limited (1, 3).
9) Therapy sessions are structured and utilize the development of a session agenda that is directly associated with the treatment plan, goals and objectives. Agendas need to be flexible, as needed.
10) From a cognitive perspective, patients are taught to identify, evaluate and respond to (modify) their dysfunctional thoughts and beliefs.
11) Therapy integrates cognitive and behavioral techniques to modify cognitive, emotional and behavioral patterns.
12) Therapy is an active process, involving both the therapist and the patient.
13) It is tailored to the specific needs of the patient.
14) Therapy requires patient's action and application in the natural environment.

In current CBT, all of the behavioral techniques described above are utilized. In the cognitive model, various techniques are specifically utilized, all based on the hypothesis that a person's emotional, physiological, and behavioral (action) reaction to a specific situation or event is affected by how the person perceives and interprets that situation or event, i.e., the meaning it is given. Thus a situation activates automatic thinking, which in turn affects the emotional-behavioral-physiological reaction (1). Specific cognitive restructuring techniques include:

1) Problem definition, case conceptualization, and goal setting (also a behavioral task),
2) Educating and socializing the patient (and family) to the cognitive model,
3) Educating and socializing the patient to the structure of the therapy session,
4) Behavioral activation,
5) Educating, explaining, and eliciting automatic thoughts and teaching the patient to identify them,
6) Helping the patient distinguish between automatic thoughts and emotions, rating intensity of emotion,
7) Identifying and focusing on the most impactful automatic thoughts,
8) Helping the patient examine and evaluate automatic thoughts,
9) Utilizing techniques to engender alternative and more effective modes of thinking,
10) Helping the patient respond to automatic thoughts in a more realistic and effective manner,
11) Helping patients identify and distinguishing healthy and unhealthy (negative) beliefs,
12) Helping patients modify negative beliefs and develop helpful, realistic and balanced beliefs, associated with healthier emotional and behavioral reactions

CONCLUSION

In summary, in applying the basic behavioral and cognitive procedures of CBT with children and adolescents, modifications need to be made. These vary as to the age, developmental stage, and cognitive and behavioral maturation of the child or adolescent. It is also very important to consider socio-cultural, economic, spiritual and religious factors in applying these procedures. CBT is consistently evolving, expanding, and integrating its field of application. It is imperative that the primary care physician and medical specialists become cognizant of the capacity and effectiveness of these procedures when applied in pediatric treatment.

REFERENCES

[1] Beck JS. Cognitive behavior therapy: basics and beyond, 2nd ed. New York: Guilford, 2011.
[2] Kendall PC. Child and adolescent therapy: cognitive-behavioral procedures, 4th ed. New York: Guilford, 2012:3-24.
[3] Bearman SK, Weisz JR. Cognitive behavior therapy: An introduction. In: Szigethy E, Weisz JR, Findling RL, eds. Cognitive-behavior therapy for children and adolescents. Washington DC: American Psychiatric Publishing, 2012:1-28.

[4] Beck AT, Rush J, Shaw BT, Emery G. Cognitive therapy of depression. New York: Guilford, 1979.
[5] Ellis A. Rational psychotherapy. J Gen Psychol 1958; 59:35-49.
[6] Beck AT. Thinking and depression: Idiosyncratic content and cognitive distortions. Arch Gen Psychiatry 1963;324-33.
[7] Meichenbaum D. Cognitive-behavior modification: An integrative approach. New York: Plenum, 1979.
[8] Bandura A. Social learning theory. Englewood Cliffs, NJ: Prentice Hall, 1977.
[9] Martin G, Pear J. Behavior modification: What it is and how to do it, 9th ed. Upper Saddle River, NJ: Prentice Hall, 2010.
[10] Antony M, Roemer L. Behavior therapy. Washington DC: American Psychological Association, 2011.
[11] Boston ME, Westbrook RF, Corcoran KA, Marne S. Contextual and temporal modulation of extinction: Behavioral and biological mechanisms. Biol Psychiatry 2006;60:352-60.
[12] Barlow DH. Anxiety and its disorders: The nature and treatment of anxiety and panic, 2nd ed. New York: Guilford, 2002:219-51,328-79.
[13] Craske MG, Barlow DH, Meadows E. Mastery of your anxiety and panic: Therapist guide for anxiety, panic, and agoraphobia. San Antonio, TX: Gray Wind/Psychological Corporation, 2000.
[14] Wolpe J. Experimental neurosis as learned behavior. Br J Psychol 1952;43:243-68.
[15] Wolpe J. Reciprocal inhibition as the main basis of psychotherapeutic effects. Arch Neurol Psychiatry 1954;72:205-26.
[16] Glick B, Gibbs J C. Aggression replacement training: A comprehensive Intervention for aggressive youth, 3rd ed. Champaign, IL: Research Press, 2013.
[17] Linehan MM. Cognitive-behavioral treatment of borderline personality disorder. New York: Guilford, 1993.
[18] Cohen AC, Mannering AP, Dubliner E. Treating trauma and traumatic grief in children and adolescents. New York: Guilford, 2006.
[19] Miller AL, Arthurs JH, Linehan MM. Dialectical behavior therapy with suicidal adolescents. New York: Guilford, 2007.
[20] Southam-Gerow MA. Emotion regulation in children and adolescents: A practitioner's guide. New York: Guilford, 2013.
[21] Cannon W. The wisdom of the body, 2nd ed. New York: Norton, 1939.
[22] Davis M, Robbins-Eshelman E, McKay M. The relaxation and stress reduction workbook. Oakland, CA: New Harbinger, 2008.
[23] Leahy RL, Tirch D, Napolitano LA. Emotion regulation in psychotherapy. New York: Guilford, 2011:177-200.
[24] Martell CR, Dimidjian S, Herman-Dunn R. Behavioral activation for depression: A clinician's guide. New York: Guilford, 2013.
[25] Maalouf FT, Brent DA. Depression and suicidal behavior. In: Szigethy E, Weisz JR, Findling RL, editors. Cognitive-behavior therapy for children and adolescents. Washington, DC: American Psychiatric Publishing, 2012.
[26] Perlis ML, Jungquist C, Smith MT, Posner D. Cognitive behavioral treatment of insomnia: A session-by-session guide. New York: Springer, 2005.

Submitted: June 05, 2015. *Revised:* July 03, 2015. *Accepted:* July 10, 2015.

In: Alternative Medicine Research Yearbook 2017
Editor: Joav Merrick
ISBN: 978-1-53613-726-2
© 2018 Nova Science Publishers, Inc.

Chapter 4

FAMILY THERAPY AS AN INTEGRATED CARE MODEL FOR PEDIATRICIANS

Galen Alessi[*], *PhD and Colleen C Cullinan, MA*

Department of Psychology, Western Michigan University,
Kalamazoo, Michigan, US

ABSTRACT

Family therapy is an important therapeutic modality for children and adolescents with behavioral health problems and disorders. Research studies have consistently demonstrated the efficacy of family therapy for select pediatric patients and their families. Principles of family therapy are presented in this discussion. Examples based on actual cases illustrate what family therapists do and how they might integrate their expertise into cases, while working side-by-side with pediatricians. It is important for primary care clinicians working with children and youth to collaborate with family therapists when their pediatric patients face behavioral or psychiatric issues.

Keywords: family therapy, behavior, pediatrics

INTRODUCTION

Pediatricians can dread questions from patient families about complex behavioral health issues. Concerns about psychosocial stresses too often are voiced just as the pediatrician is wrapping up a visit. Trying to handle these concerns during a typical pediatric visit runs over the scheduled time, and pediatricians may feel overwhelmed and unprepared to assess and navigate underlying family health dynamics. While research studies consistently demonstrate the efficacy of carefully selected family therapy interventions in treating behavioral health issues, there are many barriers in the health care system to families receiving such

---

[*] Correspondence: Galen Alessi PhD, Department of Psychology, Western Michigan University Kalamazoo, MI 49048, USA. E-mail: galen.alessi@wmich.edu.

comprehensive care. Integrated care models, which blend family therapy perspectives into pediatric visits, may offer pediatricians and their patients a solution. This review will present several key concepts in family therapy, and suggest how family therapy conceptualizations can enhance health care outcomes within the primary pediatric practice, offered in an integrated health care model. Examples based on actual cases will illustrate what family therapists do and how they might integrate their expertise into cases, while working side-by-side with pediatricians.

Danny is an eight years old boy who was just seen by you for a well-child examination. You have spent twenty minutes with Danny and his mother, reviewing his vital signs and asking questions about his physical activity, screen time, diet, sleep, and vitamin intake. Danny seems like a bright, outgoing, healthy child and there are no specific concerns that need to be addressed at this time. Just as you are about to leave and move on to the next patient in a long fully scheduled day, you hesitate and ask: "Is there anything else?" Danny's mother pauses and answers: "Well, Danny's teacher has some concerns about his behavior in class. She says he has a hard time staying in his seat, and he can be distracting to other kids. We've always struggled to get him to do as he is told at home, but now we are getting complaints from school about his lack of focus and his hyper behavior. Should we be concerned?" Danny gets quite angry that his mother has brought this up, and, suddenly, you have an apprehensive mother and a sulky child waiting for your response while you are almost late for your next scheduled patient.

This scenario is all too familiar for many busy pediatricians. These last second, "hand-on-the-door," questions can derail an entire day's schedule and leave physicians wishing they had not probed any additional concerns. Many physicians simply do not have the extra time or resources to adequately handle questions regarding psychosocial or behavioral health issues. Family therapists, however, specialize in these complicated issues that can affect health outcomes for pediatricians and their patients.

CHALLENGES OF A PEDIATRIC PRACTICE

Why family therapy? What is family therapy? Why see the whole family? What do family therapists do? How do they do it? How does family therapy fit with an integrated care model within the pediatric practice? All of these topics will be addressed, illustrating various concepts in family therapy with examples selected from interventions in actual cases.

While psychosocial issues can become crucial treatment factors within up to 70% of primary care appointments, confusion often arises about what guidance to give once the families present with concerns about various behavior problems, undifferentiated somatic complaints, or non-compliance with treatment protocols. Confusion is fostered by a healthcare system that treats behavioral and physical health care issues as separate entities. Silos in healthcare require families to seek services from multiple (uncoordinated) systems and professionals, none of which can provide, on their own, the full array of services necessary for comprehensive care.

Pediatric practices and traditional behavioral health clinics both face challenges in providing effective, comprehensive, and empirically informed care for families with behavioral health concerns. Oftentimes pediatrician referrals to behavioral health care providers do not get addressed in a timely manner. Pediatricians and behavioral health providers alike experience frustration about lack of communication and follow-through with patients, while families struggle with feelings of self-blame, shame, and helplessness regarding their child's condition and care. Stigma and doubt often prevent parents from pursuing family therapy even when pediatricians make thoughtful and well-informed referrals.

Pediatricians are placed in difficult positions in which they routinely see families that may benefit from receiving services from a behavioral health specialist, but also know that these therapists' waitlists are long and that a family's' likelihood of following-through with referrals is low. Due to time and cost constraints, as well as perceived lack of options, many pediatricians are reluctant to even inquire about additional stressors during visits for fear of stepping into this very predicament. Working in such a pressured context contributes to the under-identification of psychosocial issues by both pediatricians and their patient families. When families do bring up complex behavioral health concerns, pediatricians often feel underprepared to deal with the potential family dynamics. These complications within traditional health care delivery systems result in frustration among pediatricians, behavioral health care providers, and patients. Families often do not receive fully adequate or comprehensive care, while health care providers are left feeling dissatisfied and discouraged.

INTEGRATED CARE MODEL

Blount (1) suggested that one viable solution is to adopt an "integrated health care model," in which physical and behavioral health services are combined within the primary care pediatric practice setting. The several models of proposed integrated primary care are distinguished by their differing degrees of co-location and collaboration between the physician and the behavioral health provider. Some researchers argue that the "fully integrated care model" is ideal (2).

In a fully integrated care model, a family therapist (e.g., licensed psychologist or social worker) would be available on staff to provide consultation and follow-up care, side-by-side, with the pediatrician. The therapist ideally would accompany the pediatrician within the exam room, help quickly screen psychosocial or behavioral health issues and concerns, as well as any relevant family dynamics, consult briefly with the pediatrician, and, finally, schedule limited follow-up sessions as needed. Such integrated care models are being used increasingly today with much success in major community health centers, military branch healthcare systems, and Veteran's Administration hospitals.

The potential value of fully integrated care in a pediatric setting can be significant for both pediatricians and their patients. The longstanding, trusting relationship established between the pediatrician and the child's parents, as well as the child, provides an environment centered on family care that proves optimal for integrating family-based interventions. Primary care appointments within pediatric office settings, contrasted with appointments in mental health care settings, are associated with less stigmatization, mitigate opportunities for parents to engage in self-blame, and thus increase the likelihood of families engaging in treatment. Integrated care, within the pediatric setting, offers greater convenience to families, enhanced familiarity and communication with providers, immediate contact with services, and continuity of care for the child and family. Incorporating high quality, integrated family behavioral health care within the primary care pediatric setting also provides a unique opportunity for offering and enhancing preventive measures and anticipatory guidance.

Fully integrated care models also may be more cost efficient in the long run, in terms of health outcomes. While some pediatric practices may shy away from integrated care models due to anticipated problems with insurance billing issues, many third-party payers already reimburse for services provided by licensed psychologists billed under the CPT (current procedural terminology) Health and Behavior Codes. By illustration, an integrated family health care psychologist may be treating a child with diabetes who also exhibits behavior problems and difficulties with treatment compliance. The psychologist could work with this patient and his family to assess the problems and plan changes to the child's diet and family routine. When billing, the licensed psychologist may bill under the ICD-10 code for diabetes and under the relevant CPT Health and Behavior Codes for services provided (initial assessment and intervention) (2). When billing under this system, blending behavioral health services into the primary pediatric care practice can be managed relatively seamlessly.

INTEGRATING FAMILY THERAPY INTO A PEDIATRIC PRACTICE

Family therapy interventions have demonstrated efficacy in the very areas that are most problematic for pediatricians (e.g., diabetes, asthma, chronic childhood illness, etc.). Family therapists can also help families with a myriad of other issues that commonly present in the pediatrician's office, such as subclinical psychosocial complaints (depressed mood, anxiety, worry, aggression), ambiguous physical ailments (persistent stomachaches, headaches, chronic constipation), or other lifestyle-management concerns (obesity, sleep disturbances, severe weight loss). Research confirms that many families benefit from the intervention skills offered by family therapists.

Perspectives from family therapy can add particular health benefits in integrated care models. When family therapy health care conceptualizations and interventions are woven into pediatric visits, patients and their families receive richer and ideographically more tailored care. Similar to the pediatrician, the integrated family care psychologist's aim is to devise interventions that lead to the maximum amount of change with the minimum amount of family intervention. Integrated care models require that both pediatricians and the family care psychologists develop effective, brief, and goal-focused strategies tailored to each family. Family therapy within the pediatric setting is at its core a problem-solving therapy that begins with clear statements of the problem and the goals to be achieved. A problem well defined is considered a problem half-solved. Clear goals tell the patient and therapist when therapy is on or off-track, and when therapy has been successful.

It should be noted that most families facing medical illnesses and other life event stressors appear to cope quite well without any special therapy assistance. Most families prove quite resilient in the face of adversity and problems by themselves do not warrant therapy. As long as the family is coping and solving new problems as they arise, therapy is not indicated.

Therapy is indicated when the family keeps struggling with the same problems week after week, month after month. Therapy can help "stuck" families get "unstuck," so that they can move forward, solving future (inevitable) life problems on their own. Relevant family dynamics that block effective problem solving often involve disagreements between parents about the nature and meaning of the illness and how to deal with the issues it presents.

Some parents feel guilty about possibly contributing to (or exacerbating) their child's problem. Some feel so sad about the child's discomfort that they will do whatever they can to relieve the child's feelings in the short-term, even though that only exacerbates problems in the long-term. Some, feeling frustrated and helpless, fear that they are "bad" parents, or that they will be judged by others (professionals as well as family members) as "bad" parents, thus undermining confidence in their own parenting judgment. Others may feel inadequate to cope with medical problems, reluctant to implement treatment protocols, and wishing that some medical specialist will (magically) relieve them of that burden. While pediatricians treat the medical signs and symptoms of the child's illness, family behavioral health care therapists have the time and resources to help the family deal with the wide range of concerns, life issues and stresses generated among various family members when a (chronically) ill child lives in the family.

Why see the whole family?

Family therapists do not treat families, but rather help family members join together to help the child over a serious problem. The family is stuck, not sick. They need to get unstuck, not cured.

When a family member is sick or facing other serious problems, all family members are affected or troubled by this in some way. And although family members rarely are responsible for causing these problems, each has a responsibility to contribute what they can to help resolve the problem. Each family member provides unique perspectives, skills, and caring behaviors that can become part of the solution.

Behavioral health problems involve and affect more than one, or two, people. The child may act as he does because of the interactions among several family members. The mom may react to her child in a certain way because something grandmother has said to dad, who in turn says something to mom, who in turn acts differently with the child. Just looking at the child and mom interact may miss several key pieces in this interactive puzzle. Behaviors fly around the family system like a pin-ball around the pin-ball machine. Grandma affects dad, who then affects mom, who then affects the child. If grandma changes her interaction with dad, dad may change his interaction with mom, who in turn may change the way she interacts with child, who may in turn change his interactions with a sibling. The child's behavior is rarely restricted to a mom-child interaction pattern. The therapist traces out these family interactive sequences, and chooses at which strategic link in the chain to intervene most easily and effectively to achieve the desired change.

Family therapists usually need to see the whole family to assess family dynamics in order to identify the patterns of interaction among family members that may be helpful, or that may be contributing to, or exacerbating, presenting symptoms, or undermining compliance with treatment plans. They also examine each family member's perspectives about the nature and meaning of the medical diagnosis and accompanying symptoms in order to identify issues that may either help or hinder the family in pursuing a successful resolution of the problem. They assess the family's coping styles in order to identify strengths and weaknesses in communication and problem solving. They then help the family pull together, developing a tailored plan that incorporates each member's strengths, while avoiding their weaknesses, and focuses on resolving behavioral health care problems and issues with the least amount of stress.

How do cross-generational coalitions within families exacerbate problems?

Family members within the same generation naturally join together in healthy alliances to form functional subsystems. Two parents join together to form the "executive subsystem" managing family daily life. Problems arise, however, when members of different generations join in unhealthy coalitions against the influence or authority of another family member in authority. Mother and child may join in a coalition against father. Grandmother and child may join in a coalition against the child's parents.

Coalitions lead to triangulated patterns of interaction in which one member goes indirectly through a second member in order to influence a third member. Patterns of inappropriate coalitions across generations redraw structural boundaries around subsystems (spousal, parental, sibling, nuclear family), undermine hierarchy and authority of parents, and ultimately generate negative attitudes that stifle expressions of intimacy and caring among family members.

For example, consider a therapist helping a family cope with misbehavior of a young child. Grandmother lives with this family. Mother tells the family therapist that a previous therapist had recommended "chair time-out," but it did not work. Careful interviewing reveals that time-out was not used consistently, in large part because the grandmother viewed such a procedure as public humiliation that could damage her grandchild's self-esteem. Whenever the child was sent to time-out, the grandmother, protecting her grandchild, complained about damage to her self-esteem and consoled the child for having to put up with this indignity. She also argued with the mother or father about whether a particular infraction was severe enough to warrant "the chair."

The therapist might be tempted, invoking the expert power inherent in the therapist role, to block the grandmother's actions, which are viewed as undermining the effectiveness of the time-out procedure. Research data might be cited and the parents told tactfully that the grandmother has misconceptions about managing child misbehavior in general and self-esteem in particular. Imagine the impact when the parents arrive home to tell grandmother that a second therapist disagrees with her and that research data support their position. Imagine the impact on family structure, coalitions, and polarization ("spin-out"), and how much more difficult it may become for all to live in that home now, let alone effectively use time-out.

On the other hand, respecting the grandmother's protective concerns, and aware of potential unintended negative outcomes on family dynamics of therapeutic interventions, the family therapist asked the mother how grandmother (her mother) disciplined her when she was a child. The mother notes that she or her brothers were sent to their rooms "until they got control of themselves." The mother reports that this seemed to work well for her and her siblings. The therapist then proposed that perhaps the grandmother indeed knows this particular family very well, and has a keen sense of what will, and won't, work with this child. The child should be sent to his room to get control.

Imagine the grandmother's surprise when the parents arrive home to tell her that the family therapist (an expert) agrees with her, and that the child should go to her room instead of to the chair. In terms of family dynamics, the grandmother has now been empowered to support, rather than undermine, the parents' intervention. Not only will she back the parents when the child is sent to her room, but the grandmother herself may send the child now that precautions have been taken against public humiliation and damaged self-esteem. The emerging coalition between the grandmother and child against the parents' (and therapist's) intervention becomes transformed into an alliance among the therapist, parents and grandmother against the child's misbehavior. As consistency and adherence to therapeutic treatment plans replaces inconsistency and non-adherence, the problem is resolved.

While the solutions for many behavioral health problems are relatively simple, the reasons those solutions are not implemented are relatively complex. Family therapists work to unravel this complexity by addressing family dynamics that may be contributing factors. As part of the assessment process, family therapists may ask family members to discuss in session a sample problem issue (e.g., child non-compliance with the prescribed diabetes management protocol). The therapist then observes interaction sequences around the problem or issue.

When mother and child become involved in an issue, does dad eventually come in? When dad and mom discuss an executive subsystem issue, do children become involved or intrude? When parents discuss an issue, does one invoke the power of an absent in-law? Family functions are noted: who protects the child as another complains about him/her? Who minimizes a problem as another emphasizes it? Who interrupts whom? Who talks to whom about which issues? Who supports whom, in moving toward problem solving and resolution? Who agrees/disagrees with whom? Who praises/criticizes whom? Who accepts/denies responsibility? Does a young child tell the parents: "You're not the boss of me."

The viewing by family members can affect their doing when solving problems

An important factor to assess is whether the problem is viewed as a "can't do" or a "won't do" issue. Doing something (or not doing something) while denying control over it presents a different problem than doing it (or not doing it) while admitting control. Perceiving problems as either voluntary (or intentional) or involuntary (or unintentional) is a key distinction when dealing with behavioral health problems. When a person with a leg in a cast says she can't go hiking with friends, most accept this and are supportive and understanding. When a parent of a child diagnosed with ADHD, however, claims that the child can't control his "talking out, interrupting others, and grabbing sister's objects," others may question this "can't do" view and suggest that maybe he just does not want to do it.

One parent may view the symptom problem behavior as involuntary (or unintentional), while the other views it as voluntary (or intentional). Differences in "can't do" versus "won't do" views produce well intended proposals for different and often incompatible solutions to the same problem behavior, which can lead to increasing stress and hostility as each parent tries to convince the other to change their views. Family therapists probe such differences in perspective among family members and help plan interventions to pull members together around core areas of agreement, while avoiding divisive areas of disagreement. For example, although parents may not agree on whether a child can "control his ADHD," they may agree that regardless of the ADHD, he can and should act respectfully toward his parents, do homework, go to bed on time, and not defy parental requests.

Spin-out: How conflicting can't do and won't do views impact family dynamics

A common outcome of conflicting viewpoints and values among parents involves role "spin-out" over how to deal with a child's medical condition. For example, the pediatric endocrinologist refers the family because the young adolescent repeatedly has experienced diabetic crises and coma, for which no biological basis could be found. Suspected issues involve non-compliance with the treatment protocol and the problem is labeled "psychosomatic."

Upon observing the family in session, enacting their usual approach to trying to ensure compliance with diet, blood testing and insulin administration by their child, the therapist might note that each parent holds a different, and incompatible, view about the reasons for non-compliance by the child. The father sees the adolescent as disobedient and irresponsible, with a solution requiring stricter discipline and sanctions. Mother, on the other hand, sees the child as ill, fragile, and vulnerable, with a solution requiring more nurturing, support and understanding. Father views the child as "bad," while mother views the child as "sick." Both are highly motivated to protect the child, yet by pulling in different directions, they are "stuck" at an impasse in implementing potential solutions. The family's "parental executive subsystem" is paralyzed.

In this spin-out dynamic, both parents increasingly become polarized within their respective roles, and then may even begin to demonize each other for taking such extreme and inflexible positions. As father tries to implement his solution by invoking greater discipline, mother tries to ameliorate his influence by increasing her nurturing and support. The last thing she thinks her sick child needs is stricter discipline. Because the father thinks that the last thing his child needs is more "coddling of irresponsibility," he increases his attempt to impose greater discipline to offset mother's behavior. As they play off each other, the parents drive each other into opposing extreme positions, each feeling progressively alienated from the other. Both may question whether the other truly cares about or loves their child. As the dynamic continues, both may begin to question whether they have married the wrong person and the marriage may begin to dissolve.

Family therapists intervene to stop the polarization process, gently nudging each parent to move back toward the center, by integrating both parents' core values (nurturance and discipline) into one coherent role within which both parents can operate comfortably. The therapist might say: "You both obviously love and care very deeply about your child, and are clearly frustrated and upset that you have not been able to help him. You both have a piece of the solution for this problem (nurturance and discipline), but rather than pulling together, playing off your strengths, you are pulling in opposite directions and getting nowhere. Let's see if we can combine both your strengths in a way that you can pull together to help your child."

INTEGRATING FAMILY THERAPY: REVISITING DANNY

Revisiting the example of 8 year-old Danny from the beginning of this chapter will help illustrate how select concepts in family therapy can be applied within an integrated care pediatric practice. Danny's mother had brought up concerns during the last minute of a well-child visit about Danny's school performance, inattentive and hyperactive behavior, and general defiance across settings. The pediatrician in this scenario is caught in a tough spot in which she knows she cannot take the time to assess fully the potential issues like attention deficit hyperactivity disorder (ADHD) or oppositional defiant disorder (ODD), but she also knows that a quick referral to mental health services may not be helpful for the family either.

Danny's case provides a classic example of how an integrated care family therapist may play a helpful role in a pediatric practice. The pediatrician could introduce Danny and Danny's mother to the integrated care family psychologist while they are still in the exam room. The psychologist would have the time to spend an additional 20 to 30 minutes assessing the problems and dynamics within the family context, help them define clear goals, and link each goal to a specific intervention, and then follow up with the family for a few more (one to four) brief sessions. This "warm hand off" from physician to behavioral health care psychologist allows the family to contact appropriate services immediately and in a setting with which they are already familiar and comfortable.

In the case of Danny and his mother, the integrated care psychologist will initially spend time assessing and defining the problems within the family. The psychologist may ask questions about what the problem looks like, how the problem impacts the family, how the problem troubles various members of the family, and what the problem prevents the family from doing. Most important, the psychologist will also ask questions about how the family will recognize within a few sessions that they are on the right path to solving the (now well defined) problem.

In this case, Danny's mother describes a range of examples of Danny's non-compliance and hyperactivity at home and at school. According to mom, Danny won't sit still to do his homework, which leads to yelling and tantrums every day after school. She also reports that the teacher has been complaining that Danny does not complete class work and becomes disruptive to other students. Mom explains that she and her husband have tried yelling and screaming at Danny in the past for failing to listen, but nothing seems to work.

The integrated care psychologist, approaching problems through the lens of family therapy, might find it helpful for the parents to view Danny's various symptom behaviors as keys which function to get the parents to do what the child wants, at that moment. Such behavioral symptom keys usually follow clear and predictable sequences of interaction (3). To identify whether symptomatic behavior is acting as a key for the child to obtain some desired outcome, the therapist might have the parents describe three generic situations in which the symptom behavior potentially occurs: (a) when the parent [or teacher, peer, etc.] requests (demands) that the child *do* something the child doesn't want to do (pick up toys, start homework, clean room), or to *stop doing* something the child doesn't want to stop doing (stop watching TV, get off the phone, stop playing computer games); (b) when the child demands that the parent [or teacher, peer, etc.] *do* something that the parent does not want to do (give money, drive to movies, play games), or to *stop doing* something that the parent does not want to stop doing (end grounding of child, stop monitoring child's behavior, stop enforcing rules); and (c) all other situations in which the symptomatic behavior may occur (e.g., when the child is alone, playing with toys, watching TV or playing computer games).

When the parents reflect on these situations and note that symptomatic behavior occurs mainly in conditions (a) and (b), but not (c), the child's behavior is most likely functioning as a key to unlock opportunities to obtain some desired outcome (reward) from the parent, or as a key to avoid and/or escape some undesired outcome (relief). Further analysis identifies more precisely which specific behavior keys are acting to unlock which specific parent (or teacher) blocks to obtaining access to the child's desired outcomes. Symptom behaviors may differ widely in form (appearance) yet all function as keys to open the same outcome locks. A child may sulk, complain, whine, cry, scream or tantrum to escape doing homework. Other behaviors may appear very similar in form, yet all act as keys to release different outcome locks. A child may whine to get a piece of candy, to get a ride to the store, to get out of brushing his teeth, or to avoid taking out the garbage.

By contrast, when the parents note that most behavior episodes occur in (c) above, but not (a) and (b), these episodes are less likely functioning as behavior keys, and more likely are influenced by biological factors (e.g., ADD, seizures, BiPolar I disorder). Symptomatic behavior influenced mainly by biological factors (e.g., seizures) will not show clear patterns of functioning as behavioral keys to unlock access to desired outcomes, or avoid undesired outcomes.

With many medical conditions, however, symptomatic behavior that begins under the influence of biological factors eventually may take on functions as behavior keys that permit the child to access desired outcomes in the family (or school) setting. For example, parents of children with Tourette's syndrome may become frustrated because they suspect that at some times, in some situations, the child's tics may not be triggered by biological factors, but by certain demands or responsibilities the child wishes to escape. Tics that began under biological conditions seem to have taken on additional functions as behavioral keys that allow the child to escape or avoid unpleasant tasks (relief), or to obtain some desired outcome (reward). Family therapists help parents detect when an apparent medical behavior symptom is functioning more as a behavioral key, and help them change their reaction locks so that these keys no longer work. Plans are made to establish new, more appropriate, behavioral keys that will unlock the same outcomes, without the negative side effects. When overall symptom behavior is reduced, only the biologically based symptoms remain, as behavior keys and locks are changed to foster more healthy outcomes.

In the case of Danny's family, the integrated psychologist solicits specific examples of problem behavior from Danny's mother to determine which behavioral keys Danny might be using. Collecting particular details about the context of problem behaviors is critical. For example, at home, Danny might be watching TV when Danny's mother asks Danny to come to dinner. Danny might first engage in passive avoidance by ignoring mom's request, continuing to watch TV. A few minutes later mom notices the lack of compliance and repeats the request. Danny might then escalate to more assertive avoidance by verbal means, saying: "Just a minute," or "Wait until the commercial."

If the mother insists, perhaps raising her voice, Danny might escalate to active avoidance with motor behavior, by grabbing the remote control to prevent his mother from turning off the TV, or running to another room to continuing watching the show there. If mom continues to press for compliance, the Danny might escalate to ultimate avoidance of compliance by aggressive actions, such as threatening violence, destroying property, throwing things, and pushing, shoving and/or kicking. The aggressive outburst terminates the sequence, as mom gives up in frustration and allows Danny to escape complying with parental directives. Although the behavioral keys used by the child earlier in the sequence were not successful, the final aggressive outburst successfully unlocked mother's resistance to allowing him to escape complying with her request.

At school, Danny might sit in class as the teacher tells the group to take out their math books. Danny might first ignore the teacher's request (passive off-task), while doodling at his desk. If the teacher notices the non-compliance and repeats the request, Danny might escalate to verbal task avoidance, saying: "I can't do it," or "I don't want to," or "I need to go to the bathroom." If the teacher insists on task work and compliance, Danny might escalate to motor task avoidance, turning around in his seat, sliding onto the floor, dropping pencils, books and other objects from his desk to the floor, or getting out of his seat and walking around the desk and room. If the teacher continues to insist on compliance, Danny may escalate to ultimate avoidance or escape from compliance by aggressive actions, such as throwing objects, turning over the desk, tearing up workbook pages, or hitting another child.

Aggressive outbursts usually terminate the sequence, as the teacher gives up in frustration, sending Danny to the principal's office. Although the earlier behavioral keys applied by Danny in this sequence failed to allow escape from the task, the final outburst unlocked access to a viable escape route from class-work. While the teacher may think she has prevailed in this test of wills, Danny has escaped from math work, and instead is on a slow-walk adventure down various school hallways to the principal's office, waving to friends in other classes on his way.

Fortunately, most children will not allow themselves to escalate to the more serious aggressive acts in order to prevail in the struggle about who can tell whom what to do. At some point, doing the task seems easier than the effort in the struggle to avoid it. Those few children who do adopt these aggression escape keys, however, can present serious challenges to all involved. By the time a child reaches adolescence with well-honed patterns of anger and aggression available to control others in his or her environment, effective therapeutic options become increasingly limited.

These compliance interpersonal scenarios, and the escalating avoidance-escape termination sequences, may account for the majority of behavior problems reported to pediatricians. Consistent with Patterson's extensive research data (4-6), these modes of interpersonal non-compliance sequences may comprise core etiological factors (e.g., pathognomonic signs) responsible for the maintenance of a wide variety of conduct and oppositional behaviors, as well as many behavioral symptoms of ADHD and other childhood disorders, as reported to pediatricians (e.g., disrespect, defiance, disruption, destruction, hitting, biting, kicking, self-injurious behavior, abusive back talk, stealing, lying, etc.).

Identifying behavioral keys and locks requires assessing sequences of interaction to trace out reciprocal linkages. Interpersonal symptomatic behaviors cannot be understood in isolation from the context of their function in home and school interpersonal sequences. Behavioral key and lock functions can be changed by modifying strategic links in the sequences or by modifying key aspects in the contexts in which the sequences occur.

The integrated healthcare psychologist will attentively listen to these examples of non-compliance and ADHD-typical behaviors, analyzing the chain of the family's behaviors carefully. Once the psychologist has an understanding of the relevant problems and behavioral sequences, she may ask additional open-ended questions to focus the family on concrete goals for treatment. The psychologist might ask, "What small changes would you notice in a few weeks to tell us we were on the right track to being successful?" Danny's mother replies that Danny would do his homework as soon as arrives home after school and finish his few chores at home quickly so she could focus on other household activities like making dinner. Danny offers that progress to him would include being able to do fun things, like play video-games, and play basketball with his dad more often.

After this initial visit, the integrated care psychologist sends the family home with some brief assessments (e.g., NICHQ Vanderbilt Assessment Scale, a free, brief behavioral screener for parents and teachers). Brief screening measures can be important to tracking progress, and assessments may help the pediatrician develop a medication trial for the child if this becomes necessary. The psychologist will also set up follow-up appointments with Danny and both of his parents to discuss the family's goals and develop a more nuanced understanding of the family's behavioral sequences. Because the integrated care psychologist has the time, she may also call Danny's teacher to get her perspective on the problem behaviors, and coordinate interventions between home and school.

It is also important to note agreements and disagreements between the family's and teacher's accounts of the major issues, and their perspectives on the problems and potential solutions, before attempting to establish changes. When referrals are necessary to other mental health care specialists (e.g., child and adolescent psychiatrist, school based behavioral support team), the family psychologist can monitor patient follow-through and coordinate these services as part of the child's comprehensive health treatment plan.

Changing the links of behavioral chains and the contexts in which they occur may involve various intervention strategies. The integrated care psychologist may help Danny and his family work with the teacher to start a daily report card program. Working within the language and values system of the family, the psychologist will help the family set small goals for change, such as giving descriptive praise statements to Danny for specific desired behaviors five times a day. A mutual agreement (contract) might be developed in which dad will play basketball with Danny if he gets his homework and chores done by a set time, or that Danny can earn 15-minute blocks of "screen time" for each chore completed. As the family spends less time and negative energy struggling to get Danny to do what he needs to do, there will be more time and positive energy freed up to devote to fun family activities, like playing basketball with dad.

Other empirically-validated interventions might be of use such as The Home Chip System (7). The integrated care psychologist works with each family to develop brief and effective interventions tailored specifically to the strengths of members of the family. Once goals are met and improvements are noted, treatment is ended. However, the family may still have contact with the integrated care psychologist during future medication checks or well-child visits with the pediatrician. In this way, the integrated care psychologist never completely loses contact with the family and can continue to monitor Danny's behavioral progress.

What does the research indicate about the effectiveness of family therapy?

Research on effectiveness of family therapy has been accelerating rapidly over the past 20 years. A comprehensive sourcebook has been compiled by Douglas Sprenkle (8) in an edited book in which a panel of experts summarize and evaluate the published research in ten major problem areas. Numerous research studies have been published in peer reviewed journals on various kinds of problems treated, with various populations, as well as on the process variables that contribute to those health outcomes. Collections of detailed protocols to treat a wide range of presenting problems in behavioral pediatrics can be found in Christophersen and Vanscoyoc (9) and Watson and Gresham (10).

CONCLUSION

In summary, family therapists engage in brief therapy to help families achieve behavioral health goals based on the presenting symptoms, problems and issues which accompany a variety of medical and behavior problems. They assess family dynamics to identify potential problems with family structure and subsystems, with cross-generational coalitions, with differing viewpoints, and/or with inappropriate sequences of behavioral keys and locks operative in problem situations. They focus on the present rather than the past, on strengths rather than weaknesses, on presenting behavioral health problems rather than theoretical constructs and goals, and on pulling family members together rather than on interventions that create divisiveness.

They observe families as they enact parts of their problems in session so that they can see problems and dynamics unfold, and they ask families to take home tailored exercises and plans to practice solutions in their natural settings. They help families form clear and objective therapy goals which help the therapist know which areas to assess, which areas need not be assessed, which pieces of family history to probe and not probe, which intervention techniques to choose, when therapy is getting off track, when it has been brought back on track, and when therapy has been successful. They use empirically validated intervention components and protocols whenever available. They respect the uniqueness of each family, developing interventions tailored to each family's problems, needs, strengths and resources.

REFERENCES

[1] Blount A. Integrated primary care: organizing the evidence. Fam Syst Health 2003;21:121-34.
[2] Robinson P, Reiter J. Behavioral consultation and primary care: A guide to integrating services. New York: Springer, 2006.
[3] Alessi G. Direct observation methods for emotional/behavior problems. In: Shapiro E, Kratochwill T, eds. Behavioral assessment in schools: Conceptual foundations and practical applications. New York: Guilford, 1988.
[4] Patterson G. Coercive family processes. Eugene, OR: Castalia Press, 1982.
[5] Patterson G. Anti-social boys. Eugene, OR: Castalia Press, 1992.
[6] Reid J, Patterson G, Snyder J. Antisocial behavior in children and adolescents. Washington, DC: American Psychological Association, 2002.
[7] Christophersen ER. Pediatric compliance: A guide for the primary care physician. New York: Springer/Plenum Medical, 1994.
[8] Sprenkle D. Effectiveness research in marriage and family therapy. Alexandria, VA: American Association for Marriage and Family Therapy (AAMFT), 2002.

[9] Christophersen ER, Vanscoyoc SM. Treatments that work with children: Empirically supported strategies for managing childhood problems, 2nd ed. Washington, DC: American Psychological Press, 2013.

[10] Watson S, Gresham F, eds. Handbook of child behavior therapy. New York: Plenum Press, 1998.

Submitted: June 05, 2015. *Revised:* July 03, 2015. *Accepted:* July 10, 2015.

Chapter 5

A REVIEW ON PSYCHOPHARMACOLOGY IN CHILDREN AND ADOLESCENTS

Ahsan Nazeer[*], *MD*

Division Chief, Child and Adolescent Psychiatry, Department of Psychiatry,
Sidra Medical and Research Center, Doha, Qatar

ABSTRACT

This review considers basic principles of pediatric psychopharmacology. Important concepts that are identified include comprehensive assessment, therapeutic alliance, and establishment as well as implementation of a therapeutic plan. Antidepressants are discussed including those that are FDA-approved for pediatric use along with association with suicidal ideation, risk of cardiac arrhythmias, and risk of seizures. Antipsychotic medications are considered including those FDA-approved for pediatric use, risk of metabolic syndrome, risk of suicide, and drug-specific risks. Stimulants are mentioned including those that are FDA-approved and also risk of priapism. Atomoxetine is noted and monitoring should occur for hepatotoxicity, suicidal ideation, and priapism. Mood stabilizers are described including those that are FDA-approved along with risk of suicide and risk of teratogenicity. Pediatric psychopharmacology continues to be increasingly utilized for children and adolescents with psychiatric disorders in the 21st century.

Keywords: mental health, children, adolescents, psychopharmacology

INTRODUCTION

During the last 30 years, the treatment of psychiatric disorders in children and adolescents has seen a dramatic upswing in the use of prescription medications. This increase has been fueled by advances in our understanding of the epidemiology, etiology and neuroscience of

---

[*] Correspondence: Ahsan Nazeer, MD. Department of Psychiatry, Sidra Medical and Research Center, C2M 224, 2nd Mezzanine, OPC, PO Box 26999, Doha, Qatar. E-mail: anazeer@sidra.org.

childhood mental illnesses and by increasing social acceptance of medication as a treatment modality. Many neuropsychiatric disorders present in childhood and persist throughout life, and a significant body of literature supports the idea that earlier treatment interventions produce better long-term outcomes in these cases. Despite this evidence, large gaps exist in our understanding of the use of psychotropic medications in children. As a result, many medications lack appropriate labeling information and are used on the basis of minimal scientific data. During the last decade, the National Institute of Mental Health (NIMH) launched numerous studies focused on bridging this gap. Examples of such studies include the "Treatment of adolescents with depression study" (TADS), the "Treatment of SSRI-resistant depression in adolescents study" (TORDIA), the "Multimodal treatment of attention deficit hyperactivity disorder study" (MTA) and the "Studies to advance autism research and treatment" (STAART).

This review describes basic pediatric psycho-pharmacology concepts and treatment approaches. Further details regarding use of medications in the treatment of specific psychiatric disorders are provided within the designated chapters of this book.

GENERAL PRINCIPLES OF PEDIATRIC PSYCHOPHARMACOLOGY

There are significant differences between adults and children in the diagnosis, treatment and trajectory of their psychiatric illnesses. In addition, differences between the mature and the still-developing neurochemical and biological processes dramatically impact medication pharmacodynamics and pharmaco-kinetics. Children are not simply "young adults." Furthermore, the challenge of making a definitive diagnosis in a child prior to beginning treatment often means that the initial selection of medication must be guided by symptoms alone.

Comprehensive assessment

It is essential to conduct a thorough assessment of the child or adolescent prior to initiating pharmacotherapy (1). The presenting complaints and identified problems usually dictate the extent of the interview, as well as the need to use basic screening instruments or more specialized psychological testing. In any case, it is important to clearly understand parental concerns and to obtain collateral information from other family members and from the school whenever possible.

Conducting a joint initial interview is a helpful strategy for clearly ascertaining the chief complaint, as well as for establishing good rapport with the family. It is useful to initially characterize the presenting problem as being "internalizing" or "externalizing" in nature. Mood and anxiety disorders are usually considered to be internalizing; in these cases, it is preferable to seek further information from the child, as he is the best informant regarding his internal state. Disruptive behavioral disorders, on the other hand, present with aggression, defiance, impulsivity and thought disorganization and are considered to be externalizing disorders; in these cases, the most valuable information, including a detailed description of the behavior, usually comes from family members and others who regularly engage with the child.

One of the major challenges in the psychiatric evaluation of children is that a given presenting symptom may be common to several diagnostic categories. For example, aggression can be the result of oppositional defiant disorder, attention deficit hyperactivity disorder (ADHD) or an underlying anxiety disorder. It is because of this clinical ambiguity that symptoms must be evaluated and characterized over time. Nevertheless, symptoms may require immediate intervention, and clinical judgment must be used in providing care.

A complete medical history should be obtained, paying particular attention to conditions such as traumatic brain injury, cardiac defects, syncope, family history of sudden cardiac death, Marfan's syndrome, seizures and other neurological conditions. Any personal or family history of mental illness or substance use disorder should be noted. Gathering specific facts concerning any previous medication trials can be very helpful, especially with regard to symptom response and side effects. All of this information will be vital in selecting and monitoring medications that address the presenting problem.

Evaluation of the psychological and social aspects of the presenting situation is another facet of a thorough assessment. Gaining a sense of the youth's ability to form relationships, understand others' feelings and emotions, self-regulate behavior and demonstrate appropriate executive function is informative from a psychological standpoint. In assessing social factors, emphasis should be placed on evaluating any risk factors present in the home or at school, including familial discord, loss of a parent, pending divorce, an overly critical home or school environment, bullying and lack of close friendships.

A complete physical examination should be conducted, and observation of any focal neurologic signs should prompt consideration of further evaluation using CT, MRI and/or EEG. Laboratory testing also may be ordered, depending upon the presence of medical comorbidities and the psychotropic mediations under consideration. In an older teen, physicians always should maintain a high index of suspicion regarding substance abuse and consider urine drug testing. It is also advisable to order pregnancy testing in female youth who are of childbearing age. If a decision is made to use tricyclic antidepressants (TCA's), a baseline electrocardiogram (ECG) is recommended, and repeat ECG testing should be performed at follow-up visits for high dose TCA maintenance.

Therapeutic alliance

It is essential to establish a strong therapeutic alliance with the family, beginning with the initial assessment. Showing compassion, being attentive, making eye contact, actively listening and keeping everyone engaged in the assessment process helps to build rapport. During the evaluation, time should be set aside to answer any questions the family or youth may have; this helps to ensure that the family's understanding of the treatment plan is aligned with the provider's vision. Research suggests that having a solid treatment alliance promotes patient satisfaction, enhances adherence and is the best predictor of a good therapeutic outcome.

Establishing a treatment plan

Once target symptoms have been identified and comorbid conditions have been considered, the family and physician must review the treatment options and decide on a comprehensive plan. Treatment alternatives should be discussed, along with the advantages and disadvantages of each, and the family should be cautioned to avoid making the erroneous assumption that medication alone will transform the identified symptoms. A comprehensive treatment plan is multimodal and may consist of behavioral, psychosocial and psycho-educational interventions in addition to pharmacotherapy.

Once the family and physician agree on a treatment plan and choose to use a particular medication, formal documentation of the informed consent of the family and assent of the child should be obtained. In the case of divorced parents, temporary guardianship or foster care placement, the physician must determine which party is legally able to give consent for treatment. During the consent process, it is extremely important to discuss why a particular medication is being chosen, the risks and benefits of the proposed and alternative medications, the target symptoms that are expected to improve, the common side effects, the significance of any black-box warnings and whether the medication is FDA approved for the disorder or is being used "off-label" without a formal evidence base (2).

The FDA defines "off-label" as "not having been studied adequately in a particular population." It is important for parents to understand that lack of formal FDA approval of a particular medication for use in children or for a particular disorder does not preclude its safe and effective use. The parents' ability to understand written and verbal directions should be assessed, and appropriate written information about the medication should be given to them. They also should be encouraged to use online resources to learn more about their child's diagnosis and about the medication that has been prescribed.

Implementation of treatment plan

As always, medications must be titrated to an appropriate dose and be continued for an adequate period of time in order to be effective. Several other variables also must be considered in children, including the body fluid to tissue ratio, the hepatic capacity and the status of the developing cytochrome P450 system.

It is recommended that the expected duration of treatment, need for regular follow-up visits and importance of identifying and managing side effects be discussed with the child and family. The potential for medication non-adherence is another important issue to address with the youth and family. Reasons for non-adherence may include inconvenience, defiance, multiple daily doses, poorly understood directions, unexpected side effects and the child's perception that taking medications will make them different from their peers. Maintaining a strong therapeutic alliance, managing concerns and encouraging active participation by the family are strategies, which are usually helpful in maintaining adherence.

PSYCHOTROPIC MEDICATIONS

In the following brief discussion of psychotropic medications, the major issues pertinent to each group of medications will be highlighted. More detailed information on the dosing and titration of these medications may be found in the appropriate chapters of this book.

ANTIDEPRESSANTS

There are numerous antidepressants on the market, and they are indicated for a wide array of diagnoses, including depressive disorders, anxiety disorders, eating disorders, attention deficit hyperactivity disorder and enuresis. Antidepressants are classified according to their mechanism of action, but the choice of medication for a specific child depends upon the diagnosis, the age of the patient, the physician's level of comfort with the medication and its side effect profile. It also is important to consider whether a medication is FDA-approved for a certain diagnosis and age range or is being used off-label. In prescribing off-label, it is strongly recommended that psychoeducation provided to the parents be especially thorough. It also is advisable to carefully document having discussed with the family the reasoning underlying the choice of medication, the risks and benefits of the chosen medication and the possible alternatives. Table 1 identifies common anti-depressants and their side effects.

Table 1. *Commonly* prescribed antidepressants and their side effects

Class	Agent	Average daily dosage	Side effects
SSRIs	Fluoxetine Paroxetine Sertraline Citalopram Escitalopram Venlafaxine	5-60 mg 5-40 mg 12.5-200 mg 5-40 mg 5-20 mg 37.5-225 mg	All SSRIs may increase the risk of suicidal ideations. Sexual side effects
SNRIs	Duloxetine Bupropion Levomilnacipran (Fetzima)	20-40 mg 37.5-300 mg 20-120 mg	Lower seizure threshold, irritability, insomnia Hypotension, seizures
Atypical	Mirtazapine Trazodone (Oleptro) Vortioxetine (Brintellix) Vilazodone (Viibryd)	7.5-45 mg 150-300 mg 5-20 mg 10-40 mg	Weight gain Priapism Seizures Somnolence
TCAs	Imipramine Clomipramine Amitriptyline	25-75 mg 25-200 mg 25-100 mg	Somnolence, priapism Cardiac arrhythmias, lethal in overdose, sedation, orthostatic hypotension

FDA-approved antidepressants for pediatric use

Only two selective serotonin reuptake inhibitors (SSRIs) are FDA approved for the treatment of depression in pediatric populations. Fluoxetine is approved for children 8-18 years of age, and escitalopram is approved for children 12-17 years of age. SSRIs that are FDA approved for the treatment of obsessive-compulsive disorder (OCD) in the pediatric population include sertraline for ages 6 years and older, fluoxetine and fluvoxamine for ages 8 years and older and escitalopram for ages 12 years and older (3). Two of the tricyclic antidepressants, imipramine and clomipramine, have FDA approved indications for the pediatric population. Clomipramine is approved for OCD in 10-17 year olds and imipramine is approved for enuresis in 6-17 year olds.

According to an August 2013 Center for Medicaid & Medicare Services (CMS) Fact Sheet, the antidepressants citalopram, paroxetine, sertraline and venlafaxine do not have clinical support for their use in pediatric major depressive disorders (MDD). The FDA had already recommended in 2003 that paroxetine not be used in children and adolescents with MDD. Two placebo-controlled trials of citalopram and sertraline in pediatric populations with MDD and three placebo-controlled trials of paroxetine in similar populations failed to provide evidence supporting a pediatric indication for their use. Studies from the paroxetine group also showed an increased incidence of suicidal thoughts, agitation, mood lability and hostility as compared to the placebo group. Venlafaxine XR also was studied in pediatric (6-17 year olds) MDD and generalized anxiety disorder; however, clinical trials failed to support indications for its use in either disorder (4).

Antidepressants and suicidal ideation

In 2004, the FDA directed pharmaceutical companies to label all antidepressant medications with a "black-box warning" to draw attention to the increased risk of suicidality among children and adolescents taking these drugs. The warning came as a result of the FDA's analysis of 24 clinical trials involving 4,582 children and adolescents, in which 4% of the antidepressant group reported suicidal ideation, compared to 2% of the placebo group (5). The announcement received heavy media coverage, and SSRI prescriptions subsequently declined by 22%. During the period between 2003 and 2005, rates of youth suicide increased by 14%. Re-analysis of the original data, in conjunction with new data from 7 additional studies, failed to replicate the FDA findings, showing only a 0.7% increase in risk for suicide; nevertheless, the controversy continues, even in light of more recent evidence supporting the effectiveness of these medications.

The "Treatment of adolescents with depression study" (TADS), a multicenter clinical trial funded by the National Institute of Mental Health (NIMH), is one such example (6). In this study, combined treatment with fluoxetine and cognitive behavioral therapy (CBT) led to a 71% improvement in adolescents with MDD, in comparison to 61% improvement with fluoxetine alone and 35% with placebo. Before the start of the study, 29% of the depressed adolescents reported suicidal ideation. After treatment with the combination of fluoxetine and CBT, suicidal ideation decreased to 10% among all groups.

Antidepressants and risk of cardiac arrhythmias

In 2013, an FDA Safety Communication notified physicians and patients of cardiac arrhythmias possibly resulting from the use of fluoxetine. Reports indicated post-marketing discovery of cases demonstrating prolonged QTc interval and resultant Torsade de Pointes. Patients with hypokalemia, hypomagnesemia, underlying cardiac defects, bradycardia, congenital QT prolongation, and those also being treated with other CYP2D6 inhibitors (e.g., antipsychotics) are considered to be at increased risk for QTc prolongation.

Antidepressants and risk of seizures

Seizures have been reported with the use of clomipramine and bupropion. Bupropion lowers the seizure threshold and significantly increases the risk of seizure in patients who have a concurrent eating disorder diagnosis. Seizures reported during the pre-marketing clinical trials of clomipramine were found to be associated with both the dose and duration of treatment. Caution also is advised in using SSRIs in patients with pre-existing seizure disorders.

ANTIPSYCHOTICS

Antipsychotics are one of the most commonly prescribed medications in the pediatric population. In fact, their use in children has doubled between 2000 and 2007, and the number of prescriptions written by pediatricians has increased by 25% since 2006 (7, 8). The FDA has approved use of these medications only for schizophrenia, irritability in autism and mania among children aged 5 years and older; however, schizophrenia and bipolar disorder diagnoses are rare in the pediatric age group, and most of the antipsychotic prescriptions are being written on an off-label basis to manage disruptive behavior disorders, sometimes in children as young as 2 years of age.

There are reports indicating that the rise in use is especially notable among children of lower socioeconomic status, minorities, those in foster care, and those covered by Medicaid. A 2011 report published by the "Agency for Healthcare Research and Quality" (AHRQ) noted that among children taking antipsychotic medications, *atypical* antipsychotics were prescribed 90% of the time, mostly for off-label indications. The long-term safety and effectiveness of antipsychotics is not well established, and the current recommendation is to use these medications only in children with disabling symptoms and serious psychopathology. Table 2 identifies common antipsychotics and their side effects.

FDA approved antipsychotics for pediatric use

A few first generation antipsychotic (FGA) medications are approved for use in the pediatric population, but only haloperidol and chlorpromazine are used routinely, due to the numerous side effects of drugs in this class and concerns about QTc interval prolongation and risk of sudden cardiac death. Chlorpromazine is FDA approved for the treatment of hyperactivity, severe behavioral problems, bipolar mania and schizophrenia in children aged 1-12 years. Prochlorperazine is approved for bipolar mania in children who are older than 2 years, with a body weight > 20 lbs. FGAs approved for childhood schizophrenia include thioridazine for ages 2 years and older, trifluoperazine for ages 6 years and older and loxapine, perphenazine and thiothixene for children aged 12 or older.

The FDA has approved five atypical antipsychotics for pediatric use. Risperidone is approved for irritability in autistic disorder for ages 5-16 years, bipolar I disorder (manic or mixed state) for ages 10-17 years and for schizophrenia in 13-17 year old youth. Aripiprazole is approved for irritability in autistic disorder in youth aged 6-17 years and for bipolar disorder and schizophrenia in a similar age range as risperidone. Olanzapine is approved for schizophrenia and bipolar disorder (manic or mixed) from 13-17 years of age. Quetiapine is approved for the manic or mixed phase of bipolar disorder for 10-17 year olds and for schizophrenia in adolescents 13-17 years of age. Paliperidone is approved for schizophrenia in children who are 12-17 years of age.

Table 2. Commonly prescribed antipsychotics and their side effects

Class	Agent	Avg. daily dose	Side effects
First-generation			
Phenothiazine	Chlorpromazine	50-400 mg	Common side effects of first generation antipsychotics include: sedation, orthostatic hypotension, anticholinergic symptoms, parkinsonism, dystonia and akathisia
	Thioridazine	50-400 mg	
	Fluphenazine	2-10 mg	
	Perphenazine	5-40 mg	
	Trifluoperazine	2-20 mg	
Butyrophenone	Haloperidol	2-10 mg	
Miscellaneous	Loxapine	5-50 mg	Weight gain, hypercholesteremia, hyperprolactinemia, tardive dyskinesia
	Molindone	5-50 mg	
	Thiothixene	2-20 mg	
Second-generation			
	Clozapine*	25-300mg	Weight gain, hypercholesteremia, hyperprolactinemia, tardive dyskinesia
	Risperidone	1-4 mg	
	Olanzapine	5-20 mg	
	Quetiapine	200-600 mg	
	Ziprasidone	80-120 mg	
	Asenapine	5-20mg	
	Iloperidone	2-12mg	
	Paliperidone	3-12mg	
	Lurasidone	40-160mg	
Partial DA agonist	Aripiprazole	10-25 mg	Can exacerbate psychosis

* Side effects that are unique to clozapine: hypersalivation, tachycardia, increased risk of seizures and agranulocytosis.

Antipsychotics and risk of metabolic syndrome

The FDA has issued warnings to health care professionals that all antipsychotics have "increased potential" in children (in comparison to adults who are taking the same medications) for causing weight gain, metabolic syndrome and contributing to the precipitation of type-2 diabetes. In fact, a recent study found a threefold increase in risk for diabetes among children taking antipsychotic medications, as compared to those who were on other psychotropic medications. Olanzapine and clozapine are associated with the greatest weight gain, while ziprasidone has shown fewer side effects in this particular domain.

The American Diabetic Association (ADA) recommends measuring waist circumference and body mass index at baseline, then monthly for 3 months and quarterly thereafter. The ADA also recommends measuring fasting glucose and lipid levels at the start of therapy, after 3 months and then yearly. If impaired glucose tolerance is suspected, more aggressive monitoring is recommended, and patient care should be co-managed with a pediatric endocrinologist. Table 3 lists basic steps for the management of metabolic syndrome.

Table 3. Management of metabolic syndrome

Prevention:
- Provide education about metabolic syndrome
- Discuss the long term morbidity and mortality concerns
- Encourage a healthy lifestyle in terms of eating and exercise
- Encourage routine physical activity
- Encourage a healthy diet
- Choose medications that have a lower tendency to cause metabolic syndrome

If the patient develops metabolic syndrome:
- Change or stop the antipsychotic if clinically appropriate
- Establish a team approach to the problem
- Be aware of the risk of ketoacidosis and educate the patient about the signs and symptoms
- Closely and frequently monitor the metabolic profile

Antipsychotics and risk of suicide

Aripiprazole, quetiapine and lurasidone are FDA approved for use in the depressed phase of bipolar I disorder and as an adjunct for the treatment of major depressive disorder in adults. These medications are not approved for monotherapy of depressive disorders in either the pediatric or adult population. Despite the fact that these medications are not approved for use in pediatric depression, they can increase the risk of suicidality in children and young adults.

Drug-specific risks

An increased risk of hypertension exists with use of quetiapine in the pediatric population; therefore, baseline measurement and periodic monitoring of blood pressure is recommended. Baseline measurement of HbA1C and periodic weight monitoring is recommended with paliperidone use, because of its association with weight gain. Olanzapine use is associated with more significant weight gain and should be considered only after other antipsychotics have been tried. Aripiprazole is known to potentiate psychosis in rare cases, due to its partial dopaminergic chemical profile. Safety and efficacy in the pediatric population has not been established for lurasidone, iloperidone, paliperidone or asenapine.

STIMULANTS AND RELATED MEDICATIONS

Stimulants are considered to be the first line of treatment for management of attention deficit hyperactivity disorder (ADHD) in the child and adolescent population, but it is important to recognize that pharmacotherapy is only one part of a comprehensive treatment plan for ADHD. Other interventions include parent education programs, parent management training, social skills training and problem-solving skills training for children, group cognitive behavioral therapies and behavioral interventions in the classroom.

Before starting the treatment, it is essential to assess cardiovascular status by inquiring about any history of exercise syncope, chest pain, palpitations or family history of sudden cardiac death. Heart rate (HR), and blood pressure (BP) should be evaluated, and an ECG should be considered in individuals with any of the above risk factors. An assessment of the risk for potential drug misuse or diversion also should be a part of the comprehensive pre-treatment evaluation. The decision regarding which medication to use is based on any adverse effects experienced during previous trials, anticipated adherence issues, potential for diversion, convenience (including whether a mid-day dose will be needed at school) and presence of comorbid conditions, including tics, seizures and structural cardiac defects (9).

FDA approved indications

Stimulants are approved for the treatment of ADHD, narcolepsy and exogenous obesity (body mass index at or above 95th percentile) in pediatric patients. Methamphetamine and benzphetamine are both approved for the treatment of exogenous obesity in 12-17 year old patients. Dextroamphetamine IR (immediate release), dextroamphetamine SR (sustained release) and amphetamine mixed salts are approved for narcolepsy in 6-17 year olds. Almost all of the stimulant medications are approved for the treatment of ADHD in children aged 6-17 years old, with two exceptions: amphetamine mixed salts and dextroamphetamine IR are approved for children 3 years and older, while dextroamphetamine IR and SR do not carry FDA approval for use in adolescents older than 16 years of age. The FDA has approved three non-stimulant medications for use in children and adolescents with ADHD: atomoxetine, extended release guanfacine and extended release clonidine.

Stimulants and risk of priapism

In 2013, the FDA issued a warning regarding a possible link between the use of methylphenidate and priapism (painful erection lasting > 4 hours). There is still only limited information available, but the FDA has recommended updating drug labels to include mention of a "rare but serious risk of priapism." The FDA has identified 15 cases of priapism that occurred from 1997-2012; most cases- twelve- occurred in children younger than 18 years of age. These cases have presented under different conditions, including during use of short acting methylphenidate, after discontinuation of methylphenidate, upon restarting the medication and when there was a longer than usual interval between doses. The rarity of this side effect can be understood in light of the fact that in 2012 alone, 20 million prescriptions were written and 4 million prescriptions were dispensed. However, physicians are advised to discuss this issue with parents and youth and to recommend seeking immediate medical treatment if an erection lasts longer than 4 hours, in order to prevent long-term problems.

Stimulants and risk of cardiovascular events

In 2005, awareness of the cardiovascular impact of stimulant medications was heightened when Health Canada suspended distribution of Adderall XR, after receiving reports of sudden cardiac death among children receiving the drug. This ban was later lifted and a warning was issued regarding the possibility of sudden cardiac death among children with known cardiac anomalies who are taking Adderall XR. The FDA also issued warnings about the use of stimulants in children with underlying cardiac disease; however, a 2006 FDA review acknowledged that no definite conclusions can be made about the association of stimulant use with sudden cardiac death. In 2011, the FDA announced that a large, recently completed study had not shown an association between the use of stimulants and adverse cardiovascular events such as stroke, myocardial infarction and sudden cardiac death.

The study under discussion was one of three studies sponsored by the FDA and the Agency for Healthcare and Quality (AHRQ), published in the November 1, 2011issue of the *New England Journal of Medicine*. This study was a retrospective review of 1,200,438 children and young adults 2-24 years of age, followed for 373,667 person-years (sum of years that each person in the study was under observation) of ADHD medication use. Researchers reported no evidence of increased risk of cardiovascular events among individuals taking ADHD medications; however, the FDA continues to recommend periodic evaluation of HR and BP and advises avoiding the use of stimulants in individuals with serious cardiac problems.

Stimulants and risk of abuse and dependence

Stimulant medications are the most effective treatment for ADHD; however, their illicit use and diversion have become major public health concerns. According to the Centers for Disease Control and Prevention (CDC), more than 20% of high school students have used prescription medications, including amphetamines and methylphenidate, without a doctor's knowledge. The prevalence of misuse increases to 35% among college-age individuals. The presence of conduct disorder or partially treated ADHD, use of immediate release stimulant medications and enrollment in a competitive college program are all risk factors for misuse.

The task of detecting and treating ongoing substance abuse in patients with ADHD is challenging. It is recommended that serial assessments of symptoms be performed, noting whether they present in a consistent pattern or are sporadic. Risk factors should be evaluated, and collateral information about the patient's behavior should be gathered from family members. Some of the telltale signs of a youth who may be abusing or diverting medications are a disheveled appearance, agitated behavior during sessions, unexplained and suspicious loss of medication bottles or prescriptions, repeated requests for increases in dose, requests to switch to immediate release formulations and unexplained accidents. Close observation and monitoring of symptoms in these situations is mandatory.

Atomoxetine and risk of hepatotoxicity, suicidal ideation and priapism

Atomoxetine is a selective norepinephrine reuptake inhibitor that is FDA approved for the treatment of ADHD in the pediatric population. The FDA has issued a "black box warning" regarding the increased rate of suicidal ideation among children taking this medication. If atomoxetine is chosen for the treatment of ADHD, then parents should be warned to watch for any negative changes in behavior. Patients should be assessed at baseline and monitored at regular intervals for symptoms of worsening irritability, agitation or emerging suicidal ideation (10).

Atomoxetine also is associated with serum aminotransferase (AST) elevation (often >20 times normal) and has caused acute hepatic injury in a small number of cases. Onset of injury is usually within 3-12 weeks of medication initiation, and individuals present clinically with symptoms suggestive of acute viral hepatitis. Most cases are self-limited, but instances of acute liver failure have been noted in the literature. Atomoxetine should be discontinued if hepatic injury is suspected. Priapism is another known side effect of atomoxetine and appears to be more common among patients taking atomoxetine than among those taking methylphenidate.

MOOD STABILIZERS

Little is known about the efficacy of mood stabilizers in the child and adolescent population. Traditionally, these medications have been used to address symptoms of bipolar disorder, violent aggressive outbursts (a characteristic of numerous psychiatric diagnoses), conduct disorder, severe ADHD and as an adjunct to antidepressants for the treatment of severe depression.

Lithium and divalproex are the most widely used mood stabilizers in children, although only lithium is approved for use in pediatric bipolar disorder in adolescents who are 12 years of age or older. Other mood stabilizers are being used on an off-label basis, and their efficacy data is usually extrapolated from the adult scientific literature. It is important to note that there are numerous drawbacks to such extrapolation from adult studies. Although the course of late adolescent bipolar disorder is somewhat similar to the adult form of bipolar disorder, the nosology and phenomenology of pre-pubertal bipolar disorder is still somewhat controversial.

There also are numerous important differences between children and adults in the pharmacokinetics and pharmacodynamics of these medications. For example, children have more efficient hepatic systems and metabolize certain medications more rapidly than do adults. They also have faster renal clearance rates, causing the elimination half-life of lithium to decrease from 24 hours in adults to less than 18 hours in children. As a result of such differences, children may have higher peak levels, lower trough levels and may need higher dosages. It is because of these and other factors that caution is advised in making prescribing decisions based on empirical evidence from research on adults.

FDA approved mood stabilizers

As noted above, lithium is the only available mood stabilizer approved by the FDA for the treatment of bipolar disorder in adolescents aged 12 and older. Lithium is relatively well tolerated in children, although young children may experience more side effects than do their older peers. Beyond its use in bipolar disorder, lithium also is commonly used in the treatment of severe aggression in children with intellectual disabilities, intermittent explosive disorder, autism and other disorders.

Valproate is widely used for the treatment of seizures and has FDA approval for this indication. It also is frequently used for the treatment of bipolar disorder, although it does not have a pediatric indication for this purpose. This drug appears to be more effective in youth with rapid cycling bipolar disorder and those with mixed features.

Carbamazepine has been well studied in the neurology literature and is FDA approved for the treatment of seizure disorder. It is not approved for any psychiatric indications at this time, but is commonly used for the treatment of bipolar disorder and for severe aggression that is unresponsive to lithium and valproate. Carbamazepine is associated with serious hematological, hepatic and pancreatic side effects, somewhat limiting its usefulness.

Lamotrigine has an FDA indication for maintenance use in adult bipolar disorder, but efficacy data in the pediatric population is lacking at this time. It is commonly used in the depressed phase of bipolar disorder; however, its use is associated with Stevens-Johnson syndrome, and caution is therefore advised in titrating this medication to optimal dosage and in weaning the patient from this medication.

Mood stabilizers and risk of suicide

In 2009, the FDA required eight mood stabilizers/antiepileptics to carry a warning regarding increased risk of suicidal ideation. The mood stabilizers involved in the warning are divalproex sodium, carbamazepine, lamotrigine, gabapentin, topiramate, oxcarbazepine, tiagabine and Levetiracetam. An FDA meta-analysis of 199 clinical trials with 43,892 patients showed almost twice (0.43%) the risk of suicidal ideation among individuals taking these medications as compared to those on placebo (0.22%). In the analysis, the FDA found 4 suicides and 105 reports of suicidal ideation among patients receiving mood stabilizers, compared to no suicides and 35 reports of suicidal ideation among patients who were taking placebo. The risk of suicidal ideation emerged as early as 1 week after the start of medication and continued through 6 months (24 weeks).

Mood stabilizers and risk of teratogenicity

Any medication that increases the risk of congenital malformation over the baseline risk (2% in the U.S.) is considered teratogenic. The FDA has relegated lithium, valproate and carbamazepine to Pregnancy Category D, reflecting the fact that these medications have positive evidence of risk to the fetus. Lithium has a risk of cardiovascular malformations (Ebstein's anomaly) that is 20 times higher than the risk in unexposed mothers. Neonatal hypothyroidism, diabetes insipidus and "floppy baby syndrome" are other risks associated with the use of lithium.

Valproate also has a poor reproductive safety profile. The risk of malformation after valproate exposure is 2-3 times higher than with carbamazepine exposure. This risk is dose-dependent and appears to rise when valproate is used in combination with other drug therapies (e.g., valproate with lamotrigine). In contrast, carbamazepine was considered for years to be highly teratogenic, but has shown an overall prevalence of malformation similar to that of lamotrigine.

CONCLUSION

The last decade has seen numerous changes in the way pediatric psychopharmacology is conceptualized and practiced (11). With the advent of neuroimaging and genome mapping, the once farsighted goal of understanding the neurobiology of psychiatric disorders now appears to be within reach. There is also greater emphasis on evidence based psychiatric practice and on understanding the long-term effects of medications on the developing brain (12). There is a clear need for further research to enhance our understanding of the complex treatment of these multifaceted disorders (13).

REFERENCES

[1] AACAP Official Action. Practice parameter on the use of psychotropic medication in children and adolescents. J Am Acad Child Adolesc Psychiatry 2009;48(9):961-73.
[2] Lee E, Teschemaker AR, Johann-Liang R, Bazemore G, et al. Off-label prescribing patterns of antidepressants in children and adolescents. Pharmacoepidemiol Drug Saf 2012;21:137–44.
[3] Wagner KD, Robb AS, Findling RL, Jin J. A randomized, placebo-controlled trial of citalopram for the treatment of major depression in children and adolescents. Am J Psychiatry 2004;161:1079–83.
[4] Emslie GJ, Findling RL, Yeung PP, Kunz NR, Li Y. Venlafaxine ER for the treatment of pediatric subjects with depression: results of 2 placebo-controlled trials. J Am Acad Child Adolesc Psychiatry. 2007;46:479-88.
[5] US Food and Drug Administration. Relationship between psychotropic drugs and pediatric suicidality: review and evaluation of clinical data. URL: http://www.fda.gov/ohrms/dockets/ac/04/briefing/2004-4065 b1-10-TAB08-Hammads-Review.pdf.
[6] March JI, Silva S, Petrycki S, Curry J, Wells K, Fairbank J, et al. Treatment for Adolescents With Depression Study (TADS) Team. Fluoxetine, cognitive-behavioral therapy, and their combination for adolescents with depression: Treatment for Adolescents with Depression Study (TADS) randomized controlled trial. JAMA 2004;292:807-20.
[7] Olfson M, Blanco C, Liu SM, Wang S, Correll CU. National trends in the office-based treatment of children, adolescents, and adults with antipsychotics. Arch Gen Psychiatry 2012;69:1247–56.

[8] Harrison JN, Cluxton-Keller F, Gross D. Antipsychotic medication prescribing trends in children and adolescents. J Pediatr Health Care 2012;26(2):139-45.

[9] Greydanus DE, Nazeer A, Patel DR. Psycho-pharmacology of ADHD in pediatrics: Current advances and issues. Neuropsychiatr Dis Treat 2009;5:171-81.

[10] Kubiszyn T, Mire SS. A review of recent FDA drug safety communications for pediatric psychotropics. J Child Family Stud 2014;23(4):716-27.

[11] March JS., Szatmari P, Bukstein O, Chrisman A, Kondo D, Hamilton JD, et al. AACAP 2005 Research Forum: speeding the adoption of evidence-based practice in pediatric psychiatry. J Am Acad Child Adolesc Psychiatry 2007;46(9):1098-1110.

[12] Reeve A. Principles of psychopharmacology for the adolescent patient. Adolesc Med State Art Rev 2013; 24(2):356-70.

[13] Vitiello B. Research in child and adolescent psych-opharmacology: recent accomplishments and new challenges. Psychopharmacology 2007;191:5-13.

Submitted: June 05, 2015. *Revised:* July 03, 2015. *Accepted:* July 10, 2015.

In: Alternative Medicine Research Yearbook 2017
Editor: Joav Merrick
ISBN: 978-1-53613-726-2
© 2018 Nova Science Publishers, Inc.

Chapter 6

LONG-TERM MUSIC-LISTENING'S EFFECTS ON BLOOD PRESSURE, HEART RATE, ANXIETY, AND DEPRESSION

Taunjah P Bell[*], *PhD and David O Akombo, PhD*

Department of Psychology and Department of Music, College of Liberal Arts,
Jackson State University, Jackson, Mississippi, US

ABSTRACT

Listening to music could not only impact physiological responses but also affect psychological indicators. Extensive research has focused on the beneficial effects of music on blood pressure (BP), heart rate (HR), respiration rate (RR), anxiety, and depression in predominantly Caucasian samples; however, to date few studies have been designed to determine the influence of long-term music listening on mindfulness in minorities. The purpose of the present study was to examine the effects of long-term music listening on BP, HR, anxiety, depression, and mindfulness in African Americans. Two-hundred seventeen adults (156 females and 61 males) under age 25 were assigned at random to one of four conditions (no music, classical, classic jazz, or classic rock and roll music) using a computer-based program and were instructed to listen to music or remain silent for 30 minutes per session four times per week for 12 weeks in our laboratory. Our research findings indicated that participants in the classical music group were more likely to have lower BP and HR measurements, lower anxiety and depression scores, and higher mindfulness scores than individuals who listened to no music, classic jazz, or classic rock and roll. There was a statistically significant difference between music group means on the combined dependent variables ($F(3, 213) = 8.923$, $p = .009$; Wilk's Lambda $(6, 422) = 2.704$, $p = .006$, partial eta squared $= .733$, with a large effect size). Results supported the hypothesis tested and suggested that music can be used to promote wellness and enhance cognition.

---

[*] Correspondence: Taunjah P Bell, PhD, Department of Psychology, College of Liberal Arts, 231 Dollye ME Robinson Building, Jackson State University, 1400 John R. Lynch Street, POBox 17550, Jackson, Mississippi 39217-0350 USA. E-mail: taunjah.p.bell@jsums.edu.

Keywords: music-based interventions, blood pressure, heart rate, anxiety, depression, African Americans

INTRODUCTION

Listening to music, whether a classical symphony, a jazz ensemble, or a rock and roll band, could not only impact physiological responses including BP, HR, and RR, but also affect psychological indicators such as anxiety, mood, and cognition. Some results of published research on the physiological and psychological effects of music-based interventions suggested that listening to classical music decreases pain (1), stress (2), anxiety (3), BP (4), HR (5), and/or plasma levels of stress hormones (6) for a long duration after treatment has ended. As impressive as the evidence is, however, previous studies are limited by small sample sizes, short-term treatment programs, short follow-up durations, and the absence of underrepresented minorities, specifically African Americans. To our knowledge to date and based on the published literature reviewed, little research conducted on this topic includes predominantly African Americans recruited from the southern United States, particularly from urban communities or even historically black institutions. Thus, most of the existing studies are not adequate to establish the effectiveness of this music-based intervention across diverse populations. Therefore, the purpose of the present study is to help fill a gap in this line of research by examining the effects of listening to instrumental music on BP, HR, anxiety, depression, and mindfulness in an African American sample recruited from a population of participants residing primarily in an urban capital city in the Deep South. The strengths of this study include a large sample size, long-term music programs, and a predominantly minority sample. We proposed that long-term listening to classical music induces its beneficial effects by decreasing physiological stress responses such as BP and HR, reducing anxiety and depression, and increasing mindfulness.

In the present study, classical music is defined as music written in the European tradition during a period lasting approximately from 1750 to 1830, when forms such as the symphony, concerto, and sonata were standardized. This music genre is often contrasted with baroque (c. 1600-1750) and romantic (c. 1804-1910) music eras and includes composers such as Antonio Vivaldi, Johann Sebastian Bach, George Frideric Handel, Wolfgang Amadeus Mozart, and Ludwig van Beethoven. Classic jazz is commonly and widely defined as an American style of music characterized by a strong but flexible rhythmic understructure with solo and ensemble improvisations on basic tunes and chord patterns recorded by notable and well-renown artists such as for example Miles Davis, Duke Ellington, Louis Armstrong, Thelonious Monk, and Herbie Hancock. In the United States (US), the classic rock and roll music format commonly features music ranging generally from the late 1960s to the late 1980s and includes music by legendary bands such as The Beatles, The Rolling Stones, The Doors, Jimi Hendrix, and Led Zeppelin. Many participants indicated that they preferred listening to these music genres and numerous individuals even listed favorite songs composed by some of these musical artists.

Music may have either a calming or stimulating effect and elicits an individual reaction from each listener (5). One of the purposes and purported benefits of long-term music listening is a reduction in the stress response of the person listening to music (2). The physiological stress response propagated by the hypothalamic-pituitary-adrenal (HPA) axis in response to stress-inducing stimuli involves an elevated BP, HR, or RR, and the increased secretion of stress hormones including adrenocorticotropic hormone (ACTH), corticotrophin-releasing hormone (CRH), glucocorticoids, and cortisol (7). The HPA axis is activated in response to stress resulting in the secretion of CRH from the hypothalamus, ACTH from the pituitary gland, and cortisol combined with other neurochemicals from the adrenal gland (7). Results of music-based intervention studies in medicine indicated that slow, quiet, instrumental music lowered physiological stress responses, thereby decreasing the secretion of stress hormones; whereas fast, loud, lyrical music heightened stress responses and reduced baroreflex sensitivity (8-9). Watkins (10) reported that music-listening can be an effective nursing intervention for decreasing HR, BP, and, in some cases, RR in stressful situations. Bartlett (11) also found that listening to music induced changes in physiological reactions including changes in stress hormone secretions, HR, and RR. Similar findings suggested that anxiolytic music reduced physiological stress responses in the cardiovascular system (12). Other researchers indicated that music can be used as an adjuvant to sedation and for the relief of postoperative pain (9, 10, 13).

Various types of music have been used successfully alone or paired with other evidence-based treatments as a complementary therapeutic tool to reduce stress and stress-related problems associated with psychiatric disorders from clinical anxiety to major depression or to treat the symptoms associated with these illnesses (9). Results of clinical studies showed that effective music-based interventions decreased anxiety levels, elevated mood, reduced BP and/or HR measurements, and decreased ACTH as well as CRH levels, which attenuates the stress response (6, 10, 14). Guétin, Soua, Voiriot, Picot, and Hérisson (15) reported that music-based interventions can be used successfully to manage patients' moods, specifically those suffering from anxiety and depression, following traumatic brain injury. Kim et al. (16) found that engaging in an active music-based program elevated mood and facilitated recovery of function following stroke. Salamon et al. (17) proposed that sound therapy down regulates the stress response of the HPA axis through mediation of the complex nitric oxide system believed to be the primary and fundamental mechanism by which music induces relaxation.

Music has been a medium of therapy for centuries, and there are numerous examples of the curative or healing powers of music in the historical records of different cultures (14). Over the last fifty years, music therapy has developed as an evidence-based, clinically applied treatment administered within a therapeutic relationship created to accomplish individualized goals directed by a credentialed professional who has completed an approved music therapy program (14). Therapeutic goals can be created to help patients overcome mental, physical, emotional, intellectual, and social challenges; behavioral objectives can be geared toward promoting wellness by assisting patients with managing stress, alleviating pain, expressing emotional feelings, enhancing memory, improving communication, and engaging in physical rehabilitation exercises (9, 14). Music therapists, therefore, work in community mental health centers, medical hospitals, psychiatric institutions, schools, nursing homes, and correctional facilities as well as other settings (14). They are trained to assess cognitive skills, physical health, emotional well-being, social functioning, and communication abilities through responses to musical stimuli. These skilled professionals also are trained to design music interventions for individuals and groups based on client (children, adolescents, adults, and elders) needs as well as follow up progress (14). Clearly stated music therapy goals, measurable behavioral objectives, and observable progress are documented in a treatment plan, following client assessment, and service is delivered in accordance with the American Music Therapy Association (AMTA) Standards of Clinical Practice (18). In accordance with

AMTA standards, for example, song selections for receptive music listening programs and certain activities for active music producing and songwriting programs can be modified based on client preferences, cultural considerations, age appropriateness, physical abilities, and individualized needs (18).

Steve Porges (19) reasoned that music is intertwined with psychological processes related to physiological responses to emotional cues, environmental stimuli, interpersonal challenges, and intrapersonal demands. He uses the Polyvagal Theory to present a plausible model to explain how and why music-based interventions aid in supporting physiological health, promoting psychological well-being, and enhancing recovery of function following trauma associated with physical, mental, or emotional illness. The Polyvagal Theory even entails insights that link music-based interventions to a functioning autonomic nervous system (ANS) and a healthy endocrine system (19). To understand Porges' theory, it is necessary to investigate features of the vagus nerve, a major component of the ANS. The vagus nerve is a mixed nerve composed of 20-30% efferent motor fibers carrying information from the brain to peripheral cardiac muscles, smooth muscles, organs, and glands and 70-80% afferent sensory fibers carrying information to the brain from thoracic and abdominal regions (20). This bilateral cranial nerve has both left and right branches that exit the brain stem, regulating several organs including the heart and stomach and modulating autonomic functions including BP, HR, and gastric tone (20). Porges (21) proposed that the two branches of the vagus are related to different behavioral strategies. One vagal branch is involved in regulating an appropriate physiological state during social interactions in safe environments. The other vagal branch is involved in regulating an adaptive physiological state in response to life-threatening stimuli (21).

This theoretical perspective is vital to understanding the mechanisms underlying music-based interventions including active and receptive music therapy, which require processing auditory stimuli, engaging in appropriate social interactions, and developing a therapeutic relationship between the client and the professional in a safe environment. Porges' Polyvagal Theory might be used to explain results of the current study designed to examine the long-term impact of music-listening on participants' physiological and psychological responses as measured by BP and HR readings combined with self-report findings obtained from anxiety, depression, and mindfulness scales, respectively.

METHODS

Two-hundred seventeen African Americans (156 females and 61 males) under age 25 years were recruited to participate voluntarily in this study. During recruitment, individuals were asked to sign-up if interested in this study so a researcher could contact them to schedule the initial and subsequent data collection sessions. A majority of the participants attended a historically black university located in an urban capital city. Others lived in surrounding communities or resided in neighboring southern states. To be included in this study, individuals had to be age 18 or older, have an initial (baseline) BP <140/90 mmHg, have no hearing impairments or use no auditory aids, and be able to comply with the research protocol. Individuals with a baseline BP >140/90 mmHg (considered hypertensive according to official guidelines issued by the American Heart Association/American Stroke Association (22) were excluded from the study and referred to the University Health Center or their private physician. Prior to data collection, the research protocol and supporting documents were submitted to the Institutional Review Board (IRB) for approval. Following approval, participants were recruited and research was conducted according to the IRB standards and guidelines for studies involving human participants. This research also was conducted in adherence to the legal requirements of studies completed in the US.

Measurements

Prior to the initial data collection session, participants were asked to read and sign a consent form. During this time, individuals were permitted to ask any questions pertaining to the purpose and procedures of our study. All questions were answered by the researchers. Then, participants were asked to acknowledge that they had no hearing impairments and used no auditory devices or hearing aids and were able to comply with the conditions of the experiment. At this time, individuals also confirmed that they were able to visit the laboratory four times per week for 30 minutes per session during the course of this study. Next, using a computer-based program, each individual was assigned at random to one of four conditions (no music, classical, jazz, or rock and roll music) for 12 weeks.

After reading and signing a consent form and receiving a condition assignment, the participant was connected to an Ambulatory Blood Pressure Monitoring (ABPM) device (Microlife® WatchBP® O3, Microlife Medical Home Solutions, Inc., Golden, CO, US) so BP and HR measurements could be recorded and tracked. The individual was then given The Anxiety Study Group Demographic Questionnaire (TASGDQ), State-Trait Anxiety Inventory (STAI), the Center for Epidemiologic Studies Depression Scale Revised (CESD-R), and the trait version of the Mindful Attention Awareness Scale (MAAS) to complete. The TASGDQ is a 20-item, self-designed instrument used to collect background data (e.g., gender, ethnicity, age, academic classification, religious affiliation, and music genre preference) on our participants. The STAI is a widely used 40-item self-report inventory designed to measure the current state of anxiety induced by arousal of the ANS as well as proneness or a predisposition to developing anxiety symptoms. The CESD-R is a popular 20-item self-administered scale used to measure depression symptoms clustered in nine different domains. The well-known trait MAAS is a 15-item, self-report measure used to assess a core characteristic of mindfulness defined as a receptive state of mind in which an attentive individual, informed by a sensitive awareness of what is occurring in the present, simply observes what is taking place. This mental state is in contrast to the conceptually driven mode of processing, in which events and experiences are filtered through cognitive appraisals, judgments, evaluations, memories, beliefs, emotions, and other forms of cognitive manipulation (23).

Experimental design

After reading the informed consent form, asking any questions, and signing two copies of the document, the participant was given one copy of the consent form and the other was stored in a securely locked filing cabinet. The participant then received his or her condition assignment and was connected to the ABPM so the researcher could record and track BP and HR measurements. Next, the individual was directed to complete the demographic questionnaire (TASGDQ) and all self-report measures. The demographic questionnaire included questions about the frequency and duration, if any, of each participant's music-listening. An item that required respondents to indicate and rank their preferred music genres appeared on the demographic questionnaire as well. Definitions of various music genres including those examined in the present study were provided as references. Participants were asked to list a few of their favorite songs for each preferred genre endorsed. Information pertaining to the preferred music genre was used by other researchers who loaded instrumental samples of songs from the three target music genres on the MP3 players. The device with the downloaded music and over-the-ear headphones were given to each person in the study. There was no guarantee that an individual's favorite tunes would be included in the downloaded playlist or that participants would be randomly assigned to their preferred music genre group. To avoid violating copyright laws and paying hefty fines to recording labels/record companies, we obtained relatively lengthy samples of songs that were recorded from the internet (Pandora® Internet Radio and YouTube) and blended to make a continuous loop of songs loaded on each electronic device. The researchers who loaded the music on the MP3 players were different from those who conducted the experimental sessions. The researchers who conducted the data collection sessions and assisted with data analysis were blind to the condition to which each participant was assigned; therefore, they did not know to which type of music each individual was listening. We employed this procedure to exercise scientific control and possibly avoid any confounding factors that might interfere with the clear results of our study. All experimental data collection sessions were scheduled for 10:00AM-2:00PM. This time frame was based on the availability and schedules of both the researchers and the participants. Also, an attempt was made to schedule each participant's data collection session for the same time of day for every session whenever possible. We were successfully able to do this approximately 95% of the time.

At the start of the data collection session, each individual was provided with headphones and an MP3 player preloaded with preferred instrumental classical, jazz, or rock and roll music and instructed to sit and listen to music alone for 30 minutes in the laboratory. At the end of the 30-minute session, the researcher returned to the room to disconnect the participant from the ABPM and to request that the individual complete all self-report measures again so that we could use the results as post-test data to which pre-test findings were compared. Prior to data collection, participants in the control (no music) condition were instructed to sit quietly and remain silent without falling asleep in the laboratory for the 30-minute session. Otherwise, the same protocol was followed prior to and following the 30-minute period for the control and experimental groups. Only one participant was allowed in the laboratory during each data collection session which was videotaped with the individual's permission. At the end of this study, all data were analyzed by the researchers.

RESULTS

Descriptive and inferential statistical analyses were performed on the data using IBM® Statistical Package for the Social Sciences Predictive Analytics Software (v.20). Results of the descriptive statistical tests revealed that the majority (71.9%) of the 217 individuals who participated in this study were African American females (n = 156) and the remaining 28.1% were African American males (n = 61). There were 55 participants in the control group and 54 participants in each music group. Among the statistical analyses, a multivariate analysis of variance (MANOVA) inferential test was performed to examine the effect of 12 weeks of no music or music on BP (separated into systolic BP, or SBP, and diastolic BP, or DBP) and HR measurements as well as on STAI, CESD-R, and MAAS scores. The independent variable is music with four levels (no music, classical, jazz, and rock and roll music) and the five dependent variables are BP, HR, anxiety, depression, and mindfulness. Preliminary assumption testing was conducted to check for normality, linearity, univariate and multivariate outliers, homogeneity of variance-covariance matrices, and multicollinearity. No violations of these assumptions were noted. There was a statistically significant difference between music group means on the combined dependent variables ($F_{(3, 213)}$ = 8.923, p = .009; Wilk's Lambda $(6, 422)$ = 2.704, p = .006, partial eta squared = .733, with a large effect size).

Follow-up univariate analyses of variance (ANOVAs) indicated that SBP ($F_{(3, 213)}$ = 4.875, p = .014), DBP ($F_{(3, 213)}$ = 2.461, p = .008), and HR ($F_{(3, 213)}$ = 2.592, p = .020) measurements were significantly lowered after 12 weeks of listening to classical music compared to the other conditions. Results also showed that STAI ($F_{(3, 213)}$ = 6.317, p = .002) and CESD-R ($F_{(3, 213)}$ = 4.638, p = .001) scores were significantly reduced and MAAS ($F_{(2, 211)}$ = 2.151, p = .014) scores were noticeably improved by long-term exposure to classical music compared to the other conditions. Post-hoc comparisons using Tukey's Honestly Significant Difference (HSD) test revealed that listening to classical music resulted in a greater reduction in SBP, DBP, and HR (14.26 + 1.25 mmHg, p = .021; 11.84 + 1.73 mmHg, p = .034; and 17 + 2 bpm, p =.019, respectively) than listening to rock and roll or remaining silent. Findings from Tukey's HSD post hoc comparisons also indicated that listening to jazz music resulted in a slight reduction in SBP, DBP, and HR (4.31 + 1.01 mmHg, p = .098; 3.29 + 1.91 mmHg, p = .067; and 8 + 3 bpm, p = .161, respectively); however, these findings were not significant.

DISCUSSION

Overall, our data provided evidence to support the hypothesis tested, and we concluded that long-term, classical music-listening resulted in a significant decrease in physiological responses and psychological factors associated with stress as well as a noticeable increase in mindfulness viewed as an attentive, non-judgmental awareness of the present moment (23). The current results are consistent with those of Knight and Rickard (24) who found that music has significant effects on SBP, HR, and subjective anxiety in healthy male and female undergraduate students exposed to a cognitive stressor task involving preparation for an oral presentation either in silence or in the presence of Pachelbel's Canon in D major. Bernardi, Porta, and Sleight (12) also found a relationship between music, BP and HR. They noted that BP, HR, and ventilation increased and mid-cerebral artery flow velocity and baroreflex activity decreased when participants were exposed to fast tempo music. Bernardi and colleagues (12) also indicated that slow tempo or meditative music induced a relaxing effect in their patients. Yet, the underlying physiological bases of these phenomena are unknown.

Apparently, music induces its beneficial or arousal effects through the ANS (21), but the factors directly involved remain unclear. The implication is that anxiolytic or relaxing music evokes positive emotions and impacts cognitive function perhaps by inducing the release of neurotransmitters and other neurochemicals known to elevate mood or reduce anxiety.

As previously mentioned, music-based interventions have been used successfully in medical and clinical research to elevate mood, alleviate anxiety, and induce relaxation in a variety of patients diagnosed with conditions ranging from mental illnesses and physical disabilities to speech pathologies and behavioral disorders. Smith (25) used a single music session to induce relaxation in the workplace and reduce state anxiety levels in 80 customer service specialists (40 females and 40 males) recruited from a call center in Queensland. A randomized controlled trial was conducted comparing verbal discussion (control condition) to music relaxation (experimental condition). Smith (25) compared pre- and post-test scores on the State subscale of the STAI, and the results revealed that the single session music relaxation intervention significantly reduced anxiety levels in participants compared to the control intervention. Immediately following the music relaxation intervention, participants reported a positive increase in feelings of relaxation and pleasantness. They also indicated a reduction in tension at the end of their shift. Smith's (25) data yielded evidence to support the use of music relaxation to decrease employees' anxiety levels while at the job site. Replication of this study in different occupational environments is recommended to provide further support for the use of music relaxation in workplace settings.

In another music relaxation intervention study, John and colleagues (6) exposed pistol shooters to a four-week program prior to competitive sporting events to determine the impact of music on pre-competition stress, shooting performance, and HPA axis activity as measured by salivary cortisol secretion levels. One hundred male shooters between the ages of 25 and 33 years (M = 29.5, SD = 4.3) were included in their study comprised of two groups of 50 participants each. Fifty males were exposed to a music relaxation intervention combined with a standard sports training program while the remaining participants were exposed to the standard sports training program alone. The entire study lasted five weeks and included a four-week music relaxation intervention with a one-week follow-up. Baseline data were collected prior to the intervention to compare to post-test results obtained at the end of week four and follow-up data collected at the end of week five, one week after the study was completed. Salivary cortisol samples collected during these three phases were analyzed and post-test along with follow-up data results indicated that the experimental group experienced a statistically significant reduction in salivary cortisol secretions compared to the control group, which showed no significant reduction in salivary cortisol levels. John et al. (6) concluded that the music relaxation intervention combined with routine sports training may be an effective intervention used to reduce pre-competition stress and enhance shooting performance by suppressing HPA axis activity thereby reducing salivary cortisol secretions believed to be a reliable physiological biomarker of pre-competition stress (6).

Because previous and current findings suggested that long-term music-listening can significantly affect physiological responses as well as psychological indicators linked to autonomic function, music-based interventions appear to be non-pharmacological, non-invasive, cost-effective techniques that can be used as adjunct approaches to the traditional treatment of clinical disorders associated with stress and anxiety as well as medical conditions related to elevated BP and HR, especially in patients who believe that listening to preferred music is fun and enjoyable. Thus, directions for future research can include examining the use of music as an evidence-based, alternative strategy to complement antianxiety, antidepressant, and antihypertensive medications prescribed to relatively young minorities similar to those included in the present study. Other directions can involve exploring the effects of long-term music-based interventions on the expression and secretion of salivary, serum, and plasma concentrations of stress hormones in response to acute and chronic stressors. Finally, goals related to research on the continued investigation of the effectiveness of music-based interventions should be vigorously pursued.

ACKNOWLEDGMENTS

The authors would like to thank all individuals who volunteered to participate in this study and the research assistants in the Jackson State University Anxiety Study Group Research Laboratory who assisted with participant recruitment, data collection, and data input.

REFERENCES

[1] Ovayolu N, Ucan O, Pehlivan S, Pehlivan Y, Buyukhatipoglu H, Savas MC, et al. Listening to Turkish classical music decreases patients' anxiety, pain, dissatisfaction and the dose of sedative and analgesic drugs during colonoscopy: A prospective randomized controlled trial. World J Gastroenterol 2006;12:7532-6.

[2] Nilsson U. The effect of music intervention in stress response to cardiac surgery in a randomized clinical trial. Heart Lung 2009;38:201-7.

[3] Shabanloei R, Golchin M, Esfahani A, Dolatkhah R, Rasoulian M. Effects of music therapy on pain and anxiety in patients undergoing bone marrow biopsy and aspiration. AORN J 2010;91:746-51.

[4] Chafin S, Roy M, Gerin W, Christenfeld N. Music can facilitate blood pressure recovery from stress. Br J Health Psychol 2004;9:393-403.

[5] 5. Nakahara H, Furuya S, Obata S, Masuko T, Kinoshita H. Emotion-related changes in heart rate and its variability during performance and perception of music. Ann NY Acad Sci 2009;1169:359-62.

[6] John S, Verma SK, Khanna GL. The effect of music therapy on salivary cortisol as a reliable marker of pre competition stress in shooting performance. J Exerc Sci Physiother 2010;6:70-7.

[7] Kalat JW. Biological Psychology. Boston, MA: Cengage Learning, 2016.

[8] Altenmueller E, Schuermann K, Lim VK, Parlitz D. Hits to the left, flops to the right: Different emotions during listening to music are reflected in cortical lateralisation patterns. Neuropsychologia 2002;40: 2242-56.

[9] Trappe H-J. Music and medicine: The effects of music on the human being. Appl Cardiopulm Pathophysiol, 2012;16:133-42.

[10] Watkins, GR. Music therapy: Proposed physiological mechanisms and clinical implications. Clin Nurs Specialist 1997;11:43-50.

[11] Bartlett DL. Physiological reactions to music and acoustic stimuli. In: Hodges, DA, ed. Handbook of music psychology. San Antonio, TX: IMR Press, 1996.

[12] Bernardi L, Porta C, Sleight P. Cardiovascular, cerebrovascular, and respiratory changes induced by different types of music in musicians and non-musicians: The importance of silence. Heart 2006; 92:445-52.

[13] Nilsson S, Kokinsky E, Nilsson U, Sidenvall B, Enskär K. School-aged children's experiences of postoperative music medicine on pain, distress, and anxiety. Pediatr Anesth 2009;19:1184-90.

[14] Wigram T, Pedersen IN, Bonde LO. A comprehensive guide to music therapy: Theory, clinical practice, research, and training. Cambridge, UK: Jessica Kingsley, 2002.

[15] Guétin S, Soua B, Voiriot G, Picot M-C, Hérisson C. The effect of music therapy on mood and anxiety-depression: An observational study in institutionalised patients with traumatic brain injury. Ann Phys Rehabil Med 2009;52:30-40.
[16] Kim DS, Park YG, Choi JH, Im S-H, Jung KJ, Cha YA, et al. Effects of music therapy on mood in stroke patients. Yonsei Med J 2011;52:977-81.
[17] Salamon E, Kim M, Beaulieu J, Stefano GB. Sound therapy induced relaxation: Down regulating stress processes and pathologies. Med Sci Monit 2003; 9:RA96-RA101.
[18] American Music Therapy Association. AMTA standards of clinical practice. URL: http://musictherapy.org/about/standards.
[19] Porges SW. Music therapy and trauma: Insights from the polyvagal theory. In: Stewart K, ed. Symposium on music therapy and trauma: Bridging theory and clinical practice. New York: Satchnote Press, 2008.
[20] Foley JO, DuBois FS. Quantitative studies of the vagus nerve in the cat: I. The ratio of sensory to motor fibers. J Comp Neurol 1937;67:49-67.
[21] Porges SW. The polyvagal theory: Phylogenetic substrates of a social nervous system. Int J Psychophysiol 2001;42:123-46.
[22] Goldstein LB, Bushnell CD, Adams RJ, Appel LJ, Braun LT, Chaturvedi S, et al. Guidelines for the primary prevention of stroke: A guideline for healthcare professionals from the American Heart Association/American Stroke Association. Stroke 2011;4:517-84.
[23] Brown KW, Ryan RM. The benefits of being present: Mindfulness and its role in psychological well-being. J Pers Soc Psychol 2003;84:822-48.
[24] Knight WE, Rickard NS. Relaxing music prevents stress-induced increases in subjective anxiety, systolic blood pressure, and heart rate in healthy males and females. J Music Ther 2001;33:254-72.
[25] Smith M. The effects of a single music relaxation session on state anxiety levels of adults in a workplace environment. Aust J Music Ther 2008;19:45-66.

Submitted: July 16, 2015. *Revised:* August 20, 2015. *Accepted:* August 28, 2015.

In: Alternative Medicine Research Yearbook 2017
Editor: Joav Merrick
ISBN: 978-1-53613-726-2
© 2018 Nova Science Publishers, Inc.

Chapter 7

ANTIBACTERIAL AND ANTIOXIDANT POTENTIAL OF ORGANIC SOLVENTS EXTRACT OF MANGROVE ENDOPHYTIC FUNGUS *EUPENICILLIUM SENTICOSUM* SCOTT

Ambarish Cheviry Nair[1],,
Santhosh Goveas[2], Laveena D'Souza[3],
Flavia D'Cunha[3] and Viana D'Souza[3]*

[1]Department of Biochemistry, St Aloysius College, Mangalore, India
[2]Department of Biotechnology, St Aloysius College, Mangalore, India
[3]P.G Department of Biochemistry, St. Aloysius College, Mangalore, Karnataka, India

ABSTRACT

Endophytic fungus *Eupenicillium senticosum* Scott isolated from the stem of mangrove plant *Acanthus ilicifolius* was cultured and the crude extracts were screened for antibacterial as well as antioxidant activities. Out of different organic extracts, methanolic extract had shown promising inhibition activity against gram positive and gram negative pathogenic bacteria. Furthermore, these extracts were subjected for different *in-vitro* antioxidants activities assays and revealed that methanol extracts were found to have significantly higher total antioxidant activity ($p < 0.01$), scavenging abilities on DPPH-free radicals ($p < 0.01$), Fe^{2+} ion chelation ($p < 0.05$) and lipid peroxidation inhibition activities ($p < 0.05$) compared to DEE, CF and EA extracts. Even though their reducing powers were similar to that of Butylated hydroxy toluene, moderate ferrous ion chelating ability compared to that of the EDTA-2Na. The significance difference was observed between EC_{50} values of methanolic and other organic extracts. The results of present study indicate a significant positive correlation between antioxidant activities vs. phenolic and flavonoid contents. This attributes to high contents of bioactive compound in a sample is directly proportional to high antioxidant activity. Bioactivity profiling in the current study clearly demonstrated that endophytic fungus (*Eupenicillium*

---

* Correspondence: Ambarish Cheviry Nair, Department of Biochemistry, St Aloysius College, Mangalore, 575003, Karnataka, India. E-mail: ambarishnair84@gmail.com.

senticosum Scott) serve as a novel source of potent natural antioxidant and antibacterial agents.

Keywords: mangrove plants, endophytic fungus, phenolics, flavonoid, antibacterial activity, antioxidants activity

INTRODUCTION

Natural products discovery is a present trend of developing new drugs for various human disease and most of the drugs were of microbial origin (1). In spite of vast diversity, microbial world is much less explored in metabolite characterization as well as bioactivity profiling (2). Most of the microbes, inhabited in stressful environmental conditions are known as prolific producer of various metabolites as a part of biochemical association with the host (3). Bacteria, fungi and actinomycetes are the major organism able to produce diverse biochemical compounds having potent bioactivity (1). As reported (4) reactive oxygen species are responsible for lipid per oxidation, protein denaturation and cell death. In normal condition, natural antioxidant enzymes found in human body helps to counteract the cellular effects of highly active oxygen radicals. However, a study (5) found that intense excise may lead to production of large quantity of ROS which may overcome the scavenging effect of natural antioxidants. To decrease the harm of intensively producing ROS, exogenous intake of neutraceuticals are required.

To meet present demand of consumers from a decade's overwhelming trend to search for naturally occurring antioxidants and antimicrobial compounds from different endophytes, which inhabits varieties of ecological niche (1). With respect to the habitat, endophytes synthesize different varieties of secondary metabolites and most of the endophytes are considered as potential source of bioactive compounds (6). Novel metabolites exploited in pharmaceutical, food and agricultural industries are widespread among the endophytic fungi (7). Even though number of pharmacological compounds with antimicrobial, antitumor, anti-inflammatory and antiviral activities have been previously reported from different endophytes (1, 8, 9), but the reports related to stress tolerant mangrove plants endophytic fungi antimicrobial and antioxidant activities are very scanty (10). Very few studies were carried out on endophytic fungi of mangrove plants and most of them are confined to foliar endophytes (2, 11). In the present study stress tolerant mangrove endophytic fungus (*Eupenicillium senticosum* Scott) were subjected to antibacterial and various *in-vitro* antioxidant activity assays to assess its biopotentiality for the extraction novel therapeutic agents for better advancement.

METHODS

The plant material was collected from the mangrove of Nethravathi River, Mangalore, India (12° 50' N, 74° 50' E) and plant was identified as *Acanthus ilicifolius*. Fungus was isolated from the stem of the plant.

Endophytic fungus isolation

Pieces of plant (*Acanthus ilicifolius*) stem was rinsed with sterile water, sterilized by soaking in 70% ethanol (1min) and 3.5%NaCl solution (3min), and rinsed again with sterile water. Later on, the plant stems were excised with a sterilized scalpel into pieces of about 5mm length and plated onto the potato dextrose agar (PDA) medium which is supplemented with antibiotic streptomycin (0.1g/l) and incubated at 24°C until growth appeared. Colonies were transferred to fresh Potato dextrose agar plates for further growth and fungus was identified as *Eupenicillium senticosum* Scott.

Fermentation and extraction

The isolated endophytic fungus was grown in Erlenmeyer flasks containing 500 ml of PDB medium. The test fungus was inoculated and incubated for nearly 21 days with regular observation. After incubation the extraction was carried out by using equal amount of diethyl ether (DEE), chloroform (CF), ethyl acetate (EA) and methanol (ME) solvents respectively in order to separate nonpolar and polar substances present in the filtered fungal broth. The organic phase was collected and the solvent was then removed by evaporation under reduced pressure at 45°C using rotary vacuum evaporator. The dry solid residues were re-dissolved in respective organic solvents and crude extract were evaluated for their antibacterial and antioxidant properties.

Antibacterial activity

Antibacterial activity was assessed with disk diffusion technique (12) and dried crude extracts recovered from fractions were dissolved in respective organic solvents (diethyl ether, chloroform, ethyl acetate and methanol). Plain antibiotic disks (6 mm; Hi-Media Laboratories, Mumbai, India) were impregnated with 10µl crude extract and tested against four bacteria (*Bacillus subtilis, Escherichia coli, Staphylococcus aureus, Klebsiella pneumonia*) procured from MTCC, Chandigarh, India. Sterile nutrient agar (peptone, 5 g; sodium chloride, 5 g; beef extract, 1.5 g; yeast extract, 1.5 g; agar 15 g; distilled water, 1000 ml) served as basal medium. For the comparison, standard antibiotic discs were used according to the resistance to respective pathogenic organism. Plates were incubated at 37°C for 24 hours. Antibacterial activity was expressed as the diameter of the inhibition zone (mm) produced by the extract.

Determination of total phenolics

The total phenolics content of endophytes extracts were evaluated by using Folin-ciocalteu reagent in alkaline medium and were expressed in Gallic acid equivalents (13). The reaction mixture contained 0.1 ml of 5 mg/ml extract, 0.05 ml of freshly prepared Folin-ciocalteu reagent, and 0.15 ml of 20% sodium carbonate. The final volume of mixture was made up to 1 ml with distilled water. The mixtures were incubated in dark for about two hours. The absorbance was measured spectrophotometrically at 765 nm. Gallic acid (GA) was employed as a standard and results were calculated as Gallic acid equivalents (mg GA/g).

Determination of total flavonoid content

Total flavonoid content of the extracts was estimated as per the method of (14). The 100 µl of methanolic extract was mixed with of distilled water (300 µl) and 30 µl of Sodium nitrite (5%). 30 µl of 10% Aluminium chloride was added after 5 min and mixed well. The above mixture was incubated (5 min) and 1mM Sodium Hydroxide (0.2 ml) was added. Finally, the volume was made up to 1 ml with distilled water and mixed well. Quercetin was used as standard and absorbance was measured at 510 nm.

Antioxidant activity

Organic solvent extract of endophytic fungus (*Eupenicillium senticosum* Scott) were also subjected for *in-vitro* antioxidant activity assays.

Total antioxidant activity

Total antioxidant activity (TAA) of fungal extracts was determined as per the methodology of (15). Methanolic extract (0.1 ml) was mixed with reagent mixture of 1 ml, sulphuric acid (0.6 M), sodium phosphate (28 mM) and ammonium molybdate (4 mM). The samples were incubated at 95°C for 90 min and cooled to room temperature. Later absorbance was measured at 695 nm. TAA was expressed as µM equivalent of ascorbic acid/gram of the extract (µM AAEs/g).

2, 2'-Diphenyl-1-picrylhydrazyl (DPPH) radical scavenging assay

The DPPH radical scavenging activity of methanolic fungal extracts were performed as per the methodology of [16] with minor modification.0.004% of DPPH in methanol was prepared and 2.0 ml of this solution was added to 1.0 ml of extract solution at different concentration (200-1000µg/ml). Thirty minutes later, the absorbance was measured at 517nm. A control was prepared without adding extract and ascorbic acid served as standard. The capability to scavenge the DPPH radical reaction mixture was calculated using the following equation:

$$\text{DPPH scavenging activity (\%)} = \frac{(A_0 - A_1)}{A_0} \times 100$$

where, A_0 is the absorbance of the control reaction and A_1 is the absorbance of the samples or the extracts.

Ferrozine assay

In Ferrozine assay the ferric ions are converted to ferrous ions (17). These ions react with Ferrozine to form a violet colored complex which is measured spectrophotometrically. The absorbance is proportional to iron concentration in the sample. 5mM Ferrozine and 2mM ferric chloride is prepared. 0.1ml of ferric chloride is added to 3.8ml of extract in water in different concentration (200-1000µg/ml). After 30 seconds, 0.2ml of Ferrozine is added. Absorbance was measured at 560 nm. EDTA-2Na is used as a positive control at different concentrations (200-1000µg/ml). Lower the absorbance of the reaction mixture indicates higher the ferrous chelating activity.

$$\text{Ferrous chelating activity (\%)} = \frac{(A_0 - A_1)}{A_0} \times 100$$

where, A_0 is the absorbance of the control reaction and A_1 is the absorbance of the samples or the extracts.

Reducing power assay

The reducing power assay was performed as described by Oyaizu (18). Various concentrations of the fungal extracts in 1.0 ml of de-ionized water were mixed with phosphate buffer (1ml) and potassium ferricyanide (2.5ml). The mixture was incubated at 50°C for 20 minutes. Aliquots of tri-chloro acetic acid (1.5ml) were added to the mixture, which was then centrifuged at 5000 rpm for 10 min. The upper layer of solution (1ml) was mixed with distilled water (2.5ml) and a freshly prepared ferric chloride solution (0.5ml). The absorbance was measured at 700 nm. BHT (Butylated hydroxyl toluene) was used as standard. Increased absorbance of the reaction mixture indicates increase in reducing power.

Lipid peroxidation inhibition assay

Lipid peroxidation assay was carried out as per methodology of (19). The freshly collected sheep liver was minced and 10% (w/v) homogenate was prepared in 0.15 M KCl (0-4°C). The homogenate obtained was centrifuged at 8000×g for 15 min and clear cell free supernatant was considered for *in-vitro* lipid peroxidation inhibition assay. 200-1000µg/ml concentrations of extract were used. 0.15M KCl of 1ml and 0.5 ml of liver homogenate was added to each test tube. Peroxidation was initiated by adding 0.2mM 100 ml of $FeCl_2$. After 30 min incubation at 37°C, the reaction was stopped by adding 0.25N, 2 ml of ice cold HCl containing 15%Trichloroacetic acid (TCA), 0.38% TBA (NaOH), and 0.5% BHT. The reaction mixtures were heated at 80°C for 60 min. The samples were cooled, centrifuged and absorbance of the supernatants was measured at 532 nm. The percentage of inhibition of lipid peroxidation was calculated by formula:

$$\text{Inhibition of lipid peroxidation (\%)} = 1 - (\text{sample OD/blank OD}) \times 100$$

Statistical analysis

Each data point is the average of triplicate measurements with each individual experiment performed in duplicate. Data was compared by using One way-ANOVA with p values <0.05 were considered to be significant and p values <0.01 to be very significant (20).

RESULTS

The dry weight yield was high in methanolic extract (ME) compared to DEE (Diethyl ether), CF (Chloroform) and EA (Ethyl acetate) extracts (ME > EA > CF > DEE) (see Table 1). These different organic solvent extracts (ME, DEE, EA and CF) were subjected for bioactivity profiling like, antibacterial assay and antioxidant activities.

Table 1. Weight of samples after extraction with different solvents

Solvents used for extraction	Weight of the sample after evaporation (grams) per 250 ml of broth
Chloroform(CF)	0.11 ± 0.056g
Diethyl ether(DEE)	0.27 ± 0.08g
Ethyl acetate (EA)	0.17 ± 0.023g
Methanol (ME)	0.96 ± 0.12g

Table 2. Antibacterial activity of crude extracts derived from Endophytic fungus [Diameter in mm; n = 5, Mean ± SD). (Test organisms; Ks-*Klebsiella pneumonia*, Ec- *E. coli*, Bs-*Bacillus subtilis*, Ss-*Staphylococcus aureus*)

Fungal extracts	Bacteria (zone of inhibition in mm)			
	Gram negative bacteria		Gram positive bacteria	
	Ks	Ec	Bs	Ss
Diethyl ether extract(DEE)	0	1.6 ± 0.4	1.8 ± 0.3	3.6 ± 0.3
Chloroform extract (CE)	3.5 ± .52	0	3.6 ± 0.36	3.8 ± 0.4
Ethyl acetate extract (EAE)	10.3 ± 0.33	8.6 ± 0.6	9.1 ± 0.4	9.9 ± 02.
Methanol extract (ME)	12.21 ± 0.4	11.27 ± 0.53	14.19 ± 0.6	13.14 ± 0.4
Amphicilin	-	13.89 ± 0.6	-	14.87 ± 0.6
Tetracycline	13 ± 0.2	-	-	-
Vancomycin	-	-	15.12 ± 0.3	15.37 ± 0.3

Antibacterial activities

Disc diffusion method was exclusively used to investigate the antibacterial activity of fungal extracts in the present study. The different solvent extracts were evaluated for antimicrobial activity against four pathogenic bacteria, namely *E. coli, Bacillus subtilis; Staphylococcus aureus* and *Klebsiella pneumonia,* showed inhibition zones (see Table 2). DEE and CE extracts shown very minimum inhibition zone for selected bacteria. EAE extract showed moderate antibacterial activity when compared to standard antibiotics. Among 4 solvent extracts were tested, it was found that the methanol extract showed promising growth inhibitory activity against Gram negative and Gram positive bacteria. Methanol extracts shows ≈ 14.2mm diameter of inhibition zone for *Klebsiella pneumonia,* ≈ 15.2mm of inhibition zone for *E. coli, Bacillus subtilis* and *Staphylococcus aureus* shown nearly 16.19 and17.14 mm of inhibition zones respectively.

Antioxidant activities

The organic solvents (DEE, EA, CF and ME) extract of endophytic fungus was subjected for possible antioxidant activity assays. Five complementary test systems like, Total antioxidant activity, 2, 2'-Diphenyl-1-picrylhydrazyl (DPPH) radical scavenging assay, reducing power assay, ferrozine assay and lipid peroxidation inhibition assay were used. Total antioxidant activities (TAA) of endophytic extract were given in Figure 1a. The TAA of extract increased with increasing concentration and at the1000 µg/ml showed the highest activities. At the maximum concentration, methanolic extract showed significantly high activity (456 AAEs/g) ($p < 0.05$) compared to other solvent extracts (Diethyl ether, 119.8 AAEs/g, Chloroform 241.36 AAEs/g and Ethyl acetate 411.3 AAEs/g). The DPPH radical scavenging assay is an easy, rapid and sensitive method for the antioxidant screening of fungal extracts. The sample was tested at different concentrations ranging from (200 to 1000µg/ml) and the readings were observed
by decreasing the absorbance taken as a measure indicates the extent of radical scavenging property. The scavenging effects of the sample were evaluated along with the standard ascorbic acid. The free radical scavenging activities of samples are depicted in Figure1b. The crude methanolic fungal extracts against DPPH radical showed activity of 70.84% at the maximum concentration of 1000µg/ml, but for same concentration the activity of the standard was 84.8% and lower activities were observed for other solvent extracts (23.69% DEE, 12.9% CF and 62.36% EA). The scavenging effect of Methanolic extract was significantly higher than other extracts at maximum concentration ($p < 0.05$). EC_{50} for methanolic fungal extract was 705.8µg/ml and in comparable range with ascorbic acid (EC_{50}-589.6µg/). From the above observation the methanolic extract shows good scavenging activity compared to other extracts and synthetic antioxidants. The extract might be serves as an effective radical scavenger to react with the DPPH, converting them into stable products.

The results of fungal extract reducing power activity were given in the Figure 1c. At maximum concentration 1000µg/ml of methanolic extract shows the reducing power activity of about 1.12 in the terms of optical density, whereas standard BHT (Butylated hydroxyl toluene) was about 1.2. The activity of methanolic extract was higher at different concentrations (200-1000µg/ml) when compared to other extracts. Reducing power activity of different extracts were as follows; ME > EA > DEE > CF. In ferrous chelating activity assay the ability to chelate ferrous ion was calculated.

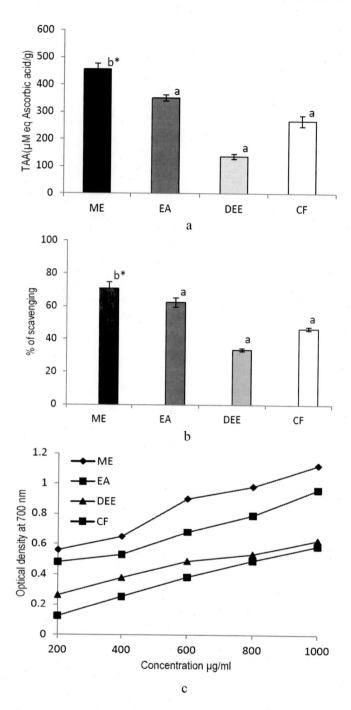

Figure 1. (a) Total antioxidant activity;(b) DPPH radical scavenging assay; (c) Reducing power assay (ME-Methanolic extract, EA-Ethyl acetate extract, DEE-Diethyl ether extract and CF-Chloroform extract; One way-ANOVA, * $p < 0.05$ ** $p < 0.01$).

Antibacterial and antioxidant potential of organic solvents extract ... 89

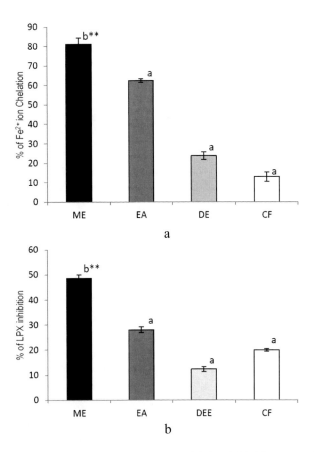

Figure 2. (a) Ferrous ion chelation activity; (b) Lipid peroxidation inhibition assay. (ME-Methanolic extract, EA-Ethyl acetate extract, DEE-Diethyl ether extract and CF-Chloroform extract; One way-ANOVA, ** $p < 0.01$).

As shown in Figure 2a, 1000μg/ml EDTA chelated almost 94.35% of Fe^{2+}, whereas the extracts ME, EA, DEE and CF were able to chelate 81.3%, 62.36%, 12.9%, and 23.69% respectively. Significantly high ($p < 0.01$) chelation was observed in ME compared to EA, DEE and CF. EC_{50} was 615μg/ml for methanolic extract, this indicated that the extract possess very good Fe^{2+}-chelating ability (EC_{50}, EDTA-549.9μg/ml). From the, total antioxidants, DPPH, ferrozine and reducing power assay we observed that extracts were found to possess good antioxidant activity and has the ability to scavenge reactive oxygen species. Therefore, extracts were further analyzed for lipid peroxidation inhibition activity assay. Figure 2b shows the result of lipid peroxidation inhibition activity of endophytes organic solvent crude extracts. LPX inhibition activity of standard ascorbic acid was 46.1% at the concentration of 1000 μg/ml similarly at that concentration the ME activity was 48.5%. Hence the Inhibition capacity of extract was significantly higher (p < 0.05) than standard ascorbic acid and other extracts (DEE, AE and CF). From the above observation, concluded that methanol extract possess promising capacity to prevent oxidative deterioration of mitochondrial membrane lipids in compared to synthetic antioxidants.

Total phenolic and flavonoid contents

Phenolics and flavonoids were the major antioxidant constituents of the endophytes. Total phenolics were expressed in equivalents of Gallic acid and were estimated by slightly modified Folin-ciocalteu reagent method. The total phenolics content of extract is 27.63 mg/g equivalents of Gallic acid. The flavonoid is the polyphenolic secondary metabolite, most widespread among different plant species and correlated with most of the bioactivity. The quantitative estimation of the total flavonoid in the current study demonstrated that endophytic fungus was able to produce flavonoid 9.3 mg/g of Quercetin equivalent. The significant positive correlation was observed between total phenolics, flavonoids and total antioxidant activities ($p < 0.05$).

DISCUSSION

In the current study, methanolic extract was exhibited maximum antibacterial activity compared to other organic extracts. As reported by different authors that endophytes are mines of novel metabolites and more than 50% of Nethravathi mangrove endophytic fungi shows antimicrobial activities (21-23). Similarly, several metabolites of the marine derived fungus *Aspergillus niger* showed anti-bacterial and anti-fungal potential (24). Endophytic fungus *Pestalotiopsis* spp, are known to generate antifungal, anti-oxidant and anti-cancer biomolecules (10, 23). Altersin, a novel antibacterial agent isolated from endophytic *Alternaria* species, exhibited a potent MIC (minimum inhibitory concentration) against several pathogenic Gram-positive bacteria (19). From the study of (25) revealed that 1% ethyl acetate extract of *Alternaria* species showed inhibition zone against *Candida albicans*. However, investigations on mangrove endophytic fungal metabolites are very minimum. The present study result indicates that methanolic crude extract of endophytic fungus (*Eupenicillium senticosum* Scott) contains different antibacterial substances which inhibit the growth of specific bacteria substantially compared to other organic extracts. The further purification and characterization work is required for the isolation of specific compound responsible for the antibacterial properties.

The measurement of total antioxidant activity of fungal extract indicates the potentiality of natural antioxidants. The total antioxidant activities of endophytic fungal extracts are promising and confirm the results of total antioxidant activities of methanolic extracts of various endophytes (24). The present study also corroborates the total antioxidant activities in endophytes isolated from plants of different habitat (25). Cellular biomolecules are the main target of hydroxyl radical and which can induce severe damage to cells (22). Methanolic extract of endophytic fungus has shown dose dependent DPPH radical scavenging activity. From earlier studies it is known that the antioxidant activity of an aromatic compound is proportional to the number of hydroxyl groups it contains (10). This probably explains the high radical scavenging activities of methanolic extracts. As reported (24) the reducing power is associated with presence of reductones and this reductones play significant role in reducing power by breaking free radical chain as a donator of hydrogen atom. The results of the present study also corroborate studies on antioxidant activity of Alpine Plants associated Endophytic Fungi (*Rhodiola angusta*, *R. crenulata*, and *R. sachalinensis*) (7). Different authors also demonstrated the ferrous ion chelation capacity of bioactive components derived from the endophytes (4, 23). Various authors opined that endophytes from different habitat poses high lipid peroxidation inhibition activity to fight against stress (1, 4). Different studies on plant extracts are also showed that methanolic extracts possess high lipid peroxidation inhibition activities (23). Most of the antioxidants studies were concentrated on medicinal plants endophytes (10), as well as (25) isolated two antioxidant novel metabolites, pestacin and isopestacin, from the endophytic fungi *Pestalotiopsis microspora*. Another study (24) reported that garcinia plant and its endophytes have exhibited remarkable antioxidant activities.

The total phenolic contents act as a key component of scavengers of free radical (4). The result of present study is compared with earlier studies on various endophytes (4, 7) and found that phenolics compounds have major role in stabilizing lipid per-oxidation and are also associated with antioxidant activity (22). Direct role of antioxidant activity of phenolics compound was also elucidated by (25). Inhibitory effect on mutagenesis and carcinogenesis are also correlated with phenolics compounds in food and vegetable (4, 7). Phenolics and flavonoids play a major role in stabilizing lipid peroxidation and antioxidant activity (4).

CONCLUSION

The current studies lead to the conclusion that endophytes can be considered as a source of novel metabolites due to their promising antibacterial and antioxidant activities. The data also reveals that antioxidant activities of methanolic extracts of endophyte (*Eupenicillium senticosum* Scott) comparable to standard antioxidant ascorbic acid and BHT. Extracts of *Eupenicillium senticosum* Scott might play an important role in free radical scavenging, inhibiting lipid peroxidation and protect living organisms from damaging effects. Considering high activity, these extracts can be utilized as alternative source for the production of therapeutic agents. Furthermore, comprehensive chemistry and bioactivity of individual molecules should be carried out in the future to develop new pharmacological agents of wide applications.

ACKNOWLEDGMENTS

The author is grateful to Department of Biochemistry, St Aloysius College for permission to carry out these studies. No conflicts of interest have been declared by the authors.

REFERENCES

[1] Lin Z, Zhu T, Fang Y, Gu Q. Polyketides from *Penicillium* sp. JP-1, an endophytic fungus associated with the mangrove plant *Aegiceras corniculatum*. Phytochemistry 2008;69:1273-8.

[2] Suryanarayanan TS, Kumaresan V. Endophytic fungi of some halophytes from an estuarine mangrove forest. Myco Res 2000;104:1465-7.

[3] Stierle A, Strobel G, Stierle D. Taxol and taxane production by *Taxomyces andreanae*, an endophytic fungus of Pacific yew. Science 1993;260:214-6.

[4]   Liu L, Tian R, Liu S, Chen X. Pestaloficiols A-E, bioactive cyclopropane derivatives from the plant endophytic fungus *Pestalotiopsis fici*. Bioorg. Med Chem 2008;16: 6021-6.

[5]   Anderson D. Antioxidant defences against reactive oxygen species causing genetic and other damage. MutaRes 1996;350:103-8.

[6]   Medved I, Brown MJ, Bjorksten AR, Murphy KT. N-acetylcysteine enhances muscle cysteine and glutathione availability and attenuates fatigue during prolonged exercise in endurance-trained individuals. J Appl Physiol 2004;97:1477-85.

[7]   Cui J-L, Guo T-T, Ren Z-X, Zhang N-S, Wang M-L. Diversity and antioxidant activity of culturable endophytic fungi from alpine plants of *Rhodiola crenulata*, *R. angusta*, and *R. sachalinensis*. PLoS One 2015;10(3):e0118204. doi:10.1371/journal.pone.0118204.

[8]   Petrini O, Sieber TN, Toti L, Vivet O. Ecology, metabolite production and substrate utilisation in endophytic fungi. Nat Tox 1992;1:185-96.

[9]   Souza AD, Rodrigues-Filho E, Souza AQ, Pereira JO. Koninginins, phospholipase A2 inhibitors from endophytic fungus Trichodermakoningii. Toxicon 2008; 51:240-50.

[10] Strobel G, Ford E, Worapong J, Harper JK. Isopestacin, an isobenzofuranone from Pestalotiopsismicrospora, possessing antifungal and antioxidant activities. Phytochemistry 2002; 60: 179-83.

[11] Suryanarayanan TS, Kumaresan V, Johnson JA. Foliar fungal endophytes from two species of the mangrove Rhizophora. Can J Microbio 1998;44:1003-6.

[12] Bauer AW, Kirby WM, Sherris JC, Turck M. Antibiotic susceptibility testing by a standardized single disk method. Am J ClinPathol1966;45:493-6.

[13] Ikawa M, Schaper TD, Dollard CA, Sasner JJ. Utilization of Folin-ciocalteu reagent for the detection of certain nitrogen compounds. J Agri Food Chem 2003;51:1811-5.

[14] Zhishen JT, Mengcheng T, Jianming W. The determination of flavonoid content in mulberry and their scavenging effects on superoxide radicals. Food Chem 1999;64: 555-9.

[15] Prieto P, Pineda M, Aguilar M. Spectrophotometric quantitation of antioxidant capacity through the formation of a Phosphomolybdenum Complex: Specific application to the determination of vitamin E. Ana Biochem 1999;269:337-41.

[16] Miliauskas G, Venskutonis PR, Van Beek TA. Screening of radical scavenging activity of some medicinal and aromatic plant extracts. Food Chem 2004;85:231-7.

[17] Viollier E, Inglett PW, Hunter K, Roychoudhury AN, Van Cappellen P. The ferrozinz method revisited:Fe (II). Fe(III) determination in natural waters. App Geochem 2000;15:785-90.

[18] Oyaizu M. Studies on products of browning reactions: Antioxidative activities of products of browning reaction prepared from glucosamine. Japan J Nutr 1999;44: 307-15.

[19] Hellwig V, Grothe T, Mayer-Bartschmid A, Endermann R, Geschke FU, Henkel T, et al. Altersin, a new antibiotic from cultures of endophytic *Alternaria* spp. taxonomy, fermentation, isolation, structure elucidation and biological activities. J. Antib2002;55:881-92.

[20] SigmaPlot. Version 11. San Jose, CA: Systat Soft Inc, 2008.

[21] Maria1 GL, Sridhar KR, Raviraja NS. Antimicrobial and enzyme activity of mangrove endophytic fungi of southwest coast of India. J Agri Tech 2005;1:67-80.

[22] Bugni, TS, Abbanat D, Bernan VS, Maiese WM, Greenstein M, Wagoner RMV, et al. Yanuthones: novel metabolites from a marine isolate of Aspergillusniger. J Org Chem 2000;65:7195-7200.

[23] Strobel GA, Daisy B. Bioprospecting for microbial endophytes and their natural products. MicrobiolMolBiol Rev 2003;67:491–502.

[24] Phongpaichit S, Nikom J, Rungjindamai N, Sakayaroj J. Biological activities of extracts from endophytic fungi isolated from garcinia plants. FemsImmunol Med Mic 2007;51:517-25.

[25] Harper JK, Arif AM, Ford EJ, Strobel GA. Pestacin: a 1, 3-dihydro isobenzofuran from Pestalotiopsis microspora possessing antioxidant and antimycotic activities. Tetrahedron 2003;59:2471-6.

Submitted: December 12, 2015. *Revised:* January 05, 2016. *Accepted:* January 10, 2016.

In: Alternative Medicine Research Yearbook 2017
Editor: Joav Merrick
ISBN: 978-1-53613-726-2
© 2018 Nova Science Publishers, Inc.

Chapter 8

EXCLUSIVE ROLE OF POTENTIZED *THUJA OCCIDENTALIS* ON MYOMA RECOVERY: CASE REPORT

Supriyo Ghosh, DHMS, Riya Dutta, BSc, Aswini K Sasmal, DHMS, Animesh Das, BHMS, Subhabrata Sinha, BHMS, Rathin Chakravarty, MD and Sandhimita Mondal*, PhD

Molecular Homeopathic Research Unit,
Dr. Bholanath Chakravarty Memorial Trust,
Kolkata, India

ABSTRACT

A myoma or uterine fibroid or uterine leiomyoma or fibromyoma or fibroleiomyoma is a leiomyoma, which is a benign tumor or monoclonal tumors and 40 to 50% show karyotypically detectable chromosomal abnormalities. Myoma originates from the smooth muscle layer (myometrium) of the uterus. A 46 years old woman reported at our clinic. Complaints were slightly coarse uterine myometrium with small myoma (77 mm X 45 mm X 39 mm) and bulkiness in left ovary (30 mm X 41 mm). According to physical and mental symptoms, potentized drug *Thuja ocidentalis (*from an evergreen coniferous tree *Thuja occidentalis)* was given. After the treatment of potentized drug, uterus (51mm X 39 mm X 22 mm) and ovaries (Left ovary: 26 mm X 12 mm; Right ovary: 24mm X 11 mm) became normal in size.

Keywords: myoma, uterine fibroid, thuja occidentalis, ovaries, case report

---

* Correspondence: Sandhimita Mondal, PhD, Molecular Homeopathic Research Unit, Dr. Bholanath Chakravarty Memorial Trust, Kolkata, India. E-mail: sandhimita@gmail.com.

INTRODUCTION

A myoma or uterine fibroid or uterine leiomyoma or fibromyoma or fibroleiomyoma is a leiomyoma, which is a benign tumor or monoclonal tumors and 40 to 50% show karyotypically detectable chromosomal abnormalities. That originates from the smooth muscle layer (myometrium) of the uterus (1). When multiple leiomyomata present in the uterus, known as diffuse uterine leiomyomatosis. The cancerous form of a fibroid is very uncommon and called leiomyosarcoma. Fibroids occur normally during the middle and later reproductive years. In general, fibroids are asymptomatic, but they can grow. Manifestations are heavy and painful menstruation, painful sexual intercourse, urinary frequency and urgency. Sometimes fibroids may interfere with pregnancy (2). The proper reasons of the fibroids are not clearly understood, but multiple fibroids occurs due to unrelated genetic defects, such as genetic predispositions, prenatal hormone exposure, effects of hormones, growth factors and xenoestrogens may be the cause of fibroid growth (3). Specific mutations of the MED12 protein have been noted in 70 percent of fibroids (4). FH mutations change the expression profiles of fibroids significantly. This mutation regulates the genes which are involved in the glycolysis (5). Uterine artery embolization and surgical options may be the option for the treatment (6). *Thuja occidentalis* (leaves) has crucial role on phytopreventive bioefficacy against 7, 12 dimethylbenz (a) anthracene (DMBA)-induced mammary carcinogenesis (7). The aim of the present study was to see the effect of potentized *Thuja* on myoma recovery.

CASE REPORT

A 46 years old woman reported at our clinic. Complaints were slightly coarse uterine myometrium with small myoma (77 mm X 45 mm X 39 mm) and bulkiness in left ovary (30 mm X 41 mm). Grandmother and paternal uncle were asthma patients. She had moderate temperament and likes dogs. She is very cravings to chili and onion. She is suffering from frontal headache and sinusitis. According to physical and mental symptoms potentized *Thuja* was given. Total prescription and follow up has shown in Table 1.

Table 1. Outcome, follow up and second prescription

Date	Follow-up
10.05.2010	*Thuja ocidentalis* 200 (12 powders) twice a day
12.07.2010	*Thuja ocidentalis* 200 (12 powders) twice a day
13.09.2010	*Thuja ocidentalis* 200 (12 powders) twice a day
22.11.2010	*Thuja ocidentalis* 200 (12 powders) twice a day
04.04.2011	*Thuja ocidentalis* 200 (12 powders) twice a day
30.05.2011	*Thuja ocidentalis* 200 (12 powders) twice a day
21.11.2011	*Thuja ocidentalis* 200 (12 powders) twice a day
16.08.2012	*Thuja ocidentalis* 200 (12 powders) twice a day
19.12.2012	*Thuja ocidentalis* 200 (12 powders) twice a day

RESULTS

After the treatment of potentized drugs uterus (51 mm X 39 mm X 22 mm) and ovaries (Left ovary: 26 mm X 12 mm; Right ovary: 24 mm X 11 mm) became normal in size.

DISCUSSION

This case is interesting from several points of view. First, effectiveness of potentized drugs on bulkiness of left ovary. Secondly, potentized drugs also effective on uterus myoma recovery.

Estrogen regulates and increase IGF-1, EGFR, TGF-beta1, TGF-beta3 and PDGF, and promotes growth. Estrogen regulates and decrease p53, increasing expression of the anti-apoptotic factor PCP4 and antagonizing PPAR-gamma signaling promotes aberrant survival of leiomyoma cells. Progesterone is the growth promoting agent of leiomyoma by regulating EGF, TGF-beta1, TGF-beta3. Progesterone also regulates Bcl-2 expression and decrease TNF-alpha and ultimately promotes survival of the leiomyoma. Progesterone is believed to neutralize growth by decreasing IGF-1 (8, 9). Expression of transforming growth interacting factor (TGIF) is amplified in leiomyoma compared with myometrium (10), where TGIF is a crucial repressor of TGF-β pathways in myometrial cells (11). *Thuja*-induced p53-dependent apoptosis in breast cancer cells mediated by oxidative stress (12). Mutation of fumarate hydratase (*FH*) at 1q43 is known to effect the uterine leiomyomata (MCL) and hereditary leiomyomatosis. *FH* mutations have been detected in some non-syndromic uterine leiomyomata also (13).

Potentized *Thuja* may alter estrogen and progesterone expression. It may reduce growth of myoma by down regulating IGF-1, EGFR, TGF-Beta and increase p53. Potentized *Thuja* may also help in the repair of FH mutation. Ultimately, bulkiness in left ovary and myoma became normal in size after the treatment of potentized *Thuja*.

ACKNOWLEDGMENTS

We are very thankful to Dr Bholanath Chakravarty Memorial Trust for providing space and infrastructure of this research and Mr. Swajjan Bhajan, Century Ply limited for the funding of this research.

REFERENCES

[1] Neiger R, Sonek J D, Croom CS, Ventolini G. Pregnancy-related changes in the size of uterine leiomyomas. J Reprod Med 2006;51(9):671–4.

[2] Wallach E E, Vlahos N F. Uterine myomas: an overview of development, clinical features, and management. Obstet Gynecol 2004;104(2):393–406.

[3] Okolo S. Incidence, aetiology and epidemiology of uterine fibroids. Best practice & research. Clin Obstet Gynaecol 2008;22(4):571–88.

[4] Mäkinen N, Mehine M, Tolvanen J, Kaasinen E, Li Y, Lehtonen HJ, et al. MED12, the Mediator Complex Subunit 12 Gene, is Mutated at High Frequency in Uterine Leiomyomas. Science 2011;334(6053):252–5.

[5] Vanharanta S, Pollard PJ, Lehtonen HJ, Laiho P, Sjöberg J, Leminen A, et al. Distinct expression profile in fumarate-hydratase-deficient uterine fibroids. Hum Mol Genet 2006; 15 (1):97-103.

[6] Gupta JK, Sinha A, Lumsden MA, Hickey M. Uterine artery embolization for symptomatic uterine fibroids. Cochrane Database Syst Rev 2014;12:CD005073.

[7] Hodge JC, Morton CC. Genetic heterogeneity among uterine leiomyomata: insights into malignant progression. Hum Mol Genet 2007;16(1):R7–13.

[8] Rein M S. Advances in uterine leiomyoma research: the progesterone hypothesis. Environ Health Perspect 2000;108(5):791–3.

[9] Maruo T, Ohara N, Wang J, Matsuo H. Sex steroidal regulation of uterine leiomyoma growth and apoptosis. Hum Reprod Update 2004;10(3):207–20.

[10] Yen-Ping Ho J, Man WC, Wen Y, Polan ML, Shih-Chu Ho E, Chen B. Transforming growth interacting factor expression in leiomyoma compared with myometrium. Fertil Steril 2009;94(3):1078–83.

[11] Ojeswi B K, Khoobchandani M, Hazra D K, Srivastava M M. Protective effect of Thuja occidentalis against DMBA-induced breast cancer with reference to oxidative stress. Hum Exp Toxicol 2010;29(5):369-75.

[12] Saha S, Bhattacharjee P, Mukherjee S, Mazumdar M, Chakraborty S, Khurana AA, et al. Contribution of the ROS-p53 feedback loop in thuja-induced apoptosis of mammary epithelial carcinoma cells. Oncol Rep 2014;31(4):1589-98.

[13] Hodge JC, Morton CC. Genetic heterogeneity among uterine leiomyomata: insights into malignant progression. Hum Mol Genet 2007;16(Spec no 1):R7-13.

Submitted: July 03, 2015. *Revised:* August 03, 2015. *Accepted:* August 20, 2015.

In: Alternative Medicine Research Yearbook 2017
Editor: Joav Merrick
ISBN: 978-1-53613-726-2
© 2018 Nova Science Publishers, Inc.

Chapter 9

GRIEF IN PRIMARY CARE PRACTICE: LOSS OF HOUSE

Mohammed Morad[1,2,3,*], *MD, FRCP (Edin), MRCPS(Glasg) and Adam Morad*[4]

[1]National Institute of Child Health and Human Development, Jerusalem, Israel
[2]Kentucky Children's Hospital, University of Kentucky, Lexington, US
[3]Yaski Medical Center, Clalit Health Services, Department of Family Medicine, Faculty of Health Sciences, Ben Gurion University of the Negev, Beer-Sheva, Israel
[4]Vrije Universiteit, Amsterdam, Netherlands

ABSTRACT

According to Wikipedia, grief or bereavement is defined as a multifaceted response to loss, particularly to the loss of someone or something that has died, to which a bond or affection was formed. Although conventionally focused on the emotional response to loss, it also has physical, mental, cognitive, behavioral, social and philosophical dimensions. Grief impacts also on health and can cause depression of variable degrees and a risk factor for suicide. Since bereavement is associated with increased morbidity and mortality it is very important that primary health care professionals identify risk and initiate intervention to prevent further deterioration of mental and health situation of their patient or client. In this case report we describe a case of grief causes by a fire that destroyed the house of our patient. It is important that primary care physicians should be trained to screen, treat and follow-up patient at high risk for adverse effects of bereavement.

Keywords: grief, primary care, general practitioner

---

[*] Correspondence: Professor Mohammed Morad, MD, FRCP (Edin), MRCPS (Glasg), Medical Director, Yaski Community Medical Center, Ben Gurion University of the Negev, Clalit Health Services, Rehov David Hamelech 24, IL-84541, Beer-Sheva, Israel. E-mail: morad62@gmail.com.

INTRODUCTION

Over the life span most people will have experienced grief. Grief can occur after any loss, like losing a job, getting another job or moving to a new location, divorce or diagnosis of a chronic illness or a terminal illness (1). Three elements are common in bereavement: 1) an attachment to a person or thing that is valued, 2) a loss of that relationship and 3) becoming a survivor of the loss (1).

Primary care physicians should be able to identify grief, develop strategies for management of the patient and his/her family and also able to recognize abnormal grief (1).

In this paper a case is described of a patient with grief due to the loss of his house.

CASE STORY

Looking neglected, although dressed in new clothes, a 50 years old man was brought by his wife to the primary health care clinic. I came out to the corridor, where he was sitting with his wife and asked them to come in. Unshaved, very quiet, looking depressed, slowly moving in the room, I did not register whether he responded to my self-introduction. When I asked: "Which way I may help," he did not respond verbally, but a very deep silence attacked the room.

His wife took the initiative, "I am worried about him, I am afraid that he is not interested in life. He is not eating, not drinking enough and not sleeping," she said. "He is not talking to anybody in the house. He has closed into himself. He refused to come to see a doctor, so I phoned and made an appointment for him."

While he was weeping tears calmly, she continued explaining to me his condition. "All was good, until two weeks ago, when our house was destroyed completely by fire. I was at home alone. He was at work. My son informed him about the catastrophe, he came and accompanied me to the hospital, because I had breathlessness and to be sure that I did not inhale the smoke, while trying to stop the fire, I was checked in the emergency room and they discharged me." "You have no problems" they said and sent me home."

"My husband was busy all the week, contacting the police, firemen and making arrangements to get new documents for us. Everything was burned in the house. Money, the whole salary, documents and valuable things stayed there and burned out. I wanted to die in the firing house, when I did not succeed to stop the fire. But, the Rabbi took me out of the house. I can manage, I suffer, I cannot sleep these days since the fire, I am not working now, I cook and clean the house and stay beside my husband and meet people, coming to visit and support us. I need some tablets to sleep. But he is not doing well. He is apathetic, not going to work, he is not leaving the house even to the synagogue, where he has friends and loved to go daily. The last week was terrifying for me. I want you to help him to eat and sleep."

To my question, where they live today, she said that transiently they live in the hired apartment of the oldest son. Two other children, a daughter and son live with relatives in another place. They are supposed to move to a hired house, that the insurance company has paid for them. Two sons and a daughter, were shocked by the accident, but they manage, they go to work, help her and the father and they are worried about the father according to her explanation. She also stated that they borrowed money from the bank to buy new clothes and things and to pay for new documents and food. The relatives come and offer help, also the friends of her husband from his previous work came and showed sympathy. But, he refuses to speak or meet relatives or friends.

I turned to him, and asked him about the cause of his suffering. Hyperventilating, weeping tears and crying loudly among sentences, he said:

> "Everything is lost; the house I worked for all my life is lost. My life has no value. I feel useless and worthless. I have no interest in life more. I am 50 years old, there is no hope to start again. I feel so bad because I lost the meaning of life after the fire. My photos, certificates, and documents were there. All my life was in this house. I need only something to sleep and to be alone. I do not need anybody."

I asked if he has any plan to kill himself or to die, and he reassured me that nothing like that is going to be. He is a Jewish man and believes in God and visit the synagogue daily and has a great respect for life and he would never think about suicide. I asked if he gets support, and he said that the family give a warm feeling and they are beside him and take care excessively for him. His relatives, friends from his previous work also offer support. He refuses to accept help and meet people. The oldest son takes care of regular and extraordinary needs of the family since one week.

The medical history

He denied suffering from depression or psychiatric diseases or taking medications for any chronic condition. He suffered from moderate hearing loss caused by noise, while he had been working at an air force base with clear cut audiometric pathologic finding in both ears. He is a former cigarette smoker. Except for a long-lasting cough with normal laryngoscopic examination and road traffic accident with soft tissue contusion, no chronic diseases were reported. Infrequently, he was seen in the primary health clinic for back pain or urinary tract infection.

The physical examination

A moderate hearing loss was noticed. He was pale, and his hands and lips were shaking. His voice was hoarse and his speech was slow. Hemodynamically he was stable. His short and past memory and orientation ability was preserved, although with some difficulty evoked. Neurologic examination was normal. No odor of alcohol came out of his mouth, but the smell of smoke was felt a few meters from his body. His electrocardiogram was normal, urine and blood sugar were normal.

Follow-up

After the examination and conversation, I prescribed him and his wife a sedative, Diazepam, 5-10 mg x 3 times daily and I also gave him my phone number and to his wife. I asked them to phone if my help would be needed. I also asked them to tell their children that they could call and talk if any need should arise.

I was disturbed by the situation of my patient and although the patient denied any suicide planning or will to die, he was functionally severely disabled and his mood very impaired. His was frustrated and mentally exhausted and the depressed mood, loss of appetite and sleep affected his physical condition. I invited him to come with the family after two days.

I contacted the social worker and agreed that we were dealing with adjustment reaction to the fire and because of functional impairment of the patient and the crisis of family without house, there was a need for family therapy, psychotherapy and medications for the couple.

Two days later they did not come, so I phoned the daughter and she was very worried about her father's health. She told me that she and her brothers are at work and they are in contact with the parents, but her father is not leaving the house and they have to encourage him to drink and eat. She will convince him to visit the clinic. It was difficult to speak to him because they moved to the house, offered by the insurance company, where no phone was available. She reassured me that they will bring him to the clinic, if his condition will worsen.

In another two days, the wife came to my office. Although she had no appointment, she asked me to be admitted immediately. She complained of headache and insomnia. But, she was not worried about herself, but rather about the husband. He does not eat, not sleeping and refuse to go out or visit the clinic. He is not working. The children are at work and she stays all the day with her husband. She asked for blood tests to find out the cause of her headache and for tablets for her husband. She complained that they have no money and they will pay a lot and they have only partial insurance certificate for the house.

After being checked, she was reassured that her headache is due to her psychological distress and that no smoke inhalation was found in the hospital. She does not blame herself and not the husband blaming or accusing her for the fire. She cannot understand why this happened to them. They are living only six months in this house. All their savings were invested in this house. This was their dream to have a house like this one. They did not receive any financial support yet.

I made a new appointment for three days later, but they did not come. He came one day later alone. He looked depressed and broken, his appearance neglected, although he had new clothes. I asked him to enter the room and be seated. He started crying and articulating nothing understandable, while his lips and hands were shaking. He was hyperventilating and coiled in his chest. He all the time mentioned the house and his bad luck. The efforts he made to build it and the years spent at overtime work to save money. "Why should that happen to him and his family?" that was his several times repeated question. He asked for help to get out of this miserable condition.

He is not back at work yet. He feels weak and unable to concentrate. He has no motivation to continue on life. Nobody asked about him from his new job, where he worked for few weeks, before the fire. He denied suicidal attempt or plans and promised to come for follow-up.

His is mentally occupied with the lost things, photos and certificates he received through life at work and the Bible and prayer books, the children photos and school certificates, his mother's photo and many valuable things were burned in the fire. The house and the lost personal property are all that has meaning for his past life and the source of his pain and sorrow.

He agreed that we could be talking about grief as the course of his situation, as I had explained. I also reassured him that time is a good healer together with medical, social support and self-encouragement.

He asked this time for a sick report for his employer and tablets. He is leaving the house in the last days frequently, but only to visit the burned house, sitting there several hours and crying. He dislikes questions of relatives and friends about the event and avoids them. He does not blame or accuse anybody for the fire. The relations with the wife and the children are very positive and supportive, he stated. He has no interest in sex or play, as before the event.

The crisis intervention plan

At the moment we found impairment in the functional status of the patient after the house fire, we decided to work with the family, by listening and giving attention to the family function and family therapy on the basis of the crisis intervention model.

The family, including the patient, his wife and two sons and daughter were invited to the clinic 10 days later. We had four meetings to allocate family resources, family dysfunction and seeking social support for the patient and his family.

Looking for resources we found that our patient has three children. The oldest, a 26-years old male, police officer, living alone outside the family, had a verbal conflict with his father a few months before the fire, but after the house fire, the relationship between the son and father has significantly improved. This son from the first moment after the fire offered his hired apartment to his family, he financially supported them, took a part in arrangements, preparing new documents and reassuring his father.

The daughter is a 24 year old secretary, successful and very discrete person, unmarried woman, described by her father and her brothers to be an ambitious person. She lives with her parents and her youngest brother. Her relationship with the parents and brothers is considered to be "fine" by both sides. She especially manages well with the youngest brother. About her intimate life, the parents have scarce information. They know that she has a boyfriend. She also offered support and care to her parents, and phoned me several times to inform about the father's health and to give me information about the family struggle with this event. She is an open person with a lot of respect for her parents. They are also satisfied with her and wish to see her married.

The youngest son, 22-years old, is a recently discharged soldier and two months before the house fire, he signed a long-term service contract with the army. He comes home every evening. He manages well and had no problems during the military service. He is also looking for good career and financially supports his family. He lives in the same house with his parents. He smokes, but not in front of his father. He respects and support his parents, although he has very little time to be with them. He refuses to speak about future plans or personal issues.

None of the children were at home, when the house fire destroyed the house and its content, including their photo albums and school certificates. They were sad and sorry for that; they also were shocked and tried to continue the routine as they said. They went to work, made arrangements, and helped their parents to overcome this crisis.

The Rabbi and one neighbor of the couple appeared at the actual fire event and the Rabbi convinced the wife to leave the burning house, when she was not able anymore to subdue the flames, coming out of her bedroom. Later he also visited several times to give support and reassure. The couple found his support very valuable help.

Our patient is a traditional and religious man. Since he retired from his work, he visited the synagogue daily to pray and to meet friends. He promised to establish a small synagogue at his big parcel beside the house in the future. His religious books and praying tools burned out in the house. When he received their remnants from the insurance company, he made a burying ceremonial for these books, as the Rabbi told him to do. Friends from synagogue visited our patient and his family and offered their support and help.

The children were also close to this religious life style and although they were less traditional than the parents, they do respect this life style. Our patient's family, brothers and sisters were available to give support and help. His father, although functionally disabled because of chronic heart disease and elderly, tried by phone to give verbal help. He also had a good relationship with his mother in law since his father married after the death of his mother, when he was only two years old. She gave the warmth to him the same way she gave to her own siblings. But, as he said, she was not considered to be as warm and supportive as his wife's mother, he adored, and was shocked deeply when she died due to diabetic complication. His mother in law is also invalid and demented and cannot offer any support.

Our patient has seven sisters and four brothers, but most live out of the city. With all of them he keep in contact, but his best relationships he has with his wife's family. The wife's father died from heart attack during the Yom Kippur war in 1973, when our patient was mobilized in the army. He had no time to grieve or think, because of the war. When his wife's mother died he felt lost and his shock was great. He lost many days of work and was involved in a car accident during the year after her death. With other members of his wife's family, he has a wonderful relationship.

His wife is a "practical" wife and mother, who takes care of the financial family issues. She takes part in all family decisions and plans. She is the initiator of family projects. While speaking about her husband, she said that she respect him for his efforts and work to assure good life for the family and her. She is proud of him, because he fulfilled her dream to have her own house and happy family. Both of them had only elementary education, and were born in Morocco. They married, took care of children and changing apartments several times in their life till they found their loved warm shelter, but alas lost a few months after they entered. Describing her emotional and sexual life with her husband, she said it is normal and sufficient for her. She denied troubles in this intimate side of their life. When asked to give details, she refused to comment.

During thirty years of work at an air-force factory as manual worker, the patient had a good and non-problematic career. Although noise of planes affected his hearing, he was satisfied with his work there and with his former colleagues, his past and present friends, who gave him support and encouragement. When he has retired, because of a progressing hearing loss, he got a good financial compensation. All savings were invested in the house and with the compensation money he bought a new car. All papers documenting his professional career including photos were lost in the fire. So, he felt as a man with a worthless life.

He is also very distressed, because the neighbor, whose house was damaged by the fire, is now demanding repair or financial compensation. Our patient, who has not been working for three months since the house fire and his wife does not earn much money to pay the compensation.

Summary

At this point it was obvious, that we were dealing with a 50 years old man, who lost his house, the fruit of his whole life project. He complains of insomnia and decreased concentrating ability, feeling worthless and depressed. Weak and broken, again and again visiting his burned house. Denying suicide planning or intention to die, he feels empty and blames some unspecified "authority" for this arranged fate.

Crying, suffering loss of interest in what is happening around him, he is feeling stagnated and devastated. Loss is the hallmark of his life. He lost his mother, as a child. He was brought to a new environment as his family immigrated to this country. He had to work as a very young man, to help his father, bringing income to feed his siblings. So, he had no opportunity to get the care and the education, as other children. When he became a man and wanted to get closer to his father, the heart attack killed him, and he had no time for mourning, because of the war. When he found the woman, that played the mother's role, he lost her. The diabetes was stronger. He felt so broken, and impaired physically. He was sick and started looking for medical care.

He lost his job, but felt compensated well till he lost all he invested during the house fire. He lost all valuable things attaching him to the successful years of his life. Thirty years of work at the moment the house burned were lost.

He is now unemployed, non-productive, alone at home, he feels he lost himself, when his house burned. He did not see any chance to bring it all back together.

He has nobody to blame or accuse.

DISCUSSION

At this point we realized that we have a patient undergoing the process of grief while loss as a prominent life event penetrates his whole life. I asked myself, whether the loss of the house is a possible cause for a grief reaction. The broad definition of grief as 'being robbed of anything we value' (2), made my mind more open to accept the loss of house as the cause.

The premorbid conditions such as unemployment and the loss of loved persons he was dependent on, disturbed me because they signaled that there was a possibility that the patient could suffer from pathologic grief with severe physical and mental impairment (3, 4). The possibility of developing pathologic grief was the alarm that promoted us to give him medical intensive attention. We tried to reveal medical uncovered conditions, threatening his life, because of reported increased mortality and morbidity with pathologic grief, especially when the initial reaction also is severe and physical or mental impairment is additive to the grief.

Sudden, unexpected loss increases the chance of poor outcome. The same thing happens when grief is associated with social withdrawal. An ongoing sense of loneliness, anxiety and depression also predicts bad outcome of grief. The intense yearning also contributes to the poor outcome of grief, when the patient is dependent on the lost.

The family was functioning well and used the available resources in the core and extended family and services needed in this particular crisis. So, our effort was directed to mobilize social support, medical attention and psychiatric therapeutic modes for the grieving and functionally and socially impaired patient, the father. We intended to release some of the pressure that the family faced, due to its managing adaptation to crisis and put the father in a specialized circle of care. At this point, when the patient was in our care and receiving psychotherapy the patient's family felt relief and went back to work and daily routine without being anxious about the father.

In his first visit the patient and his wife asked for tablets to help him eat and sleep. They recognized that this depression and ill condition was related to the loss of the house. Both, the patient and his wife were treated with Diazepam, reassured that time will bring the improvement. When medical record, history or physical examination revealed no medical conditions, the patient was sent home and asked to come back in few days. The drug therapy brought some improvement in sleep, but the patient did not go back to work, and did not show functional betterment. So, he was referred for psychiatric evaluation. Diagnosed as a depressed patient without mental disorder, he started taking Prozac (Fluoexetine) 20 mg daily and Valium (Diazepam) 10 mg in the evening.

Slight improvement was noticed, but no return to work was planned by the patient. He continued to complain of weakness, impaired concentration, and lack of initiative work. His wife came again after one week from her first visit and complained of headache and weakness,

An evaluation of the past history of the patient and his family including reviewing genogram and life events of the patient's family as extensive family work up was aimed to find out family dysfunction, adaptive mechanisms and social support available and offering crisis intervention to the whole family with the house loss (5). The patient was seen on a regular basis twice weekly for one month and once every two weeks later on. Then we saw him every two months for six months. The patient was seen by a psychotherapist during short sessions at the Mental Health Center and the drugs were dosed according to his functional and affective situation.

The short psychotherapy objectives were limited to the enhancement of self-esteem and diminution of anxiety and a therapeutic alliance encouraging ventilation and offering a shared awareness and a reassuring guidance. No significant improvement was observed after one month of drug therapy and sessions of psychotherapy. The mood was depressed, but there was less functional impairment. He was able to sleep, eat and take care of himself, while other members of the family were at work. A diagnosis of adjustment disorder was established and previous therapy with Prozac discontinued.

New drug therapy including Elatrol (Amitriptyline) 50-100 mg was started. No adverse effects were reported and with Diazepam at evening time and psychotherapy his condition has significantly improved.

This case and a literature review improved our knowledge about dealing with survivors of a house fire and giving psychological support.

CONCLUSION

Grief and bereavement are part of human life, that occasionally affects mental and physical health status and physicians should be aware of it significance, to screen for high risk and train to manage these cases.

In our times of war or massive immigration, the losses that a person can experience is hard to comprehend and what we see in Europe these days will have long term effects on those families and also on public health in societies that receive the current day refugees.

We still need to learn about palliative care, bereavement and also look at the neuroscience to explain and understand the health consequences of grief and the neurobiology of attachment (6, 7).

REFERENCES

[1] Zeitlin SV. Grief and bereavement. Prim Care 2001;28(2):415-25.
[2] Charlton R. Bereavement. A protocol for primary care. Br J Gern Pract 1995;45:427-30.
[3] McAvoy. Death after bereavement. BMJ 1986;293 (6551):835-6.
[4] Preston J. The consequences of bereavement. Practitioner 1989;233:137-9.
[5] Rynearson EK. Psychotherapy of pathological grief. Psychiatr Clin North Am 1987;10(3):487-99.
[6] Kissane DW, McKenzie M, Bloch S, Moskowitz C, McKenzie DP, O'Neill I. Family focused grief therapy: A randomized, controlled trial in palliative care and bereavement. Am J Psychiatry 2006;163(7):1208-18.
[7] Gündel H, O'Connor MF, Littrell L, Fort C, Lane RD. Functional neuroanatomy of grief: An fMRI study. Am J Psychiatry 2003;160(11): 1946-53.

Submitted: February 02, 2016. *Revised:* March 06, 2016. *Accepted:* March 12, 2016.

Section two - Virtual reality technologies for rehabilitation

In: Alternative Medicine Research Yearbook 2017
Editor: Joav Merrick

ISBN: 978-1-53613-726-2
© 2018 Nova Science Publishers, Inc.

Chapter 10

A PARTICIPATORY DESIGN FRAMEWORK FOR THE GAMIFICATION OF REHABILITATION SYSTEMS

Darryl Charles[1,], BSc, PGCE, MSc, PhD and Suzanne McDonough[2], BPhysiotherapy, HDip, PhD*

[1]Computer Science Research Institute,
School of Computing and Information Engineering,
University of Ulster, Northern Ireland
[2]Centre for Health and Rehabilitation Technologies, School of Health Sciences,
Institute of Nursing and Health Research, University of Ulster, Northern Ireland

ABSTRACT

In recent years games and game technology have been used quite widely to investigate if they can help make rehabilitation more engaging for users. The underlying hypothesis is that the motivating qualities of games may be harnessed and embedded into a game-based rehabilitation system to improve the quality of user participation. We present here the PACT framework which has been created to guide the design of gamified rehabilitation systems; placing emphasis on people, aesthetics, context, and technology from the beginning of a design and development process. We discuss the evolution of PACT from our previous GAMER framework, which was used to develop a range of games for upper arm stroke rehabilitation with natural user interfaces. GAMER was established to guide the design of rehabilitation games from the viewpoint of a designer, whereas with PACT greater emphasis has been placed on an inclusive design process. We provide a detailed work flow illustration for the use of PACT in the development of rehabilitation systems and provide examples of practical design and analysis tools that improve the quality of workflow in PACT.

Keywords: gamification, rehabilitation, games, design framework

---

[*] Correspondence: Dr. Darryl Charles, BSc, PGCE, MSc, PhD, Senior Lecturer of Computing, Computer Science Research Institute, School of Computing and Information Engineering, University of Ulster, Northern Ireland. E-Mail: dk.charles@ulster.ac.uk.

INTRODUCTION

PACT (People, Aesthetics, Context, and Technology) may be described as a participatory design framework for the gamification of rehabilitation systems. Inclusive participation from the beginning of a rehabilitation design process has been raised as an increasingly important experimental methodology (1). Influence from games in the design of engaging rehabilitation software has also received a lot of recent attention (2). Though only a few papers make explicit reference to gamification, e.g., (3), there is often an implicit application of simple gamification techniques in the design of bespoke rehabilitation. The focus is often on inclusion of fun user feedback for the completion of tasks, with points, badges, high score tables, and leader boards being typical design patterns used. There is a danger, however, in taking too narrow a focus in the application of gamification to the design of systems. If the design focuses too much on task completion and rewards then there may be an over emphasis on extrinsic motivation, which may have less impact on long term behaviour and attitude change. Behavioural change is central to the goals of a well-designed rehabilitation system (4).

There are several definitions for gamification that vary depending on context, but most focus on engagement or motivation (5). For example, the influential company Badgeville states that "gamification is the concept of applying game-design thinking to non-game applications to make them more fun and engaging' (6). We prefer a broader definition in its application to rehabilitation software, considering gamification as the application of game elements and metaphors, game design patterns, or game technology to the design of systems that can positively influence behaviour, and improve motivation and engagement of people with non-game tasks and processes. We therefore view gamification as taking any influence from games and applying it to a non-game context. In this way a serious game, game-based learning, simple reward based feedback, and a walk in a virtual world can all be thought of as subsumed by the gamification label. In the PACT framework we endorse a system of gamification that can account for variation in motivational factors amongst different individuals and we illustrate this with a workflow diagram.

GAMER FRAMEWORK

The GAMER framework (see Figure 1) was developed to guide the design of rehabilitation games (see (7) for an expanded version) that help motivate people to engage with their required exercise regime in the home. It has been successfully utilised in the creation of several webcam (8) and augmented reality games (9) for upper arm stroke rehabilitation, the latter being licensed to US robotics company Myomo in 2011. GAMER was developed after extensive investigation of game design theory from leading game designers and in collaboration with physiotherapy researchers to map therapy goals to tailored, motivating physical gameplay. Our approach was similar to Goude et al. (10) who also used the comprehensive collection of game design patterns by Björk and Holopainen (11) as a central design inspiration. GAMER maps key game design or gameplay elements that have been identified as being specifically relevant to physical gameplay via a natural user interface to core therapy goals. The framework can be used to aid a designer in creating varying forms of gameplay that emphasises different aspects of therapy by choosing a suitable subset of game design elements/patterns in the design and directing of the choice of interaction hardware. Burke (7) provides detailed worked examples on how we evaluated GAMER through the design of several rehabilitation games over two case studies.

PACT GAMIFICATION FRAMEWORK

GAMER demonstrated the potential of a structured approach in the design of usable, engaging, and effective rehabilitation games. It is particularly useful in mapping therapy goals to physical gameplay elements and embedding positive reinforcement feedback aesthetics. Our PACT framework evolved from GAMER to increase our focus on stakeholder involvement and place a stronger emphasis on personal motivation of users. The PACT framework (Figure 2) has four dimensions, People, Aesthetics, Context, and Technology, which form the focus for the design of gamified rehabilitation systems. Unlike GAMER, PACT has an implicit focus on participatory design and involvement with all of the relevant stakeholders from the beginning of a rehabilitation design process. The emphasis on gamification within the PACT framework has a number of significant advances. Firstly, the outcome of a gamification process may not be an obvious game but may simply result in the addition of fun feedback (e.g., points and badges) to a non-game context (e.g., physical movements round the home), could recommend the use of gaming hardware in a non-game context (e.g., digital painting), or the use of game worlds to immerse and inspire (e.g., walks with friends in virtual game worlds). Secondly, new advanced gamification approaches can help tailor system design to account for diversity in motivation between different people. The emphasis on behavioural change correlates with other framework designs in the research area (4).

Figure 3 provides a typical workflow diagram for the implementation of the PACT framework in practice. This resembles the practice that we undertook in the design of our recent upper arm stroke rehabilitation simulations with the Leap Motion controller (12). We can split the PACT design process into three phases:

Phase 1 is essentially a requirements gathering phase and involves a dialog between clinicians, researchers, users/patients and other stakeholders from the community to establish the basis for system design founded on therapy goals and on specific user and carer needs. Capability of the target group will be accounted for at this stage and temperament models and personal interest of users may be taken into account in order to tailor the design more effectively.

Phase 2 is the core design phase and in our new model includes both an underpinning of game design and gamification. In the work flow example shown in Figure 3 we utilise the set of comprehensive game design patterns from Goude et al. (10) and list the key pattern group headings (NB other references may also be used). The gamification technique that we propose is based on Marczewski's Hexad gamification typology (13). This model has its origins in Bartle's player types (14) and RAMP intrinsic motivation model. Effective gamification can engage individuals by tapping into particular aspects of their intrinsic motivational psychology. The RAMP model outlines four key motivational drivers for people:

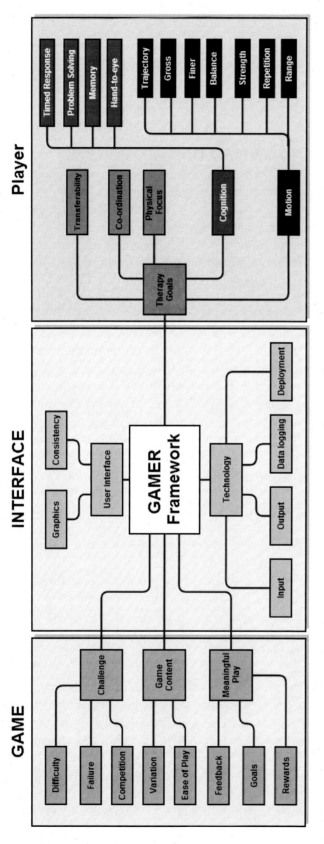

Figure 1. The GAMER framework is designed to guide the design of rehabilitation games.

A participatory design framework for the gamification of rehabilitation systems 113

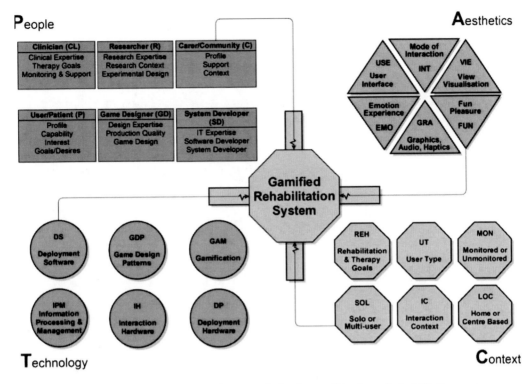

Figure 2. PACT is a participatory design framework for the gamification of rehabilitation systems.

Relatedness, autonomy, mastery and purpose

Relatedness equates to social connections and a feeling of belonging (feeling safe and cared for in one's interpersonal relationships); autonomy is about facilitating choice to engage in certain behaviours and creativity; mastery relates to the provision of opportunities to learn and improve knowledge or a skill; and purpose recognises that people are more motivated when they understand the context for their efforts. The Hexad (13) suggests six basic types of user, each being motivated by different intrinisc or extrinsic motivational priorities. The outcome from Phase 2 is a system design developed in partnership with key stakeholders (defined under people in Figure 2).

Phase 3 is essentially an evolutionary protyping phase where system software is created and integrated with required hardware. In the workflow example provided we suggest a structured approach for the analysis of the design based on the evolving system prototypes. As a 1st stage of the evaluation process we suggest rigorous evaluation of the design by a research and development team using a tool such as Schell's game design lenses to focus on core design topics (15). A 2nd evalution stage involves play and usability testing by users and other stakeholders using techniques developed during our GAMER experiments (or similar). During a 3rd stage of the system evaluation, the gamification system is analysed and redesigned on the basis of user feedback. A structured method such as the use of Marczewski's gamification cards can aid this process. The eventual outcome from Phase 3 will be a completed gamified rehabilitation system.

114 Darryl Charles and Suzanne McDonough

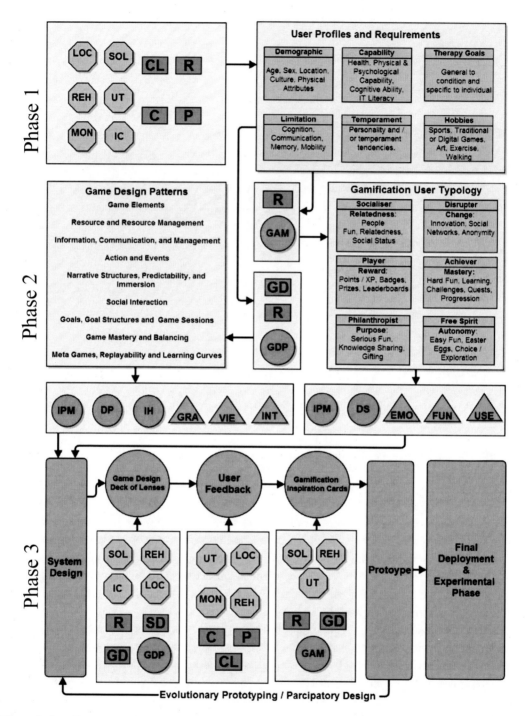

Figure 3. Sample PACT Rehabilitation System Design Workflow (see Figure 2 for symbol meaning).

The development of the PACT workflow was informed by the recent development of an upper arm rehabilitation systems using a virtual reality based approach and Leap Motion depth sensing controllers for a natural user interface (12). Physiotherapy and computing researchers, clinical physiotherapists and occupational therapists from the Northern Ireland Regional Acquired Brain Injury Unit (RABIU) at Musgrave Hospital in Belfast (n=8), and game designers/developers from a commercial company (SilverFish Studios) were engaged in the appropriate phases of PACT (though not patients in this initial proof of concept process). The outcome was very positive and the software is currently under development (PACT Phase 3) for use in clinical trials.

CONCLUSION

In this paper we introduced our PACT framework, a participatory design oriented process for gamifying rehabilitation systems. To explain its use in practice we provided a detailed work flow diagram that included specific suggestions for analysis and design with key stakeholders. Early and structured ongoing involvement of key stakeholders within the system design process is central to PACT. A core recommendation for the realisation of PACT is the separate consideration of the influence of game design patterns and gamification best practices for rehabilitation system design. This allows us to separate functional aspects of game design from motivational qualities of game interaction and can enhance the quality of design. A novel approach in our PACT work flow illustration is the use of Marczewski's gamification Hexad to help identify ways in which different people can be motivated to participate. PACT has been developed ahead of a new three year project which seeks to design and develop motivating game-based exercise systems for people affected by Stroke, Multiple Sclerosis, and those at risk of falls.

REFERENCES

[1] Gooberman-Hill R, Jinks C, Bouças SB, Hislop K, Dziedzic KS, Rhodes C, et al. Designing a placebo device: involving service users in clinical trial design. Health Expect 2013;16(4):e100–10.

[2] McNeill MDJ, Charles DK, Burke J, Crosbie J, McDonough S. Evaluating User Experiences in Rehabilitation Games. J Assist Technol 2012 Jul;6(3): 173–81.

[3] López-Rodríguez D, García-Linares A. Spare: Spatial rehabilitation with learning, recommendations and gamification. ICERI2013 Proc, 2013.

[4] Michie S, van Stralen MM, West R. The behaviour change wheel: a new method for characterising and designing behaviour change interventions. Implement Sci 2011;6(1):42.

[5] Deterding S, Björk SL, Nacke LE, Dixon D, Lawley E. Designing gamification. CHI '13 Extended Abstracts on Human Factors in Computing Systems – CHI EA '13. New York: ACM Press, 2013:3263.

[6] Gamification Wiki. What is gamification? Gamification .org [Internet]. 2014 [cited 2014 May 21]. Available from: http://badgeville.com/wiki/Gamification.

[7] Burke J. Games for upper-limb stroke rehabilitation. Dissertation. Univerity of Ulster; 2011. Available from: http://goo.gl/O56mnE.

[8] Burke JW, Morrow PJ, McNeill M, McDonough S, Charles D. Vision Based Games for Upper-Limb Stroke Rehabilitation. IMVIP '08: Proceedings of the 2008 International Machine Vision and Image Processing Conference. Washington, DC, 2008:159–64.

[9] Burke J, McNeill MDJ, Charles DK, Morrow PJ, Crosbie J, McDonough S. Augmented reality game design for upper-limb stroke rehabilitation, 2nd IEEE International Conference on Games and Virtual Worlds for Serious Applications (VS-GAMES 2010). IEEE, 2010:75–8.

[10] Goude D, Björk S, Rydmark M. Game design in virtual reality systems for stroke rehabilitation. Stud Health Technol Inform 2007;125:146–8.

[11] Björk S, Holopainen J. Games and design patterns. Salen K, Zimmerman E, Editors. The game design reader. Cambridge, MA: MIT Press, 2006.
[12] Charles D, Pedlow K, McDonough S, Shek K, Charles T. An evaluation of the leap motion depth sensing camera for tracking hand and fingers motion in Physical Therapy. ITAG: Interactive Technologies and Games – Education, health and disability. Nottingham: Nottingham Trent University,2013.
[13] Marczewski A. User types hexad. URL: gamified.co.uk. 2014.
[14] Bartle R. Hearts, clubs, diamonds, spades: Players who suit {MUDs}. J {MUD} Res [Internet]. 1996;1(1). Available from: http://web.cs.wpi.edu/~ypisan/virtual worlds/readings/hearts-clubs.pdf.
[15] Schell J. The art of game design: A book of lenses. Boca Raton, FL: CRC Press; 2008.

Submitted: July 01, 2015. *Revised:* August 05, 2015. *Accepted:* August 10, 2015.

In: Alternative Medicine Research Yearbook 2017
Editor: Joav Merrick
ISBN: 978-1-53613-726-2
© 2018 Nova Science Publishers, Inc.

Chapter 11

EVIDENCE-BASED FACIAL DESIGN OF AN INTERACTIVE VIRTUAL ADVOCATE

Wendy Powell[1,], PhD, DC, BSc, BA,*
Tom A Garner[2], PhD, PGCE, MA, BA,
Daniel Tonks[1], MSc, BSc and Thomas Lee[1], BSc

[1]School of Creative Technologies, University of Portsmouth,
Winston Churchill Avenue, Portsmouth, United Kingdom
[2]Centre for Child Protection, University of Kent,
Giles Lane, Canterbury, United Kingdom

ABSTRACT

RITA (Responsive InTeractive Advocate) is the vision for a computer software-based advocacy and companion service to support older adults and provide an alternative to institutional care. The RITA service will offer a preventative care approach, creating a digital champion who will learn an individual's needs and preferences over time, and be a friendly interface between users, family and professionals. This will involve the integration of a variety of technical components: (i) *The Face*, a realistic and emotionally expressive avatar, encouraging communication and interaction; (ii) *The Mind*, a repository to store, organise and interpret personal and memory-related information representing the 'essence' of a person, with user-defined access controls; and (3) *The Heart*, an empathetic sensory interface which is able to understand and respond to the physical, emotional and psychological needs of the user. Each of these aspects presents a series of technical challenges, which will be addressed by combining existing state-of-the art techniques from a variety of disciplines, together with innovative processes and algorithms, to improve and extend functionality. RITA is being designed in consultation with user groups and service providers, drawing extensively on existing research to inform the design and functionality of the system. We introduce here the design and development of the face of RITA.

---

[*] Correspondence: Wendy Powell, PhD, School of Creative Technologies, University of Portsmouth, Winston Churchill Avenue, Portsmouth, United Kingdom. E-mail: wendy.powell@port.ac.uk.

Keywords: avatar, facial animation, intelligent agent, virtual companion, elderly

INTRODUCTION

Around 3 million over 65s in England and Wales live alone (1), with over half suffering from long-term health or mobility issues. Increasingly pressured lifestyles place burdens on extended family, restricting the opportunities for care and support (2, 3), and increasing demands on the social care system mean that it is unable to address many of the issues associated with social isolation. Frequent changes between carers, alongside poor communication (across a fragmented healthcare system) presents a significant challenge in the provision of personalised support which is responsive to the needs, preferences, history and personality of an individual.

RITA (Responsive InTeractive Advocate) is the vision for a computer software-based advocacy and companion service that brings together three elements: (1) a 3D virtual avatar and conversational agent, (2) an 'essence' repository for storage and organisation of various forms of information pertaining to the user, and (3) an empathetic communication system that is capable of understanding and responding to the psychological, social and emotional needs of the individual user. It is the design of the first of these elements with which we are concerned here.

AVATAR CHARACTERISTICS: REQUIREMENTS AND EVIDENCE

Although it is recognised that visual rendering of an avatar influences the user's perception of the character's personality (4), there is often a lack of systematic and informed design of virtual agents (5,6). Perception of character is subject to multiple and diverse influences, ranging from character type to clothing, facial expression to body language (5) and thus it can be challenging to decide on individual characteristics for any given avatar. However, a clearly defined purpose, together with elicitation of user requirement, can facilitate the process of meaningful and effective avatar design. The RITA animation team worked closely with health care service designers in order to identify the key personality characteristics required for the RITA avatar. The main characteristics identified were *trustworthiness* and *competence*.

The first consideration was whether the avatar should be human or non-human, and the level of realism necessary. Whilst animal or other non-human characters can be perceived as friendly and engaging, human characters are considered to be more attractive (7). Research within this area is currently lacking in fully evidenced conclusions with regards to the more highly-specific questions, such as: *What are the advantages of using a human avatar within a healthcare and wellbeing context? Does a human avatar evoke a greater sense of professionalism and competence?* We can make a certain degree of inferences from the various existing healthcare-associated avatar products, the majority of which are human in design.

The Uncanny Valley theory (8–10) suggests a danger in that increasing the human realism of a character may lead to a sense of discomfort if the end result looks almost, but not quite, human. In light of this, the avatar is based on a human character but using techniques to maximise the realism and visual fidelity, in order to reduce the sense of discomfort whilst optimising the required characteristics.

There are a number of factors which have been identified as being key elements defining the character of virtual agents, including movement and hand gestures (11), voice and verbal communication (12, 13), facial and emotional expression (11), and facial characteristics (5). The notion that perception of character can be drawn from the face has remained a popular cultural belief over the centuries (14) and it could be asserted that a personality profile can be projected onto a person based upon an observer's perception (physiognomic stereotyping (15)). The face is a powerful communication tool in which the majority of human expressions are formed during conversation (16). Consequently, the RITA avatar will initially be displayed from the neck upwards. This maintains the key features necessary for engaging interaction, whilst reducing the computational load required for high fidelity realistic animation of a full-body avatar. In light of this, the key features for consideration in avatar design will be facial characteristics, voice and facial expression.

Facial characteristics

It is clear that people make enduring judgements of character based on less than one second of exposure to a face (17). The perception of trustworthiness and competence appears to be based on variations in a few key facial features, summarised in Table 1.

Table 1. Facial features associated with trustworthiness and competence

Feature	Competence/Dominance	Trustworthiness/Honesty
Face shape	Not too round (18, 19) Angular or square face (20)	Round or baby face (22) Smooth smaller face (23) Fatter face (24) Pronounced cheekbones (23)
Chin	Wider chin, not too round (20)	Wide chin (23) Rounder broad chin (22) Shorter chin (22)
Nose	Bridge not pronounced (20)	Slim nose with shallow nose sellion (23)
Mouth	Thinner lips (20)	Broad mouth (22) Smiling or upward corners (22)
Eyebrows	Lower brows (20)	High inner eyebrows (23) Eyebrows closer together (22)
Eyes	Not too round (20)	Brown eyes (22) Large, open eyes (23)
Hair	Brunette (21)	

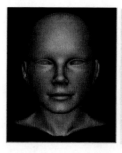 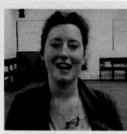 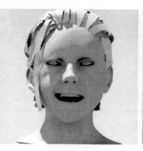 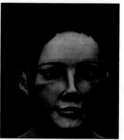

Figure 1. (left to right): the base facial mesh designed for competence and trustworthiness; an actor engaging in the motion capture process; emotions from the actor animated on the base mesh; and the textured avatar.

Based on combining the key attributes from the available evidence, the initial facial mesh was constructed with a fairly round face shape, but with a wider than average jaw, slightly pronounced cheekbones and with the more angular features slightly softened. The mouth is slightly broad, with an upward turn at the corners. The nose is slim and with a shallow sellion. The inner brows are slightly higher than average and not too far apart, with the brow ridge being less pronounced, resulting in less shadow on the eyes, creating an impression of brighter and more open eyes (Figure 1, left). The base mesh for the face was built in Autodesk Maya. A bone-based animation system drives the movements of the neck, jaw and eyelids, and blend shapes applied to simulate the macro and micro movements of the facial musculature. Once the mesh was fully rigged, the team used specialist facial capture software (Faceshift) to record facial movements and emotional expression from the actress. Animations were split into core speech and emotional state segments, before being imported into Maya and applied to the facial rig and refined by hand to optimise the fidelity (see Figure 1, centre right).

Voice

The RITA avatar voice has two elements to consider: accent and tonal quality. The latter is dependent on context, emotional overlay and speech elements, but the characteristics of the accent persist through all dialogue and therefore warrant some consideration. The cultural variation that would likely dictate users from alternative ethnic backgrounds would possess different vocal preferences for their RITA (25) suggests that, in an ideal scenario, the vocal characteristics of RITA would need to be fully customisable to best suit the individual user. Within the current stage of development however, we are required to focus upon a single accent. Research by Tamagawa and colleagues (26) suggests that, within healthcare robotics, there is a significant user-preference towards regional-sounding accents. Within the UK, a 2009 survey (27) reported Received Pronunciation as the most appealing when speaking to a call centre, followed closely by a Scottish accent. Specifically, the Edinburgh accent has been associated with pleasantness and prestige (28). The British Broadcasting Corporation (29) concluded that the Scottish accent is the 'most reassuring' during an emergency and accents from this region are largely connotative of competence, trustworthiness and friendliness. In light of this evidence, a Scottish actress was employed to provide source recordings as the basis for the voice of the avatar (Figure 1, centre left).

INTERACTION AND ONGOING DEVELOPMENT

The animated avatar is deployed in the Unity engine to allow real-time control of the avatar in response to signals from the control software. In order to build a modular and adaptable system, the "heart" and "mind" software send information to a decision-making system which will interpret the information relating to the user's emotional and physiological state, personality and preferences, sending instructions to Unity to trigger the avatar's response. Animation segments are coded and can be dynamically blended with emotional expression and audio files in order to generate appropriate speech, facial expression and synchronised speech (see www.rita.me.uk).

The essence database is being developed and extended, and will be integrated with learning algorithms in order to populate itself over time as it interacts with the end-user. The modular RITA system can evolve over time, integrating developments in natural speech synthesis, data interpretation and emotional and physiological sensing.

The project team engage regularly with service providers and service users in order to refine the capabilities and potential of the RITA advocate. Further work will report on the findings.

ACKNOWLEDGMENTS

This research was supported by a grant from the Technology Strategy Board (Long Term Care Revolution). We thank our colleagues on the RITA project, Dr Jane Reeves (University of Kent), Dr Blair Dickson (Affective State Ltd) and Dr Valerie Carr (Snook) who provided insight and expertise to support the design of the avatar.

REFERENCES

[1]   ONS. 2011 Census analysis: Internal and international migration of older residents (aged 65 and over) in England and Wales in the year prior to the 2011 census. London: Office of National Statistics, 2014.
[2]   Merrill D. Caring for elderly parents: Juggling work, family, and caregiving in middle and working class families. Westport, CT: Auburn House, 1997.
[3]   Silverstone B, Hyman H. You and your aging parent: A family guide to emotional, social, health, and financial problems. New York: Oxford University Press, 2008.
[4]   Dryer D. Getting personal with computers: How to design personalities for agents. Appl Artif Intell. 1999; 13(3):273–95.
[5]   Gulz A. Social enrichment by virtual characters – differential benefits. J Comput Assist Learn 2005;21(6): 405–18.
[6]   Gulz A, Haake M. Design of animated pedagogical agents–A look at their look. Int J Hum-Comput Stud 2006;64(4):322–39.
[7]   Schneider E, Wang Y, Yang S. Exploring the uncanny valley with Japanese video game characters. In Proceed Situated Play, DiGRA Conference, 2007:546-9.
[8]   Mori M. The uncanny valley. Energy 1970;7(4):33–5.
[9]   Mori M, MacDorman K, Kageki N. The uncanny valley [From the Field]. IEEE Robot Automat Mag 2012; 19(2):98–100.

[10] Tinwell A, Grimshaw M, Nabi D, Williams A. Facial expression of emotion and perception of the Uncanny Valley in virtual characters. Comput Hum Behav 2011; 27(2):741–9.
[11] Johnson W, Rickel J, Lester J. Animated pedagogical agents: Face-to-face interaction in interactive learning environments. Int J Artif Intell Educ 2000;11(1):47–78.
[12] Nass C, Steuer J, Tauber E. Computers are social actors. CHI 94 Proceed SIGCHI Conference Human Factors Computing Systems, 1994:72-8.
[13] Cassell J. Embodied conversational interface agents. Commun ACM 2000;43(4):70–78.
[14] Berry D, McArthur L. Perceiving character in faces: The impact of age-related craniofacial changes on social perception. Psychol Bull 1986;100(1):3–18.
[15] Hummert ML. Age changes in facial morphology, emotional communication, and age stereotyping. In: Verhaeghen P, Hertzog C, eds. The Oxford handbook of emotion, social cognition, and problem solving in adulthood. New York: Oxford University Press, 2014: 47.
[16] Argyle M. Bodily communication. London: Methuen, 2013.
[17] Todorov A, Baron S, Oosterhof N. Evaluating face trustworthiness: a model based approach. Soc Cogn Affect Neurosci 2008;3(2):119–27.
[18] Oosterhof N, Todorov A. The functional basis of face evaluation. Proceed Natl Acad Sci 2008;105(32): 11087–92.
[19] Poutvaara P, Jordahl H, Berggren N. Faces of politicians: Baby facedness predicts inferred competence but not electoral success. J Exp Soc Psychol 2009; 45(5):1132–5.
[20] Zebrowitz L, Montepare J. Social psychological face perception: Why appearance matters. Soc Pers Psychol Compass 2008;2(3):1497–1517.
[21] Kyle D, Mahler H. The effects of hair color and cosmetic use on perceptions of a female's ability. Psychol Women Quart 1996;20(3):447–55.
[22] Kleisner K, Priplatova L, Frost P, Flegr J. Trustworthy-looking face meets brown eyes. PLoS One 2013; 8(1):e53285.
[23] Todorov A, Dotsch R, Porter J, Oosterhof N, Falvello V. Validation of data-driven computational models of social perception of faces. Emotion 2013;13(4):724–38.
[24] Van Vugt M. Evolutionary origins of leadership and followership. Pers Soc Psychol Rev 2006;10(4):354–71.
[25] Khooshabeh P, Dehghani M, Nazarian A, Gratch J. The cultural influence model: when accented natural language spoken by virtual characters matters. J Artic Intell Soc 2014.
[26] Tamagawa R, Watson C, Kuo I, MacDonald B, Broadbent E. The Effects of Synthesized Voice Accents on User Perceptions of Robots. Int J Soc Robotics 2011; 3(3):253–62.
[27] Casciato P. Revealed: the perfect telephone call center accent. Reuters [Internet]. 2009.
[28] BBC. Attitudes towards accents. Accessed June 2014. URL: http://www.bbc.co.uk/voices/yourvoice/
[29] BBC. Scottish accent 'most reassuring'. BBC News Online. 2009. Accessed June 2014. URL: http://news.bbc.co.uk/1/hi/scotland/7754111.stm.

Submitted: July 01, 2015. *Revised:* August 05, 2015. *Accepted:* August 10, 2015.

In: Alternative Medicine Research Yearbook 2017
Editor: Joav Merrick
ISBN: 978-1-53613-726-2
© 2018 Nova Science Publishers, Inc.

Chapter 12

REFLECTIONS AND EARLY EVIDENCE OF THE IMPORTANCE OF PRESENCE FOR THREE TYPES OF FEEDBACK IN VIRTUAL MOTOR REHABILITATION

Thomas Schüler[1],*, Dr Rer Nat,
Luara Ferreira dos Santos[2], Dipl-Psych
and Simon Hoermann[3], PhD

[1]Institute of Computer Science, University of Osnabrück, Osnabrück, Germany
[2]Rehabilitation Robotics Group (Fraunhofer IPK/TU Berlin),
Technische Universität Berlin, Berlin, Germany
[3]Department of Medicine (DSM) and Department of Information Science,
University of Otago, Dunedin, New Zealand

ABSTRACT

The experience of presence has been shown to be important for virtual motor rehabilitation. Despite its importance, current research and therapy systems often make only limited use of it. This paper introduces a conceptualization of presence that provides a guideline for the implementation of virtual rehabilitation environments. Three types of feedback in virtual rehabilitation systems are linked to three dimensions of presence. In particular it is shown how movement representation, performance information and instructions, and context information correspond to the presence dimensions: spatial presence, involvement and realness. In addition, practical implications are discussed to support the development of future virtual rehabilitation systems and to allow better use of the experience of presence for virtual motor rehabilitation after stroke.

Keywords: stroke, virtual reality, movement visualization, performance feedback, context information

---

* Correspondence: Thomas Schüler, Dr Rer Nat, Institute of Computer Science, University of Osnabrück, Osnabrück, Germany. E-mail: t.schueler@posteo.de.

INTRODUCTION

Virtual reality (VR) systems have been shown to be effective for the treatment of patients with motor impairments; however, the exact characteristics that lead to improvements are not well understood and more research is needed to optimize therapeutic outcomes and VR systems (1). In VR systems patients interact with virtual environments: their movement is tracked with specific devices and is often visualized as movements of a virtual avatar. The virtual worlds include game components and are designed so that patients need to perform therapeutically relevant movements to achieve goals and successfully complete challenges to reach a new level of the game.

Today it is not known exactly how features of a virtual environment impact upon treatment outcomes. However, a key role for motivation and general effectiveness has been assigned to the experience of presence. Presence is defined as the illusion of nonmediation and the feeling of "being there" in the virtual environment (2). Consequently patients who experience presence during VR-based treatment focus on the game world that demands active participation. Therefore effective training may be supported through presence, yet few studies have examined this in therapeutic VR application.

With this paper we attempt to clarify the importance of presence for VR-based treatment of motor disabilities after stroke. We identify three distinct feedback types that are provided by virtual rehabilitation systems. These types match well with the three dimensional model of the presence experience proposed by Schubert et al. (3). We discuss how the feedback types and presence dimensions may foster recovery of motor function and suggest practical implications that guide future development of virtual rehabilitation systems.

Dimensions of presence

Schubert et al. (3) proposed a three dimensional model of the presence experience. They identified three distinct factors contributing to an overall experience of presence. These factors were spatial presence (construction of a spatial mental model of the VR), involvement (attention allocation and concentration on the VR) and realness (comparison of the VR experience against one in a physical world).

Spatial presence has been linked with embodied theories of cognition (4). Specifically the ability of a subject to act within a virtual environment (agency) is thought to determine a coherent spatial mental model of that environment. Importantly it is the subject's individual perception of action potentials rather than an objective availability per se that constitutes spatial presence.

Factors that contribute to involvement include technical and human conditions (3) as well as the attention towards a virtual environment. It can be influenced through the choice of hardware components, but it is also dependent on the subjects' motivation and interest. This interest can be stimulated by VR-design considerations, e.g., through presenting skill-matched tasks and providing motivating feedback about the subject's performance. Usually the interaction will take place in a setting where the subject has to suppress conflicting information from the real world (e.g., sounds from other persons, the physical boundaries of the used hardware), therefore the circumstances of interaction within a VR are also important for involvement.

The realness dimension represents a comparison of the experience made in the virtual environment with its counterpart in the real world (3). The realness judgment is influenced by the level of detail and the vividness of the VR. Background objects and the general situation that the environment displays define the physical world context with which the experience will be compared. Note that a realness judgment may also be made about fictive environments, but with an additional need for imagination. A fictive environment will be compared against a mental picture of how a physical materialization of the environment would look/feel/sound. Generally adding coherent sensory stimuli that enable a more "complete" experience will enhance the realness judgment.

Presence has been described as a multi-dimensional structure by other authors too (2, 4, 5). Usually the above mentioned concepts behind spatial presence, involvement and realness are identified similarly. Some conceptualizations also consider social components, but these seem to be less informative for contemporary virtual rehabilitation settings. However, in situations where groups of patients interact together, or where VR-systems provide a story-based game with multiple characters, social dimensions may be important.

Motor rehabilitation after stroke

Stroke is a cerebral-vascular disease of which neurologic damage is a consequence. Often cortical motor areas are affected, leading to serious behavioral impairments and stroke is one of the main causes of acquired adult disability (6). Motor impairments following stroke are treated mostly with physical and occupational therapy. The goal is to enhance cortical plasticity and motor (re)learning to restore motor function and to acquire coping skills.

Traditional therapy approaches focus on peripheral sensorimotor stimulation using active and passive movements of the affected limb. Within these approaches, practice is the most important factor for learning motor skills and a combination of repetitive and variable movement execution is required (7). Intensive training needs high patient motivation and adherence, which is often difficult to achieve with neurologic patients due to rather high demands for little progress. Informing the patients about their performance and the overall rehabilitation progress therefore is an important feature of practice. Using virtual rehabilitation, this challenge can be mitigated due to the possibility to include performance information in a motivating game experience.

Recent therapy approaches focus on central sensory stimulation of the impaired brain areas and make use of a neurologic mechanism, which activates cortical motor areas by observation or imagination of movements. This allows patients after stroke to activate neuron pathways similar to those recruited to execute movements that they are physically not able to perform. Though details about the underlying cortical mechanism are still under debate, the effectiveness of observing movements in a mirror for motor learning after stroke has been proven (8). Virtual reality systems can replicate and even exceed the capabilities of a traditional optical mirror and produce a stronger illusion of actions for central sensory stimulation (9–11).

INFLUENCING THE EXPERIENCE OF PRESENCE WITH VIRTUAL FEEDBACK

Only limited evidence about features of the VR design for specific rehabilitation effects can be drawn from the literature today (1, 12). So far no design standards have evolved. Furthermore, the applied VR-systems are often considered as a whole technology and not examined in detail during clinical studies, which makes it hard to draw conclusions about the individual design features. However a need for shared design considerations has been stated before and research towards this has been presented by Doyle et al. (13).

Virtual rehabilitation systems provide different types of information to the patients. In our view, the features of a virtual environment can be separated into distinct groups of feedback. Each of these groups corresponds primarily to a certain presence dimension (see Table 1). The three types of feedback will not always be used in virtual rehabilitation systems, but usually they will be implemented to enable a complete game experience.

Table 1. Types of feedback with their corresponding presence dimension

Type of Feedback		Presence Dimension
Movement representation	‹-›	Spatial presence
Performance information	‹-›	Involvement
Context information	‹-›	Realness

Movement representation and spatial presence

The patients' movements are represented in VR, such that motor actions are captured and transferred to e.g., a graphical object that is synchronously animated. In many cases this object will take the form of an anthropomorphic avatar that is observed from a first- or third-person perspective. However, fictive or abstract objects, as well as representations in other modalities, can also be used. In order to orient themselves in the virtual world, patients need to identify with the representation. Since the action potential of the environment is experienced through this representation, spatial presence will be evoked when the patients are able to enact their intentions with the movement representation.

Considering the visual modality, the observation of movement visualizations in virtual rehabilitation systems can have a direct effect on motor learning since it can lead to central stimulation of cortical motor areas. Neurophysiological studies have shown that observing virtual limb movements stimulates cortical activity similar to the observation of real limbs in a mirror (14). It has been postulated that observation of virtual limbs can facilitate the functional reorganization of the neuronal systems directly or indirectly affected by stroke (15). Thus an additional motor learning effect may be achieved when performing and observing movements during training.

We furthermore postulate that the experience of spatial presence modulates central stimulation of motor areas during observation of movement visualizations. When experiencing spatial presence, the subject attributes the observed virtual motor actions to itself and corresponding cortical areas will be stimulated. We hypothesize a positive correlation between spatial presence and central stimulation. Therefore spatial presence is of high importance for motor learning in virtual rehabilitation.

Performance information and involvement

Performance information such as e.g., instructions is usually considered one of the key features increasing the involvement in virtual environments. During the treatment, patients have to accomplish tasks and when they are successful they gain points or proceed to a more difficult level. The task as well as the points or level will be presented in some way in order to add meaning to the patient's exercises and inform them about their progress.

In terms of its relevance for motor learning, performance information can be further differentiated into knowledge of performance and knowledge of results (7). In traditional therapies, feedback is often given in terms of knowledge of performance, leading to an internal focus on the correct limb positions and movements during task execution. However, Wulf (16) demonstrated that an external focus on the effects that the trained movements should have in the environment is more effective for motor learning. Thus feedback on performance should also focus on providing knowledge of results.

Virtual environments are well suited to provide both, information about the performance and about the results, within a game experience. In this way performance information can be regarded as a motivational factor and may foster the patients' adherence to the training. By means of performance information, the attention of the patients will be drawn towards the VR and, assuming the patients are willing to succeed in the game, will increase their engagement and involvement. Thus the presence dimension of involvement is linked with the effectiveness of performance information by motivating and engaging the patients.

Context information and realness

Finally, context information will be displayed that pictures the virtual world. This information may resemble a naturalistic place or a fictive environment in which the patients' representative and the tasks are conceivable. Background objects and animations give the VR system the impression of a real environment that is not just a technical artefact for therapeutic purposes. Atmospheric sensory stimuli in form of sounds can add to the vividness of the experience.

An important goal of therapeutic treatment is the transfer of learned behaviour to everyday activities, which patients should be confident enough to perform. Virtual environments can display real world contexts and objects used in everyday tasks so that the patients can associate the learning with situations from their daily life.

The realness presence dimension relates to this kind of vividness of a VR environment. Depending on the treatment approach, virtual rehabilitation systems may display various types of contexts: naturalistic or fictive. However in each case the realness presence dimension will be determined by the amount and coherency of the provided context information and thus affect how well the therapy system establishes a real experience. If an everyday task should be learned the realness dimension may even point towards the possibility of transferring the training situation to daily life.

EXAMPLE OF PRACTICAL APPLICATION

In a first prospective study the assumption that presence is important for motor learning was tested (17). The "abstract virtual environment for stroke therapy" (AVUS) was used for the treatment of 5 upper-limb hemiparetic patients. The AVUS system visualizes movement in an engaging way with different levels of abstraction from human upper-limb representations (see Figure 1). The therapeutic goal with this system is to support self-regulatory training and the exploration of motor patterns while at the same time aiding motor learning through central stimulation. To achieve this, the system offers an optional mirror therapy mode, in which only the movements of the patients' healthy limbs are tracked and the information is used to manipulate both sides of the virtual environment. While training with the system atmospheric background music is played and its features (rhythm, volume) influence the visualizations too.

The patients trained with the AVUS in the different modes for approximately 30 minutes on 5 successive days. After each intervention the experienced sense of presence was evaluated using a modified version of the Igroup Presence Questionnaire (IPQ, (3)); here, the realness dimension was excluded to reduce the cognitive load of the questionnaire. A set of other clinical (Fugl-Meyer assessment, coloured analogue scale, motor imagery ability) and qualitative measures (guided interviews) was applied pre- and post-treatment to test for the rehabilitation effect and ask for subjective opinions on the AVUS therapy.

The research approach made possible a correlation between the experienced sense of presence and the rehabilitation outcome. Indeed an increased training effect was found when presence was high, as shown by correlating the IPQ data with the Fugl-Meyer improvement. Also the subjective reactions of the patients supported this correlation. Those patients who scored high on the IPQ reported to be highly engaged and stimulated by the system. They were able to identify their body with the visualizations and expressed to have experienced a positive sense of enhanced motor skills in their affected limb during the mirror therapy mode. Statistical evidence cannot be drawn from these results due to the small sample size, however the importance of the presence experience for the treatment of stroke patients with the AVUS system was indicated.

AVUS focuses on movement representation in the visual modality and its design is based on the assumption that observing abstract visualization of movements supports spatial presence and thus central stimulation of motor areas. The results of the preliminary study therefore point towards the soundness of our above given hypothesis.

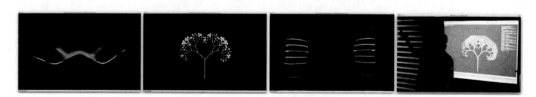

Figure 1. Movement visualization with the AVUS system.

DISCUSSION

With this paper, we introduced a conceptualization of virtual rehabilitation systems that distinguishes between three types of feedback and attributed these to three presence dimensions. We suggested how the feedback types and presence dimensions may aid motor rehabilitation after stroke. We presented theories and preliminary study results that point towards the importance of presence for virtual rehabilitation and support our hypothesis that spatial presence modulates central stimulation of motor areas when observing movement visualizations.

Some practical implications can be drawn from our conceptualization. Movement representation seems to play an important role for motor rehabilitation and should therefore be designed with special caution. However, there is no systematic knowledge about which representation strategy is best to date (12). While in the visual modality anthropomorphic shapes are used predominantly, there is also scientific rational to use more abstract forms and objects in order to develop a strong sense of spatial presence (17). Future research should focus on clarifying the effects of movement representation on the experience of presence and motor learning.

Some kind of performance information is incorporated in most virtual rehabilitation systems. There are varied ways to frame the game experience during the treatment and available systems use the full scale of options from sport activities over spaceship flights to manipulating cartooned objects. Levels and points are displayed on head-up display or indicated by sound or avatar changes. However, since involvement in a VR-experience requires concentration, performance information should not be overloaded or distract the attention of the patients. Moreover, what is judged to be motivating feedback is dependent on personality traits. This type of information should therefore be made adaptable.

With regard to context information, the provided information should place the treatment in an appropriate context and allow the patients to have an optimized experience of the VR. Patients may associate physical world experiences with the VR when context information is delivered carefully. Besides the visual vividness, auditory context information and background sound should also be considered to stimulate active motor behaviour.

Even though each of the three feedback types individually is suggested to have an influence on motor learning or transfer, combining them together will probably be most effective for therapeutic VR applications. Therefore we assume that a consideration of all interrelationships between feedback types and an optimized support of the sense of presence in the virtual environment is important for a holistic realisation of motor learning.

ACKNOWLEDGMENTS

We thank Holger Regenbrecht for his feedback that helped to improve this manuscript.

REFERENCES

[1] Laver KE, George S, Thomas S, Deutsch JE, Crotty M. Virtual reality for stroke rehabilitation. Cochrane Database Syst Rev 2011;(9):CD008349.
[2] Lombard M, Ditton T. At the heart of it all: The concept of presence. J Comput Mediat Commun 1997;3(2):0.
[3] Schubert T, Friedmann F, Regenbrecht H. The experience of presence: Factor analytic insights. Presence (Camb) 2001;10(3):266–81.
[4] Riva G, Waterworth JA, Waterworth EL, Mantovani F. From intention to action: The role of presence. New Ideas Psychol 2010;29(1):24–37.
[5] International Society for Presence Research. The concept of presence: Explication statement, 2000. URL: http://ispr.info/
[6] Langhorne P, Bernhardt J, Kwakkel G. Stroke rehabilitation. Lancet 2011;377(9778):1693-702.
[7] Carr JH, Shepherd RB. Neurological rehabilitation: optimizing motor performance. New York: Churchill Livingstone, 2010.
[8] Thieme H, Mehrholz J, Pohl M, Behrens J, Dohle C. Mirror therapy for improving motor function after stroke. Cochrane Database Syst Rev 2012;(3): CD00 8449.
[9] Regenbrecht H, Franz EA, McGregor G, Dixon BG, Hoermann S. Beyond the looking glass: Fooling the brain with the augmented mirror box. Presence (Camb) 2011; 20(6):559–76.
[10] Hoermann S, Franz EA, Regenbrecht H. Referred sensations elicited by video-mediated mirroring of hands. PLoS One 2012;7(12):e50942.
[11] Regenbrecht H, Hoermann S, Ott C, Muller L, Franz E. Manipulating the experience of reality for rehabilitation applications. Proceed IEEE 2014;102(2):170–84.
[12] Ferreira dos Santos L, Schmidt H, Kruger J, Dohle C. Visualization of virtual reality neurological motor rehabilitation of the upper limb – a systematic review. Int Conf on Virtual Rehabilitation (ICVR) 2013:176-77.
[13] Doyle J, Kelly D, Caulfield B. Design considerations in therapeutic exergaming. 5th Int Conf Pervasive Computing Technologies for Healthcare 2011:389–93.
[14] Dohle C, Stephan KM, Valvoda JT, Hosseiny O, Tellmann L, Kuhlen, T, Seitz RJ, Freund HJ. Representation of virtual arm movements in precuneus. Exp Brain Res 2011;208(4):543–55.
[15] da Silva Cameirão M, Bermúdez i Badia S, Duarte E, Verschure PF. Virtual reality based rehabilitation speeds up functional recovery of the upper extremities after stroke. Restor Neurol Neurosci 2011;29(5):287–98.
[16] Wulf G. Attentional focus and motor learning: A review of 10 years of research. E-J Bewegung Training 2007; 1:4–14.
[17] Schüler T, Drehlmann S, Kane F, von Piekartz H. Presence and motor rehabilitation in an abstract virtual environment for stroke patients. Proceedings Presence Conference 2014.

Submitted: July 01, 2015. *Revised:* August 05, 2015. *Accepted:* August 10, 2015.

In: Alternative Medicine Research Yearbook 2017
Editor: Joav Merrick
ISBN: 978-1-53613-726-2
© 2018 Nova Science Publishers, Inc.

Chapter 13

CHALLENGES IN DEVELOPING NEW TECHNOLOGIES FOR SPECIAL NEEDS EDUCATION: A FORCE-FIELD ANALYSIS

Patrice L (Tamar) Weiss[1,*], PhD, OT, Susan VG Cobb[2], PhD, Massimo Zancanaro[3], MSc, Nirit Bauminger-Zviely[4], PhD, Sigal Eden[4], PhD, Eynat Gal[1], PhD, OT and Sarah J Parsons[5], PhD

[1]Department of Occupational Therapy and ICORE Learning in a NetworKed Society, University of Haifa, Haifa, Israel
[2]Human Factors Research Group, University of Nottingham, University Park, Nottingham, United Kingdom
[3]FBK – Fondazione Bruno Kessler, Italy
[4]School of Education, Bar–Ilan University, Ramat-Gan, Israel
[5]Southampton Education School, University of Southampton, Highfield, Southampton, United Kingdom

ABSTRACT

Introduction of new technologies for use in special needs education requires careful design to ensure that their use is suitable for the intended users in the context of use and that learners benefit from the experience. This paper discusses issues that influence implementation of collaborative technologies designed to support learning of social communication skills in young people with autism. Taking a reflective view of lessons learned during the COSPATIAL project, a force-field analysis was applied to identify positive factors contributing to successful application development and negative factors that disrupted progress and implementation of the software. On the basis of our experience in the COSPATIAL project, recommendations for future projects are made.

---

[*] Correspondence: Patrice L (Tamar) Weiss, Department of Occupational Therapy and ICORE Learning in a NetworKed Society, University of Haifa, Haifa, Israel. E-mail: tamar@research.haifa.ac.il.

Keywords: autism spectrum disorders, social competence, multi-user surface, cognitive behavioural therapy, force field analysis, collaborative virtual environments

INTRODUCTION

Autism spectrum disorders or conditions (ASC) affect behaviour and the ability to communicate and interact socially (1). Social competence, entailing a child's capacity to integrate behavioural, cognitive and affective skills in order to adapt flexibly to diverse social contexts and demands is one of the core skills that is impaired in children with high functioning autism. Social incompetence adversely affects a child's ability to learn in formal and informal educational settings, and to interact appropriately with other children (2). A variety of technologies have been used to train social competence of children with ASC. These include video modeling (3), virtual reality (4), socially assistive robots (5), and multi-user or multi-touch tabletop surfaces (6). To date, well-established practices for the design of technology to support therapeutic and educational interventions for these children are lacking (7).

A "force field" analysis is a framework for looking at the factors (forces) that influence the achievement of a designated objective and has recently been applied to the field of virtual reality for motor rehabilitation (8). It identifies the positive forces that help an application to move towards achieving its goal (driving forces) and the negative forces causing it to become more distant from its goal (restraining forces). This article presents a retrospective force-field analysis on COSPATIAL (http://cospatial.fbk.eu/), an EU-funded project whose goal was designing and creating collaborative technology applications to improve social competence of children with High Functioning Autism. The project investigated two categories of technologies for collaborative interaction: Collaborative Virtual Environments (CVE) and Shared Active Surfaces (SAS). Over a three year period, multidisciplinary design teams comprising technology developers, autism specialists, human factors researchers, teachers, and young people with autism located in three countries (Italy, Israel and UK) were brought together to develop software applications to support learning of social communication skills using each technology. 43 teachers from eight schools and 85 children (48 typically developing and 37 with ASC) were involved in participatory design and evaluation of CVEs and a further 12 teachers from five schools and 24 children with ASC were involved in the formative SAS studies.

The analysis was based on examination of the accumulated evidence and lessons learned throughout the three-year project with the purpose to reflect upon the causes of specific design outcomes and generate recommendations for future technologies. Four major driving forces and four major restraining forces relating to the field of collaborative technology-based social competence training for children with ASC (as well as other related applications) were identified.

DRIVING FORCES OF COLLABORATIVE TECHNOLOGIES

CVEs and SASs offer affordances that facilitate the design of collaborative activities. CVEs permit distributed synchronous communication, enabling children to talk directly to each other and work collaboratively but without physical proximity; SASs provide co-located, action-level collaboration (e.g., touching together). These technologies may be designed to empower teachers, allowing them the flexibility of controlling the pace of a session. They can also empower children by enabling them to become actively involved in the educational activities.

Use of a strong theoretical model to inform design of learning tasks

COSPATIAL used the principles of Cognitive-Behavioural Therapy to inform the design of technology applications, and their intended mode of use with children. Although COSPATIAL adhered to CBT principles, our prototypes did not require a fully compliant CBT intervention model. Nevertheless, care was taken to abide by the model's tenets in order to remain consistent with its underlying assumptions as well as the evidence that supports its use.

User involvement in the design process

Co-design and participatory design are needed to develop prototypes that are likely to be more acceptable to target users, even if they sometimes present significant challenges (due to constraints related to time, effort and technical complexity). It is crucial to implement the process in a manner that ensures sufficient time to involve all stakeholders so that they can achieve a comprehensive understanding of the applications and can learn to interact with each other. Since participatory design processes are not always feasible, different levels of feedback from users may need to be elicited. In addition, it is important to recognize the challenge of the design process when co-designing with a group of people with different backgrounds, levels of involvement, geographical locations.

Personalisation of educational technology

There is a strong need for teachers and therapists to be able to personalize technology tools. There will be less chance of adoption of a given technology if the design process produces a tool that is too specific to the original design objective (e.g., only social collaboration) or does not enable sufficient variations in levels of ability or styles of practice. Embracing a tactic of personalization will ensure a much wider usage in terms of educational objectives, target problems and the age and abilities of the children. Although personalization should aim to adapt features of the tool to meet a child's skills, it should also provide a truly flexible tool for the teachers to custom-build learning experiences.

RESTRAINING FORCES OF COLLABORATIVE TECHNOLOGIES

Technologies (particularly large tabletops or complex virtual reality systems) may be too cumbersome and expensive for daily use. This will likely limit and even impede their implementation in the school system. In educational frameworks that are dedicated specifically to children with ASC, the purchase and installation of specialized equipment and software may be feasible. However, in settings where mainstreaming is provided via special classes for children with ASC, the use of cumbersome equipment is less feasible. It is necessary to continue to explore lost-cost, low-encumbrance platforms to deploy the prototypes, for example, use of the multi-mice version of two of the COSPATIAL SAS applications that had originally been designed for a multi-touch tabletop (9) and COSPATIAL CVEs Block Challenge and Talk2U running on standard laptops (10). Educational software must take into account requirements related to the context of use (e.g., a classroom); constraints (e.g., cost, size) should be identified at an early development stage. Nevertheless, in the context of COSPATIAL, the possibility of experimenting with expensive and cutting-edge devices allowed us to identify and explore patterns of use (i.e., constraining the interaction via multiple, simultaneous actions) that were then scaled down to more affordable solutions (e.g., multi-mice approach).

Need for on-site instruction and support in technology usage

Despite widespread positive expression of interest in using collaborative technologies on the part of teachers, clinicians and parents, actual usage will only take place with on-going, on-site instruction and support. It is necessary to accompany the transition between research efforts (such as the COSPATIAL project) and actual use in everyday practice by means of projects that are more oriented toward development of learning resources and best-practices. It is necessary to identify constraints within the special education sector for children with ASC that facilitate the adoption of technology. For example, adoption of cumbersome systems in mainstream schools will be more difficult than in specialised schools or after-school centres. Successful adoption of technology will be more likely if they are tailored to the constraints of the setting in which they will be used. In planning the transition from a research prototype to a system actually used in real settings, the robustness of the software itself is not enough. Deploying the technology depends on maintenance and support which can only be assured by a commercial company. Such involvement need not happen from the outset; indeed, not having to satisfy the interests of specific companies gave COSPATIAL greater flexibility in exploring different platforms without being committed at too early a stage. However, commercial support for full exploitation is essential.

False expectations and misunderstandings during the design process

Although participatory design is a potentially effective approach for creating collaborative technologies, care must be taken throughout the entire process in order to avoid false expectations which can impede any positive effect. Thus, co-design must be implemented with emphasis on communication and clarification, especially when the teams are geographically distributed and have different backgrounds and languages. The judicious use of tools to trace decision-making and concept clarification help track when and why decisions are taken. In the case of ASC, including children in the design process is problematic because of their difficulties with Theory of Mind (understanding what the others think). Although rapid prototyping is often suggested as a remedy to enhance visualisation of the proposed design, the notion of "rapid" is very subjective; it may be too long relative to the overall length of the project where evaluation cannot commence until the software is more advanced.

Insufficient evidence-based practice

The lack of conditions that favour optimal research designs holds back progress by reducing the impact of a technology's results. Formative studies should be initially favoured in design-oriented projects especially when the duration is limited to three years and less. However, it is essential to fund longer-term intervention studies in order to achieve a solid base of evidence for the practice of novel technology applications. The experience with COSPATIAL is that the scientific community (both in the field of autism and in the field of human-computer interaction) is keen to accept results of small studies and these forums may help to fund the type of pilot and single case study design research that will lead to the funding of full, evidence-based research designs.

RECOMMENDATIONS

The difficulties experienced by COSPATIAL in aiming to both develop and evaluate software prototypes is not unique to autism research. Although a project evaluation plan needs to be realistic and adaptable during its lifecycle, it can be difficult to anticipate problematic issues when working with new design teams to develop novel applications that have not previously been used in an educational setting. Retrospective use of the force-field analysis of the COSPATIAL project enabled us to identify positive and negative factors that influenced project progress and outcome. On the basis of this reflective review, a number of recommendations are suggested that may facilitate future development of educational software using new technologies, intended both for special needs and mainstream educational contexts:

Establish a core design team representing key stakeholder groups

The use of a co-participatory design is not a trivial undertaking. In order to fully take advantage of this approach, it should be seriously applied from the beginning of the project by using appropriate methodological approaches (which may differ for individual users or groups of users) and explicitly controlling the process. The participation of all the stakeholders is fundamental but we have learned the presence of a core team of experts that helps to liaise with the core users (teachers and children) is essential.

Include all stakeholders in the design process

Input from the target users (in this case children with high functioning ASC together with teachers/therapists) was vital for promoting greater acceptance of the developed software. Thus, co-/participatory design should be employed in projects even if the target population has significant disabilities. Children with ASC can be included in the participatory design process, although it is necessary to adapt the activities to suit their unique characteristics as well as their individual needs (11). Moreover, there should be appropriate expertise represented within the research team to enable such participatory design processes to take place.

Do not assume shared understanding between design partners

In any multi-disciplinary co-design team, it is essential to manage the interactions and the expectations, to be clear about the goals and the procedures, to negotiate the level of participation and the different responsibilities of the people involved and to effectively, but precisely, trace the decisions taken during the process.

Base learning task design on learning theory but do not be afraid to apply 'cautious flexibility' and adapt it to suit user needs

CBT proved to be an effective theoretical framework to guide the design of the prototypes by providing a context to conceptualise the affordances offered by the CVE and SAS prototypes and to explore the advantages and limitations of those affordances in meeting the requirements of the CBT principles (e.g., dividing the session into two interleaved parts for learning (cognition) and experiencing (behaviour)). The CBT model also provided us with specific techniques and procedures, such as concept clarification and role-playing.

Conduct technology development and testing in the context of use

Implementation of new technology on the classroom or other learning environment beyond the lifetime of the project is more likely to be successful if all considerations relating to the context of use have been properly taken into account (12). Setting up demonstrations of pre-configured technology developed in the research lab is not sufficient; the equipment must be set up and used by teachers and other stakeholders *in situ*.

Utilise affordances of the technology that directly address core learning needs

The cost and inconvenience of using new technologies in education will be worthwhile if the added value to students is evident. Exploiting the affordances of CVE and SAS related to their inherent collaboration dimensions for tasks directly related to the core diagnostic difficulties of autism, offers learning tools that may not be available through other means and, in COSPATIAL, led to additional applications for other children with special needs.

ACKNOWLEDGMENTS

COSPATIAL (2009-2012) was funded under the Seventh Framework Programme of the European Commission (http://cospatial.fbk.eu/). We thank our project partners and also thank the students and teachers of our collaborating schools in the United Kingdom and Israel.

REFERENCES

[1] Bailey A, Phillips W, Rutter M. Autism: towards an integration of clinical genetic, neuropsychological, and neurobiological perspectives. J Child Psychol Psychiatry 1996;37:89–126.
[2] Bauminger N. The facilitation of social-emotional understanding and social interaction in high functioning children with autism: intervention outcomes. J Autism Dev Disord 2002; 32:283–98.
[3] Nikopoulos CK, Keenan M. Effects of video modeling on social initiations by children with autism. J Appl Behav Anal 2004;37(1):93-6.
[4] Parsons S, Cobb SVG. Reflections on the role of the 'users': challenges in a multi-disciplinary context of learner-centred design for children on the autism spectrum. Int J Res Method Educ 2014;37,421-41.
[5] Dautenhahn K, Werry I. Towards interactive robots in autism therapy: Background, motivation and challenges. Pragmatics Cogn 2004;12(1):1-35.
[6] Giusti L, Zancanaro M, Gal E, Weiss PL. Dimensions of collaboration on a tabletop interface for children with autism spectrum disorder. In: Proceedings of CHI 2011. Vancouver, Canada, ACM Press, New York, 7–12 May 2011.
[7] Davis M, Dautenhahn K, Powel SD, Nehaniv CL. Guidelines for researchers and facilitators designing software and software trials for children with autism. J Assist Technol 2010;4:38-48.
[8] Weiss PL, Keshner EA, Levin MF. Current and future trends for VR and motor rehabilitation. In: Weiss PL, Keshner EA, Levin MF, eds. Virtual reality technologies for health and clinical applications. Vol 1: Applying virtual reality technologies to motor rehabilitation. Dordrecht: Springer, 2014.
[9] Weiss PL, Cobb SVG, Gal E, Millen L, Hawkins T, Glover T, Sanassy D, Eden S, Giusti L, Zancanaro M. Usability of technology supported social competence training for children on the autism spectrum. International conference on virtual rehabilitation. Zurich, Switzerland, June 2011.
[10] Cobb SVG, Hawkins T, Millen L, Wilson JR. Design and development of 3D interactive environments for special needs education. In: Hale KS, Stanney KM, eds. Handbook of virtual environments: Design, implementation and applications, 2nd ed. Boca Raton, FL: CRC Press, 2014.
[11] Millen L, Cobb SVG, Patel H, Glover T. Collaborative virtual environment for conducting design sessions with students with autism spectrum conditions. Proceed 9th Intl Conf. on Disability, Virtual Reality and Assoc Technologies. France, 2012; 269-278.
[12] Parsons S, Guldberg K, Porayska-Pomsta K, Lee R. Digital stories as a method for evidence-based practice and knowledge co-creation in technology-enhanced learning for children with autism. Int J Res Method Educ 2015;38:247-71.

Submitted: July 01, 2015. *Revised:* August 05, 2015. *Accepted:* August 10, 2015.

In: Alternative Medicine Research Yearbook 2017
Editor: Joav Merrick
ISBN: 978-1-53613-726-2
© 2018 Nova Science Publishers, Inc.

Chapter 14

GRID-PATTERN INDICATING INTERFACE FOR AMBIENT ASSISTED LIVING

Zeeshan Asghar[1,*], MSc, Goshiro Yamamoto[2], PhD, Yuki Uranishi[3], PhD, Christian Sandor[2], PhD, Tomohiro Kuroda[3], PhD, Petri Pulli[1], PhD and Hirokazu Kato[2], PhD

[1]Department of Information Processing Science, University of Oulu, Oulu, Finland
[2]Graduate School of Information Science, Nara Institute of Science and Technology, Ikoma, Nara, Japan
[3]Kyoto University Hospital, Kyoto University, Sakyo-Ku, Kyoto, Japan

ABSTRACT

This study proposes a grid-pattern indicating interface to provide instructions remotely for supporting the daily activities of elderly people living in their homes independently. Our aim is to realize smooth and easy telecommunication between supported senior citizens at their local site and supporting caregivers who are at a remote site. Although we have used a monitoring method with video streaming where the remote caregivers indicate work steps in a conventional way, occlusion and depth perception problems were occurring. Our proposed method can provide a grid-pattern interface to remote caregivers, which could be a solution for the occlusion and depth perception problems by indicating the spatial instruction easily on a 2D input interface. In this study, a prototype has been implemented with a colour camera, a range image sensor, and projector. It also demonstrated that the proposed grid-pattern indicating interface can help caregivers show an instruction easily and intuitively.

Keywords: ambient assisted living, senior citizen, projector camera system, caregiver

---

[*] Correspondence: Zeeshan Asghar, MSc, Department of Information Processing Science, University of Oulu, 90014, Oulu, Finland. E-mail: zeeshan.asghar@oulu.fi.

INTRODUCTION

Most countries around the world are facing serious aging situations nowadays. It has been estimated by the year of 2050 in Finland and Japan, the proportion of people over the age of 65 years will cover 27% and 33% of the total population, respectively. The number of senior citizens who suffer from varying memory impairments is also going to double during the next 30 years (1). The increase in senior population requires more caregivers inevitably and pressure on the health care system. However, most of the caregivers have already reported physical and mental problems (2, 3). We need to consider the balance between the supporting generation and the supported generation, and avoid from making negative feedback loops by increasing the numbers of heavily supported persons. On the other hand, those persons who have mild cognitive impairment just need a small amount of assistance to avoid deterioration in memory. One of our goals is to realize the ambient assisted living environment that allows 5 to 10 caregivers to support 10 to 30 senior citizens remotely via the Internet. Here, we propose a grid-pattern indicating interface as an easy instruction system to make the burdens of caregivers as moderate as possible.

We focus on a kitchen workspace, because cooking is an important part of daily life for elderly people living independently in their homes. Generally a cooking process consists of a series of steps and completing a step requires various kitchen items. A kitchen assistive system must know the location of the items in advance; those items might be found in an open or a closed place in a kitchen. Finding and working with the exact items plays an important role in the completion of a cooking step. If a user is unable to find an exact item, the cooking step will not be completed. Our challenge is to create a remote collaborative situation in the kitchen, paying special attention to how easily the remote caregiver can provide better instructions to a senior citizen at the local site. Here, we propose a grid-pattern interface solution for remote caregivers to indicate points in the space at the local site.

RELATED RESEARCH

Recent development in information and communication technologies can be used to develop smart living tools to assist elderly people in their daily activities, in both known and unknown environments. In addition, the availability of small, powerful and bright video projectors enables the augmentation of real objects with non-invasive displays. By adding a camera and using computer vision techniques, a projector system can also dynamically detect and track objects, correct for object surface geometry, varying surface colour and texture and allow the user to interact directly with the projected image (4). In a recent study, Yamamoto et al. (5) described the need for novel user interfaces for senior citizens to help in their daily lives and developed a projection based display system which can display information on physical surfaces according to markers. Suzuki et al. (6) have demonstrated that the visual presentation of cooking instructions was more effective than text based instruction using a projector camera system. Ikeda et al. (7) have developed a smart kitchen system in which visual prompts are displayed on a plane surfaces such as counter tops and door of cabinets using a projector and a camera. Bonanni et al. (8) have developed the 'augmented reality kitchen', which includes illuminating drawer handles to guide users to the location of utensils. In another study, Yamamoto et al. (9) have implemented 'PiTaSu,' a direct input interface system which offers visual and tactile feedback to assist memory impaired senior citizens in their daily task.

As described in the previous studies, there have different types of intervention that can be used to assist elderly people, but fewer systems have been developed which can assist elderly and caregivers in a smart living environment. Our solution is based on a projector-camera system which is a combination of a camera and projector, to assist remote caregivers in order to find an object in an unknown environment and also provide visual information as guidance or as a set of instructions on a physical surface to the elderly person.

METHODS

We propose a grid-pattern indicating interface for remote caregivers to assist local persons remotely. The whole system consists of two sites: a local site where assisted persons are performing some activity, e.g., cooking, and a remote site, where caregivers are guiding them to perform that activity. Figure 1(a) shows the overview of our conceptual system. The remote site has a remote monitoring view and grid interface on the computer screen. At the local site, in the kitchen workspace, a camera, a range image sensor, and a projector are installed. The camera captures a scene from the workspace, including the objects and the surfaces. In order to realize our system, we need to calibrate geometrical relations between each device as shown in Figure 1(b). Using the result of the calibration, we can keep the correspondence between the grid-pattern interface view and the real workspace.

System calibration

There are three coordinate systems: a camera coordinate system; a range image sensor coordinate system; and a projector coordinate system as shown in Figure 1(b). We can develop the geometric relationship within in the target scene by calculating each transformation matrix between each coordinate system in advance. The transformation matrices can be obtained by using a referential coordinate system.

First, the transformation matrix between the range image coordinate system and the referential coordinate system is estimated. The range image sensor captures the scene with the referential object as range data, and then three plane surfaces of the referential object are detected. The three normal vectors corresponding to the three plane surfaces are used as basis vectors, and in the referential object coordinate system the intersection of three plane surfaces is used as the origin.

Second, we can estimate the transformation matrices corresponding to the colour camera and the projector by applying a Gray code pattern projection (10). The basis vectors and the origin of the referential object that is represented in the camera or projector coordinate system are estimated according to the measured geometry of the scene which includes the referential object. As a last step in the main calibration process, we need to compute the transformation matrices between each device. For example, the transformation matrix M_{rc} is computed by simple multiplication, where only the relative positions between the devices need to be maintained during use. In other words, a simultaneous movement of the devices is allowed. It indicates that the system can be moved freely if the devices are fixed in their locations.

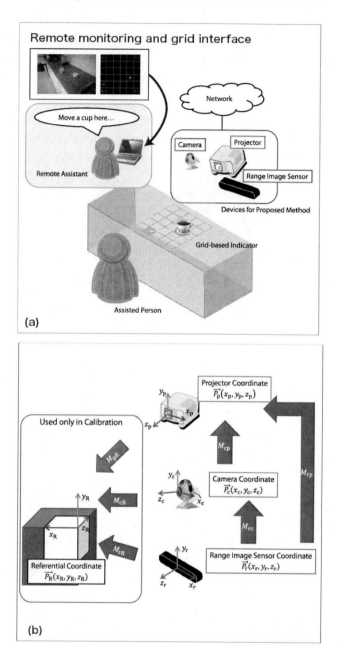

Figure 1. Our conceptual system and the coordinate systems of the devices. (a) The remote caregiver can monitor the local site remotely with a grid-pattern indicating interface via the Internet. (b) Geometrical relations between each device need to be calibrated in advance.

Target surface estimation and object locating

There are mainly two steps. First is the estimation of a parameter of the target planar for fixing the grid-pattern area in the workspace and the second is visualizing a position and a colour of the target objects on the grid-pattern view for the remote caregivers.

First, we estimated the dominant plane from the range image that has a certain colour. The colour of each pixel in the range image is given from the converted camera image via M_{cr}, where $M_{cr} = M_{rc}^{-1}$. Second, the pixels extracted as the target planar surface are clustered according to the distance between each point. Finally, each cluster is projected onto the two dimensional coordinate system of the target planar surface after the centre of gravity has been calculated. Then the average colour and the position of each cluster (with greater than a certain number of points) are shown in the grid-pattern view.

Grid pattern indications

We assume a situation where a remote caregiver gives some instructions to a senior citizen in his/her home. The simple instruction can be for example to find an item from the kitchen cabinet and place it on the worktop. When the caregiver gives these instructions, communication of spatial information of where the remote caregiver is indicating will be important for the senior citizen. In the conventional way, the remote caregiver monitors the senior with video streaming and indicates a location by speaking or clicking on the monitoring view. The monitoring makes it easier to understand in terms of spatial information. Nevertheless, there is still the remaining problem of occlusion and depth perception, which can cause mistakes in a remote caregiver's judgment. A grid-pattern indicating view for a remote caregiver is one possible solution that can avoid such occlusion and depth perception issues.

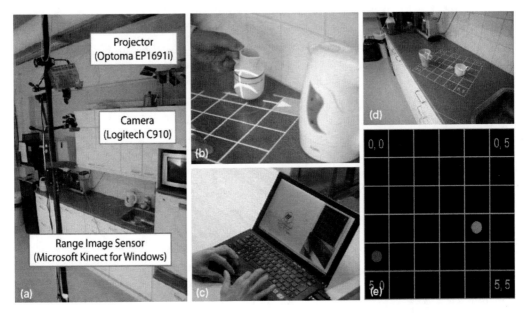

Figure 2. Our prototype system: (a) overview of the prototype system that mainly consists of a colour camera, a range image sensor, and a projector on the pole to project visual instructing information onto the kitchen workspace, (b) the scene of local site with projected lights, (c) the scene of remote site with grid-pattern indicating interface on a computer screen, (d) the view of local site and (e) the grid-pattern interface, respectively, that are shown on the computer to the caregivers at the remote site.

IMPLEMENTATION

We implemented a prototype system as shown in Figure 2. The camera is a Logitech C910 which captures 640 × 480 pixel images. The range image sensor was a Microsoft Kinect for Windows which outputs 320 × 240 pixel range images. The projector is an Optoma EP1691i Digital Light Processing Projector which projects a 1280 × 768 pixel image in onto a physical surface. Additionally, we applied Point Cloud Library 1.5.1, OpenCV 2.4.0, and Microsoft Kinect for Windows 1.5 to our prototype system.

We demonstrated the implemented system with several test users briefly, observing that most of the remote caregivers could indicate where he/she wanted to indicate in the space of the local site. However, we did not confirm how precisely they could indicate with the grid-pattern interface. On the other hand, visualizing the projected grid-pattern onto the local site would not be really needed for the senior citizen to understand where the remote caregiver indicates. Projection with infrared lights could be a method to make invisible and visible grid-patterns on the target surface simultaneously for the local and the remote person, respectively.

CONCLUSION

We have proposed a grid-pattern indicating interface for remote caregivers in ambient assisted living. Our method was implemented by installing a colour camera, a range image sensor, and a projector on the local site. The grid interface could have corresponded to the real workspace of the local site with calibration between each device. Finally, we briefly confirmed how the implemented prototype operated while the test users indicated remotely. Future work includes a user test to confirm the accuracy or ease of use of our method, making the available workspace bigger, and improving object recognition for representing the real situation into the grid-pattern interface.

ACKNOWLEDGMENTS

We are thankful to Academy of Finland-Japan Science and Technology Agency (AF-JST) as the Japan-Finland Research Cooperative Program.

REFERENCES

[1] Ferri CP, Prince M, Brayne C, Brodaty H, Fratiglioni L, Ganguli M, et al. Global prevalence of dementia: a Delphi consensus study. Lancet 2005;366:2112–7.
[2] Schulz R, Visintainer P, Williamson GM. Psychiatric and physical morbidity effects of caregiving: Prevalence, Correlates, and Causes. Gerontologist 1995; 35(6):771-91.
[3] Rabins PV, Mace NL, Lucas MJ. The impact of dementia on the family. JAMA 1982;248:333-5.
[4] Molyneaux D, Gellersen H, Kortuem G, Schiele B. Cooperative augmentation of smart objects with projector-camera systems. Proceed Ubicomp 2007; 4717:27–39.

[5] Yamamoto G, Hyry J, Pouke M, Metso A, Hickey S, Pulli P. Senior citizens' interaction with smart ambient environment. 16th International ICE-Conference on Engineering, Technology and Innovation, 2010.

[6] Suzuki Y, Morioka S, Ueda H. Cooking support with information projection onto ingredient. Presented at the Proceedings of the 10th Asia Pacific conference on Computer human interaction 2012:193-8.

[7] Ikeda S, Asghar Z, Hyry J, Pulli P, Pitkanen A, Kato H. Remote assistance using visual prompts for demented elderly in cooking. Proceed of the 4th International Symposium on Applied Sciences in Biomedical and Communication Technologies 2011;46:5.

[8] Bonanni L, Lee CH, Selker T. Counter intelligence: Augmented reality kitchen. Proceed CHI 2005, ACM Press, 2005.

[9] Yamamoto G, Kuroda T, Yoshitake D, Hickey S, Hyry J, Chihara K, Pulli P. PiTaSu: wearable interface for assisting senior citizens with memory problems. Int J Disabil Hum Dev 2011;10(4):295-300.

[10] Sato A, Watanabe K, Rekimoto J. MimiCook: A cooking assistant system with situated guidance. Proceed TEI 2014:121-4.

Submitted: July 05, 2015. *Revised:* August 09, 2015. *Accepted:* August 14, 2015.

In: Alternative Medicine Research Yearbook 2017
Editor: Joav Merrick

ISBN: 978-1-53613-726-2
© 2018 Nova Science Publishers, Inc.

Chapter 15

REALISTIC AND ADAPTIVE COGNITIVE TRAINING USING VIRTUAL CHARACTERS

Daniel Sjölie[*], PhD
Department of Computer Science and Engineering, University of Gothenburg, Gothenburg, Sweden

ABSTRACT

Computer-aided cognitive training has the potential to be an important tool in the fight against dementia and cognitive decline but there are many challenges. This article presents an example of how realistic and adaptive training can be used to address these challenges. Virtual characters were used as stimuli in a dual n-back working memory task in a realistic 3D-environment. Support for continuous adaptation was a priority, including adaption based on affective states such as arousal.

Keywords: cognitive training, virtual environments, virtual characters, brain-computer interface, adaptive training

INTRODUCTION

An aging world population makes the need for methods to combat dementia and age-related cognitive decline increasingly urgent. Computer-aided cognitive training has been championed as one such method with great potential (1, 2). Unfortunately, recent research has shown that it is very difficult to achieve general cognitive improvements with cognitive training, i.e., transfer effects (3). In this contribution we provide an example of how solutions building on an understanding of human brain function in realistic environments can be used to meet this challenge. The importance of realistic interaction and the ecological validity of

---

[*] Correspondence: Daniel Sjölie, PhD, Department of Computer Science and Engineering, University of Gothenburg, S-412 96 Gothenburg, Sweden. E-mail: daniel.sjolie@cse.gu.se.

training are fundamental motivations for the use of virtual reality (VR) for rehabilitation and training (4, 5).

The difficulty to gain general improvements from cognitive training is commonly described in terms of a distinction between near transfer and far transfer. Training a particular task often leads to improvements on similar tasks (near transfer). Transfer to tasks with no clear similarity to the trained task, however, (far transfer) has proved difficult (2, 6). Much recent work on cognitive training has been focused on trying to get general improvements related to, e.g., attention or working memory. Such general improvements should result in improved performance in everyday tasks, such as remembering what to shop for, but they require far transfer. One response to this difficulty of achieving far transfer is to focus on near transfer and on the need to train the right thing by, for example, using interactive systems with high ecological validity. Reality-based human-computer interaction (HCI) in general and virtual reality (VR) in particular provides a foundation for ecologically valid computer applications by building on the user's skills and experiences from reality (7, 8).

Previous work

One form of cognitive training that has attracted much attention is working memory (WM) training. Working memory capacity predicts performance in a wide range of cognitive tasks, and many neuropsychiatric conditions such as stroke or attention-deficit hyperactivity disorder (ADHD) coincide with impaired WM (1). Several studies have shown that performance on specific WM tasks such as 2-back (comparing the last number in a sequence to the one presented 2 steps before) does improve with training and that this effect does transfer to similar (near-transfer) tasks (1–3, 6). However, the magnitude and range of transfer, in particular the potential for far-transfer, remains disputed. Studies comparing transfer effects in old and young adults have presented seemingly conflicting results. A study by Dahlin et al. concluded that while transfer to untrained tasks is possible for both young and old the magnitude varies and it is often harder to demonstrate transfer in old adults (6). In other studies, transfer effects in young and old have been compared without any reliable differences (2). More generally, Owen et al. (3) failed to show any general cognitive improvements for 11,430 participants training on cognitive tasks online for several weeks. Suggested reasons for such results include variations in the amount and intensity of the training (sometimes with significant individual variance) as well as differences in the overlap between trained tasks and the evaluated transfer task.

One common working memory training task is n-back. In a basic implementation of the n-back task the subject may be presented with a series of numbers and asked to compare each new number to the one seen n steps before. e.g., with $n = 1$ the question is if the new number is the same as the last, with $n = 2$ if it is the same as the number before the last, etc. This requires the subject to constantly remember n previous numbers and to update this list each time a new number is presented. The numbers can be exchanged for any stimuli. In the spatial n-back version subjects need to remember where a stimulus was presented n steps back, and compare it to the location of new stimuli. If the stimulus itself is also varied this becomes a dual *n*-back task, where the subject must remember and compare both position and identity. This is a very demanding cognitive task, providing one way to increase the intensity of the training. Training on a dual spatial *n*-back test with sound as the second stimuli has been shown to improve measures of fluid (i.e., general) intelligence (9).

Presence and synchronization for virtual rehabilitation

Presence has traditionally been described as the sense of "being there" in a virtual environment (10), but recent elaborations have a closer connection to cognition and the human brain. An emphasis on presence as hypothesis selection (11) connects to the importance of predictions and prediction errors in recent theories of brain function and presence as "the ability to act there" connects to the use of existing motor representations (12). The concept of mental simulations can be helpful in understanding why existing expectations and representations are so important and in getting a handle on how cognitive training can be designed with this in mind. Mental simulation includes unconscious and flexible reactivation of memories, employed to recognize the current context and to simulate, or predict, possible actions and expected results (13). The idea that predicting future events based on previous experience is a critical aspect of how the brain works has gathered increasing support in recent years. It is prominent in recent theories of cognition and brain function by Hawkins (14), Friston (15) and others. A recent paper by Clark (16) provides a broad introduction.

Particularly interesting for presence and virtual rehabilitation is how this framework suggests that the brain essentially implements a running simulation of reality. This has prompted descriptions of presence as related to the synchronization between an external environment (real or virtual) and the subjective mental reality simulated by the brain (17). Related theories of brain function provide a basis for understanding how such synchronization develops and how we may design a virtual environment to facilitate synchronization of specific mental simulations, corresponding to cognitive skills. For example, the combination of familiar stimuli with a familiar context should provide an optimal foundation for internalization and adaptation of a specific task (i.e., learning).

REALISTIC COGNITIVE TRAINING

We have implemented a version of the dual *n*-back task using a realistic 3D-environment with animated characters in order to increase the familiarity and realism of both the stimuli and the environmental context (Figure 1). The task is transformed to remembering which characters have made which movements over the last few steps. The moving character corresponds to the position and the different animations correspond to the second stimuli. Based on the reasoning presented above, learning to keep track of who did what just a minute ago, in a realistic 3D-environment, should have a greater chance of producing transfer to similar everyday situations than training using, for example, *n*-back with arbitrary images at different 2D positions.

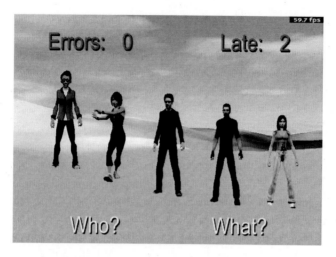

Figure 1. This task was inspired by the dual n-back task used by Jaeggi et al. (9). The stimuli to keep track of is who (which of the characters) is/was doing what (which animation) n steps back.

Much effort was spent on making it possible to balance the difficulty of the training. A gamepad was used to provide a clear and simple interface with few buttons. Buttons on the front of the gamepad were used to answer the repeated n-back question of whether the stimuli were the same or not, with buttons on the right and left respectively for each question (what/who, see figure 1). Normally, new stimuli is presented at regular time intervals but in order to reduce the risk of subjects giving up completely if they get behind we introduced an optional mode to wait for the subject to respond. This was coupled with feedback on late responses and a count of late responses. The feedback was very noticeable as the lighting in the entire virtual environment changed. Similar feedback was given in response to wrong answers. The duration of the regular time interval could also be changed to adapt the level of stress in the task. The application has been implemented using Panda3D, a full featured 3D game engine.

Adapting to affective state

Synchronization and optimal training depends on a suitable level of prediction errors. According to activity theory (18), any human activity is driven by a need to change something in the environment. Something important that is not as we would prefer it to be, or it does not match our "prediction" of the ideal world, then the mismatch arouses us to action. Based on such reasoning we attempted to measure the subject's level of arousal throughout the training using Self-Assessment Manikin (SAM, Figure 2) questions at regular intervals.

In an attempt to provide automatic adaptation of the cognitive training, we used a commercial EEG headset (Emotiv EPOC) to try to measure mental workload related to arousal. Data was collected over 13 trials with 4 subjects before data collection was aborted because of poor classification performance. The classification of the EEG data was not good enough to enable successful automatic adaptation for most users, but trends for selected subjects suggest that such adaptation may be possible given optimal conditions (see Figure 3).

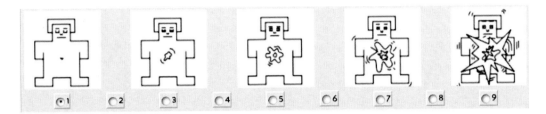

Figure 2. The Self-Assessment Manikin (SAM) may be used to present a visual scale of affective dimensions to users to get quick responses. We used scales for arousal (shown here) and valence with 5 manikin images plus in-between scale steps.

FUTURE WORK

In order to further investigate the effect of the realistic and adaptive cognitive training presented here it needs to be compared to solutions with varying degrees of realism and adaptively. Our system already implements more traditional *n*-back tasks such as images shown on different locations, in 2D- or 3D-space. This makes it possible to evaluate training with logically identical tasks while stimuli and environments vary in familiarity and realism. It is also possible to increase the realism of the environment and context by immersing the subject in the virtual environment using traditional VR technologies such as head-mounted displays (HMDs). The recent development of affordable HMDs (Figure 3) suggests that such systems may indeed become common in the near future. Support for the Oculus Rift is under development for the Panda3D engine used to build our application. Ideally, such different setups should be used to train a large number of subjects over a significant period of time, followed by an evaluation of the resulting transfer to different tasks, including everyday activities.

While the automatic adaptation using EEG failed initially, the basic motivations for implementing such functions are valid and much remains to investigate. Alternative psychophysiological measures such as galvanic skin response (GSR) or functional near-infrared spectroscopy (fNIRS) would be interesting to evaluate, and a combination of new headsets and improved training protocols may give EEG a new chance.

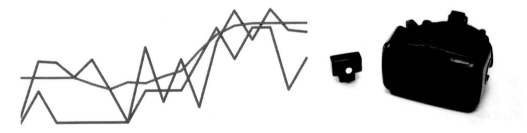

Figure 3. Left: Example of classified arousal (red) and reported arousal (blue) based on EEG measurements. The Y-axis is arousal (on a 0.0-1.0 scale) and the X-axis is consecutive 1-minute task blocks over one trial. Notice the trend when classified arousal is smoothed (green). Right: The recent DK2 version of the commercial and affordable Oculus Rift HMD.

ACKNOWLEDGMENTS

Thanks to Lars-Erik Janlert and Johan Eriksson for comments on the development of the prototype. Thanks to Kempe Foundations and Umeå University for funding.

REFERENCES

[1] Klingberg T. Training and plasticity of working memory. Trends Cogn Sci 2010;14(7):317–24.
[2] Li S-C, Schmiedek F, Huxhold O, Röcke C, Smith J, Lindenberger U. Working memory plasticity in old age: Practice gain, transfer, and maintenance. Psychol Aging 2008;23(4):731–42.
[3] Owen AM, Hampshire A, Grahn JA, Stenton R, Dajani S, Burns AS, et al. Putting brain training to the test. Nature 2010;465(7299):775–8.
[4] Pugnetti L, Mendozzi L, Motta A, Cattaneo A, Barbieri E, Brancotti A. Evaluation and retraining of adults' cognitive impairments: Which role for virtual reality technology? Comput Biol Med 1995;25(2):213–27.
[5] Rizzo AA, Buckwalter JG, McGee JS, Bowerly T, Zaag C van der, Neumann U, et al. Virtual environments for assessing and rehabilitating cognitive / functional performance. A review of projects at the USC Integrated Media Systems Center. Presence Teleoperators Virtual Environ 2001;10(4):359–74.
[6] Dahlin E, Neely AS, Larsson A, Backman L, Nyberg L. Transfer of learning after updating training mediated by the striatum. Science 2008;320(5882):1510–2.
[7] Jacob RJK, Girouard A, Hirshfield LM, Horn MS, Shaer O, Solovey ET, et al. Reality-based interaction: a framework for post-WIMP interfaces. Proc CHI 2008, ACM Press, 2008.
[8] Rizzo AA, Schultheis M, Kerns KA, Mateer C. Analysis of assets for virtual reality applications in neuropsychology. Neuropsychol Rehabil 2004;14 (1): 207–39.
[9] Jaeggi SM, Buschkuehl M, Jonides J, Perrig WJ. Improving fluid intelligence with training on working memory. Proc Natl Acad Sci 2008;105(19):6829–33.
[10] Slater M. Presence and the sixth sense. Presence Teleoperators Virtual Environ 2002;11(4):435–9.
[11] Sanchez-Vives MV, Slater M. From presence to consciousness through virtual reality. Nat Rev Neurosci 2005;6(4):332–9.
[12] Jäncke L, Cheetham M, Baumgartner T. Virtual reality and the role of the prefrontal cortex in adults and children. Front Neurosci 2009;3(1):52-9.
[13] Barsalou LW. Grounded Cognition. Annu Rev Psychol 2008;59(1):617–45.
[14] Hawkins J. On Intelligence. New York: Owl Books, 2005.
[15] Friston K. The free-energy principle: a unified brain theory? Nat Rev Neurosci 2010;11(2):127–38.
[16] Clark A. Whatever next? Predictive brains, situated agents, and the future of cognitive science. Behav Brain Sci 2013;36(03):181–204.
[17] Sjölie D. Presence and general principles of brain function. Interact Comput 2012;24(4):193–202.
[18] Kaptelinin V, Nardi B. Activity theory in HCI: Fundamentals and reflections. Synth Lect Hum-Centered Inform 2012;5(1):1–105.

Submitted: July 07, 2015. *Revised:* August 10, 2015. *Accepted:* August 15, 2015.

In: Alternative Medicine Research Yearbook 2017
Editor: Joav Merrick
ISBN: 978-1-53613-726-2
© 2018 Nova Science Publishers, Inc.

Chapter 16

CONDUCTING FOCUS GROUPS IN SECOND LIFE® ON HEALTH-RELATED TOPICS

Alice B Krueger[1,*], MS, Patrice Colletti[1], SDS, MA, MS, Hillary R Bogner[2], MD, MSCE, Frances K Barg[2], PhD, MEd and Margaret Grace Stineman[2], MD

[1]Virtual Ability® Inc., Aurora, Colorado
[2]University of Pennsylvania Perelman School of Medicine, Philadelphia, Pennsylvania, US

ABSTRACT

The "Mrs. A and Mr. B" research project uses focus groups conducted in the virtual world Second Life® to collect qualitative data on healthcare equitability as experienced by persons with and without disabilities. Novel methodological adaptations to traditional focus group methods include avatar consent, text discussion, participant advance preparation and disability accommodation. In this project, focus group findings are used to enrich and clarify results obtained from the analysis of a quantitative administrative dataset derived from Medicare data. Advantages and challenges of using virtual world focus groups are highlighted.

Keywords: focus groups, qualitative methodology, persons with disabilities, disability, virtual world, Second Life, avatar consent, participant advance preparation, healthcare equity, health care

INTRODUCTION

The "Mrs. A and Mr. B" project (www.healthcare equitability.org) examines disparities in healthcare from the perspectives of persons with disabilities. While disparities have been

---

[*] Correspondence: Alice B Krueger, Virtual Ability® Inc, 2220 S Fraser, Unit 1, Aurora, CO 80014, United States. E-mail: akrueger@virtualability.org.

examined related to gender, racial/ethnic group, economic status and education level, less is known about the quality of healthcare received by persons with disabilities and the effects this has on their life outcomes. The "Mrs. A and Mr. B" project (1), funded by the Patient-Centered Outcomes Research Institute (PCORI) in 2013, uses a mixed methods approach to address this question. A parallel mixed methods design is being used to quantify how access and quality of health care impacts the progression of disabilities and survival alongside a qualitative exploration of ways that people with and without disabilities experience healthcare in their daily lives. The quantitative portion of the study includes an in-depth analysis of ten years of administrative data from more than 41,000 adult Medicare beneficiaries. The qualitative arm of the study includes focus groups conducted in the virtual world Second Life® and in a face-to-face format. People with a wide range of disabilities add a stakeholder voice to the interpretations. The purpose of this article is to highlight the novel features of virtual world focus group functioning. Improved understanding of disparities related to disability from multiple perspectives may inform public policy and clinical practice.

METHODS

A team-based approach to research involving multiple stakeholder groups is recommended in order to increase the likelihood of improving healthcare. The "Mrs. A and Mr. B" project team involves members from the University of Pennsylvania Perelman School of Medicine and the Virtual Ability community in Second Life. Stakeholders are involved in all aspects of the research. The project team has worked to adapt the focus group methodology to the virtual world setting. Novel adaptations include: tailoring focus group facilitator training to fit an on-line format in a way that accommodates all persons with disabilities, establishing recruitment and consent procedures that assure protection of confidentiality, avoid coercion and enhance opportunities for participation, and developing procedures to facilitate participation for persons with all forms of disability.

Focus groups in virtual worlds

Traditionally, focus groups have been used in business for feedback on perceptions, attitudes, and opinions toward products or services being proposed or offered. During the introductory cycle of Second Life, when mainline businesses such as Nike and Nissan were exploring virtual worlds for traditional marketing purposes, virtual world focus groups were tried and found to be less effective than face-to-face market test groups, although some industry professionals still recommend them, with appropriate modifications. Focus groups are particularly useful when the purpose of the research is to observe in real time how participants interact around a given topic. The focus group facilitator creates a script with open-ended questions to guide the discussion. The role of the facilitator includes generating discussion, encouraging participation from all members, preventing monopolization by one individual and protecting all members from risks of breaches of confidentiality, premature disclosure or dysfunctional group dynamics. Recently, focus groups with an academic focus have been attempted in the virtual world Second Life. Stendal (2) conducted usage studies with persons with disabilities to determine level of participation and interest in virtual worlds. Input into the Access Board's public commentary about accessibility of medical diagnostic equipment was collected from focus groups in Second Life (3). The "Mrs. A and Mr. B" project will hold 4-6 virtual focus groups regarding disability and healthcare during each of the three years of the study.

Focus group facilitator selection and training

Focus group facilitators are trained in the virtual world Second Life by project staff. Criteria for selection include having previous experience as a researcher using Second Life and having excellent written English language skills. Facilitators must be comfortable working with diverse people, able to think quickly in social situations, and willing to act with discretion regarding personal health information.

All current trainees and trainers are very familiar with communicating through an avatar in a virtual world, with no less than 62 months of experience. All staff participated in an online Collaborative Institutional Training Initiative (CITI) course ("Biomedical Research, Basic Course"). Facilitators received training specific to their role. Task-specific training includes generic focus group facilitation knowledge and skills for roles both as a focus group leader and as an assistant. Trainees develop knowledge of common virtual world disability-related accommodations. The final steps in facilitator training involve conducting mock focus groups with participants. The actions of the trainees are observed and evaluated by project staff. At the end of each training session, project staff debrief both the trainees and the mock participants, allowing further modification of the procedures to improve virtual world focus group processes.

Virtual world focus group procedures

The project design includes both face-to-face and virtual focus groups. While these two types of focus groups cover identical content, the procedures for the two formats vary. Recruiting and consenting for participation in focus groups in Second Life is initiated through multiple means including the exchange of on-line Project Information notecards, the virtual world equivalent of text documents. The notecard presented to potential participants explains the research process and describes what research participation means to the potential focus group member. The information may also be provided orally in a group or individual setting. Project staff are available through instant messaging (IM) or email to answer questions before consent is obtained.

Potential participants give their consent by typing their avatar name of choice and the date on a notecard that is attached to the Project Information notecard. Demographic information (but not participant name) about the participant behind the avatar is maintained in a database separate from the focus group information. The necessity to obtain and type on this notecard and return it to a project staff member mitigates unintentional consent. These research protocols were approved by the University of Pennsylvania Institutional Review Board (IRB).

Focus group meetings take place in a secure location, 1000 meters in the sky above a Second Life island designated for research, see Figure 1. The virtual land that the meeting space is over can be made private so that only specified avatars (focus group facilitators, participants, and project staff) can enter the area. The virtual space is set up similar to a physical focus group space, see Figure 2.

The focus group facilitator has the text of the focus group script on a notecard, from which individual segments can be copy/pasted into the text chat stream. This allows the facilitator to follow the IRB-approved script while still maintaining the flexibility to insert additional probes, clarifications, or other material as needed, akin to the flexibility of a face-to-face facilitator.

As of the end of June 2015, eight virtual world (Second Life) groups (37 participants) and two face-to-face group (9 participants) have been run. Transcripts from all focus groups are de-identified to remove all names and potential personally identifiable health data.

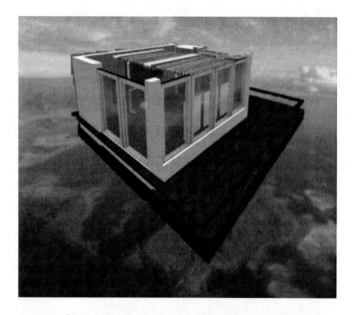

Figure 1. Focus group room, floating far above the virtual land surface.

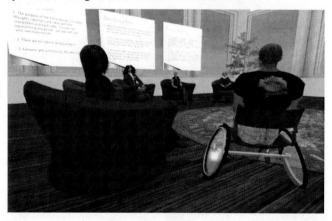

Figure 2. Focus group session showing interior of virtual focus group room and posters of expectations of participants.

The Mixed Methods Research Lab at the University of Pennsylvania receives the de-identified transcripts, enters the transcripts into NVivo 10.0 software (a qualitative data management program) and applies codes to the transcripts in order to identify themes across focus groups. Initial analysis indicates emerging ideas of patients' perceptions about their healthcare. Trends include the importance of self-advocacy, the impersonal nature of doctor-patient interactions, and the lack of communication among healthcare providers indicating system fragmentation.

RESULTS

Conducting focus groups in a virtual world setting requires some additional adaptations beyond those needed for face-to-face focus group facilitation. Both formats confront similar barriers: recruitment of an appropriate representative pool of participants, the need to support candor in participant responses, and concerns about privacy, confidentiality, and the potential for revealing personally identifiable health data.

Dealing with generic issues specific to virtual worlds (Second Life)

Within Second Life, it is possible to identify peer support communities of persons with disabilities from which to recruit a population similar to the population from which the quantitative Medicare data was drawn. The use of avatars to conceal actual identity has been known to increase candor (4). Privacy is ensured by conducting the sessions in a physically isolated skybox. Two methods are employed to deal with concerns about personally identifiable data: collect demographic data on participants separately from their focus group contributions; and de-identify focus group transcripts before submission for analysis.

Novel features of virtual world functioning

Several significant adaptations occur because these focus groups are held in a virtual world. First, the consent process is significantly different from those in face-to-face groups, as described above. Also, the focus groups are conducted entirely in text. Some individuals participating in the focus groups require Americans with Disabilities Act (ADA) accommodations in order to participate. The participants experience some advance preparation.

The facilitator and participants communicate by typing rather than orally, as text is more readily accessible by most participants, including those who access their computers using assistive technologies. Individuals for whom typing or reading is impaired by their disability request accommodations ahead of time. We assign a typist for persons wishing to give their input orally. Similarly, a reader is assigned to persons who cannot see or read the text chat. These helpers are all CITI certified.

Participants are given a notecard with the questions to be addressed when meeting arrangements are made. They are encouraged to type out responses to these questions on the notecard in advance, so that they can easily copy/paste them as appropriate. Of course they can also then type additional comments or responses to what others shared. Advance preparation accommodates those for whom typing is laborious, or who require additional time to think through their responses. It also allows more time for discussion, since spontaneous typed responses take more time to transmit than do spoken responses. Moreover, responses prepared in advance can be submitted after the focus group has been completed so that ideas that did not have a chance to emerge during discussion may still be captured.

Advantages of conducting focus groups in virtual worlds

The advantages and disadvantages of collecting qualitative data through face-to-face focus groups are well documented. Virtual world focus groups have a somewhat different set of advantages and disadvantages.

For the "Mrs. A and Mr. B" project, the major advantage of conducting focus groups in a virtual world is that it allows much easier access to our target audience – people with disabilities. People with disabilities make up a significant portion, perhaps as high as 20% (5), of those in virtual worlds. In virtual worlds, they can participate more freely in public events such as focus groups. In a virtual setting, they do not face logistical issues to attend meetings, such as transportation or the need for meeting organizers to provide medical or assistive technology equipment. Additionally, international participation is much easier, and the facilities for conducting research in virtual worlds are inexpensive. The existence of dialog as text is helpful, as no audio-to-text transcription is necessary.

Disadvantages of conducting focus groups in virtual worlds

One disadvantage of conducting focus groups in a virtual world is that the population accessed must be both computer literate and possess a high-end computer. This population is not representative of disabled people at large, nor is it representative of the population in the Medicare administrative dataset that we are using in the quantitative arm of the project. To mitigate this in the "Mrs. A and Mr. B" project, we include face-to-face focus groups with members of an urban community who have lower literacy skills and are not computer users.

Avatars do not provide nonverbal information such as gestures or tone of voice. These sources of information, often gleaned from face-to-face focus group meetings, are missing, but with the topic we are interested in, we feel that this is less important than the text content.

DISCUSSION

Overall, the advantages of using virtual world focus groups outweigh the disadvantages. People with disabilities like to help others and wish to give back to their communities. Many participants welcome the ability to be able to be heard in a forum in which issues about which they care deeply are discussed. The focus groups held in Second Life effectively involve them in academic research. The "Mrs. A and Mr. B" project is demonstrating the utility of this novel method of collecting qualitative healthcare data.

With increasing use of virtual worlds for product design, testing, and prototyping, as well as educational and therapeutic endeavors, collection of data by focus groups in virtual worlds will also increase. To fully leverage the unique affordances of a virtual world setting, typical face-to-face focus group protocols must be modified (6). Therefore our experiences with focus groups for the "Mrs. A and Mr. B" project can help improve the quality of data collected in future virtual world projects.

ACKNOWLEDGMENTS

This project was funded by the Patient-Centered Outcomes Research Institute (PCORI), PCORI contract number AD-12-11-4567.

REFERENCES

[1] Penn Medicine. Penn Medicine receives award from Patient-Centered Outcomes Research Institute to study health care disparities among people with disabilities 2013. Accessed 2014 Jul 14. URL: http://www.uphs.upenn.edu/news/News_Releases/2013/10/stineman/.

[2] Stendal K. Virtual world affordances for people with lifelong disability. Dissertation. Agder, Norway: University of Agder, 2014.

[3] US Access Board. MDE Public Information Meeting 2010. Accessed 2014 Jul 14. URL: https://www.access-board.gov/guidelines-and-standards/health-care/about-this-rulemaking/background/public-information-meeting.

[4] Broitman A. Focus groups get a Second Life 2007. Accessed 2014 Jul 14. URL: http://www.imediaconnection.com/content/13875.asp.

[5] Information Solutions Group. Survey: 'Disabled gamers' comprise 20% of casual video games audience 2008. Accessed 2014 Jul 14. URL: http://www.prnewswire.com/news-releases/survey-disabled-gamers-comprise-20-of-casual-video-games-audience-57442172.html.

[6] Houliez C, Gamble E. Augmented focus groups: On leveraging the peculiarities of online virtual worlds when conducting in-world focus groups. J Theor Appl Electron Commer Res 2012;7:2:31-51.

Submitted: July 01, 2015. *Revised:* August 05, 2015. *Accepted:* August 10, 2015.

In: Alternative Medicine Research Yearbook 2017
Editor: Joav Merrick
ISBN: 978-1-53613-726-2
© 2018 Nova Science Publishers, Inc.

Chapter 17

SELF-MANAGEMENT INTERVENTION FOR AMPUTEES IN A VIRTUAL WORLD ENVIRONMENT

Sandra L Winkler[1,2,], PhD, OTR/L, Robin Cooper[3], PhD, Kurt Kraiger[4], PhD, Ann Ludwig[5], Alice Krueger[5], Ignacio Gaunaurd[2], PhD, PT, Ashley Fisher[6], MS, John Kairalla[7], PhD, Scott Elliott[8], Sarah Wilson[1], OTR/L and Alberto Esquenazi[9], MD*

[1]Department of Occupational Therapy Department,
Nova Southeastern University, Ft Lauderdale, Florida, US
[2]Miami Department of Veterans Affairs Medical Center, Miami, Florida, US
[3]Conflict Analysis and Resolution Department,
Nova Southeastern University, Florida, US
[4]Department of Psychology, Psychology Department,
Colorado State University, Fort Collins, Colorado, US
[5]Virtual Ability Inc., Aurora, Colorado, US
[6]US Army Telemedicine and Advanced Technology Research Center (TATRC),
Fort Detrick, Maryland, US
[7]College of Public Health and Health Professions and College of Medicine,
University of Florida, Gainesville, Florida, US
[8]Scott Elliott e-learning Solutions, Chicago, Illinois, US
[9]Moss Rehab Einstein Healthcare Network, Philadelphia, Pennsylvania, US

ABSTRACT

Amputees who feel well-educated about their prosthesis care are more likely to adhere to treatment recommendations and have improved health outcomes. Few studies have tested

---

[*] Correspondence: Sandra L Winkler, PhD, OTR/L, Assistant Professor of Occupational Therapy, College of Health Care Sciences, Nova Southeastern University, Fort Lauderdale, FL, United States. E-mail: swinkler1@nova.edu.

the efficacy of using virtual worlds as a patient intervention and dissemination environment. The objective of this project was to compare dissemination of a self-management intervention for amputees under two conditions: e-learning and virtual world (SecondLife®). During the development phase, the intervention was developed using Microsoft (MS) PowerPoint® then imported into articulate e-learning software. Prior to creating the virtual world, the intervention was beta-tested (in Articulate) for content and usability. Focus groups of clinicians and amputees were conducted and the results were analysed qualitatively. Focus group findings were implemented by editing the MS PowerPoint® and Articulate accordingly. The SL® was created using the edited MS PowerPoint®. Here we concentrate on the focus group findings; the creation of the experimental, SL® condition is in progress in preparation for the clinical trial. Focus group results identified the self-directed structure and video presentation aspects of the intervention as strengths and were less enthusiastic about use of text. Research team experiences, beta-test results, and available technology suggest the need to rethink traditional textual presentation of declarative knowledge in order to meet the needs of the modern learner and create more modern learning environments. More specifically, findings prompted this research team to develop innovative techniques to render typically textual, declarative knowledge in an interactive format.

Keywords: virtual world, amputees, self-management, qualitative analysis

INTRODUCTION

Amputation is a life-long condition. Although acquiring current and evolving prosthetic- and health-related information will be an on-going process throughout the lifespan of the amputee, amputees report a lack of information available on new prosthetic devices (1). Amputees who feel well-educated about their prosthesis care are more likely to adhere to treatment recommendations and have improved health outcomes.

This project used a self-management approach to build an intervention that provides evidence-based health information for amputees regarding their prosthesis(es) and their health. The effectiveness of self-management programs is attributed to enhanced self-efficacy. The approach is based on Bandura's social cognitive and self-efficacy theories where evidence-based knowledge of risks and benefits creates a pre-condition for change, but must be coupled with a self-influence, e.g., self-efficacy or belief, before desired physical, social, and emotional outcomes can be achieved, or knowledge translated into action (2). Bandura's four sources of self-efficacy were used to guide the development of this intervention: performance accomplishment/mastery, modeling/vicarious experience, verbal persuasion/ interpretation of symptoms, and social persuasion (2). The five core skills of self-efficacy identified by Lorig and Holman (3) were also taken into consideration: problem solving, decision-making, resource utilization, forming a patient/health care provider partnership, and taking action. While Bandura's theories guided the nature of the content, Kraiger's Decision-Based Evaluation Model (4, 5) guided the presentation of the content. Kraiger's model posits that learning in training consists of affective (self-efficacy), cognitive, and behavioural change. Using Kraiger's model, we provided declarative knowledge to facilitate cognitive change and procedural knowledge to facilitate the potential for behavioural change.

A limitation of the more traditional mass communication of health information is that it is not individualized; yet individualization, social support, and guidance impact the success of health programs (2). Few studies have tested the effectiveness of using a virtual world environment to disseminate evidence-based information while at the same time building self-management skills. Virtual world environments such as SL® have been used to enhance patient experiences and increase engagement in their healthcare (6–8). Virtual worlds allow users to "explore, create, imagine, collaborate, role play, interact, socialize, learn, and experience events in a safe and vivid manner" (9). A transfer of behaviour from a virtual world to the real world has been documented (10–12).

The purpose of our three-year project, which is still in progress, is to test the effectiveness of delivering evidence-based health information to amputees in a virtual world environment. Specifically, the dissemination of evidence-based self-management information in the SL® virtual world and e-learning environments are being compared on the following outcomes: use of prosthetic devices, self-efficacy, psychosocial status, pain interference, and function. Prior to implementing the intervention in a clinical trial, we beta-tested the intervention with expert clinicians and amputees. As the clinical trial is still in progress, this manuscript describes the development of the intervention and provides the results of the beta-testing that were used to refine the intervention for the randomized clinical trial.

METHODS

The self-management intervention was created by the research team over a one-year period using MS PowerPoint®. The intervention was organized into four sections: History of Prosthetics; Epidemiology of Amputation; Phases of Rehabilitation (13); and Current Technology. The history, epidemiology, and current technology sections were declarative knowledge based, that is, learners are expected to be able to recognize or recall propositional knowledge or new information presented during training. Declarative information was presented as text and still graphics. The phases of rehabilitation section included declarative and procedural knowledge. For the latter, procedural knowledge, learners are expected to apply rules or implement procedures covered in training. Procedural knowledge was presented as video. Three amputee actors whose amputations were combat related, two lower limb and one upper limb, were issued video cameras to capture spontaneous video of what life is like as an amputee. This raw footage was edited and integrated into the MS PowerPoint®.

Once the research team had reviewed and edited each section as a group, Articulate software (www.articulate.com) was used to convert the MS PowerPoint® version of the intervention to a Flash, asynchronous (self-paced) e-learning experience, which serves as the control condition in the currently on-going randomized clinical trial. In order to keep content constant across the two conditions, the MS PowerPoint® version of the intervention was used to create the SL® experimental condition. Figures 1, 2, and 3 compare the same content presented in e-learning and SL® conditions.

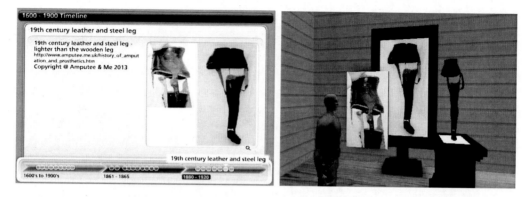

Figure 1. History of prosthetics in the e-learning and SL® environments.

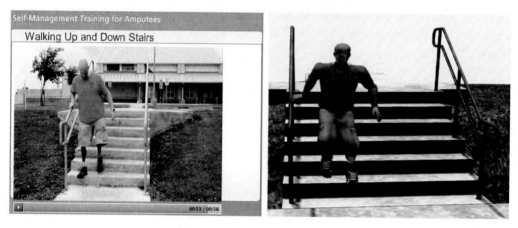

Figure 2. Stair training in the e-learning and SL® environments.

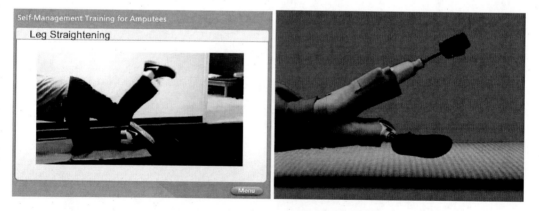

Figure 3. Conditioning exercises in the e-learning and SL® environments.

Unique to the SL® condition was the option of the subject's avatar performing the same action as in the video. For example, Figure 2 shows a bilateral lower limb amputee going down the stairs. Viewing the video and reading the accompanying text is the extent of the learning in the e-learning condition. The SL® condition adds the option of the subject seeing themselves via their avatar doing the same task that they are viewing in the video. This is accomplished by having the avatar perform an animation. The movements of the subject on the video were translated into a virtual world animation. This involved detailed analysis of the movement of the torso and all four limbs or prostheses, in relationship to the movement environment (such as chair or stairs). Then the virtual animation was produced to be as accurate a model of the subject's movements as is possible given constraints of avatar motion. The surroundings in the virtual world were created to mimic those in the video. This involved creating chairs, stairs, etc. that appear as they do in the videos. Figure 2 (right) shows an avatar going down stairs wearing the bilateral lower limb amputee gait pattern demonstrated in the video (Figure 2, left). Similarly, Figure 3 shows a demonstration video of conditioning exercises followed by the animation where the subject views his avatar performing the exercise.

Subjects

The beta-test subjects were recruited using convenience sampling. Four women and five men participated, including six occupational and physical therapy clinicians, who were colleagues of members of the research team with expertise in treating amputees, and three amputees who were also the three amputee actors in the training videos. Following signing of informed consent, the beta testers completed the e-learning version of the intervention. Focus groups were then held online using Adobe Connect software and were conducted as audio interviews supported by synchronous chat. The interview questions were organized around three main topic areas: overall impressions, style and format of the intervention, and the content of the intervention. Questions were open-ended to elicit descriptive, detailed responses. Data was collected via in-depth notes taken during the focus group interviews and digital recording. Following the interviews, the recordings were played back and additional notes were taken to capture all relevant content of the interviews as well as direct quotes illustrative of the subjects' feedback.

Analysis

Qualitative content analysis was used to analyse the complete set of detailed interview notes. Descriptive coding was used to highlight the experiences and perceptions of the beta-test subjects, followed by pattern coding to identify key themes emerging across the focus group interviews. These findings were summarized in a report, which included quotes as exemplars of the key points shared by the subjects.

RESULTS

Data were analysed by summarizing common points from all three focus groups. The common points from all three focus groups are presented here.

- Overall impression: The self-directed structure of the intervention was highly regarded. The navigation could be clarified. All web links should be active.

- Style and format: Subjects reported the sections were visually pleasing but some slides included too much textual information. The videos received universal acclaim.
- Content: Subjects reported the information was accurate and would be useful to new amputees. Several subjects felt there was too much historical information while at least one subject valued the depth of the historical information. Subjects recommended a section that targeted family members.

Not all the subjects were interested in the history section. Some clinicians expressed concern that including evidence would be overwhelming for amputees, but amputees did not share this view.

DISCUSSION

The purpose of this three-year study was to compare dissemination of health-related evidence-based information via e-learning and a SL® virtual world. An evidence-based self-management intervention for amputees was created and then beta-tested prior to using the intervention in a randomized clinical trial. The beta-test evaluated the overall impression, style and format, and context of the self-management intervention. Clinician and amputee subjects reviewed the intervention on the e-learning development server. Data were collected via focus groups. Qualitative methods were used to analyse the date. Beta-test subjects expressed high regard for the self-advocacy approach, which is characteristic of the self-management approach. The subjects praised the videos (procedural knowledge) with less appreciation of the text (declarative knowledge). Perhaps the declarative knowledge was not appreciated because the beta-test subjects were already either clinical experts or well-adjusted amputees; subjects did comment that this would be useful information for new amputees. The findings prompted the research team to add instructions to the randomized clinical trial stating that sections could be completed in any order and that not all sections need to be completed. The researchers could then use Internet tracking mechanisms to examine the order in which users view sections, which sections were viewed most often, and how long each section was viewed. Most important, the beta test results prompted the research team to rethink how and when to mix declarative and procedural knowledge in future projects, to meet the needs of the modern learner.

ACKNOWLEDGMENTS

This project is supported by Agency for Healthcare Research and Quality Grant # R1R24HS022021, PI Sandra Winkler, 2013-2016.

REFERENCES

[1] Berke GM, Fergason J, Milani JR, Hattingh J, McDowell M, Nguyen V, et al. Comparison of satisfaction with current prosthetic care in veterans and service members from Vietnam and OIF/OEF conflicts with major traumatic limb loss. J Rehabil Res Dev 2010;47(4):361-71.

[2] Bandura A. Health promotion by social cognitive means. Health Educ Behav 2004;31(2):143-64.

[3] Lorig KR, Holman H. Self-management education: History, definition, outcomes, and mechanisms, Ann Behav Med 2003;26(1):1-7.

[4] Kraiger K, Ford JK, Salas E. Application of cognitive, skill-based, and affective theories of learning outcomes to new methods of training evaluation. J Appl Psychol 1993;78(2):311-28.

[5] Kraiger K. Decision-based evaluation. In: Kraiger K, ed. Creating, implementing, and managing effective training and development. San Francisco, CA: Jossey-Bass, 2002:331-75.

[6] Hoch DB, Watson AJ, Linton DA, Bello HE, Senelly M, Milik MT, et al. The feasibility and impact of delivering a mind-body intervention in a virtual world. PloS One 2012;7(3):e33843.

[7] Johnson C, Feinglos M, Pereira K, Hassell N, Blascovich J, Nicollerat J, et al. Feasibility and preliminary effects of a virtual environment for adults with type 2 diabetes: pilot study. JMIR Research Protoc 2014;3(2):e23.

[8] Cantrell K, Fischer A, Bouzaher A, Bers M. The role of E-mentorship in a virtual world for youth transplant recipients. J Pediatr Oncol Nurs 2010;27(6):344-55.

[9] Ghanbarzadeh R, Ghapanchi AH, Blumenstein M, Talaei-Khoei A. A decade of research on the use of three-dimensional virtual worlds in health care: a systematic literature review. J Med Internet Res 2014; 16(2):e47.

[10] Bayraktar F, Amca H. Interrelations between virtual-world and real-world activities: comparison of genders, age groups, and pathological and nonpathological Internet users. Cyberpsychol Behav Soc Netw 201215 (5):263-9.

[11] Fox J, Bailenson JN. Virtual self-modeling: The effects of vicarious reinforcement and identification on exercise behavior. Media Psychol 2009;12:1-25.

[12] Napolitano MA, Hayes S, Russo G, Muresu D, Giordano A, Foster GD. Using avatars to model weight loss behaviors: participant attitudes and technology development. J Diabetes Sci Technol 2013;7(4):1057-65.

[13] Esquenazi A. Amputation rehabilitation and prosthetic restoration. From surgery to community reintegration. Disabil Rehabil. 2004;26(14):831-6.

Submitted: July 01, 2015. *Revised:* August 05, 2015. *Accepted:* August 10, 2015.

In: Alternative Medicine Research Yearbook 2017 ISBN: 978-1-53613-726-2
Editor: Joav Merrick © 2018 Nova Science Publishers, Inc.

Chapter 18

VIDEO-BASED QUANTIFICATION OF PATIENT'S COMPLIANCE DURING POST-STROKE VIRTUAL REALITY REHABILITATION

Matjaž Divjak[*], PhD, Simon Zelič, BSc and Aleš Holobar, PhD

System Software Laboratory,
Faculty of Electrical Engineering and Computer Science,
University of Maribor, Slovenia

ABSTRACT

We present a video-based monitoring system for the quantification of a patient's attention to visual feedback during robot assisted gait rehabilitation. The patient's face and facial features are detected online and used to estimate the approximate gaze direction. This gaze information is then used to calculate various metrics of the patient's attention. Results demonstrate that such unobtrusive video-based gaze tracking is feasible and that it can be used to support the assessment of patient's compliance with the rehabilitation therapy.

Keywords: video-based attention monitoring, gaze estimation, stroke rehabilitation, user compliance

INTRODUCTION

Stroke is the third most common cause of death in Western society, with about 4.7 million stroke survivors alive today. One of the hallmark residual impairments of stroke is post-stroke

---

[*] Correspondence: Matjaž Divjak, PhD, System Software Laboratory, Faculty of Electrical Engineering and Computer Science, University of Maribor, Smetanova ulica 17, SI-2000 Maribor, Slovenia. E-mail: matjaz.divjak@um.si.

walking disability, which creates a stigma for patients, makes them more susceptible to injury and directly affects their quality of life. Early rehabilitation therapy is crucial for significant improvements (1). In recent years, robotic systems have been widely tested and employed to retrain stroke patients. By imposing gait-like movements at a comfortable speed, such robotic devices are thought to provide many of the afferent cues regarded as critical to the retraining of locomotion (2).

However, a major problem with existing stroke therapies is patient non-compliance (3). Many stroke patients abandon the therapy because the process is too long, repetitive, and/or does not provide immediate results (4). The European project BETTER (5) recently addressed a new approach to gait rehabilitation by employing non-invasive brain-neural computer interaction (BNCI) based assistive technologies based on EEG (Electroencephalography), EMG (Electromyography) and IMU (Inertial Measurement Unit) sensors. In this article, we extend the BNCI-based modalities with a video-based attention monitoring system that allows automatic quantification and long-term monitoring of user attention. Such attention tracking does not require any sensors to be attached to the patient, making this method easy and fast to apply in stroke rehabilitation. Our main objective is to quantify the patient's attention to visual feedback, i.e., the amount of time the patient's gaze is actively following the displayed visual feedback and to inspect the possible impact of visual feedback on motor planning, as well as its short- and mid-term benefits.

Several studies have already examined the impact of visual feedback on stroke rehabilitation, but they mostly reported inconclusive results. They focused on quantification of results of rehabilitation, enhanced with different kinds of visual feedback, but their experimental designs did not allow for a reliable quantification of the attention a person is paying to stimuli. To the best of our knowledge, only psycho-physiological measures of a patient's attention to visual feedback has been reported in (6), while video-based assessment of attention has not been proposed in the field of rehabilitation.

Methods for real-time detection of the face, facial features, eye movements and gaze direction from video have attracted a lot of research in the past decade (7). Numerous algorithms for facial feature extraction have been proposed, mostly in the context of face detection and recognition (8). Currently, the most promising approaches rely on fusing multiple visual cues, such as combining local feature matching with intensity-based methods (9). Existing methods for the quantification of user attention to visual feedback have mostly been developed for Human-Computer Interaction applications and in order to help severely disabled people (10).

METHODS

An overview of our approach is depicted in Figure 1. The patient is fixed in a robotic gait trainer, which moves the patient's legs according to predefined rehabilitation scenarios, and is adapted to the patient's current walking abilities. In front of the patient is a large TV screen showing various types of visual feedback. A high speed video camera is mounted above the TV. The camera captures HD video of the patient's face, while simultaneously EEG data are recorded from 51 scalp sites and EMG data are recorded from both legs (tibialis anterior muscle).

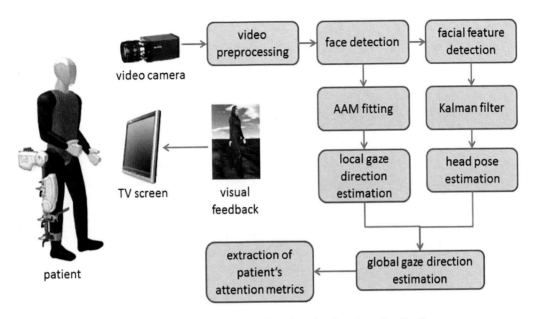

Figure 1. Overview of the proposed approach for video-based estimation of patient's attention/compliance during robot-enhanced rehabilitation.

The video streams are processed by our algorithms. First, frontal faces are detected and main facial features are extracted (corners of the eyes, pupil centers, mouth, tip of the nose). To suppress jitter from detection errors and body swings during walking, a Kalman filter is applied to the locations of the extracted facial features. Next, an active appearance model (AAM (11)) of the face with 59 facial landmarks is used to more accurately represent the current facial pose/expression. The relative distances between extracted landmarks are used to calculate the head pose and gaze direction. Finally, different metrics of the patient's attention/compliance are computed: the percentage of time the patient is observing the visual feedback, the spatial gaze distribution maps, the responses to actions in the virtual reality (VR) environment, etc.

We tested five different types of visual feedback (see Figure 2): a calibration screen for the initialization of our algorithms; 2D plots of current leg positions; 2D plots of muscle activations; and two realistic VR environments (walking in a park from 1st and 3rd person perspectives). The VR environments were created in OpenGL 3.3 and consist of ground, sky dome and male/female avatars. The avatars were created in Mixamo Pro Character Creator Tool and animated with AutoDesk 3DS Max 2012. Both avatars have an underlying bone structure with all major joints modeled, allowing animation of almost all human movements. The actual avatar movement within the VR environment is controlled by kinematic data from the robotic trainer, so leg movements in VR world correspond with leg movements in real life.

The whole video processing system was designed for real-time operation, but the current version of the software is a mix of C++ and Matlab routines and runs at approximately 1 frame per second. Therefore, all video processing is currently performed offline, but (near) real-time operation is possible with further optimization of the code.

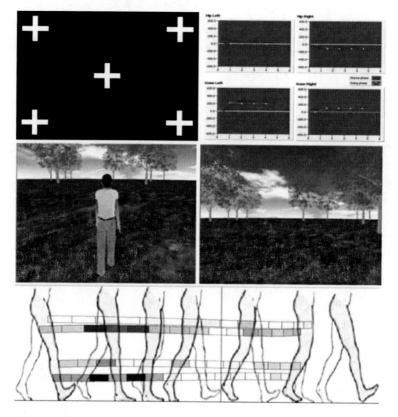

Figure 2. Five different types of visual feedback that are shown to the patient during therapy. Top row: the calibration screen for gaze direction estimation, and gait trainer's plots of current leg positions. Middle row: realistic VR environment from 1st and 3rd person perspective. Bottom row: special feedback displaying muscle activations.

EXPERIMENTAL RESULTS

The proposed system was evaluated in an experiment that involved 4 stroke patients and consisted of 5 runs of robot assisted walking with different forms of visual feedback. In all runs, the patients were instructed to walk actively, maintaining a constant speed, and applying minimum force on the robot. A 42″ screen was placed in front of the patient, 1.4 m away from his face. Each run lasted 4 minutes. For all types of visual feedback the walking speed remained constant. During the experiments videos of the patient's face were recorded to disk in HD resolution and later processed offline.

On average, the face was detected in 93% of video frames recorded (i.e., in practically all the frames with frontal faces whereas the profile faces were not detected). Eyes, mouth, nose, and pupils were accurately detected in more than 99% of detected faces (see Table 1). Detection of facial features was skipped in video frames where no face was detected. The average jitter of detected facial features was 1.0 ± 0.4 pixels. The AAM was successfully fitted to all frontal faces. The average jitter of AAM landmarks was estimated at 0.6 ± 0.4 pixels.

Table 1. Facial feature detection performance, estimated on three test videos

	Video 1 (gaze targets)		Video 2 (gaze targets)		Video 3 (VR 3rd person)	
	Frames	%	Frames	%	Frames	%
Whole video	9999	100%	13391	100%	10551	100%
Face detection	9833	93.7%	13193	98.5%	10427	98.8%
Detection of left eye	9805	99.7%*	13174	99.9%*	10419	99.9%*
Detection of right eye	9769	99.3%*	13179	99.9%*	10408	99.8%*
Detection of left pupil	9800	99.9%#	13191	99.9%#	10419	100%#
Detection of right pupil	9769	100%#	13187	100%#	10408	100%#
Detection of nose	9827	99.9%*	13150	99.8%*	10423	99.9%*
Detection of mouth	9742	99.1%*	13174	100%*	10414	99.8%*

* Values normalized by the number of face detections.
# Values normalized by the number of eye detections.

Videos recorded during sessions with the screen displaying calibration targets were inspected by an expert and 9 approximate gaze directions (top-left, top-centre, top-right, bottom-left, bottom-centre, bottom right, left-centre, right-centre and centre of the screen) were manually annotated. The time periods corresponding to eye movements or eye blinks were ignored and were not annotated. Gaze direction was then calculated automatically by our algorithm and compared to the manually annotated gaze directions. The gaze directions were identified with average accuracy of 94% ± 6%. Most errors originated from distinguishing between top-left vs. bottom-left and top-right vs. bottom-right gaze directions.

Figure 3 shows an example of a patient's detected level of attention to visual feedback, estimated as percentage of time, in 1 second intervals, with gaze fixed to the TV screen; all gazes outside the screen were classified as non-attention. Figure 4 presents an example of the estimated spatiotemporal gaze distribution metric. This metric shows relative frequency of identified gaze locations over a 4 minute long gait rehabilitation session. Brighter spots in the gaze distribution plots indicate areas with more frequent attention. Such maps support the identification of gaze targets (i.e., gaze hot-spots) and the assessment of spatiotemporal correlation between a patient's attention to visual feedback and other BNCI-based performance indices of gait rehabilitation.

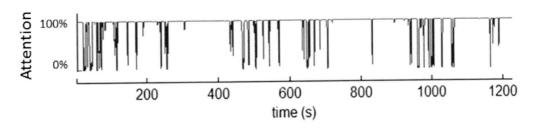

Figure 3. An example of estimated level of a patient's attention to visual feedback during a 20 minutes long rehabilitation session (5 × 4 minutes).

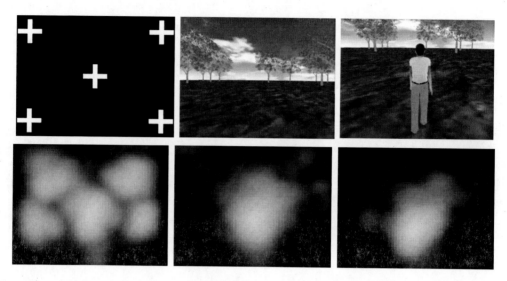

Figure 4. An example of spatial gaze distribution plots (bottom row) for three different types of visual feedback (top row) shown to a patient during 4 minutes long gait rehabilitation sessions.

CONCLUSION

We developed and validated a video-based system for the robust tracking of a patient's face pose and gaze direction during robot-assisted lower limb rehabilitation therapy. The results (see Figures 3 and 4) show that such a system can be used to unobtrusively analyze patient's attention to displayed visual feedback and to provide a means for long-term quantification of visual feedback effects on the rehabilitation progress. It can also serve as an additional feature for other BNCI performance indices, such as similarity of motor modules, kinetic and kinematic profiles and brain patterns. For example, preliminary results show a significant correlation between attention to muscle activation plots and improvements in muscle activations during walking.

ACKNOWLEDGMENTS

This work was supported by the Commission of the European Union within Framework 7, grant agreement FP7-2009-7.2–247935 - "BETTER – Brain-Neural Computer Interaction for Evaluation and Testing of Physical Therapies in Stroke Rehabilitation of Gait Disorders." The authors would like to thank the personnel of Fondazione Santa Lucia in Rome, Italy, for organizing and performing the experimental recordings.

REFERENCES

[1] Kollen B, Kwakkel G, Lindeman E. Functional recovery after stroke: A review of current developments in stroke rehabilitation research. Rev Recent Clin Trials 2006;1:75-80.

[2] Mehrholz J, Werner C, Kugler J, Pohl M. Electro-mechanical-assisted training for walking after stroke. Cochrane Database Syst Rev 2007;17:4.
[3] Matarić MJ, Eriksson J, Feil-Seifer DJ, Winstein CJ. Socially assistive robotics for post-stroke rehabilitation. J Neuroeng Rehabil 2007;4:5.
[4] Teasell R, Kalra L. What's new in stroke rehabilitation: Back to basics. Stroke 2005;36:215-7.
[5] Project BETTER. Accessed 2015 Jan 20. URL: http:// www.car.upm-csic.es/bioingenieria/better/
[6] Bakker M, de Lange FP, Stevens JA, Toni I, Bloem BR. Motor imagery of gait: a quantitative approach. Exp Brain Res 2007;179:497–04.
[7] Hansen DW, Ji Q. In the eye of the beholder: A survey of models for eyes and gaze. IEEE Trans Pattern Anal Mach Intell 2010;32:478-00.
[8] Bagherian E, Rahmat, RWOK. Facial feature extraction for face recognition: a review. International Symposium on Information Technology 2008;1-9.
[9] Liao WK, Fidaleo D, Medioni G. Robust, real-time 3D face tracking from a monocular view. EURASIP J Image Video Process 2010;2010:183605.
[10] Poole A, Ball LJ. Eye tracking in human-computer interaction and usability research: Current status and future. In: Ghaouli C, ed. Encyclopedia of human-computer interaction. Hershey, PA: Idea Group, 2005.
[11] Matthews I, Xiao J, Baker S. 2D vs. 3D deformable face models: representational power, construction, and real-time fitting. Int J Comput Vis 2007;75:93-13.

Submitted: July 02, 2015. *Revised:* August 07, 2015. *Accepted:* August 12, 2015.

In: Alternative Medicine Research Yearbook 2017
Editor: Joav Merrick
ISBN: 978-1-53613-726-2
© 2018 Nova Science Publishers, Inc.

Chapter 19

PUTTING IMMERSIVE THERAPIES INTO PRAXIS: TOWARDS HOLISTIC WELLBEING MULTISENSORY MEDITATION ENVIRONMENTS

Henry J Moller[1-3],*, MD, MSc, DABIHM, Lee Saynor[2,3], Harjot Bal[2], Kunal Sudan[3] and Lee Jones[2,3]

[1]Faculties of Medicine, Knowledge Media Design,
Music and Health Research Collaboratory,
University of Toronto, Toronto, Canada,
Faculty of Applied Health Sciences, Department of Recreation
and Leisure Studies, University of Waterloo, Waterloo, Canada
[2]Digital Futures Initiative, OCAD University, Toronto, Canada
[3]PRAXIS Holistic Health, Toronto, Canada

ABSTRACT

A core focus for PRAXIS Holistic Health is the facilitation of stress reduction techniques and to provide a variety of environments, both geophysical and virtual-immersive that are conducive to a patient's wellbeing. Through continuous seamless patient feedback via tablet-based Electronic Medical Record (EMR), we have been able to customize and provide innovative inclusive health care design while ensuring that each patients needs are addressed. Our "Wellpad" EMR also allows us to seamlessly glimpse at patient progress, allowing us to continuously taper technologically enhanced multimodal meditation (TEMM) treatment and learn what therapeutic programs are most effective for that particular patient. The growing palate of customized programs available through TEMM treatment allow us to target various medical and psychosomatic conditions while continuously adjusting target programs and parameters, marking PRAXIS Holistic Health's unique inclusive health care design for mental health. It is important to note that with iterative patient feedback, recorded every time a patient is treated, we are able to

---

* Correspondence: Henry J. Moller, MD, MSc, DABIHM, PRAXIS Holistic Health, 785 Carlaw Ave, Suite 101, Toronto, Ontario, Canada. E-mail: drmoller@praxisholistic.ca.

observe trends to inform which TEMM programs fit optimally for particular medical conditions, promoting optimized patient health care. Increasingly, virtual meditative experiences are also employed to inspire patients towards health- and wellness-oriented praxis, i.e., action. We touch upon seamless diagnostic evaluation and clinical utility of Wellpad, our EMR system developed using an iterative inclusive design approach. We place our multisensory meditation therapy within the scope of Virtual Environment Therapy (VET) and suggest the mechanism of action as an induced leisure or flow state to potentiate relaxation, stress-reduction, resilience and personal transformation.

Keywords: virtual environment therapy, technology-enhanced multimodal meditation, mindfulness based stress reduction, vibro-acoustic therapy, workplace wellness, inclusive design, holistic health, mental health

INTRODUCTION

It is fair to say that VET-based therapies have struggled to integrate into mainstream mental healthcare, yet the opportunity in the current era to demonstrate relevance in the healing arts is greater than ever. For some time, there has been promise that media technologies such as VETs could provide effective and standardized health delivery options (1). Holistic healthcare paradigms incorporating media technology may now play a role in delivering on this promise. In an era where there is a crisis of confidence among the public and academia in scientific reporting of biomedical healthcare studies (2), informed patients now often seek wellbeing restoration rather than illness treatment as a true healthcare goals (3); given this trend, the opportunity has arisen for immersive technologies to clinically deliver longstanding health claims of representing a pathway towards credible, safe and effective therapeutics. Many patients, skeptical of biomedical risk-benefit ratios, gravitate to holistic and/or "natural" health and wellness models, such as meditation, yoga, naturopathy, or massage therapy (to name a few). Particularly in mental health care, conventional therapeutic options are often ineffective and/or limited by undesirable iatrogenic side effects, leading to non-compliance. Ideal VETs that seek to improve upon this track record of biomedical therapies need to be salient, aesthetically pleasing and hedonically rewarding, causing patients to seek them out, rather than enduring them through cumbersome tasks or aversive stimuli such as typical VET phobia protocols.

At PRAXIS, reproducible technology-enhanced multimodal meditation (TEMM) protocols are gradually being developed into therapeutic programs to meet the needs of patients seeking mental health care for safe and effective symptom relief of stress-related symptoms such as anxiety, insomnia and depression. As boundaries between real and virtual, technologically mediated and "organic" states of consciousness continue to blur with the march of media technology, the need to address this convergence in a therapeutic paradigm is increasingly relevant and warranted (4). In parallel to this, the fast pace of technology in work environments, and the impact of this on health is being described (5). We have recently advocated for the public health implementation of more accessible leisure opportunities (6) to create a healthier and productive society via personalized, immersive and standardized media-based therapeutics.

TEMM programs seek to tap into the health benefits of leisure, which within a neuropsychiatric paradigm we define as freely chosen, intrinsically motivated and self-directed "flow states," often environment-directed and quite probably with the potential to enact potent changes of consciousness. Optimal leisure experiences are thought to result in enhanced mental wellbeing, positive affect and transformational learning states that carry over into effectively coping with daily routines, stresses and roles. Leisure has also been defined as "perceived freedom." We have developed and researched the medically supervised administration of standardized simulated leisure-state TEMM meditation experiences in the context of pleasant, hedonic sensory input incorporating multiple sensory channels (visual, auditory, haptic) to promote broad-spectrum wellbeing in mental health care.

We review a prospective study investigating clinical outcomes for a case series of patients undertaking a therapeutic protocol of a TEMM-based medically supervised meditation program. We suggest that TEMM is a promising therapeutic avenue for virtual/immersive therapies, with a broad-spectrum mental health benefit, analogous to conventional Mindfulness Based Stress Reduction (MBSR) programs, and a therapeutic risk-benefit margin possibly superior and often preferred by patients to medication therapy.

METHODS

The PRAXIS team has developed and researched the medically supervised administration of synthetically "packaged" leisure-state meditation experiences in the context of pleasant, relaxing, hedonic sensory input incorporating multiple sensory channels (visual, auditory, haptic). Detailed psychobiological models have been previously reported (6–8). As outlined above, the overarching goal of our meditation protocols is to simulate or "recreate" leisure states as per Mihaly Csikszentmihalyi's description of "flow" as an immersive, often hedonic, state of absorption and peak performance with positive psychological outcomes (9). Also described as "inner presence," (10), this complex consciousness process involves the processing of sensory stimuli and consolidation with previously integrated information, very similar to that described in our neurobiological process of dreaming (8), and in Csikszentmihalyi's flow model of highly memorable and meaningful peak states, using immersive simulated environments to approximate the best experiences of people's lives.

We will now review briefly the clinical protocol for medical patients who have undertaken a standardized course of regularly scheduled (weekly or biweekly) medically supervised 20-40 minute multisensory technology-enhanced multimodal meditation (TEMM) sessions to therapeutically address stress-related symptoms in a psycho-supportive paradigm. TEMM's multimodal nature consists of visual, auditory and haptic sensory cues to users.

Visual cues in our current TEMM model are recurrent light pulses via specialized glasses using built-in light emitting diodes (LEDs), at a frequency between 2 and 12 Hz, corresponding to the electroencephalographic (EEG) rhythm ranging from delta (1-4Hz), through theta (4-8 Hz) and alpha (8-12 Hz) brain activity, to entrain a calming and relaxed user state, compared to higher frequencies common in chronic high stress-states.

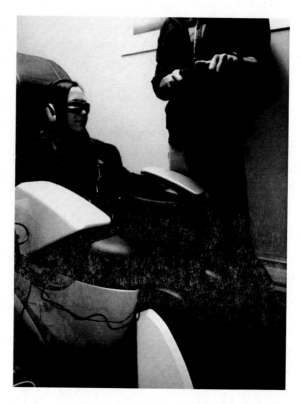

Figure 1. A patient relaxing in our Medically-Supervised Meditation/TEMM therapy program.

The audio component typically involves exposure to a standardized guided meditation invoking a relaxing scenario such as a nature experience (e.g., walking in a meadow or sitting on a beach) accompanied by repetitive positive affirmations and mantras to enhance a participant's self-esteem or psychological outlook. Themes addressed within the meditation sessions include "dealing with stress," "relax," "balancing your moods" and "creative problem solving." The intent of the standardized audio content of the immersive TEMM-based meditation scenarios is to mimic, and on a therapeutic level reprogram autonomous thought processes.

Haptic sensory stimulation (gentle massage, heat, vibration) occurs through a specialized chair that the patient rests in during the meditation process, where multimodal visual, auditory and haptic elements are synergistically combined within a therapy session to create an integrative and transformative therapeutic experience (see Figure 1). Pre- and post-treatment core psychosomatic self-states are assessed to track response.

RESULTS

In our recently reported clinical study of twenty consecutive fully consenting patients seeking medically supervised meditation in a holistic healthcare centre setting using the above protocol (7), participants were invited to complete a feedback form in which they were asked to describe the following: (i) initial symptoms/concerns which led to treatment; (ii) overall impression of the treatment; and, using 5-point Likert scales ratings, (iii) effectiveness of the

TEMM treatment for initial symptoms or concerns; (iv) adequacy of the duration of sessions; and (v) adequacy of the number of sessions. Another set of 5-point Likert scales were also used to allow patients to rate symptom-based self-states before and after the treatment plan, including the following: (i) tension/relaxation level; (ii) stress level; and (iii) mood state. Open-ended qualitative feedback regarding therapy experience was also solicited.

On average there was a noticeable decline in perceived levels of tension ($p < 0.001$) and stress ($p < 0.001$), before versus after the program, as reported by study subjects. Over 50% of individuals specifically commented on the capacity for TEMM to help them relax and better deal with their stress and anxiety. For changes in mood states of patients there was a similarly positive shift ($p = 0.019$); the TEMM therapy program was found to be significantly effective in addressing the symptoms and concerns of subjects, with a mean rating of 4.15 points on the 5-point Likert scale. The layout of the treatment was favourably evaluated, with mean ratings for both individual session and program duration near the "neutral" 3 points on the 5-point Likert scale, i.e., close to the "just right" point.

Some individuals also articulated their appreciation of the design of the TEMM program; using different sensory and psychological elements integratively seems to create a complete and powerful wellbeing experience. TEMM was consistently reported to have helped initiate an introspective dialogue for a select number of users – these individuals reported more self-awareness of emotions and anxieties and being better able to cope with them outside of the sessions, implying an experiential shift in consciousness. We have dubbed this transformative clinical outcome as a "vacation effect." Flow-related engagement with the therapy experience across multiple senses was described by many patients, despite some variation in awareness and recollection of the specifics of the guided meditation they had experienced. This is reminiscent of the residual leisure experience of a vacationer returning from a journey or trip and being able to remember and integrate novel thought patterns and/or behaviours observed and experienced into their daily routine.

A helpful approach to reliably track patient progress is to make this process easy, usable and even enjoyable for patient and provider. In this sense, to complete a holistic immersive therapeutic experience, the gathering of clinical data should ideally be non-obtrusive and facilitate patient-doctor communication across a wide clinical population base. Our tablet-based Wellpad electronic medical record (EMR) tool (see Figure 2) represents our team's commitment to Inclusive Design principles (11, 12) in gathering quantitative and qualitative results by establishing "a universal language that bridges the gap between patient and doctor/circles-of-care, while accommodating the growing reality of technological and ethnic diversity in a global community with common health concerns but often differing language and culture" (13). Patients of varying cultures, and varying cognitive and physical abilities have self-reported using Wellpad's novel Happy- and Frowny-face touch-based sliders to be a significant improvement over complex, lengthy and confusing paper-based questionnaires, and also have given feedback that Wellpad's easy-to-understand data visualization display is helpful to summarize their clinical progress during appointments.

A related immersive meditation-based therapy that shows promise for our patient group is Vibro-Acoustic Therapy (VAT). Conceptually similar to TEMM, VAT utilizes loudspeaker transducers, positioned throughout an adjustable bed, providing somatic/haptic stimulation with low frequency sound waves (usually at 40 Hz or less, most often between 20 and 40 Hz). While the body is subjected to these low frequency sound wave pulsations, patients are also immersed in binaural pulsatile musical relaxation soundscape programs through headphones.

This induces a pleasant wellbeing state for patients, which alleviates pain and/or reduces nociception (14). Operationalization and optimization are still core areas of focus for this therapy, but it shows much promise in the further design of multisensory meditative therapies facilitating stress, pain and tension reduction.

Furthermore, PRAXIS is also currently testing VET leisure experiences that integrate heart rate biofeedback data for mindfulness-based stress reduction. The system called *Your Body of Water* visualizes a user's heart rate as water. As heart rate increases, the body of water grows, the water flow increases in speed and the installation emits louder wave sounds. As heart rate decreases, the water flow becomes calm. The project takes a psycho-physiological approach to the body, focusing on how mood and emotional state influence bodily functions such as heart rate. The visualisation in *Your Body of Water* represents these emotional states through the liveliness of the water, and in doing so aims to get patients more in touch with the physiological responses to their emotional states, and therefore better able to deal with daily stress. This project expands upon previous research done in the field such as *The BrightHearts Project* developed by paediatrician Dr Angie Morrow and designer George Khut, which used abstract visualizations of heart rate biofeedback data to help children regulate stress and cope with anxiety (15). Ultimately, *Your Body of Water* asks how combining VET with biofeedback data might give patients a way to connect to how they are feeling and their bodily responses to those feelings.

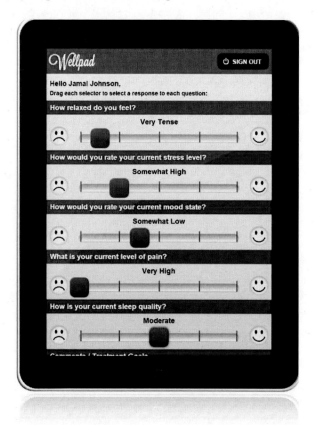

Figure 2. Our inclusively designed Wellpad EMR app makes tracking patient symptoms easy.

DISCUSSION

We have described a theoretical framework, rationale and early user feedback for standardized therapeutic VET leisure experiences packaged as medically-supervised mediation. We wish to point out the potential societal benefit of health promotion on a preventative level through TEMM therapy, for example, if more closely linked to workplace health management services. Specifically, with difficulty in regularly scheduling predictable vacations or other leisure events, the notion of "bringing leisure into the workplace" may be a promising avenue to pursue for employee wellbeing and productivity. The acute as well as residual effects of such simulated leisure states appears able to approximate real experiences, and perhaps even deliver these more efficiently and predictably. While similar outcomes might ordinarily occur with conventional leisure activities such as play, enjoyment of outdoor nature experiences or cultural activities, it is intriguing to consider that immersive media technologies might be able to operationalize these experiences in a standardized format, which would allow essentially a supervised "prescription" of leisure-based multimodal meditation experiences by healthcare professionals trained in this paradigm. This could have significant health policy implications as well as reinventing service delivery in workplace wellbeing initiatives (16). Clarifying differences between individuals and linking qualitative "lived experience" reports to clinical data and robustness/durability of wellbeing states would be a welcome next step. Certainly, in comparison to many pharmaceutical alternatives, the lack of adverse effects seem to offer favourable risk-benefit, and therefore, risk management profile to cautious clinicians. The possibilities of personalized immersive wellbeing environments currently appear wide open for future discovery and implementation. To this end, PRAXIS Holistic Health will continue to explore new opportunities in consumer-level virtual reality technology, panoramic video development tools, and relaxation technologies for maximal patient wellbeing with minimal risk, as per the Hippocratic "Above all, do no harm" mantra sworn by physicians.

ACKNOWLEDGMENTS

PRAXIS Holistic Health appreciates the daily feedback from patients enrolled in our Medically-Supervised Meditation program.

REFERENCES

[1] Gregg L, Tarrier N. Virtual reality in mental health: A review of the literature. Soc Psychiatr Psychiatric Epidemiol 2007;42(5):343-54.
[2] Pashler H, Wagenmakers EJ. Editors' introduction to the special section on replicability in psychological science: A crisis of confidence? Perspect Psychol Sci 2012;7:528-30.
[3] AHHA. Wellness from within: The first step. Anaheim, CA: American Holistic Health Association, 2003.
[4] Moller HJ. From Absence to Presence: Blurred consciousness and sleep states. PRESENCE 2008, the 11th Annual International Workshop on Presence, Padova, Italy, 2008.

[5] Heusser M. M&M's, stress and the quest for a sustainable pace in the tech rat race. Biztech Magazine 2003;8. Accessed 2014 Aug 20. URL: http://www.biztechmagazine.com/article/2013/08/mms-stress-and-quest-sustainable-pace-tech-rat-race.
[6] Moller HJ, Bal H, Sudan K, Potwarka LR. Recreating leisure. How immersive environments can promote wellbeing. In: Riva G, Waterworth J, Murray D, eds. Interacting with presence: HCI and the sense of presence in computer-mediated environments. London: Versitas, 2014. Accessed 2014 Aug 20. URL: http:// www.presence-research.com.
[7] Moller HJ, Bal H. Technology-enhanced multimodal meditation: Clinical results from an observational case series. Proc 10th International Conference on Virtual Rehabilitation, Philadelphia, PA 26-29 Aug, 2013: 1-9.
[8] Moller HJ, Barbera J. Media Presence, dreaming and consciousness. In: Riva G, Anguera MT, Wiederhold BK, Mantovani F, eds. From communication to presence: The integration of cognition, emotions and culture towards the ultimate communicative experience. Amsterdam, NL, IOS Press, 2006.
[9] Csikszentmihalyi M, Kleiber DA. Leisure and self-actualization. In: Driver BL, Brown PJ, Peterson GL, eds. Benefits of leisure. State College, PA: Venture Publishing, 1991:91-102.
[10] Revonsuo A. Inner presence: Consciousness as a biological phenomenon. Cambridge, MA: MIT Press, 2006.
[11] Nussbaumer LL. Inclusive design: A universal need. New York: Fairchild Books, 2001.
[12] Marti P. Enabling through design: Explorations of aesthetic interaction in therapy and care. Eindhoven, Holland: Technische Universiteit Eindhoven, 2012.
[13] Moller HJ, Saynor LJ. Wellpad: An inclusively designed tablet-based digital medical record with optimized efficiency and usability. MobileHCI 2014, Sept 23-26, 2014, Toronto, Canada.
[14] Wigram T, Saperston B. The art and science of music therapy: A handbook. New York: Routledge, 2013.
[15] Khut GP, Morrow A, YouguiWatanabe M. The BrightHearts Project: A New Approach to the Management of Procedure-Related Paediatric Anxiety. Proceedings for OzCHI, Canberra, ACT, 2011. Accessed 2015 Apr 20. URL: http://khut2011.anat.org.au/files/2011/10/Body-in-Design-Position-Paper-OZC HI-KHUT-20110926.pdf.
[16] Peters T, Ghadiri A, Kohl M. Betriebliches Gesundheitsmanagement: audio-visuelle Entspannung kann Krankenstand senken. CO-MED 2013;19(4):40-43. [German].

Submitted: July 02, 2015. Revised: August 07, 2015. Accepted: August 12, 2015.

Chapter 20

ASSESSMENT OF MOTOR FUNCTION IN HEMIPLEGIC PATIENTS USING A VIRTUAL CYCLING WHEELCHAIR

Remi Ishikawa[1,]*, MS, Norihiro Sugita[2], PhD, Makoto Abe[1], PhD, Makoto Yoshizawa[3], PhD, Kazunori Seki[4], MD, PhD and Yasunobu Handa[4], MD, PhD

[1]Department of Electrical Engineering, Graduate School of Engineering, Tohoku University, Sendai, Japan
[2]Department of Management Science and Technology, Graduate School of Engineering, Tohoku University, Sendai, Japan
[3]Cyberscience Center, Tohoku University, Sendai, Japan
[4]Sendai School of Health and Welfare, Sendai, Japan

ABSTRACT

A cycling wheelchair (CWC) is a rehabilitation tool for hemiplegic patients. In previous studies, our group developed a virtual reality system that allows patients to practice driving a CWC. This study proposes a new method to estimate the torque of each leg extension of a hemiplegic patient while driving the virtual CWC. Experimental results from four healthy subjects and four hemiplegic patients showed the usefulness of the proposed method in evaluating the motor function of the patients.

Keywords: force sensing, cycling wheelchair, rehabilitation

INTRODUCTION

Stroke is a common disorder among the elderly in Japan, and it often causes paralysis of the legs. In general, people who have difficulties walking use wheelchairs in daily life. However,

---

* Correspondence: Remi Ishikawa, Department of Electrical Engineering, Graduate School of Engineering, Tohoku University, Research Building 1, Room 521, Sendai, Japan. E-mail: r-ishikawa@yoshizawa.ecei.tohoku.ac.jp.

while moving with wheelchairs, they do not use their legs because wheelchairs are operated by their hands or an electric motor. Typically, when the legs perform work, blood is returned to the heart. Therefore, people who do not use their legs for a long period of time risk suffering from disuse syndrome, causing muscle weakness and a fall in cardiopulmonary functions.

To solve this problem, a cycling wheelchair (CWC) has been developed and explored as a new rehabilitation tool for hemiplegic patients, see Figure 1 (1). These individuals can drive the CWC by rotating the pedals with their non-paralyzed feet. CWCs allow hemiplegic patients to move quicker and travel longer distances without fatigue in comparison to conventional wheelchairs (2). Moreover, they can use their hands freely while using a CWC.

However, CWCs require patients to pedal and steer simultaneously while changing direction. Therefore, driving a CWC is difficult for patients who are not accustomed to its operation. Patients must practice driving the CWC to avoid the danger of falling and becoming stranded. A large and safe area is required to practice driving the CWC. Additionally, to ensure safety, assistants must be present to monitor patients using a CWC.

In previous studies, a virtual reality (VR) system was developed, which allows patients to safely practice driving a CWC, as shown in Figure 2 (3, 4). By applying VR technology, patients can practice driving in a narrow place. To confirm the efficacy of rehabilitation using the system, Suzuki evaluated the input torque generated by the user's legs to move the CWC (4). However, it was difficult to evaluate whether the paralyzed leg recovered because they were not able to extract the torque of the paralyzed leg from the entire input torque. Since the torque of each leg includes gravity effects, the influence of gravity must be considered. Therefore, it is necessary to improve the method to analyze the motor performance of the patients.

In this study, we proposed a new method to estimate the torque produced by the power of each leg separately when the user is driving the virtual CWC. To calculate the torque of each leg, we attached force sensors to each pedal. Additionally, we estimated the torque produced by the power of each leg by assuming the gravity effects and devised a new evaluation index using the estimated torque. The efficacy of the proposed method was tested experimentally.

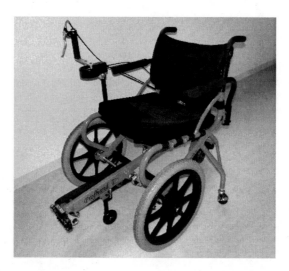

Figure 1. Cycling wheel chair (CWC).

Assessment of motor function in hemiplegic patients ... 187

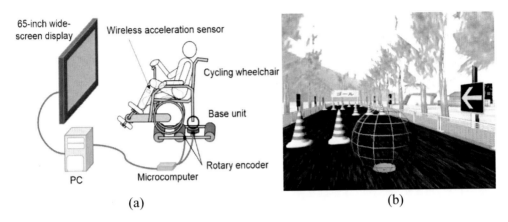

Figure 2. Virtual reality system developed in previous study. (a) Outline of system (b) Screenshot of VR (3).

METHODS

Figure 3 shows the system developed in this study. The user sits on the virtual CWC, which is fixed to the base unit, and rotates the pedals while measurements are taken. In reality, the measurement is influenced by the change in road surface conditions. Using the virtual CWC, a user can rotate the pedals in fixed conditions. The angle of the crankshaft is measured by a rotary encoder (E6A2-CWZ3C; Omron Corp.) and the data are transmitted to a personal computer (PC) using a microcomputer (Arduino; Arduino Software Corp.). To measure the forces applied to the left and right pedals, wearable force plates (M3D-FP-U; Tec Gihan Corp.) are attached to both pedals. The force plates contain three-axis force sensors, an accelerometer, and a gyroscope. To observe the change in torque produced by the user's legs, a brake system that changes the load required to drive the virtual CWC is introduced.

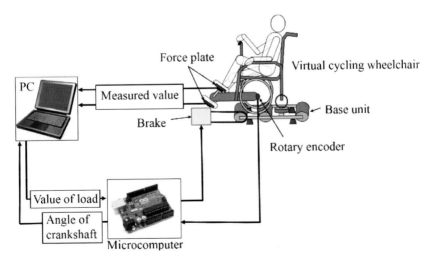

Figure 3. System developed in this study.

Leg torque estimations

The torque of each leg, τ_{pedal}, is calculated using the forces applied to the pedals as follows:

$$\tau_{pedal} = L \times (F_y \cos \theta_t + F_z \sin \theta_t), \qquad (1)$$

where F_z is the force perpendicular to the pedal, F_y is the force parallel to the pedal, L is the length of the crankshaft, and θ_t is the angle consisting of the angle of the pedal, θ_{pedal}, and the angle of the crankshaft, θ_{crank}. These forces and angles are represented in Figure 4. To calculate the torque of each leg, it is necessary to acquire the angle of pedal. Therefore, we use the Kalman filter.

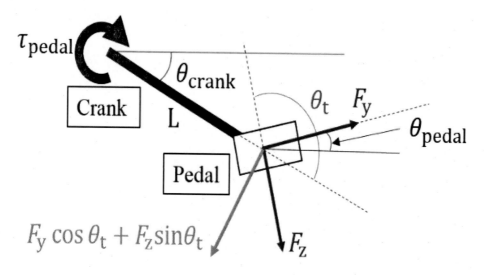

Figure 4. Torque estimation in the pedal.

Pedal angle estimation using the Kalman filter

To acquire the angle of the pedal, we applied the steady-state Kalman filter (5). This method uses the outputs of both an accelerometer and a gyroscope. The angle of the pedal is obtained by integrating the gyroscope outputs, and including the error caused by the offset drift of the gyroscope. Figure 5 shows a block diagram of this method, where θ_{gyro} is the angle obtained by the gyroscope outputs, θ_{acc} is the angle obtained by the accelerometer outputs, and Δy is difference between θ_{gyro} and θ_{acc}. We acquire θ_{pedal} by reducing the error of the angle, $\Delta \hat{\theta}$, which is estimated from θ_{gyro} using the Kalman filter. To apply this method, we determined the Kalman gains, which were required to estimate the error of the angle, using a preliminary experiment.

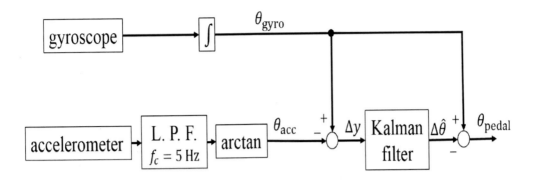

Figure 5. Block diagram of angle measurement using the Kalman.

Elimination of leg gravity effects

To estimate the torque produced by the power of each leg, we must eliminate the gravity effects on the legs. The torque of the gravity effects on the leg consists of the torques of the hip, knee, and ankle joints, which are caused by the gravity effect on the thigh, shin, and ankle, respectively. Kaisumi estimated the leg gravity effects by applying a model of the human leg (6). However, the previous study assumed that the hip and knee joints are active joints that exert torques, but the ankle joint is not. In this study, we consider the ankle as an active joint with torque. Thus, this study estimates the effect of gravity on the leg by applying a model of the human leg that has not only hip and knee joints, but also an ankle joint. The torque produced by the power of each leg is given by:

$$\tau_{human} = \tau_{pedal} - \tau_{gravity}, \tag{2}$$

where τ_{human} is the torque produced by the power of each leg, and $\tau_{gravity}$ is the torque arising from the gravity effects on the leg.

Index to evaluate user's motor performance

A new evaluation index using the torque produced by the power of each leg was proposed as follows:

$$\tau_{left} = \tau_{lpedal} - \tau_{lgrav}, \tag{3}$$

$$\tau_{right} = \tau_{rpedal} - \tau_{rgrav}, \tag{4}$$

$$T_{diff} = \frac{1}{360} \sum_{\theta=0}^{359} |\tau_{left}(\theta_{crank}) - \tau_{right}(\theta_{crank} + 180)|, \tag{5}$$

where τ_{left} and τ_{right} are the torques produced by the power of the left and right legs, respectively; τ_{lpedal} and τ_{rpedal} are the torques of the left and right legs, respectively; and

τ_{lgrav} and τ_{rgrav} are the torques arising from gravity effects on the left and right legs, respectively. All torques are the mean values for 10 rotations of the crankshaft. T_{diff} is the difference in the torque produced by the power of the healthy leg and that of the paralyzed leg. We expect that if the motor function of the patient is recovered, the value of T_{diff} will become smaller.

Experiment

An experiment was performed to test the efficacy of the evaluation index using the torque estimated by the proposed method. Four healthy subjects (three males and one female) and four hemiplegic patients (four males; Brunnstrom stages II to IV; two right-side impaired, two left-side impaired) participated in this experiment. The age range for the healthy subjects was 18 to 22 and for the hemiplegic patients was 46 to 83. All subjects had previously used a CWC.

In the experiment, the subjects sat on the virtual CWC and rotated the pedals for 30 seconds. The speed of pedaling was controlled at 30 rpm. The conditions of the load were changed in two steps: 0 Nm and 2 Nm. Prior to measurement, subjects practiced pedaling at each load condition and measurement was aborted if the subject could not rotate the pedals because of the excess load. The torque produced by the power of the leg and the value of T_{diff} were calculated using MATLAB.

RESULTS

All subjects could rotate the pedals at both load conditions. Figure 6 shows the mean values of T_{diff} for the healthy subjects and the hemiplegic patients. For both load conditions, the values of T_{diff} for the hemiplegic patients were larger than those of the healthy subjects. Independent t-test analysis showed that these differences are significant. These differences occurred because the paralyzed leg was not able to generate the same torque as the healthy leg. Figures 7 (a) and (b) show examples of the torque produced by each leg for the healthy subject and the hemiplegic patient, respectively. For the healthy subject, the torque of each leg is similar. However, the hemiplegic patient results show that the paralyzed leg produced a negative torque because it hardly moved and did not rotate the crankshaft. In addition, the healthy leg needed to generate a larger torque to compensate for the shortage of torque from the paralyzed leg. Thus, the value of T_{diff} for the hemiplegic patients is larger than that for the healthy subjects. Also, as load increased, the difference of the values of T_{diff} between hemiplegic patients and healthy subjects became large. This result is because the hemiplegic patients had to apply a stronger force to the pedal of the healthy leg when the condition of the load was 2 Nm. Therefore, only the value of T_{diff} for the hemiplegic patients became large. This means that applying an additional load can be used to estimate the motor function in more detail.

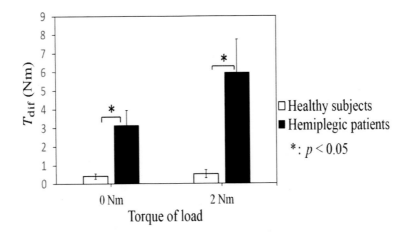

Figure 6. Results comparison between the healthy and hemiplegic subjects.

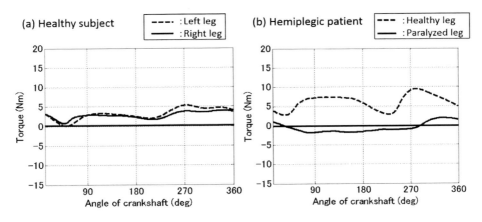

Figure 7. Torque produced by the power of the leg for (a) a healthy subject and (b) a hemiplegic patient.

DISCUSSION

In this study, we proposed a new method to estimate the torque produced (and hence the power of) each leg separately for a hemiplegic patient driving a virtual CWC. Moreover, we evaluated the motor function by an evaluation index using the torque, which is estimated by the proposed method. The experimental results show that the torque difference for the hemiplegic patients is significantly larger than that for the healthy subjects. These results indicate that the proposed method is useful in evaluating the motor function of the patient.

In the future, we plan to evaluate the motor function of patients driving the CWC while viewing the VR. To raise motivation for patient rehabilitation, patients must know the evaluation results using the VR. Therefore, we will develop a rehabilitation system that enables the patients to undergo rehabilitation and obtain feedback about their motor function. Moreover, we will collect long-term experimental results for the patients to evaluate the validity of the system.

ACKNOWLEDGMENTS

The authors wish to thank the staff and patients of the Miki Hospital and the staff of TESS Co., Ltd., for their technical contributions. This study was supported by JST Revitalization Promotion Program.

REFERENCES

[1] Suzuki K. The law of the medical innovation studied to a "cycling wheelchair". J Industry Acad Govern Collaboration 2012;8(6):20-3. [Japanese].

[2] Seki K, Sato M, Handa Y. Increase of muscle activities in hemiplegic lower extremity during driving a cycling wheelchair. Tohoku J Exp Med 2009; 219(2):129-38.

[3] Sugita N, Kojima Y, Yoshizawa M, Tanaka A, Abe M, Homma N, et al. Development of a virtual reality system to evaluate skills needed to drive a cycling wheel-chair. IEEE International Conference on Engineering in Medicine and Biology Society 2012: 6019-22.

[4] Suzuki S. Rehabilitation system for patients with leg paralysis using virtual reality. Dissertation. Sendai: Department Elect Common Engineering, Tohoku University, 2005. [Japanese].

[5] Saito H, Watanabe T, Arifin A. Ankle and knee joint angle measurements during gait with wearable sensor system for rehabilitation. Proceeding of World Congress on Medical Physics and Biomedical Engineering 2009; 25(9):506-9.

[6] Kaisumi A. A pedaling-assistive control method of a cycling-wheelchair. Dissertation. Sendai: Department Mech Engineering, Tohoku University, 2014.

Submitted: July 04, 2015. *Revised:* August 08, 2015. *Accepted:* August 14, 2015.

Chapter 21

LOW-COST ACTIVE VIDEO GAME CONSOLE DEVELOPMENT FOR DYNAMIC POSTURAL CONTROL TRAINING

Annie Pouliot-Laforte[1,2,3], MSc, Édouard Auvinet[2,4], PhD, Martin Lemay[1,2,3], PhD and Laurent Ballaz[1,2,3],*, PhD

[1] Department of Kinanthropology, Université du Québec à Montréal, Montreal, Canada
[2] UHC Sainte-Justine Research Center, Montreal, Canada
[3] Quebec Rehabilitation Research Network, Montreal, Canada
[4] Department of Mechanical Engineering, École Polytechnique de Montréal, Montreal, Canada

ABSTRACT

Weight shifting is a key ability to both train and monitor in rehabilitation processes. In the last decade, active video game consoles (AVGC) have been viewed as a promising and appealing way to facilitate weight shifting ability. However, to date, no commercially available AVGC have been specifically developed for balance and postural control throughout rehabilitation processes. The present study aims to establish a proof of concept about the possibility to integrate into a unique AVGC, a board, monitoring the player centre of pressure, and a Kinect, which takes into account the postural movement and player motor function capacity.

Keywords: active video games, dynamic postural control, rehabilitation, Kinect, Wii balance board

---

* Correspondence: Professor Laurent Ballaz, Department of Kinanthropology, Université du Québec à Montréal, 141 av. President-Kennedy, Montreal, Canada. E-mail: laurent.ballaz@gmail.com.

INTRODUCTION

Dynamic balance is particularly relevant in rehabilitation because of its importance in daily life activities (1). The ability to initiate and control weight shifts have been reported as a prerequisite for independent walking in various populations with motor disability (2). Performing weight shifting in response to a visual stimulus is a key ability to train and monitor in many motor impaired individuals (3, 4). More specifically, visually guided weight shifting is often required in everyday life situations. However, most tests currently used by clinicians and researchers involve self-generated weight shifting in which a person is asked to shift his or her weight within his or her stability limits (5) and do not require responses to any visual stimulus.

The lack of evidence concerning visually guided weight shifting ability could be related to the difficulty to adequately evaluate and train this complex ability. Active video game consoles (AVGC) have been used in people with motor impairment to solicit M/L (medial/lateral) weight shifting in the context of visually guided and task-oriented movements (6). AVGC based on centre of pressure (CoP) displacement measurement could therefore be viewed as a promising and appealing way to induce such movements. Ballaz et al. (7) evaluated the postural movement during a Nintendo Wii™ game (Nintendo, Kyoto, Japan) in children with cerebral palsy. They reported inappropriate trunk movements when participants with cerebral palsy shifted their weight from one leg to the other. This result highlighted the limit of this game controller, based on CoP displacement, to solicit adequate M/L weight shifting. Indeed, it is known that optimal weight shifting should be mainly performed with minimal trunk inclination (8). Therefore, a video based controller should be added to take into account postural movements of the participants. Also, the base of support width affects weight shifting and can vary greatly between participants, especially in a rehabilitation context. It is therefore crucial to consider this parameter to make sure that game requirements are adapted to the participant's weight shifting capacity.

In the next few years, we intend to develop and validate an AVGC dedicated to dynamic postural control rehabilitation. A first version of the AVGC is proposed here. The aim of the present study is to establish a proof of concept using different low-cost technologies to develop an innovative AVGC, which take into account the player weight transfer performance and the player postural movement. More specifically, this present study provides preliminary results on a) trunk inclination and b) base of support width measured using a video controller.

METHODS

An AVGC was developed combining the Nintendo Wii Fit board (Nintendo, USA) and the Kinect (Microsoft, Redmond, Washington, USA), to solicit M/L weight shifting in response to visual stimuli in a functional context. The association of the Wii Fit board and the Kinect allows quantifying both the CoP displacement (9) and the postural strategy (10) used by the player. The goal of the game is to catch water drops with a bowl that the player controls by lateral movement of their CoP (i.e., performing M/L weight shifting). The Kinect provides the opportunity to: (a) quantify the weight shifting strategy used by the player; and (b) provide a visual feedback about the adopted posture. More specifically, when the player shifts their weight with an excessive lateral trunk bending, the bowl topples (see Figure 1). Based on previous work (7) the trunk inclination required to make the bowl topple was set at a 20° angle. The amplitude of weight shifting and the velocity of the water drops are adjustable depending on the functional level of the player.

Participants

A convenience sample of four healthy adults, aged between 24 and 38 years old (2 males and 2 females; mean age [SD]: 30.5 [6.8] years; body mass: 65.3 [14.0] kg; height: 175 [9] cm) were recruited from our research center. A child of 6 years old with cerebral palsy (CP) was also recruited to test the AVGC (Gross Motor Function Classification System level I; body mass: 24 kg; height: 117.3 cm).

Procedure

Evaluation of the Kinect system
Healthy participants were asked to stand on the Wii Fit board at a distance of 2.7 meter from the Kinect. They were asked to place their feet following verbal instructions given by the examiner and to keep the same feet placement during a 5 seconds period. Participants were asked to simultaneously place their right and left foot as follow: left side, middle and right side. By combining the left and right foot positions, a total of 9 positions were tested. Thereafter, the participants were asked to shift their weight by bending the trunk laterally. They had to complete a set of 10 weight shifting at different amplitude, i.e., small, medium and maximal amplitude. This procedure was implemented to report the parameters using the usual game configuration.

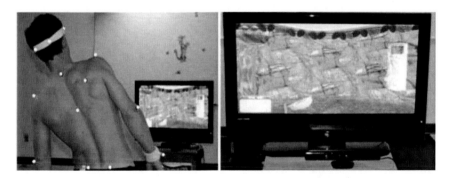

Figure 1. The visual feedback of trunk movement in the developed active video game.

Evaluation of the AVGC
A child with CP was asked to play the game as described above, namely "Choplo," for a duration of 5 minutes. The game parameters were defined as follows: maximal tolerated trunk inclination of 20 degrees; water drop fall frequency of 0.3 Hz; maximal horizontally water drop distance of 20 cm (related to the ankle distance). Here, we wanted to test the

performance of this integrated multi-sensor system. No measurements were performed with this participant.

Measurements

For all tests, the data were recorded synchronously by the Kinect and a 12-camera motion analysis system (ViconMX, Oxford Metrics, Oxford, UK) sampled at 100 Hz. Reflective markers, placed over several anatomic landmarks according to a slightly modified full body plug-in gait kinematic model, were tracked (see Ballaz et al. (7) for details). Kinematic data were exported from the Vicon workstation software and subsequently analysed using MatLab 7.4 (The MathWorks Inc., USA). The Kinect data were recorded and analysed with Microsoft NUI library (Microsoft, Redmond, USA). The Kinect frame rate was established at 30 Hz. To characterize the trunk inclination during M/L weight shifting, the trunk was modeled as a one-segment rigid linked system. The trunk segment was defined by the C7 marker and the middle of the posterior pelvic markers. With the Kinect, the trunk inclination was defined as the angle between the spine and the shoulder center markers (as defined by the Kinect kinematic model) versus the world vertical axis. To quantify the foot position and thereby the base support width, the ankle joint centre position was estimated by averaging the position of the internal and external malleolus Vicon markers. The ankle distance measured by the Kinect was calculated based on the ankle joint center marker.

Statistics

Pearson correlation coefficients were calculated to quantify the relationship between the Kinect and the motion analysis measurement for the distance between the ankle and the trunk inclination angle. Individual correlation was assessed for the two variables on all four participants.

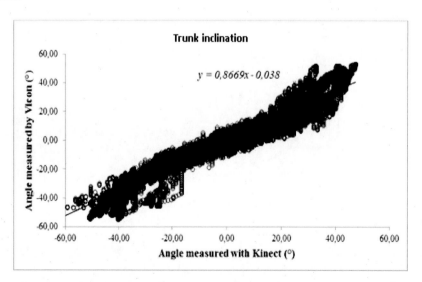

Figure 2. Pearson correlation for the trunk inclination angle measured with the Kinect and the motion analysis system.

RESULTS

The trunk inclination angle measured with the Kinect and the motion analysis system correlate highly ($r = 0.96$; $p < 0.05$). Individually, the correlations were similar ($r = 0.97$; $r = 0.98$; $r = 0.97$ and $r = 0.97$ for participants 1, 2, 3 and 4 respectively) with $p < 0.001$ for all correlations. No correlation was found between trunk angular velocity and measurement differences between the two systems.

A good correlation ($r = 0.85$; $p < 0.05$) was observed between the ankle distance measured with the Kinect and with the motion analysis system. Individually, correlations were high ($r = 0.86$; $r = 0.85$; $r = 0.88$ and $r = 0.98$, $p < 0.05$). The child with CP who played the AVG verbally reported that the game was a little difficult. The child reported that the water drops were falling too far on each side to be able to catch them and that they were falling too fast.

DISCUSSION

This study presents a new AVGC combining the Wii Fit board and the Kinect to elicit M/L weight shifting in response to visual stimuli in a functional context. The AVGC use the CoP measured by the Wii Fit board as a controller to move the bowl from one side to the other; the Kinect allows the quantification of trunk movement during M/L weight shifting. To our knowledge this is the first active video game combining these two devices.

The lateral trunk inclination was measured using a Kinect. Our results showed a high association between the motion analysis system and the Kinect measurements. The trunk inclination threshold was fixed, based on previous results comparing strategy of M/L weight shifting in children with CP and typically developing children (7). Our data demonstrated a high correlation in a range of 40 degrees of trunk inclination. Our results supports the results from Clark et al. (10) who compared the maximal trunk inclination measured with the Kinect and an optoelectronic motion capture system during functional reach tests.

The experiment with the CP participant showed the ability of this integrated multi-sensors system to function in a gaming context. The child with CP reported that the water drops were too far to the sides and that this parameter increased the difficulty of the game. It is important to note that the game was not calibrated to take into account the participant base of support width. As mentioned previously, the width of the participant's base of support can greatly vary in a rehabilitation context. Furthermore, weight shifting amplitude is related to the base of support width, a larger base of support allows a greater weight shifting amplitude. The participant's feedback highlights the importance of taking in account the base of support width in the game setting.

The high correlation reported in the present study between the ankle positions defined with the Kinect and the ankle positions defined with the optoelectronic motion capture system allow us to consider the Kinect as an efficient tool to quantify base of support width. Further studies are required to confirm this point and also to establish a relation between ankle distance and base of support width. Indeed, depending on the foot shape, the ankle position does not exactly represent the limit of the base of support. Eventually, it would be pertinent to calculate the base of support width continually while participants play on the AVGC, because foot movements are expected during the game. On the other hand, our results should be taken cautiously; the correlation coefficients do not allow quantifying systematic bias with Kinect measurement. Further analysis should be performed to answer those limitations.

Further research should validate the estimation of distance between the ankles in children with CP. They often have foot deformities and joint contractures in the lower limbs that may compromise the estimation of ankle distance by the Kinect. Moreover, the child with CP reported, after playing at the game, that the water drop falls were too fast. The game was developed to alter the velocity of the water drops depending on the functional level of the player. This result put in perspective that further studies should be performed to define the optimal speed or frequency of visual stimuli to allow adaptation of the game for people with impaired motor function.

An active video game combining the Wii Fit board and the Kinect is a promising way to assess visually guided weight shifting ability. This project also demonstrated that the Kinect is an effective tool to measure the distance between the ankle and the trunk inclination.

REFERENCES

[1] Brouwer B, Culham E, Liston R, Grant T. Normal variability of postural measures: implications for the reliability of relative balance performance outcomes. Scand J Rehabil Med 1998;30(3):131-7.

[2] Eng JJ, Chu KS. Reliability and comparison of weight-bearing ability during standing tasks for individuals with chronic stroke. Arch Phys Med Rehabil 2002; 83(8):1138-44.

[3] Dault MC, de Haart M, Geurts ACH, Arts IMP, Nienhuis B. Effects of visual center of pressure feedback on postural control in young and elderly healthy adults and in stroke patients. Hum Movement Sci 2003; 22(3):221-36.

[4] Laufer Y, Dickstein R, Resnik S, Marcovitz E. Weight-bearing shifts of hemiparetic and healthy adults upon stepping on stairs of various heights. Clin Rehabil 2000;14(2):125-9.

[5] de Haart M, Geurts AC, Dault MC, Nienhuis B, Duysens J. Restoration of weight-shifting capacity in patients with postacute stroke: A rehabilitation cohort study. Arch Phys Med Rehabil 2005;86(4): 755-62.

[6] Snider L, Majnemer A, Darsaklis V. Virtual reality as a therapeutic modality for children with cerebral palsy. Dev Neurorehabilitation 2010;13(2):120-8.

[7] Ballaz L, Robert M, Parent A, Prince F, Lemay M. Impaired visually guided weight-shifting ability in children with cerebral palsy. Res Dev Disabil 2014; 35(9):1970-7.

[8] Michalski A, Glazebrook CM, Martin AJ, Wong WWN, Kim AJW, Moody KD, et al. Assessment of the postural control strategies used to play two Wii Fit™ videogames. Gait Posture 2012;36(3): 449-53.

[9] Bartlett HL, Ting LH, Bingham JT. Accuracy of force and center of pressure measures of the Wii Balance Board. Gait Posture 2014;39(1):224-8.

[10] Clark RA, Pua Y-H, Fortin K, Ritchie C, Webster KE, Denehy L, et al. Validity of the Microsoft Kinect for assessment of postural control. Gait Posture 2012; 36(3):372-7.

Submitted: July 05, 2015. *Revised:* August 08, 2015. *Accepted:* August 14, 2015.

Chapter 22

IMPROVED MOBILITY AND REDUCED FALL RISK IN OLDER ADULTS AFTER FIVE WEEKS OF VIRTUAL REALITY TRAINING

Shirley R Shema[1], BPT, Pablo Bezalel[1], MSc, Ziv Sberlo[1], BSc, Orly Wachsler Yannai[2], MHA, Nir Giladi[1,3,4], MD, Jeffrey M Hausdorff[1,4,5,6], PhD and Anat Mirelman[1,], PhD*

[1]Center for the study of Movement, Cognition, and Mobility (CMCM),
Department of Neurology,
Tel Aviv Sourasky Medical Center, Tel Aviv, Israel
[2]Department of Physical Therapy, Tel Aviv Sourasky Medical Center,
Tel Aviv, Israel
[3]Sackler Faculty of Medicine, Tel-Aviv University, Tel Aviv, Israel
[4]Sagol School of Neuroscience, Tel-Aviv University, Tel Aviv, Israel
[5]Department of Physical Therapy, Tel-Aviv University, Tel Aviv, Israel
[6]Harvard Medical School, Boston, Massachusetts, US

ABSTRACT

The aim of this analysis was to assess whether five weeks of training with virtual reality (VR) in a clinical setting can reduce the risk of falls in a variety of older adults. Thirty-four participants attending the VR clinic were studied. Participants underwent 15 training sessions consisting of walking on a treadmill with a VR simulation. Significant improvements were observed in gait speed, the Four Square Step Test and the Timed Up and Go. Treadmill training with VR appears to be an effective and practical clinical tool to improve mobility and reduce fall risk in older adults.

Keywords: executive function, treadmill training, virtual reality, fall risk

---

[*] Correspondence: Anat Mirelman, PhD, Associate Director, Center for the Study of Movement, Cognition, and Mobility (CMCM), Department of Neurology, Tel Aviv Sourasky Medical Center, 6 Weizmann Street, IL-64239 Tel Aviv, Israel. E-mail: anatmi@tlvmc.gov.il.

INTRODUCTION

Normal and safe mobility depends on intact sensory and motor systems, but there is a growing body of research that specifically links the cognitive sub-domains of attention and executive function (EF) to gait alterations and fall risk (1, 2). EF apparently plays a critical role in the regulation of gait especially under challenging conditions where decisions need to be made in real-time and constant adaptation is required to manage internal and external factors (3). External factors can include, for example, obstacle crossing or attending to multiple tasks during walking. The performance during more demanding daily activities, such as walking while performing a simultaneous task (i.e., dual or multi task) or obstacle negotiation, plays a key role in the safety and well-being of a variety of individuals with either motor and cognitive dysfunctions (4, 5). Thus, interventions which focus on a combined motor-cognitive approach may improve gait and decrease the risk of falls.

Previous studies on the use of virtual reality (VR) for training of balance, gait and fall risk in older adults and individuals with neurological disorders have shown positive effects on walking speed, stride time and step length as well as in the ability to perform dual task and obstacle negotiation as compared to training in conventional balance training groups (6–8). Studies have also shown improved dual task ability and cognitive function after the use of motor-cognitive rehabilitation using VR (9, 10). Recently we have also shown positive effects of using VR as a clinical service (11). The effects of VR on the risk of falls in older adults are unknown.

The 'timed up and go' test (TUG) (12) is a quick and widely used performance-based measure of mobility. The TUG has been extensively studied in older adults (13, 14) and recommended as a simple screening test of fall risk. TUG duration has also been associated with cognitive function (15, 16). More specifically, older adults with better executive function and attention performed the TUG more quickly (16, 17). Previous work has demonstrated the added value of using body-worn sensors to augment the traditional TUG (18). Thus the aim of this analysis was to assess whether five weeks of training with VR in a clinical setting can reduce the risk of falls as measured using the instrumented TUG and other tests of mobility in a variety of older adults with gait impairments.

METHODS

The current retrospective data analysis reviewed the medical records of 34 participants (mean age 74.51 ± 10.51 years, 56% women) attending a gait rehabilitation program at the VR clinic in the Tel Aviv Sourasky Medical Center. The study was approved by the local institutional human studies committee. All participants were referred to the clinic by their physicians. Indications for referral included recurrent falls, fear of falling, complaints of gait instability or recent deterioration of gait, mainly but not exclusively due to neurological etiology. Participants were eligible for the training program if they were: (i) able to walk independently for at least 5 minutes with or without walking aids; (ii) did not have any cardiac contra-indication for moderate training intensity; and (iii) did not have severe visual loss that could interfere with their ability to see the VR simulation. Participants who could not follow simple instructions and those with dementia (as per DSM IV guidelines) or diagnosed psychiatric disorders were not eligible for the training program.

Training

Training was provided three times per week for five weeks with each session lasting about one hour. During the training, patients walked on a treadmill with a safety harness which did not provide body weight support. Two light emitting diodes (LEDs) were attached to the lateral side of the patients' shoes which served as the interface to the VR simulation that was projected on a screen in front of the treadmill. The virtual environment (VE) simulation included an obstacle course situated along different pathways in an outdoor scene. The various pathways differed in duration, number of intersections, and challenging segments which included bifurcations and walking on a bridge over a river. The virtual obstacles required negotiation in two planes: (i) vertical, to increase step clearance; and (ii) horizontal, to increase step length (see Figure 1). Difficulty levels were graded based on obstacle size and frequency of appearance as well as time of appearance requiring the participants to plan ahead, adapt their steps and select the correct negotiation strategy to avoid a collision. Feedback was provided by the simulation and consisted of knowledge of performance and knowledge of results. Training parameters were gradually increased from week 1 to week 5. Motor load was increased by adapting the treadmill speed, prolonging walking duration and decreasing the participants' hand support on the treadmill bars while walking. The VE parameters were progressed by presenting a wider range of obstacle sizes, increasing obstacle frequency of appearance, disrupting visual clarity and the addition of virtual distracters. Cognitive load progression was achieved by challenging sustained and divided attention, planning and reaction time.

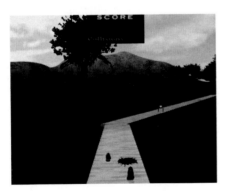 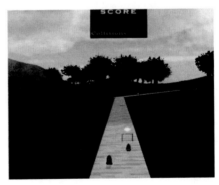

Figure 1. Two types of virtual obstacles were used, requiring patients to adjust proper step length and step clearance.

Clinical evaluation and assessment

Gait speed was assessed before and after the training by measuring the time walk 10 meters. Obstacle negotiation was assessed using the Four Square Step Test (FSST). The instrumented Timed Up and Go (TUG) test was used to evaluate functional mobility, dynamic balance and fall risk (14). Participants wore a small, portable, light-weight body-fixed sensor (DynaPort, McRoberts BV, The Hague, the Netherlands) on their lower back secured using a neoprene belt. The sensor includes a triaxial accelerometer and gyroscope. Acceleration signals were derived from three axes: vertical, mediolateral, and anterior posterior. Angular velocities were derived from the gyroscope as yaw (rotation around the vertical axis), pitch (rotation around the mediolateral axis), and roll (rotation around the anterior-posterior axis). After testing was completed, data were transferred to a personal computer for further analysis. The TUG subtasks (sit-to-stand and stand-to-sit transitions, walking, and turning) were analyzed using an automated algorithm based on the anterior-posterior axis that was used for detecting the start and end times of the TUG (19).

Data analysis

Data was examined for normality and descriptive statistics were extracted for all clinical measures. Data was compared across time (i.e., before vs. after the 5 weeks of training) using paired t-tests or Wilcoxon Signed Rank test, as appropriate. Analyses were performed using SPSS version 21 with an alpha level of 0.05.

RESULTS

All participants finished all 15 sessions of training. No adverse events were reported. All subjects had a history of falls (mean 2.82 ± 4.16 falls in the 6 months prior to the study) and demonstrated a high risk of falls as reflected by the TUG pre-training (18.53 ± 9.08 sec). Gait speed improved after training (0.97 ± 0.26 m/s to 1.03 ± 0.28 m/s; $p = 0.025$). Similarly, dynamic balance and obstacle negotiation (FSST) improved after training by 14% (from 17.34 ± 6.77 sec to 14.92 ± 4.99 sec; $p = 0.014$).

Time to complete the TUG significantly improved demonstrating a decrease in fall risk (18.53 ± 9.08 sec to 16.77 ± 7.63 sec; $p = 0.008$). Analysis of the subtasks of the instrumented TUG demonstrated that improvements in TUG duration stem from faster walking speed during the walking subtask of the TUG (10.5 ± 6.07 sec vs. 9.48 ± 5.57 sec; $p = 0.019$), with decreased number of steps taken (20 ± 13.48 vs. 17.38 ± 11.61; $p=0.009$). In addition, the duration of the turn-to-sit was reduced after training (2.38 ± 0.89 sec vs. 2.12 ± 0.62 sec; $p = 0.043$), reflecting lower angular velocity during the turns.

DISCUSSION

The study demonstrates that after 5 weeks of intensive treadmill training with VR, the participants preformed the TUG and the FSST faster, suggesting improved functional mobility. The improvements observed in after training further reflect an important decrease in the risk of falls at a group level. The use of wearable sensors to quantify the TUG and its subtasks provided insights into gait performance and the specific effects of the VR training. The results demonstrated that the subjects walked faster with an increased step length as reflected by the decreased number of steps taken. This finding is directly related to the trained tasks and demonstrated transfer of training effects. However, the results also revealed additional benefits in dynamic stability and planning as observed by the reduced turn duration.

Training with VR differs from usual gait training, as it contains cognitive aspects of planning, constant adaptation and shifting of attention under challenging motor conditions. As a combined approach, it promotes motor learning through problem solving, thus enhancing executive. The TUG and FSST present short yet relatively complex motor-cognitive tasks, demanding rapid changes in body alignment (i.e., turns or step direction) while maintaining balance. These tests are associated with cognitive processes, since they require subjects to remember and execute a timed motor sequence, involving motor planning and shifting, attributes that are needed for maintaining safe gait in daily living. Thus the present findings suggest that training with VR can promote both motor and cognitive function that can transfer to daily living activities and promote health.

We believe that the use of different virtual obstacles promoted greater clearance and increased step length contributing to the improved gait pattern. The virtual environment enabled a challenging training in a functional context, while maintaining patient safety which is valuable for the patient and the trainer. The ecological validity of the virtual simulation promoted motor learning as well as transfer of gains into real world performance. The findings suggest that after training, participants had better functional mobility and had decreased risk of falls. The study further demonstrates the utility of VR in a clinical setting in improving functional abilities and gait performance in a variety of older adults. A future analysis of a larger cohort, including subjects with additional musculoskeletal pathologies, may help to identify further indications for this program.

ACKNOWLEDGMENTS

We would like to thank the participants of this study as well as Eran Gazit, Inbal Maidan, Moran Dorfman, Lior Yeshaayahu, Ricki Turgeman for their assistance in this study. This research was supported in part by the European Commission (FP7 project V-TIME-278169) and by the Tel Aviv Sourasky Medical Center Grant of Excellence.

REFERENCES

[1] Springer S, Giladi N, Peretz C, Yogev G, Simon ES, Hausdorff JM. Dual-tasking effects on gait variability: the role of aging, falls, and executive function. Mov Disord 2006;21(7):950–7.

[2] Yogev-Seligmann G, Hausdorff JM, Giladi N. The role of executive function and attention in gait. Mov Disord 2008;23(3):329–42.

[3] Ble A, Volpato S, Zuliani G, Guralnik JM, Bandinelli S, Lauretani F, et al. Executive function correlates with walking speed in older persons: the InCHIANTI study. J Am Geriatr Soc 2005;53(3):410–5.

[4] Beauchet O, Dubost V, Herrmann F, Rabilloud M, Gonthier R, Kressig RW. Relationship between dual-task related gait changes and intrinsic risk factors for falls among transitional frail older adults. Aging Clin Exp Res 2005;17(4):270–5.

[5] Shumway-Cook A, Woollacott M. Attentional demands and postural control: the effect of sensory context. J Gerontol A Biol Sci Med Sci 2000;55(1):M10-6.

[6] Buccello-Stout RR, Bloomberg JJ, Cohen HS, Whorton EB, Weaver GD, Cromwell RL. Effects of sensorimotor adaptation training on functional mobility in older adults. J Gerontol B Psychol Sci Soc Sci 2008;63(5): 295–300.

[7] de Bruin ED, Schoene D, Pichierri G, Smith ST. Use of virtual reality technique for the training of motor control in the elderly. Some theoretical considerations. Z Gerontol Geriatr 2010;43(4):229–34.

[8] Mirelman A, Patritti BL, Bonato P, Deutsch JE. Effects of virtual reality training on gait biomechanics of individuals post-stroke. Gait Posture 2010;31(4):433–7.

[9] Mirelman A, Maidan I, Herman T, Deutsch JE, Giladi N, Hausdorff JM. Virtual reality for gait training: can it induce motor learning to enhance complex walking and reduce fall risk in patients with Parkinson's disease? J Gerontol A Biol Sci Med Sci 2011;66(2):234–40.

[10] Mirelman A, Raphaely-Beer N, Dorffman M, Brozgol M, Hausdorff JM. Treadmill training with Virtual Reality to decrease risk of falls in idiopathic fallers: a pilot Study. International Conference on Virtual Rehabilitation (ICVR) 2011:1–4.

[11] Shema SR, Brozgol M, Dorfman M, Maidan I, Sharaby-Yeshayahu L, Malik-Kozuch H, et al. Clinical experience using a 5-week treadmill training program with virtual reality to enhance gait in an ambulatory physical therapy service. Phys Ther 2014;94(9):1319-26.

[12] Podsiadlo D, Richardson S. The timed 'Up & Go': a test of basic functional mobility for frail elderly persons. J Am Geriatr Soc 1991;39(2):142–8.

[13] Hatch J, Gill-Body KM, Portney LG. Determinants of balance confidence in community-dwelling elderly people. Phys Ther 2003;83(12):1072–9.

[14] Shumway-Cook A, Brauer S, Woollacott M. Predicting the probability for falls in community-dwelling older adults using the Timed Up & Go Test. Phys Ther 2000; 80(9):896–903.

[15] Donoghue OA, Horgan NF, Savva GM, Cronin H, O'Regan C, Kenny RA. Association between timed up-and-go and memory, executive function, and processing speed. J Am Geriatr Soc 2012;60(9):1681–6.

[16] Herman T, Giladi N, Hausdorff JM. Properties of the 'Timed Up and Go' test: more than meets the eye. Gerontology 2011;57(3):203–20.

[17] Donoghue OA, Horgan NF, Savva GM, Cronin H, O'Regan C, Kenny RA. Association between timed up-and-go and memory, executive function, and processing speed. J Am Geriatr Soc 2012;60(9):1681–6.

[18] Mirelman A, Weiss A, Buchman AS, Bennett DA, Giladi N, Hausdorff JM. Association between performance on Timed Up and Go subtasks and mild cognitive impairment: further insights into the links between cognitive and motor function. J Am Geriatr Soc 2014;62(4):673–8.

[19] Weiss A, Herman T, Plotnik M, Brozgol M, Giladi N, Hausdorff JM. An instrumented timed up and go: the added value of an accelerometer for identifying fall risk in idiopathic fallers. Physiol Meas 2011;32(12):2003–18.

Submitted: July 05, 2015. *Revised:* August 08, 2015. *Accepted:* August 14, 2015.

In: Alternative Medicine Research Yearbook 2017
Editor: Joav Merrick
ISBN: 978-1-53613-726-2
© 2018 Nova Science Publishers, Inc.

Chapter 23

THE POTENTIALITY OF VIRTUAL REALITY FOR THE EVALUATION OF SPATIAL ABILITIES: THE MENTAL SPATIAL REFERENCE FRAME TEST

Silvia Serino[1,]*, Francesca Morganti[2], PhD, Pietro Cipresso[1], PhD, Erika Emma Ruth Magni[2], MS and Giuseppe Riva[1,3], PhD

[1]IRCCS Istituto Auxologico Italiano, Milan
[2]Department of Human and Social Sciences,
University of Bergamo, Bergamo, Italy
[3]Università Cattolica del Sacro Cuore, Milan, Italy

ABSTRACT

In recent decades, the use of virtual reality (VR) in the context of cognitive evaluation of dementia has considerably increased. The main objective of this preliminary study is to assess the feasibility of a VR-based tool for detecting deficits in using different spatial reference frames by comparing the performances of patients with probable Alzheimer's disease with cognitively healthy controls. Although preliminary, our results showed the potentiality of using this VR-based tool to evaluate the ability in encoding and using different spatial reference frames.

Keywords: virtual reality, allocentric reference frame, egocentric reference frame, Alzheimer's disease

INTRODUCTION

The ageing population (aged 65 years and over) is projected to increase to 1.2 billion in 2025. Consequently, the prevalence of dementia will significantly increase. Alzheimer's disease

---

* Correspondence: Silvia Serino, IRCCS Istituto Auxologico Italiano, Via Pellizza da Volpedo 41, 20149 Milan (MI), Italy. E-mail: s.serino@auxologico.it.

(AD) is the most common type of dementia, and it is estimated that the number of elderly affected will reach 81.1 million by 2040 (1). Thus, the identification of early markers of cognitive decline in the elderly population is now a worldwide health policy priority.

In recent decades, the use of virtual reality (VR) in the context of cognitive evaluation of dementia has considerably increased (2). VR technologies may be integrated in clinical and research settings to support the detection of early cognitive deficits by offering enriched environments with ecological but controlled demands (3, 4). Specifically, digital environments, perceived as comparable as real ones, may overcome the limits of traditional tests used to measure spatial abilities. Precisely, VR offers the chance to easily control and manipulate the egocentric point of view to investigate the ability to encode and use different spatial reference frames. Indeed, spatial cognition may be defined as a high-level cognitive process based on two different spatial reference frames: an egocentric spatial frame in which object locations are represented relative to the individual and an allocentric spatial frame in which object locations are represented irrespective of the individual (5). Specifically, within the hippocampus, the CA3 region, receiving input from the entorhinal cortex, constitutes a cognitive model of the scene towards which the individual is drawn (namely, an allocentric view-point dependent representation) while the CA1 neurons, receiving input from the CA3 via Schaffer's collaterals, quickly encode abstract object-to-object information (namely, an allocentric view-point independent representation) (6, 7). Accordingly, VR may be particularly useful for evaluating the cognitive profile of AD, since deficits in spatial cognition distinguish the first stages of this disease (8–10).

Nestor and colleagues (11) developed and tested a virtual navigation test – the Virtual Route Learning Test (VRLT) – for investigating spatial abilities in AD patients, and this provides an interesting example. In this virtual test, participants are invited to learn four routes of increasing complexity. They are then required to retrieve the same route from memory but in reverse. The results showed that the VRLT is able to detect spatial impairment in very early AD, as well as discriminate the AD patients from patients with Semantic Dementia. On these premises, we developed a VR-based tool – the Mental Spatial Reference Frame Test – to specifically evaluate the ability to encode and use different spatial reference frames. The main objective of this preliminary study is to assess the potentiality of utilizing this virtual tool to detect deficits in the use of different spatial reference frames by comparing the performances of patients with probable AD with cognitively healthy controls.

METHODS

Overall, 16 participants, eight cognitively healthy participants (CG, control group), and eight participants suffering from probable AD (probable AD) according to NINCDS-ADRDA criteria, participated in the study (12). The probable AD group comprised two women and eight men while CG included four women and four men. CG and probable AD participants were recruited from different social senior centers located in Lombardy, Italy. Individuals did not receive monetary reward for their participation in the study and was asked to sign the informed consent to participate in the study.

Spatial neuropsychological assessment

To evaluate the cognitive functioning of the participants in the study, the Mini Mental State Examination (MMSE) (13) was administered. Moreover, the probable AD group was also assessed using Milan Overall Dementia Assessment (MODA) (14), a brief neuropsychological test developed to evaluate dementia.

In order to evaluate the spatial abilities of the participants of the study, the following neuropsychological tests were administered:

- Corsi Block Test (15, 16): The test material consists of nine wooden blocks (1.25 inch cubes) unevenly distributed over a flat board. Once the experimenter taps different sequences of blocks, the participants are invited to tap out the same sequences. It is used to measure short-term spatial memory (Corsi – Span) and long-term spatial memory (Corsi – Supraspan);
- Money Road Map (17): This is a paper and pencil assessment of left-right discrimination that requires an egocentric mental rotation in space;
- Manikin's Test (18): This test is used to evaluate general mental rotation abilities by asking participants to evaluate in which hand a "little man" (shown from different view-points) was holding a ball;
- Benton Judgment of Line Orientation Test (19): This is a common neuropsychological test to assess visuo-spatial judgment.

All scores obtained from these neuro-psychological tests have been corrected for age, education level, and gender according to Italian normative data. Mean scores of these tests are summarized in Table 1.

Table 1. Mean scores at neuropsychological spatial assessment tasks reported by the two groups in the study

	Group	
	Probable AD	**Control Group**
Age	82.2 (6.69)	82.9 (9.12)
Years of Education	6.13 (2.8)	9.38 (4.81)
MMSE	23.1 (1.49)	28.7 (.965)
MODA	66.2 (9.66)	
Corsi Block Test – Span	4.19 (.91)	4.75 (.5)
Corsi Block Test – Supraspan	5.58 (1.24)	9.61 (2.86)
Money Road Map	17.6 (3.70)	19.4 (6.02)
Manikin's Test	17.00 (3.07)	26.00 (3.55)
Judgment of Line Orientation	6.38 (5.63)	15.63 (5.75)

Mental spatial reference frame test

The "Mental spatial reference frame test" consists of two main tasks that assess the abilities to encode and use different spatial reference frames. In the encoding phase, the participant is asked to navigate in a virtual room that includes two objects, that is, starting from the center of the room oriented toward North, he/she has to memorize the position of two objects. On the first task (Task 1), she/he is asked to indicate the position of one object on a real map (namely, a retrieval with spatial allocentric information independent of point of view). On the second task (Task 2), she/he is asked to enter an empty version of the same virtual room. The participant has to indicate the position of the object, starting from the position of the other object (namely, a retrieval without any spatial allocentric information). In both tasks, the accuracy of the answer is the dependent variable [1 = poor answer, for example, choosing the opposite side of the virtual room (i.e., choosing the southern side when the object in the learning phase was in the northern part); 2 = medium answer, for example bad left-right discrimination (i.e., the eastern part of the virtual room, when the object in the learning phase was in the western side); 3 = correct answer)].

The entire procedure was repeated across three different trials. In the first trial, the object in the learning phase was on the East side, in the second trial the object was on the West side, in the third trial the object was on the South side. From a technical point of view, the Mental Spatial Reference Frame was created using NeuroVirtual 3D, a recent extension of the software NeuroVR (20, 21), which is a free virtual reality platform for creating virtual environments that are useful for neuropsychological assessment and neurorehabilitation. The virtual environments was rendered using a portable computer (ACER ASPIRE with CPU Intel® Core™i5 and Nvidia GeForce GT 540M graphic processor). Participants also had a gamepad (Logitech Rumble F510), which allowed them to explore and to interact with the environment.

RESULTS

The data were entered into Microsoft Excel and analyzed using SPSS version 18 (Statistical Package for the Social Sciences–SPSS for Windows, Chicago, IL, USA). First, differences in neuropsychological tests of spatial abilities between groups (CG vs. Probable AD) were calculated using one-way ANOVAs. The results showed significant differences between the two groups in all tests, with the exception of the Corsi Block Test – Span and the Money Road Map. Specifically, when compared to CG, probable AD participants showed poorer spatial abilities. Then, differences in the scores on the Mental Spatial Reference Frame Test were calculated using a repeated measure ANOVA (Bonferroni's adjustment): 2 Tasks (Task 1 vs. Task 2) × 3 Trials as within factors, and Group (CG vs. probable AD group) as between variable.

The results showed a significant effect of Trials, $F(2, 26) = 5.48$, $p < .05$, $\eta p2 = .301$. Specifically, pairwise comparisons indicated that the average scores were significantly lower on the third trials (M = 1.99, SD = 0.11) compared to the first trials (M = 2.55, SD = .12).

Second, the results showed significant differences between the two different Tasks, $F(1, 13) = 20.30$, $p < .001$, $\eta p2 = .610$. In particular, pairwise comparisons revealed that the average scores were significantly lower in Task 2 (M = 1.96, SD = 0.13) compared to Task 1 (M = 1.96, SD = .13). Although we found no significant differences between Groups, it is possible to observe a trend toward significance in the interaction Trials × Tasks × Groups $F(2, 26) = 2.70$, $p = .086$, $\eta p2 = .176$. In particular, probable AD participants performed poorer on the third trial of Task 2 (see Figure 1).

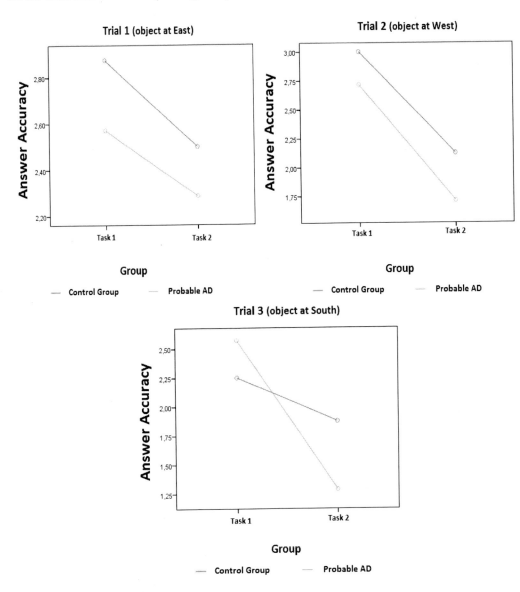

Figure 1. Probable AD group performed poorer on the third trial (object in the South of the virtual room), especially in the Task 2.

CONCLUSION

Due to the impressive growth in the ageing population, the identification of cognitive markers to characterize the profile of AD has been recently the focus of considerable research interest. In this direction, our main objective was to investigate the potentiality of using the Mental Spatial Reference Frame Test in the traditional neuropsychological evaluation of spatial abilities in patients suffering from probable AD.

First, as expected, our results confirmed that probable AD patients were impaired in the traditional neuropsychological evaluation of spatial functions when compared with the control group. Concerning the results from the Mental Spatial Reference Frame Test, our findings showed that all participants were less accurate in completing the third trial, significantly when compared to the first one. The third trial may have been more difficult since the object was presented at the South end of the virtual room in the encoding phase, requiring a complete spatial rotation to retrieve it. Moreover, our results showed that all participants performed poorer on Task 2 when compared to Task 1. While Task 1 measured the ability to encode and store an allocentric reference frame by asking participants to retrieve the position of the object on a real map, Task 2 evaluated a more complex spatial ability, since the participants were required to indicate the position of the object in an empty virtual room without any spatial allocentric information. Indeed, to solve Task 2, it was necessary to retrieve the object-to-object abstract cognitive representation of the scene and impose on it a new egocentric view-point. According to Byrne and colleagues (22) an effective spatial orientation in the surrounding environment requires a translation from a long-term allocentric reference frame to an egocentric one.

Starting from this model, Serino and Riva proposed that, for an effective translation between allocentric and egocentric spatial reference frames, it is crucial that allocentric view-point independent representation has to be synced with the allocentric view-point dependent representation (23, 24). From this perspective, our findings showed that probable AD participants performed poorer on the third trial of Task 2, that is, when they were required a complete mental rotation, they showed a deficit in the synchronization between the allocentric view-point independent representation and the allocentric view-point dependent representation. A break in the "mental frame syncing", underpinned by damages to the hippocampus, may be a crucial cognitive marker both for early and differential diagnosis of AD (23). The findings of this preliminary study are interesting, although some limitations should be acknowledged. First, the sample size was very small. Moreover, it would be interesting to replicate this study using an immersive VR set-up. Future studies should investigate whether the detection of subtle spatial deficits could be used to identify individuals most at risk for progression to AD.

ACKNOWLEDGMENTS

This study was partially supported by the research project "NeuroVirtual 3D" funded by Regione Piemonte (Grant No. FA 211-432C- 2012).

REFERENCES

[1] Ferri CP, Prince M, Brayne C, Brodaty H, Fratiglioni L, Ganguli M, et al. Global prevalence of dementia: a Delphi consensus study. Lancet 2006;366(9503): 2112-7.
[2] Bohil CJ, Alicea B, Biocca FA. Virtual reality in neuroscience research and therapy. Nature Rev Neurosci 2011;12(12):752–62.
[3] Rizzo AA, Schultheis M, Kerns KA, Mateer C. Analysis of assets for virtual reality applications in neuropsychology. Neuropsychol Rehabil 2004;14 (1-2):207–39.
[4] Riva G. Virtual reality: an experiential tool for clinical psychology. Br J Guidance Couns 2009;37(3):337–45.
[5] Klatzky RL. Allocentric and egocentric spatial representations: definitions, distinctions, and interconnections. In: Freksa C, Habel C, eds. Spatial cognition. An interdisciplinary approach to representing and processing spatial knowledge. Dordrecht: Springer, 1998:1–17.
[6] Robertson RG, Rolls ET, Georges-François P. Spatial view cells in the primate hippocampus: effects of removal of view details. J Neurophysiol 1998;79(3): 1145-56.
[7] Behrendt RP. Conscious experience and episodic memory: hippocampus at the crossroads. Front Psychol 2013;4:304.
[8] Gazova I, Vlcek K, Laczó J, Nedelska Z, Hyncicova E, Mokrisova I, et al. Spatial navigation – a unique window into physiological and pathological aging. Front Aging Neurosci 2012;4.
[9] Lithfous S, Dufour A, Després O. Spatial navigation in normal aging and the prodromal stage of Alzheimer's disease: insights from imaging and behavioral studies. Ageing Res Rev 2013;12(1):201–13.
[10] Serino S, Cipresso P, Morganti F, Riva G. The role of egocentric and allocentric abilities In Alzheimer's disease: A systematic review. Ageing Res Rev 2014;16: 32–44.
[11] Pengas G, Patterson K, Arnold RJ, Bird CM, Burgess N, Nestor PJ. Lost and found: bespoke memory testing for Alzheimer's disease and semantic dementia. J Alzheimers Dis 2010;21(4):1347–65.
[12] McKhann G, Drachman D, Folstein M, Katzman R, Price D, Stadlan EM. Clinical diagnosis of Alzheimer's disease Report of the NINCDS-ADRDA Work Group* under the auspices of Department of Health and Human Services Task Force on Alzheimer's Disease. Neurology 1984;34(7):939–44.
[13] Folstein MF, Folstein SE, McHugh PR. "Mini-mental state": a practical method for grading the cognitive state of patients for the clinician. J Psychiatr Res 1975;12(3): 189–98.
[14] Brazzelli M, Capitani E, Della Sala S, Spinnler H, Zuffi M. A neuropsychological instrument adding to the description of patients with suspected cortical dementia: the Milan overall dementia assessment. Journal of Neurology, Neurosurg Psychiatry 1994;57(12):1510–7.
[15] Corsi PM. Human memory and the medial temporal region of the brain. Dissertation. Montreal: McGill University, 1972.
[16] Spinnler H, Tognoni G. Standardizzazione e taratura Italiana di test neuropsicologici. Italian J Neurol Sci 1987;6(Suppl 8):47-50. [Italian].
[17] Money I, Alexander D, Walker HT. Manual: A standardized road-map test of direction sense. Baltimore, MD: Johns Hopkins Press, 1965.
[18] Ratcliff G. Spatial thought, mental rotation and the right cerebral hemisphere. Neuropsychologia 1979;17(1): 49–54.
[19] Benton AL, Varney NR, Hamsher KS. Visuospatial judgment Arch Neurology 1978;35:364–7.
[20] Riva G, Gaggioli A, Grassi A, Raspelli S, Cipresso P, Pallavicini F, et al. NeuroVR 2-A free virtual reality platform for the assessment and treatment in behavioral health care. Stud Health Technol Inform 2011;163: 493-5.
[21] Cipresso P, Serino S, Pallavicini F, Gaggioli A, Riva G. NeuroVirtual 3D: A multiplatform 3D simulation system for application in psychology and neuro-rehabilitation. In: Ma M, ed. Virtual, augmented reality and serious games for healthcare 1. Dordrecht: Springer, 2014:275–86.
[22] Byrne P, Becker S, Burgess N. Remembering the past and imagining the future: a neural model of spatial memory and imagery. Psychol Rev 2007;114(2):340.

[23] Serino S, Riva G. Getting lost in Alzheimer's disease: A break in the mental frame syncing. Med Hypotheses 2013;80(4):416–21.
[24] Serino S, Riva G. What is the role of spatial processing in the decline of episodic memory in Alzheimer's disease? The "mental frame syncing" hypothesis. Front Aging Neurosci 2014;6:33.

Submitted: July 08, 2015. *Revised:* August 18, 2015. *Accepted:* August 16, 2015.

In: Alternative Medicine Research Yearbook 2017
Editor: Joav Merrick

ISBN: 978-1-53613-726-2
© 2018 Nova Science Publishers, Inc.

Chapter 24

VIRTUAL SPATIAL NAVIGATION TESTS BASED ON ANIMAL RESEARCH: SPATIAL COGNITION DEFICIT IN FIRST EPISODES OF SCHIZOPHRENIA

Iveta Fajnerová[1,2,*]*, MSc, MA, PhD, Kamil Vlček*[2]*, MSc, PhD, Cyril Brom*[3]*, MSc, PhD, Karolína Dvorská*[1]*, MA, David Levčík*[2]*, MSc, PhD, Lucie Konrádová*[1]*, MA, Pavol Mikoláš*[1]*, MD, Martina Ungrmanová*[1]*, Michal Bída*[3]*, MSc, Karel Blahna*[2]*, MD, PhD, Filip Španiel*[1]*, MD, PhD, Aleš Stuchlík, RNDr, PhD, Jiří Horáček*[1]*, Prof, MD, PhD and Mabel Rodriguez*[1]*, PhDr, PhD*

[1]Department of National IT System of Mental Health and Brain Monitoring, National Institute of Mental Health, Klecany, Czech Republic
[2]Department of Neurophysiology of Memory, Institute of Physiology, Czech Academy of Sciences, Prague, Czech Republic
[3]Department of Software and Computer Science Education, Faculty of Mathematics and Physics, Charles University, Prague, Czech Republic

ABSTRACT

The impairment of cognitive functions represents a characteristic manifestation in schizophrenia and related psychotic disorders, together with positive and negative symptoms. Cognitive symptoms offer very useful methodological approach for comparative studies in schizophrenia research. Both animal models of schizophrenia and schizophrenia patients have demonstrated behavioral changes in several spatial

---

* Correspondence: Iveta Fajnerová, MSc MA, PhD. National Institute of Mental Health (NIMH), Klecany, Czech Republic. E-mail: iveta.fajnerova@nudz.cz.

navigation tasks; assessment of spatial cognition can be therefore applied in comparative studies. To demonstrate the deficit of spatial cognition in schizophrenia, and to test the validity of pharmacological animal models of schizophrenia, we designed two virtual navigation tasks inspired by previous animal research: the virtual Morris water maze and the virtual Carousel maze. Both virtual tests consisting of four phases have been tested in a group of 30 first episode schizophrenia patients and a group of healthy volunteers matched for age, sex and education. In both tests, subjects were required to navigate towards several hidden goal positions placed on the floor of an enclosed stable arena or a rotating arena. Data obtained using these virtual tests show a decline in the cognitive performance of schizophrenia patients in comparison to matched healthy volunteers. Our findings thus support the validity of the animal model of cognitive deficit in schizophrenia and the presence of measurable impairment of cognitive functions in first episode schizophrenia patients.

Keywords: cognitive functions, spatial navigation, schizophrenia, virtual reality environment, Morris water maze, Carousel maze

INTRODUCTION

Schizophrenia is manifested in positive, negative and cognitive symptoms. Cognitive deficit is considered a characteristic and permanent manifestation accompanying schizophrenia and related psychotic disorders, affecting several cognitive domains (1, 2). The MATRICS (Measurement and Treatment Research to Improve Cognition in Schizophrenia) initiative identified seven crucial cognitive areas typically influenced in schizophrenia: attention, psychomotor speed, working memory, logical thinking, problems solving, social cognition, verbal memory and visuo-spatial learning (3).

Impairment of visuo-spatial abilities has been already demonstrated in animal models of schizophrenia (4–6) and in schizophrenia patients by application of complex virtual environments (7, 8) and various virtual tasks developed based on the original paradigm used in animals (9–11). Tasks used to test spatial skills thus have the potential to assess similar cognitive abilities in humans and animals.

To assess these complex spatial abilities in schizophrenia and compare our results with the data obtained previously in animal models of this disease, we have designed two virtual reality tests adopted from the original animal research. The first Morris water maze (12) paradigm was designed for rats to test their ability to search for a hidden platform in a circular pool filled with water and surrounded by several orientation cues. The second Carousel maze paradigm, the Active Allothetic Place Avoidance task (13), was designed for rats to test avoidance of the punished sector on the rotating arena defined by the room-bound orientation cues. Experiments in our study have been conducted in virtual reality (VR) environments that allowed us to build large-scale and dynamic environments with variable orientation cues. In addition, the VR technology allowed us to easily record precise information about the subjects' rotation and position, in order to measure their behavior in the virtual environments in a similar fashion as the camera tracking the behavior of animals in original animal tasks.

METHODS

A study group of 30 (17 males and 13 females, age 18-35) first-episode schizophrenia patients (SZ, diagnosed as acute psychotic episode or schizophrenia according to DSM-IV) and a control group of healthy volunteers (HC) were recruited and matched for age, sex, education level and gaming experience.

Apparatus and software

The game engine Unreal Tournament (UT2004; Epic Games) was used to visualize the virtual scene to the respondents, presented in a first-person view on a 24" LCD monitor. The custom-made Java software toolkit called "SpaNav" was connected to the game engine to control the experiment and collect online data. Subjects controlled their movements in the virtual environment using only one joystick of the gamepad device and one gamepad button marked by a green color to mark their orientation while pointing towards the target position.

Design and procedure

Clinical and Neuropsychological Assessment
To confirm the cognitive impairment in our group of first episode schizophrenia patients in comparison to the healthy controls, overall cognitive performance was measured with a battery of neuropsychological tests compatible with the MATRICS battery that assess psychomotor speed, mental flexibility, learning, memory and executive functions (see Table 1). In addition, all patients completed a psychiatric interview prior to the experiment in order to obtain information about their current symptomatology using the Positive and Negative Symptoms Scale – PANSS (14), and the Global Assessment of Functioning scale – GAF (15). All the patients were treated by second generation antipsychotics (olanzapin, risperidon and amisulpirid). The dose of antipsychotic medication was calculated in chlorpromazine (CPZ) equivalents (according to 16, 17).

Pre-training of motor control
Prior to the experiment all participants underwent a short pre-training of movement control via the gamepad device in a complex virtual maze. Consecutively all participants performed the experiment in two virtual tests, which both required the subject to navigate towards one of the 4 hidden goal positions placed on the floor of an arena, either stable or rotating. Each single trial started with pointing towards the goal and was followed by navigation towards the goal using three visible orientation cues.

Test on the stable arena
The virtual task with the hidden goal paradigm was inspired by the Morris water maze – MWM (12) and was performed in a large-scale enclosed virtual arena, see Figure 1B. This virtual test, called the virtual Four Goals Navigation – vFGN task (18), requires the participant to find and remember the hidden goal position on the floor of an enclosed virtual

tent using three visible orientation cues. Four separate phases of the vFGN task represent the analogies of the MWM protocol variants: (i) *Training* – a reference memory protocol with a stable goal position; (ii) *Acquisition* – a reversal protocol with a changing goal position; (iii) *Recall* – a delayed matching-to-place protocol; and (iv) *Probe* – trials with an inactivegoal position (without feedback).

Table 1. Group differences obtained in the battery of standard neurocognitive tests

Neurocognitive Assessment	Group Differences (SZ and HC)	
	Mann-Whitney U Test	p-value
Perceptual Vigilance task (PEBL)	111	0.0001
Verbal fluency	142	0.0001
Categorical fluency	152.5	0.0001
Trail making test (TMT)		
TMT - A	131.5	0.0001
TMT – B	82	0.0001
Auditory verbal learning test (AVLT)		
AVLT –I-V	156	0.0001
AVLT-VI after interference	125	0.0001
AVLT – after 30 min	116	0.0001
Spatial Span (WMS-III)		
forward	281.5	0.42
backward	218.5	0.046
Digit Span (WAIS-III)		
forward	296.5	0.078
backward	143.5	0.0001
Similarities (WAIS-III)	74	0.0001
Key Search test	314.5	0.143
Money Road map test - errors	243	0.0071

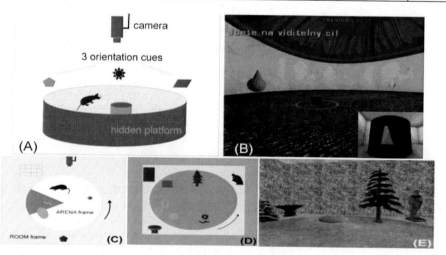

Figure 1. Illustration of the two virtual tasks (adjusted according to Fajnerova et al. (18): (A) The model of the original MWM apparatus for rats; (B) Virtual version – the vFGN task performed in an enclosed dry circular arena with visible goal position and two of the three orientation cues; (C) The original Carousel maze task; (D) Schematic view of the virtual AAPP tasks in Training conditions with two goal positions placed in two different reference frames – Room frame (square shaped goal position) and Arena frame (circular goal position); and (E) Rotating arena from the first-person view.

Test on the rotating arena (dynamic environment)

The second virtual test was inspired by the dynamic Carousel maze – Active allothetic place avoidance (AAPA) task – performed on a rotating arena (13). Notice, the original avoidance task was modified to a preference version k, as a virtual arena called the Active Allocentric Place Preference task (AAPP, Vlček et al. unpublished). The same hidden goal principle as in the previous task was used to test spatial abilities in subjects standing on a rotating arena. The hidden goal positions were either attached: (i) to the ARENA frame and rotated together with the tested individual; or (ii) to the ROOM frame and were stable throughout the experiment (and therefore moving with respect to the subject/arena, see Figure 1D). The time limit for each trial was set to 20 seconds. The task was divided to four separate phases: (i) *Training* – searching for two goals, one in the arena frame and one in the room frame; (ii) *Arena frame* – navigation towards two goals both attached to the arena frame; (iii) *Room frame* – navigation towards two goals that are both stable in the room frame; and (iv) *Frame switching* – alternated search between all 4 previously learned goals attached either to the arena frame or to the room frame.

Measured parameters and data analysis

The spatial performance measured in the *Stable arena* was, in all except probe trials, evaluated using two parameters: the *pointing error* (absolute angular difference between the pointed and correct linear direction towards the goal position); and the *path efficiency* (range 0 to 1, calculated as a ratio between the minimal path length and the real distance travelled by the subject). In probe trials, the *goal quadrant preference* (proportion of the trial time spent in the correct arena quadrant) was evaluated.

The performance in the *Rotating arena* was measured using the previously described *pointing error* parameter. The second applied *trial time* parameter represents the time needed to enter the goal position. Only selected parameters are presented in this paper. To analyze the data a custom-made PHP program called drf2track was used to produce primary data tables and trajectory pictures; further statistical analysis was performed in Statistica 11. The group differences in the standard test battery were calculated using the Mann-Whitney U test and differences in the repeated trials of virtual tests were calculated using the repeated measures ANOVA. The overall level of significance was set to 0.05.

RESULTS

The results of both virtual tests confirmed the deficit of cognitive abilities in the group of first episode schizophrenia patients.

Neurocognitive battery

A battery of standard neurocognitive tests, performed to determine the cognitive deficit in the group of schizophrenia patients, showed significant group differences, as expected according to the previous studies (2, 3). These results suggest that the first episode schizophrenia patients tested in our study are impaired in all assessed cognitive domains (see Table 1).

Stable arena

All phases of the vFGN task show a decline in the spatial abilities of schizophrenia patients in comparison to healthy volunteers, see (18) for further details. The first Training phase demonstrates learning difficulties presented in pointing error (see Figure 2A) and navigation accuracy ($p < 0.01$) in schizophrenia patients. The subsequent Acquisition phase, with changing goal position (A>B>C) as a measure of mental flexibility, showed only mild group differences in pointing ($p < 0.01$) but not in navigation accuracy (see Figure 2B – gray area), probably due to the skill learning effect (as all three goal positions were spatially identical). The recall of the three previously learned goal positions sequence (ABC) in the later Recall phase showed deficits of spatial working/long-term memory, demonstrated in significantly decreased navigation performance ($p < 0.001$), more so in the first repetition round, see Figure 2C. The last Probe phase, without feedback about the correct position, showed significantly disturbed spatial bias in schizophrenia patients ($p < 0.001$), demonstrated by a lower proportion of time spent in the correct arena quadrant where the hidden goal position was present (see Figure 2C).

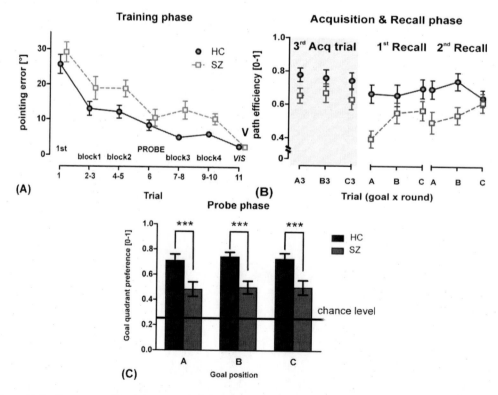

Figure 2. Performance of both groups in the vFGN task: (A) the Training session performance expressed using the pointing error parameter; (B) the path efficiency in the Acquisition phase (the last trial for each goal position) and in all Recall trials; and (C) the time proportion spent in the correct arena quadrant in the last Probe phase.

Rotating arena

Similarly, all phases of the virtual AAPP task show a decline of spatial performance in schizophrenia. The first Training phase showed impaired learning abilities on the rotating arena ($p < 0.01$, see Figure 3A). The second phase performed in the 'rotating (subjectively) stable' Arena frame showed only a mild decrease in measured parameters ($p < 0.01$), less clearly evident in the second half of trials (see Figure 3B). However, the third phase with navigation towards the goals connected to the stable (subjectively moving) Room frame (see Figure 3C) showed a strongly profound decline of spatial abilities in schizophrenia ($p < 0.001$). The last phase, created to assess the cognitive flexibility and coordination, as it required repeated switching between the two reference frames (switching between two mental maps or two sets of orientation cues specific for arena or room frame), shows a substantial deficit in schizophrenia patients ($p < 0.001$, see Figure 3D).

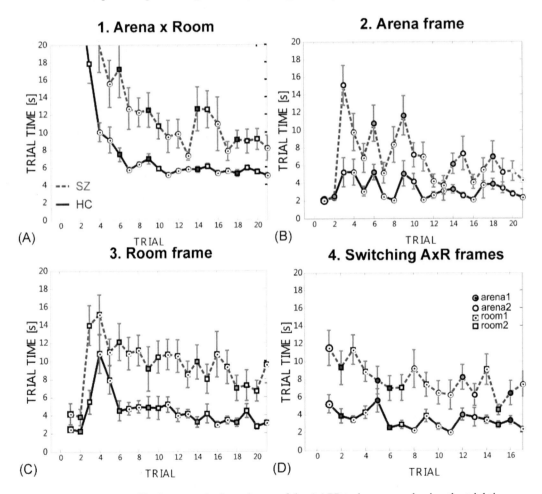

Figure 3. Performance of both groups in four phases of the AAPP task expressed using the trial time parameter: (A) the Training phase with simple frame switching (arena x room); (B) the Arena frame performance; (C) the Room frame performance; and (D) the alternation between all 4 previously acquired goal positions placed in one of the two reference frames.

DISCUSSION

Data obtained in the presented study show significant decline of visuo-spatial functions in first episode schizophrenia patients in comparison to healthy controls. Impaired spatial performance was present in all four phases of both tested virtual paradigms (navigation to the hidden goal on a stable and on a rotating arena). These findings support our results obtained using the battery of standard cognitive tests and results of previous studies in schizophrenia patients (2, 9) showing the necessity for remediation of spatial learning and memory after the first episode of psychosis.

Even though both methods used the same hidden goal paradigm and the same amount of orientation cues (three objects) for each hidden goal position, the dynamic environment of the rotating arena shows more pronounced decline of the spatial performance in schizophrenia than the paradigm in stable environment. This is not surprising as, due to the rotation of the arena, the task demands attentional shifts and navigation in changing conditions of the two reference frames, in contrast to the stable environment.

Considering that our results support the findings of visuo-spatial deficits observed in the animal model of schizophrenia (4–6), both tasks could be used as useful tools for future comparative studies transferring observations from the animal model of neuropsychiatric disorder to the simulated disease. In addition, we do believe that both virtual tasks could be useful in the measurement of cognitive enhancement as an outcome of pharmacological or non-pharmacological treatment in neuropsychiatric disorders, as they address complex cognitive functions.

Importantly, individual phases of both virtual tests demonstrated a variable extent of sensitivity towards the cognitive deficit in schizophrenia, supporting our assumption that particular parts of each test examine distinct visuo-spatial functions (e.g., learning, working memory, mental flexibility and coordination etc.). The first test on the *stable arena* showed that the performance in later recall and probe phases was more impaired than the performance measured during the acquisition process and reference memory phases. Similarly, in the experiment on the *rotating arena* the navigation towards goals defined in the room reference frame (perceived as moving goals) was more affected than the search for goal positions rotating together with the subject in the arena frame. These findings indicate that individual parts of these virtual tasks could form suitable tools for future virtual remediation of impaired visuo-spatial abilities in schizophrenia applying growing difficulty concept, e.g., by switching from stable to unstable reference frame.

Due to the potential of VR to easily modify the environmental stimuli, modified versions of the presented tests could be later applied in longitudinal clinical studies, such as the non-pharmacological intervention in schizophrenia patients provided by the National Institute of Mental Health. This computer-based and individually oriented cognitive remediation for psychotic patients combines several cognitive rehabilitation methods over 8 weeks (19) and could later proceed in a form of online training (neurokog.pcp.lf3.cuni.cz). Retest variants of the presented tests could be applied either to test the outcome of the remediation therapy by monitoring of complex spatial behavior, or as methods directly applicable in the neurocognitive training.

The future analysis will be aimed at clarifying the relationships between the two newly-developed virtual tasks and the battery of standardized tests used in this study. In addition, we currently also perform repeated assessment of schizophrenia patients one year after their first hospitalization, in order to test the presence of the cognitive deficit in full remission. This measurement also addresses the possible sensitivity of the newly developed methods towards the future course of illness in individual patients, either in the full remission of symptoms or potential relapse of the illness.

ACKNOWLEDGMENTS

We are grateful to Prof. Jan Bureš and Věra Bubeníková-Valešová for their scientific inspiration and valuable advice at the beginning of the project. We thank all ESO team members (study of first episodes of schizophrenia at NIMH) for their assistance in the collection of clinical data and Zbyněk Krulich for VE design. The study was supported mainly by IGA MZ CR grant No. NT13386, and partially by projects No. NT14291 and NT13843. The institutional support from the Academy of Sciences of the CR (RVO: 67985823) and the project Nr. LO1611 with a financial support from the MEYS under the NPU I program covered the salaries and other institutional costs.

REFERENCES

[1] Andreasen NC. A unitary model of schizophrenia: Bleuler's "fragmented phrene" as schizencephaly. Arch Gen Psychiatry 1999;56:781-7.
[2] Keefe RS, Eesley CE, Poe MP. Defining a cognitive function decrement in schizophrenia. Biol Psychiatry 2005;57:688-91.
[3] Green MF, Kern RS, Heaton RK. Longitudinal studies of cognition and functional outcome in schizophrenia: implications for MATRICS. Schizophr Res 2004;72:41-51.
[4] Lobellova V, Entlerova M, Svojanovska B, Hatalova H, Prokopova I, Petrasek T, Vales K, Kubik S, Fajnerova I, Stuchlik A. Two learning tasks provide evidence for disrupted behavioural flexibility in an animal model of schizophrenia-like behaviour induced by acute MK-801: a dose-response study. Behav Brain Res 2013;246:55-62.
[5] Vales K, Bubenikova-Valesova V, Klement D, Stuchlik A. Analysis of sensitivity to MK-801 treatment in a novel active allothetic place avoidance task and in the working memory version of the Morris water maze reveals differences between Long-Evans and Wistar rats. Neurosci Res 2006;55:383-8.
[6] van der Staay FJ, Rutten K, Erb C, Blokland A. Effects of the cognition impairer MK-801 on learning and memory in mice and rats. Behav Brain Res 2011; 220:215-29.
[7] Landgraf S, Krebs MO, Olie JP, Committeri G, van der Meer E, Berthoz A, Amado I. Real world referencing and schizophrenia: are we experiencing the same reality? Neuropsychologia 2010;48:2922-30.
[8] Weniger G, Irle E. Allocentric memory impaired and egocentric memory intact as assessed by virtual reality in recent-onset schizophrenia. Schizophr Res 2008; 101:201-09.
[9] Hanlon FM, Weisend MP, Hamilton DA, Jones AP, Thoma RJ, Huang M, Martin K, Yeo RA, Miller GA, Canive JM. Impairment on the hippocampal-dependent virtual Morris water task in schizophrenia. Schizophr Res 2006;87:67-80.
[10] Spieker EA, Astur RS, West JT, Griego JA, Rowland LM. Spatial Memory Deficits in a Virtual Reality Eight-Arm Radial Maze in Schizophrenia. Schizophr Res 2012; 135(1-3):84–9.
[11] Folley BS, Astur R, Jagannathan K, Calhoun VD, Pearlson GD. Anomalous neural circuit function in schizophrenia during a virtual Morris water task. Neuroimage 2010;49:3373-84.

[12] Morris R. Developments of a water-maze procedure for studying spatial learning in the rat. J Neurosci Methods 1984;11:47-60.
[13] Cimadevilla JM Fenton AA, Bures J. Continuous place avoidance task reveals differences in spatial navigation in male and female rats. Behav Brain Res 2000; 107:161-9.
[14] Kay SR, Fiszbein A, Opler LA. The positive and negative syndrome scale (PANSS) for schizophrenia. Schizophr Bull 1987;13:261-76.
[15] Jones SH, Thornicroft G, Coffey M, Dunn G. A brief mental health outcome scale-reliability and validity of the Global Assessment of Functioning (GAF). Br J Psychiatry 1995;166:654-9.
[16] Andreasen NC, Pressler M, Nopoulos P, Miller D, Ho BC. Antipsychotic dose equivalents and dose-years: a standardized method for comparing exposure to different drugs. Biol Psychiatry 2010;67:255-62.
[17] Woods SW. Chlorpromazine equivalent doses for the newer atypical antipsychotics. J Clin Psychiatry 2003; 64: 663-7.
[18] Fajnerová I, Rodriguez M, Levčík D, Konrádová L, Mikoláš P, Brom C, Stuchlík A, Vlček K, Horáček J. A virtual reality task based on anímal research – spatial learning and memory in patients after the first episode of schizophrenia. Front Behav Neurosci 2014; 8:157. doi: 10.3389/fnbeh.2014.00157.
[19] Rodriguez MV. Feasibility of Non-Pharmacological Intervention in Therapy of Cognition Deficit in Czech Schizophrenia Patients - Computer-assisted Cognitive Remediation. Dissertation. Prague: Charles University Prague, 2013. URL: https://www.is.cuni.cz/webapps/ zzp/detail/104163/.

Submitted: July 09, 2015. *Revised:* August 09, 2015. *Accepted:* August 17, 2015.

In: Alternative Medicine Research Yearbook 2017
Editor: Joav Merrick
ISBN: 978-1-53613-726-2
© 2018 Nova Science Publishers, Inc.

Chapter 25

ENHANCING BRAIN ACTIVITY BY CONTROLLING VIRTUAL OBJECTS WITH THE EYE

Cristián Modroño[1,*], PhD, Julio Plata[2], MD, PhD, Estefanía Hernández[1], Iván Galván[1], Sofía García[1], Fernando Zelaya[3], PhD, Francisco Marcano[1], Óscar Casanova[1], PhD, Gorka Navarrete[4], PhD, Manuel Mas[1], MD, PhD and José Luis González-Mora[1], MD, PhD

[1]Department of Physiology, University of La Laguna,
Campus de Ciencias de la Salud, Tenerife, Spain
[2]Department of Neurosurgery, Hospital Universitario de Canarias, Tenerife, Spain
[3]Centre for Neuroimaging Sciences, King's College London,
London, United Kingdom
[4]Laboratory of Cognitive and Social Neuroscience,
Diego Portales University, Santiago, Chile

ABSTRACT

Stimulation of the damaged neural networks is a key factor for the reorganization of neural functions in the treatment of motor deficits. This work explores, using functional MRI, a system to activate motor regions that does not require voluntary limb movements. Healthy participants, in a virtual environment, controlled a virtual paddle using only their eye movements, which related to an increase of the activity in frontoparietal motor regions. This may be a promising way to enhance motor activity without resorting to limb movements that are not always possible in patients with motor deficits.

Keywords: fMRI, eye control, motor system, neurorehabilitation, virtual reality

---

[*] Correspondence: Cristián Modroño, Department of Physiology, University of La Laguna, Campus de Ciencias de la Salud, La Laguna, 38071, Tenerife, Spain. E-mail: cmodrono@ull.edu.es.

INTRODUCTION

Physical therapy is a common treatment for motor deficits but it is not always possible because of limitations in the affected limbs. Thus, alternative approaches have been used to support the recovery of motor functions by generating an activation of the sensorimotor system without resorting to overt voluntary movements (1). One approach is based on passive movements caused by an external agent. Another approach is based on motor imagery, i.e., the mental rehearsal of motor acts in the absence of actual movement production (2). There is a third approach (action observation therapy), based solely on the visual presentation of actions, which may facilitate the reorganization of the affected motor areas, and has demonstrated good therapeutic results (3).

Several basic imaging studies, outside the field of the neurorehabilitation, comparing different kinds of limb and eye movements have supported the idea that the cortical representations for diverse movements, specifically frontal and parietal circuits for limb and eye movements, are highly distributed and overlapping in the human brain (4). This overlap, which may seem surprising at first, is not so surprising if one takes into account that limb and eye movements are naturally coupled in daily life (5). Thus, it would not be unreasonable to think that eye movements could be used in some way to generate brain activity related with limb movements.

Considering the results of such basic studies, this work explores a new system to activate sensorimotor regions in healthy participants that does not require voluntary limb movements. The idea is to use the eye (instead of the limb) to control objects in a virtual environment. Here, the object is a virtual paddle that is controlled by the participants in the context of a digital game. Participants in a functional MRI experiment move the virtual paddle to hit a ball using their eyes (with an eye tracking system) or just observe the game (baseline). An increase of frontoparietal activation might be expected when participants are using the eye as effector because of the overlapping of brain circuits for limb and eye movements. If this expectation is confirmed, it could have a potential application in the field of the virtual reality neurorehabilitation.

METHODS

The study recruited 15 right-handed neurologically healthy subjects (10 female, 5 male) between 19 and 21 years of age (mean = 20.8; SD = 0.6). They had normal or corrected-to-normal vision. The study was approved by the local Ethics Committee (University of La Laguna) and was conducted in accordance with the Declaration of Helsinki.

Virtual environment

A virtual 3D environment, using Visual C# and DirectX, was developed where the subjects play a paddle and ball game from an egocentric perspective. Participants had to prevent the ball entering the space behind them by trying to hit the approaching ball back towards the opponent (the computer), who controlled its own paddle (see Figure 1). The paddle had one degree of freedom (left-right) and was cuboid in shape.

Participants used their gaze to control the virtual paddle. This was done by using an MRI-compatible eye tracking system (MReyetracking, Resonance Technology Company, Northridge, CA), which obtains the participant's gaze point in real-time. This system includes a Software Developer's Kit (SDK) that allows programs like the virtual game to interface with the eyetracker. The gaze point horizontal coordinates were transformed into positions of the virtual paddle using this SDK, which allowed the participant to control it in real-time.

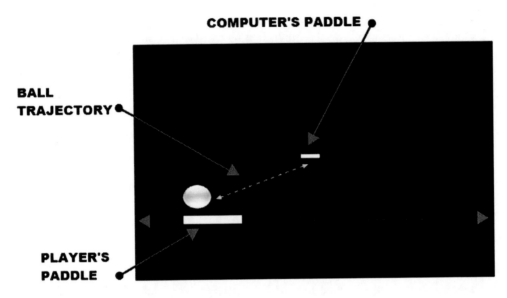

Figure 1. The virtual game. Participants used their eyes to control a paddle to hit an approaching ball. The paddle had one degree of freedom (left-right). The display has a 3D feel, so the more distant the computer's paddle was, the smaller its representation.

Data acquisition

The fMRI run consisted of three conditions: *play*, *observation* and *fixation*. The *play* condition consisted of six 20 second blocks where the participant was playing against the computer using gaze. During the *observation* condition, the participants just watched another six games. These observed games were similar to the executed games, but in this case the two paddles were controlled by the computer. The *play* and *observation* blocks were presented in random order and were preceded by a *fixation* task where the player stared at a grey cross in the middle of a black screen. The participants were instructed to focus on the game during the *observation* periods. Visual stimuli were given via MRI compatible eyeglasses (Visuastim, Resonance Technology, Northridge, CA).

Axially oriented functional images were obtained by a 3T Signa HD MR scanner (GE Healthcare, Milwaukee, WI) using an echo-planar-imaging gradient-echo sequence and an 8 channel head coil (TR = 2000 msec, TE = 22 msec, FA = 75°, matrix size = 64×64 pixels, 36 slices, 4×4 mm in plane resolution, spacing = 4 mm, ST = 3.3 mm, interleaved acquisition). The slices were aligned to the anterior commissure-posterior commissure line and covered the whole brain. High resolution sagittally oriented anatomical images were also collected for anatomical reference. A 3D fast spoiled-gradient-recalled pulse sequence was obtained (TR = 6 msec, TE = 1 msec, FA = 12º, matrix size= 256 × 256 pixels, 0.98 × 0.98 mm in plane resolution, spacing = 1 mm, ST = 1 mm).

Data analysis

Data were preprocessed and analyzed using the software SPM8 (www.fil.ion.ucl.ac.uk/spm/). The images were spatially realigned, unwarped, normalized and smoothed using standard SPM8 procedures. The three conditions were modelled in the design matrix for each participant. Activation maps for the contrast *play > observation* were generated for each subject by applying t statistics. These first level contrast images were used in a random effects group analysis. Statistical maps were set at a voxel-level threshold of $p < 0.05$, FDR corrected for multiple comparisons, and a minimum cluster size of 25 voxels.

RESULTS

Figure 2 shows the brain regions that were more activated when participants played the game using their gaze than when they were just observers. Many of the activations appear located in areas related with motor aspects (6). It is worth mentioning here the extended, bilateral activity that was found in a region centred in the Brodmann area 6 (premotor cortex and supplementary motor area). Bilateral activity was also found in several regions of the inferior and superior parietal lobules (such as the supramarginal gyrus, the angular gyrus and the precuneus). The occipital lobe and the cerebellum were also bilaterally activated, and, to a lesser extent, some temporal areas.

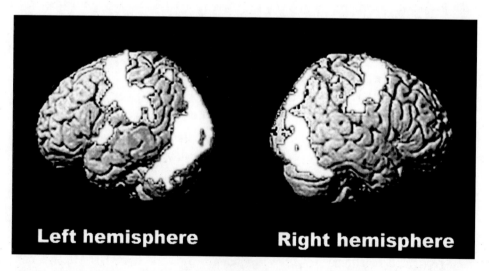

Figure 2. Results of the play > observation contrast. When compared with an observation task (with a similar visual input), controlling the virtual paddle using eye movements was associated with an increase of the activity (white areas) in frontoparietal motor regions (group analysis, N = 15, threshold: $p < 0.05$ at the voxel level, false discovery rate [FDR] corrected for multiple comparisons; minimum cluster size = 25 voxels).

DISCUSSION

In line with our expectations, when compared with an observation task with a similar visual input, using gaze to control a virtual object is associated with an increase of the activity in frontoparietal motor regions. A key factor influencing reorganization of function in damaged neural networks is stimulation (7), and the method presented here may be a promising approach to enhance motor activity without resorting to voluntary limb movements. Another advantage of this approach is that the control of a virtual object with gaze may be more entertaining for the patients than other kinds of tasks used in rehabilitation, which therefore may help the patient to adhere to the therapy. In the future, attractive neurorehabilitation gaze-based systems could be developed for the users, which may be especially useful in the case of children and adolescents. Therefore, the results presented here can be of interest for researchers, developers and medical professionals working in the field of the neurorehabilitation.

ACKNOWLEDGMENTS

We acknowledge the support of Servicio de Resonancia Magnética para Investigaciones Biomédicas de la Universidad de La Laguna and the following national competitive programs: Ministerio de Ciencia e Innovación [PTA2011-4995-I, TIN2011-28146]; Ministerio de Industria, Turismo y Comercio [TSI-020100-2011-189, TSI-020100-2010-346]; Ministerio de Economía y Competitividad [IPT-2012-0961-300000]. We also thank Miguel Angel León Ruedas for his assistance with data acquisition.

REFERENCES

[1] Szameitat AJ, Shen S, Conforto A, Sterr A. Cortical activation during executed, imagined, observed, and passive wrist movements in healthy volunteers and stroke patients. Neuroimage 2012;62(1):266-80.
[2] Zimmermann-Schlatter A, Schuster C, Puhan MA, Siekierka E, Steurer J. Efficacy of motor imagery in post-stroke rehabilitation: a systematic review. J Neuroeng Rehabil 2008;5:8.
[3] Carvalho D, Teixeira S, Lucas M, Yuan TF, Chaves F, Peressutti C, et al. The mirror neuron system in post-stroke rehabilitation. Int Arch Med 2013;6(1):41.
[4] Filimon F. Human cortical control of hand movements: Parietofrontal networks for reaching, grasping, and pointing. Neuroscientist 2010;16(4):388-407.
[5] Levy I, Schluppeck D, Heeger DJ, Glimcher PW. Specificity of human cortical areas for reaches and saccades. J Neurosci 2007;27(17):4687-96.
[6] Kandel ER, Schwartz JH, Jessell TM, Siegelbaum SA, Hudspeth AJ. Principles of neural science. New York: McGraw-Hill, 2013.
[7] Johnson-Frey SH. Stimulation through simulation? Motor imagery and functional reorganization in hemiplegic stroke patients. Brain Cogn 2004;55(2): 328-31.

Submitted: July 10, 2015. *Revised:* August 19, 2015. *Accepted:* August 20, 2015.

In: Alternative Medicine Research Yearbook 2017
Editor: Joav Merrick

ISBN: 978-1-53613-726-2
© 2018 Nova Science Publishers, Inc.

Chapter 26

COLOUR-CHECK IN STROKE-REHABILITATION GAMES

Veronika Szücs, MSc, Cecília Sik Lanyi, PhD, Ferenc Szabo, PhD and Peter Csuti, PhD*

Department of Electrical Engineering and Information Systems,
University of Pannonia, Veszprém, Hungary

ABSTRACT

This article presents the colorimetric testing of rehabilitation games designed for the StrokeBack project. In this testing, the main subject of the investigation was how the people with different colour-blindness types can perceive the games. Many programmers and game designers do not pay attention to the accessible aspect of games. This accessibility implies that users who are colour-blind should be able to use the games the same way as the people with no vision impairment.

Keywords: colour-check, rehabilitation game, stroke

INTRODUCTION

The purpose of the research described here is to investigate the colour palette of virtual reality (VR) based rehabilitation games (1), as designed for the 'StrokeBack' (2) project. The goal of the StrokeBack project is to improve the speed and quality of stroke recovery through the development of a telemedicine system which supports ambulant rehabilitation in home settings for stroke patients with minimal human intervention. During our investigation we designed our VR based rehabilitation games in such a way that they would also be enjoyable for people who have colour-blindness.

---

[*] Correspondence: Veronika Szucs, Department of Electrical Engineering and Information Systems, University of Pannonia, Veszprém, Hungary. E-mail: szucs@virt.uni-pannon.hu.

The disorders in colour vision can be inherited and acquired. The cones' red and green colour specific paint cell's genes are linked to the X chromosome. Because of the gender-linked inheritance, this type of impairment is 20 times more prevalent in men. About 8% of Caucasian males and 0.4–0.5% of females are "red-green" colour-blind. Inherited blue-blindness (tritanopia) is much rarer – only about 0.05% of the population can be detected. Some colour vision disorders are not inherited, they are so called "acquired"; several ophthalmological diseases can result in colour perception disorders (e.g., retinal diseases, glaucoma, cataracts, etc.) (3).

Stroke is a leading cause of death in the United States, killing nearly 130,000 Americans each year – that is 1 of every 20 deaths (4). Every year, about 800,000 people in the United States have a stroke. About 610,000 of these are first or new strokes; 185,000 are recurrent strokes. Evidence from opticians indicates that about 10% of the male population are colour-blind. This, together with stroke incidence rate, leads to a statistically important problem.

STATE OF THE ART

The harmony of colours and proportions play an essential role in the appearance. Although many tend to neglect these issues, numerous scientific research studies are concerned with this field. All this is based on the colour perception of the eye, which, however unconsciously, may have an influence on patients' decisions.

Scientists and artists over the last centuries (5–7) and nowadays (8) developed colour order systems where they defined rules to establish harmonic sets of colours. These colour harmony studies were based on the orderly arrangement of colours in the colour order system. The second group of authors (9, 10) defined colour harmony as an interrelationship of colours. The main principles of these studies are "complementary" and "analogous" but these concepts are not consistent among the studies. Also, the colour wheel was often adopted as a tool to define these basic relationships. Judd and Wyszecki (11) define colour harmony as a more universal concept: "when two or more colours seen in neighbouring areas produce a pleasing effect, they are said to produce colour harmony." In addition, there is no consistency among the principles and the keywords of colour harmony: it is *completeness* according to Goethe (9), *order* according to Nemcsics (8) and Chevreul (10), and *balance* according to Munsell (6). A quantitative model for two-colour combinations based on the CIECAM02 colour appearance model was developed by Szabó et al. (12). Many other effects (i.e., age, cultural background) of colour harmony feeling have yet to be investigated.

In visual experiences, harmony is something that is pleasing to the eye. It engages the viewer and it creates an inner sense of order, a balance in the visual experience. When something is not harmonious, it is chaotic. At one extreme is a visual experience that is so bland that the viewer is not engaged. The human brain will reject under-stimulating information. The human brain rejects what it cannot organize, what it cannot understand. The visual task requires that we present a logical structure. Colour harmony delivers visual interest and a sense of order. Extreme unity leads to under-stimulation, extreme complexity leads to over-stimulation. Harmony is a dynamic equilibrium (13).

Colour deficiency is often neglected, as most people do not consider colour deficiency as a serious problem. Up to 15% of the population being affected by one form or another of colour deficiency (13). It is quite common to see combinations of background and foreground colours that make web-pages, software, games etc. virtually unreadable for colour deficient users. Background, text, and graphics colours should be carefully chosen to allow understanding for people with colour deficiency. Designing for colour deficient people is complicated. It is not simply a matter of green/red or yellow/blue combinations (13).

The most important issue in designing for colour deficient users is not to rely on colour alone to convey information and not to use colour as a primary means to impart information (14).

METHODS

Currently 3 games are built in the StrokeBack project:

- Break the Bricks game: practices horizontal (right-left) wrist movements – the player's task is to control the object at the bottom of the monitor;
- Birdie game: practices vertical (up-down) wrist movements – the player's task is to make a little bird fly and not let it fall;
- Gardener game: practices finger extension movements – the player's task is to pump a virtual sprinkler to make the plants grow by watering them.

These games can be used during the home rehabilitation process by the patients or replacing/enhancing clinical rehabilitation, thereby speeding up the process of recovery. These games are single player games which the patient can play by himself/herself. It is expected that the patients will play more with the games than they would do exercises. To these games several 'locations' were developed:

- Break the Bricks: default bricks, car, cake, duck, ship, train.
- Birdie: default meadow, cave (played with a bat), circus, forest, jungle, mountain, sea, town, winter.
- Gardener: bluebell, carrot, currant, geranium, grape, pepper, rose, strawberry, tomato, tulip.

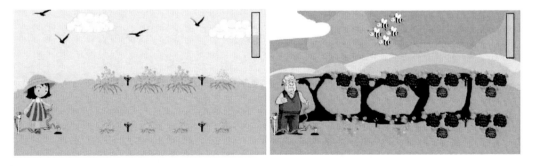

Figure 1. Gardener's "Bluebell" and "Grapes" themes as seen by a person with good vision.

Besides the 24 backgrounds for the 24 themes, more than 170 different objects had to be inserted, each of which had to be clearly visible. These were tested by different colour-blindness simulators and automatic testers.

Figure 1 shows two themes of Gardener as seen by a person with a good vision. Figure 2 presents the jungle theme of game Birdie and the objects that can be inserted as obstacles in the theme.

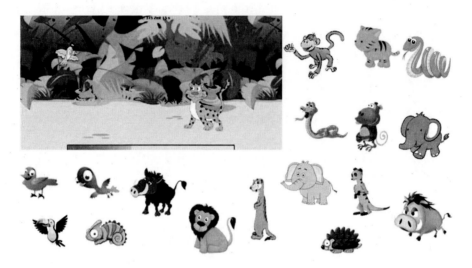

Figure 2. Jungle theme of "Birdie" game and the objects that can be inserted.

RESEARCH AND DEVELOPMENT

For the investigation four different colour-blindness simulators were used, which are accessible on the Internet and where pictures can be uploaded (15–17), and a downloadable software, ColorOracle (18), with which we could test the pictures appearing on the screen on the developer computer to find out how the users of different types of colour-blindness – deuteranopia, protanopis, tritanopia – see the colours.

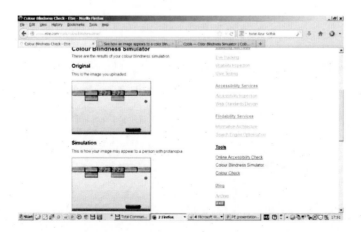

Figure 3. (Continued).

Colour-check in stroke-rehabilitation games 233

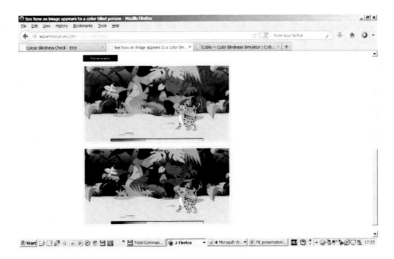

Figure 3. Testing of "BTB basic brick" theme with ETRE simulator (left) and "Birdie jungle" theme with ASP.NET based online simulator (right).

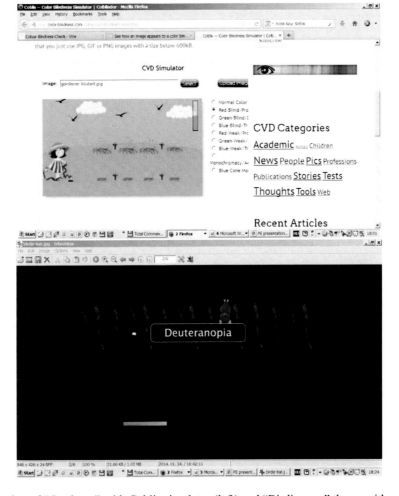

Figure 4. Testing of "Gardener" with Coblis simulator (left) and "Birdie cave" theme with ColorOracle tester.

Testing and contribution to the field

Testing has been completed not only with the *ETRE-*, *ASP.NET based-*, and *Coblis-* simulators and the *ColorOracle* tester, but also with Variantor's special glasses (19), with two individuals with good vision, and two persons with colour-blindness. Based on prevalence (10%) of colour-blindness in the male population, and the case that colour-blindness is aggravated by stroke (20), individual tests using a standard colour chart display has been conducted. Figure 5 shows the difference between normal colour vision (Figure 5a) and colour blindness in the red tone (Figure 5b).

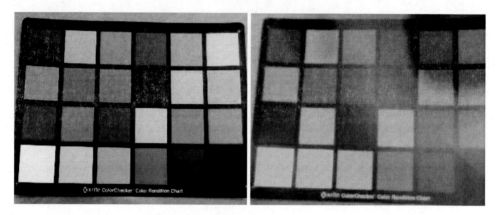

Figure 5. Original colour chart (left). Colour chart vision with Variantor glasses (right).

The tests were completed by people with normal vision and those with colour-blindness. The visual elements of the games were not just tested with online applications. Out of the possible test subjects, we filtered for colour-blindness by applying the Farnsworth-Munsell 100 HueColor Vision test (21).

During the test, the subjects had to look at some parts of images taken from the games and were then asked questions regarding them. The questions concentrated on visibility and perceptibility, and the elements disturbing or obstructing visibility and perceptibility. Example questions are:

- *Jungle theme*: What kind of fruits could you see on the tree? How many? Which animal has a darker colour?
- *Cave theme*: How many bats have been in the cave? What objects could you see on the ground beneath the crab?
- *Forest theme*: Was there a wooden high-stand in the picture? What colour are the mushroom caps? How many separate clouds are visible?
- *Winter theme*: How many white animals could you see in the picture? From which direction did the bird (if there has been) fly to the image?
- *General questions*: What value did the achievement bar show on the right hand side?

Based on the test subjects' opinion, the achievement bar has been placed on the periphery of the screen and for the most of the time they have not even noticed that it is placed there. In the test subjects' judgement, the games' visibility and perceptibility is good, although they have indicated that, in the circus theme, the white and red stripes of the circus tent have been disturbing, which generated the vibrating effect. In the case where the recurrence of some image elements have been questioned, the elements have been recognized in the pictures and the subjects have even been able to determine the correct number, but the colours of the elements could not be recalled. As an example, in the garden topic the subjects were able to tell how many tulips have there been on the picture, but they could not tell the colours of the flowers. Responses to questions on colour balance include remarks that the plants in the picture mostly fade into the greenish hue background and, in case of the jungle theme, the green parrot can hardly be noticed between the leaves of the tree.

For some of the users and test subjects the noisiness and pixel problems due to the low image resolution were disturbing. The test subjects have also emphasized some situations that had disconcerting effects, for example when combinations of colours have been shown which physically interrupted the focusing of the eyes, as in the case of combination red-blue colours.

The results of the tests have shown that the observers – despite their colour vision deficiency – have seen picture elements taken from the game appropriately, the small details having been recognized and identified. The separation, observation and recalling of the games' image elements did not cause any problems for the validly colour-blind test subjects.

CONCLUSION AND PLANNED ACTIVITIES

We have not found any publications that consider the testing of colours of rehabilitation games, lending credence to our view that developers do not think about the colour-blind people. As a result of our testing, we reached the conclusion that, within the StrokeBack games, the objects are clearly visible, so the colour-blind patients can practice in the same way as the normal sighted. In future, games should not only be tested with the software, but also with other simulation goggles (tunnel-vision, macula or lens degeneration). Clinical tests of efficiency (which refer to the colour testing and efficiency of the rehabilitation) were started in June, 2014, and future reporting will detail these results.

ACKNOWLEDGMENTS

The StrokeBack research project (20) is supported by the European Commission under the 7th Framework Programme through Call (part) identifier FP7-ICT-2011-7, grant agreement no: 288692.

REFERENCES

[1] Sik Lányi C, Szűcs V, Dömök T, László E. Developing serious game for victims of stroke, Proceed 9th Intl Conf on Disability, Virtual Reality and Assoc. Technologies, Laval, 2012:503-6.
[2] StrokeBack project. Accessed 2015 Feb. 19. URL: http://www.strokeback.eu/.
[3] Colour-blindness simulator. Accessed: 2015 Feb 01.
[4] URL: http://www.encyclopedia.com/topic/color_blind ness.aspx.
[5] Centre for Disease Control and Prevention. Stroke Statistics. Accessed 2015. June 6. URL http://www.cdc.gov/stroke/statistics_maps.htm.

[6] Itten J. The Art of Color. Translation by Ernst van Haagen from German "Kunst der Farbe." New York: Van Nostrand Reinhold, 1961.
[7] Munsell RVN. A grammar of colour. New York: Reinhold, 1969.
[8] Ostwald W. The color primer. New York: Van Nostrand Reinhold, 1969.
[9] Nemcsics A. Farbenlehre und Farbendynamik, Budapest: Akadémiai Kiadó, 1993.
[10] Goethe JW. Theory of colours. Cambridge, MA: MIT Press, 1970.
[11] Chevreul ME. The principles of harmony and contrast of colours. New York: Van Nostrand Reinhold, 1981.
[12] Judd DB, Wyszecki G. Colour in business, science and industry, Third ed. New York: John Wiley, 1975.
[13] Szabó F, Bodrogi P, Schanda J. Experimental modelling of colour harmony. Color Res Appl 2010;35(1):34-49.
[14] Sik Lányi C. Choosing effective colours for websites, In: Best J, ed. Colour design theories and application. Cambridge: Woodhead Publishing Limited, 2012:600-21.
[15] Karagol-Ayan B. Universal usability in practice, Colour vision confusion. 2001. Accessed 2015 Feb. 19. URL: http://www.otal.umd.edu/uupractice/color/.
[16] ASP.NET colour-blindness simulator. Accessed 2015 Feb 19. URL: http://aspnetresources.com/tools/color blindness.
[17] ETRE colour-blindness simulator. Accessed 2015 Feb. 19. URL: http://www.etre.com/tools/colourblind simulator//.
[18] Coblis by Colblindor. Accessed 2015 Feb. 19. URL: http://www.color-blindness.com/coblis-color-blindness-simulator/.
[19] ColorOracle. Accessed 2015 Feb. 19. URL: http://www. colororacle.org/.
[20] Variantor – an experience based tool to aid universal design. Accessed 2015 Feb. 19. URL: http://variantor.com.
[21] Szücs V, Sik Lanyi C, Szabo F, Csuti P. Color-check in the the Stroke-rehabilitation games, Proceed 10th Intl Conf. Disability, Virtual Reality & Associated Technologies Gothenburg, Sweden, 2014 Sept 2–4. ICDVRAT, 2014:68-73.
[22] Farnsworth-Munsell 100 Hue Colour Vision test. Accessed 2015 Feb. 19. URL: http://www.color-blindness.com/farnsworth-munsell-100-hue-color-vision-test/.

Submitted: July 11, 2015. *Revised:* August 10, 2015. *Accepted:* August 20, 2015.

Chapter 27

PERCEPTION OF MULTI-VARIED SOUND PATTERNS OF SONIFIED REPRESENTATIONS OF COMPLEX SYSTEMS BY PEOPLE WHO ARE BLIND

Orly Lahav[1],*, PhD, Jihad Kittany[1], Sharona Tal Levy[2], PhD and Miriam Furst[3], PhD

[1]School of Education, Tel Aviv University, Tel Aviv, Israel
[2]Faculty of Education, University of Haifa, Haifa, Israel
[3]Faculty of Engineering, Tel Aviv University, Tel Aviv, Israel

ABSTRACT

Listening to complexity is a long-term research project, which addresses a central need among people who are blind: providing equal access to the science classroom, by allowing them to explore computer models, independently collect data, adapt and control their learning process. The innovative and low-cost learning system that is used in this project is based on the principle of perceptual compensation via technologies, by harnessing the auditory mode to transmit dynamic and spatial complex information, due to its unique affordances with respect to vision. Sonification of variables and events in an agent-based NetLogo computer model is used to convey information regarding both individual gas particles and system-wide phenomena, using alerts, object and status indicators, data representation and spatial audio displays. The paper describes two experiments: (i) auditory perception of varying types of auditory representations, spatial trajectories of a modeled object's motion, relative intensity, and frequency; and (ii) auditory perception of complex sound patterns, exploring detection and recognition of multiple sound channels at different complexity levels of sound patterns. The research would serve to improve our understanding of the auditory processes by which perception of sound patterns takes place and transforms into a conceptual model. The long-term practical benefits of this research are likely to have an impact on science, technology, engineering and mathematics (STEM) education for students who are blind.

---

* Correspondence: Orly Lahav, PhD, School of Education, Tel Aviv University, Room 419, POB. IL-39040, Ramat Aviv, Tel Aviv 69978, Israel. E-mail: lahavo@post.tau.ac.il.

Keywords: blindness, learning, STEM, computer models, sonification

INTRODUCTION

The project addresses a central need among students who are blind: that of accessing information in exploratory learning of science. Students who are blind have been integrated into public schools for more than 60 years and are required to complete the same curriculum and assessments as sighted students. However, they are prevented from access to firsthand information, as many science education resources are based on the visual channel (1). In the past 40 years several manuals have been written on how to teach science to students who are blind and visually impaired (2-4). However, research into their application and impact on learning is sparse. Few learning environments based on assistive technologies have been created to support science learning, such as the use of a force-feedback mouse to learn physics (5, 6).

Auditory information technologies for people who are blind

The learning process of people who are blind is based on gathering information through perceptual and conceptual tools (7). At the perceptual level, the shortage in visual information is compensated for by other senses such as the haptic, auditory and olfactory senses. Similar to other supportive environments, the Listening to Complexity (L2C) system is based on the principle of perceptual compensation via technologies (8). L2C harnesses the auditory mode to transmit dynamic complex information. The choice of an auditory display results from three considerations: (a) the auditory mode transmits information that changes both in space and time, similar to the visual mode and different from the haptic mode; (b) the auditory mode easily interfaces with large bandwidths at fine frequency-discrimination and intensity-discrimination thresholds (9); and (c) the auditory system is used to dealing with complex and rapidly changing sound patterns (10). In fact, it has been found that individuals who are blind can recognize 2D shapes through audition that activates the right dorsal extrastriate visual cortex (11). Sonification is the presentation of information using non-speech sound (12).

Over the years, it was found that congenitally blind subjects were able to recognize auditory coded visual patterns related to hand movement (13). Subjects not only memorized simple associations between sounds and patterns, but also learned the relationship between the auditory code and spatial attributes of the patterns. Research into the impact of different components of sound on auditory perception has shown that increasing the number of channels beyond three causes degradation in comprehension (14) and that a greater frequency separation between sound streams results in better stream segregation (15).

In the current project, we go beyond these studies in several ways. On one hand, we use sound to represent a dynamic rather than a static array. Moreover, the referents of the dynamic representation are multiple and operate at two system levels. Finally, we test how systematic variation of several different sound pattern features impacts detection and recognition of multiple channels, extending research into auditory perception. Some systems were developed to support Science, Technology, Engineering and Mathematics (STEM) education among students who are blind, such as the Talking Tactile Tablets (16) based on audio and 2D tactile materials, supporting interaction with 2D images for learning mathematical and science diagrams. The Line Graphs technology is based on auditory and haptic feedback and is geared to learning mathematics (17). The reported studies continue to research into auditory compensation for visual information among students who are blind and extend it to both perception of dynamic and complex displays and learning about dynamic complex systems. The two experiments tackle a major challenge and require a leap above the current state-of-the-art in several research disciplines such as Computer Science, Learning Sciences, Auditory Perception, and Human-Machine Interaction. We seek a deeper understanding of the neuroscientist Bach-y-Rita's phrase on brain plasticity: 'We see with the brain, not the eyes' (18). To reach this overall goal we focus on two main experiments:

- Auditory perception of varying types of auditory representations, the spatial trajectory of a modeled object's motion, relative intensity and frequency of sound.
- Auditory perception of complex sound patterns, varying the number of sound streams, identity of the sonification components, their number, relative intensity and frequency.

METHODS

The study included ten participants selected through snowball sampling for both experiments. A severe limitation is the small number of blind students in the proposed age bracket in Israel, resulting in a relatively small sample. They were chosen based on six criteria: at least 15 years old; comfort in use of computers; not multi-handicapped; normal hearing; total blindness; and onset of blindness at least two years prior to the experimental period. The participants' age range was 15-36, an average of 24 years old, five participants were female, eight were congenitally blind, five participants had residual vision but none used this in their everyday life. All the participants are proficient computer users, all learned STEM in their preliminary and high schools. All participants were with normal hearing, four participants played a musical instrument and one was member in a choir. The researchers obtained a sample of ten students, with similar proportions in terms of gender, age, and musical knowledge. The consenting guardians were made fully aware of the research framework and the specific experiments.

Variables

Nine independent variables were defined. The first three variables are connected to the research participants: age of onset of blindness; gender; and musical background. The next three variables are related to Experiment One: sonification type (musical instruments, inanimate objects' sounds, man-made sounds, and animal's sounds); spatial trajectory of the modeled object's motion; and sound frequency. The last three variables are associated with Experiment Two: sound intensity (loudness); complexity of sound pattern (event frequency and complexity); and number and type of sound streams. Three dependent variables are defined: preferences among sonified representations (rating of the pleasantness of the sound – Most disliked (1); Dislike (2); Neutral (3); Like (4); and Most liked (5)); response time; and error rate in sound pattern recognition.

Research instruments

This research included four implementation tools, and four data collection tools. The four implementation tools were the following:

Research apparatus. The recorded sounds were played through an Excel file running under Windows 7 on a personal computer equipped with stereo headphones (Sennheiser, HD580). All the sounds were played at 50% of the PC volume capability.

Set of sound patterns Experiment One. A set of 31 sound patterns, developed with experts of dynamic sound patterns, include: object-object collision (7 patterns), object-wall collision (7 patterns), speed was represented in three different ways – dashed speed represented speed by creating sound at regular distance intervals resulting in more frequent sound when the object was faster (4 patterns), sound pitch-as-speed, with pitch height representing speed (4 patterns), pitch space speed represented is based on the stereo sound (right left) and intensity (loud-close, soft-far) according to the speed and the particle's location in the space (4 patterns); each of these representations with varied frequency (5 patterns). All the sounds were based on earcon (associative auditory feedback used to represent an event), or created by the computer's MIDI musical instruments, or recordings of inanimate objects' interactions and man-made sounds, or animal sounds. For example: object-object collisions were represented by a hand clap; air bubbles passing through water; glass tapping on glass; metal tapping on metal; billiard ball hit by the cue. We examined these sounds at five different frequencies: 500; 1000; 2000; 4000; and 5000. This set of sounds meets requirements regarding frequency range (500-5,000 Hz) and loudness (75dB) with respect to sensitivity of the human auditory system, duration (200 millisecond), wave structure, 16 bit per sample, and stereo stream.

Sound tests for Experiment One. All the 31 sound patterns were tested twice by using different recorded scenarios in two different tests: comparison tests (e.g., which sound is preferred to represent speed? Sound A vs. Sound B) and scale – preferences among sonified representations (Most disliked (1); Dislike (2); Neutral (3); Like (4); and Most liked (5).

Sound tests for Experiment Two. Based on results from Experiment One, five sound representations were chosen for Experiment Two. 36 combinations of these five sounds were created, meeting the requirements regarding frequency range (4,000 Hz) and with respect to loudness sensitivity of the human auditory system (75dB), duration (30 second), wave structure, and stereo stream.

In addition to the above, four tools were developed for the collection of quantitative and qualitative data: (i) Background questionnaire (15 items): personal information, science education, computer technology use, musical background, and information about hearing ability; (ii) Research protocol: two research protocols were developed, one for each experiment. These were structured as described in the procedure section below. The Research protocols for Experiment One and Experiment Two; (iii) Observations: participants' behaviors were video-recorded (Experiment Two only); and (iv) Excel file structuring and accessing the design of the sounds in the research protocol.

Data analysis

To evaluate the participants' performance in the two experiments, the results were coded directly by the researcher into an Excel file. These results were analyzed using quantitative software (Excel) to determine the relative preferences regarding sounds for each referent.

Procedure

All participants were examined individually in their home. In the first session the participants completed consent forms and a background questionnaire. Next, they were tested with Experiment One. After six months they were tested with Experiment Two. Each experiment included five parts: a short verbal explanation about the experimental process; researcher demonstration; practice and training by the participant; experiment part 1 (20 minutes); intermission (30 minutes); and experiment part 2 (20 minutes). Each of these protocols was conducted twice, 1 to 2 weeks apart.

DISCUSSION

In the described experiments ten participants took part in two experiments: Experiment One, auditory perception in which auditory representations were varied along various dimensions and Experiment Two, auditory perception of complex sound patterns, recognition of the sonified referents. The results of these experiments have important implications for continued research, and impact learning of people who are blind learning via sonified learning materials.

Some of the Experiment One results highlight the importance of sonifying with sounds that are semantically related to the referent. For example, billiard ball collisions were preferred for sonifying object-object collisions (two billiard balls, of the same material, collide with each other) with respect to glass tapping on glass. The Navajo drum-beat was preferred for representing the object-wall collisions (an object (one material) collides with a wall (leather drum-head)). The participants didn't select animal or digital sounds and preferred recorded real life objects with related meanings. Also, as a speed representation, most of the participants selected the dashed sound, for which frequency of the dashes corresponds to the speed, and not the pitch-space sound that requires additional cognitive processing for aligning the representation (pitch) with the referent (speed). The 2×2 methodology, using the two sessions (data collection sessions) with two tests (comparison and scale tests) aided the researchers in reliably determining the selected sounds.

Finally, we test how systematic variation of several different sound pattern features (type, number of audio streams, correctness of sound pattern recognition, and auditory perception tools) impacts detection and recognition of multiple channels, extending research into auditory perception, furthering support of the learning process of people who are blind based on auditory feedback. The research results show that the participants were able to handle up to three events and audio graph sounds at the same time. It proved difficult, however, to identify four and five sounds (events and audio graphs) concurrently, so it is preferable to avoid this level of complexity in a sonified learning process. Experiment Two examined different components of sound that might affect identification ability. Research into the impact of different components of sound on auditory perception has shown that a greater frequency separation between sound streams results in better stream segregation (15). Surprisingly, we found that when hearing heterogeneous sound, the participants identified fewer sounds compared to when hearing homogenous sounds. However, with gradual exposure to new sounds 60% of the participants were able to identify four and five sounds.

ACKNOWLEDGMENTS

This research was partially supported by a grant from The Israel Science Foundation (ISF) Individual Research Grant (2011-2015), (Grant No. 06070 15102). We thank our anonymous participants for their time, efforts, and ideas.

REFERENCES

[1] Beck-Winchatz B, Riccobono MA. Advancing participation of blind students in science, technology, engineering, and math. Adv Space Res 2008;42:1855-8.
[2] Hadary D, Cohen S. Laboratory science and art for blind, deaf and emotionally disturbed children. Baltimore, MD: University Park Press, 1978.
[3] Kumar D, Ramassamy R, Stefanich G. Science for students with visual impairments: Teaching suggestions and policy implications for secondary learners. Electr J Sci Educ 2001;5(3):1-9.
[4] Willoughby D, Duffy S. Handbook for itinerant and resource teachers of blind and visually impaired students. Baltimore, MD: National Federation of the Blind, 1989.
[5] Farrell B, Baldyga DD, Erlandson R. Force feedback mouse used for a physics experiment. NSF 2001 report: Engineering Senior Design Projects to Aid Persons with Disabilities, Chapter 21, Wayne State University, 2001:308-9. Accessed 2015 May 25.
[6] URL: http://nsf-pad.bme.uconn.edu/2001/Wayne%20State%20University.pdf.
[7] Wies EF, Gardner JA, O'Modhrain MS, Hasser CJ, Bulatov VL. Web-based touch display for accessible science education. In: Brewster S, Murray-Smith R, eds. Proceedings of Haptic HCI 2000, LNCS 2058, 2001:52-60.
[8] Passini R, Proulx G. Wayfinding without vision: An experiment with congenitally blind people. Environ Behav 1988;20:227-52.
[9] Lahav O, Levy ST. Listening to Complexity: Blind people's learning about gas particles through a sonified model. In: proceedings ICDVRAT (International Conference Series on Disability, Virtual Reality and Associated Technologies), Vina del Mar/Valparaiso, Chile, 2010.
[10] Capelle C, Trullemans C, Arno P, Veraart C. A real-time experimental prototype for enhancement of vision rehabilitation using auditory substitution. IEEE Trans Biomed Eng 1988;45:1279-93.
[11] Hirsh IJ. Auditory perception and speech. In: Atkinson RC, Hernstein RJ, Lindzey G, Luce RD. Handbook of Experimental Psychology. New York: John Wiley, 1988: 377-408.
[12] Collignon O. Lassonde M. Lepore F. Bastien D. Veraart C. Functional Cerebral Reorganization for Auditory Spatial Processing and Auditory Substitution of Vision in Early Blind Subjects. Cerebral Cortex 2007;17:457-65.
[13] Kramer G. An Introduction to auditory display. In: Kramer G. Auditory Display: Sonification, Audification, and Auditory Interfaces. Santa Fe Institute Studies in the Sciences of Complexity, Proceedings vol. XVIII. Reading, MA: Addison-Wesley, 1994.
[14] Arno P, Streel E, Wanet-Defalque MC, Sanabria-Bohorquez S, Veraart C. Auditory substitution of vision: Pattern recognition by the blind. Appl Cogn Psychol 2001;15:509-19.

[15] Stifelman LJ. The Cocktail Party Effect in Auditory Interfaces: A Study of Simultaneous Presentation. Technical Report. Cambridge, MA: MIT Media Lab, 1994.
[16] Bregman AS. Auditory Scene Analysis: The Perceptual Organization of Sound. Cambridge, MA: MIT Press, 1990.
[17] Landau S, Russell M, Erin J, Gourgey K. Use of the talking tactile tablet in mathematics tests. J Visual Impair Blindness 2003;97:85-96.
[18] Ramloll Y, Brewster R, Burton D. Constructing Sonified Haptic Line Graphs for the Blind Student: First Steps. In: proceedings of ASSETS'00, Arlington, Virginia, 2000.
[19] Bach-y-Rita P. Brain mechanisms in sensory substitution. New York: Academic Press, 1972.

Submitted: July 11, 2015. *Revised:* August 10, 2015. *Accepted:* August 20, 2015.

In: Alternative Medicine Research Yearbook 2017
Editor: Joav Merrick
ISBN: 978-1-53613-726-2
© 2018 Nova Science Publishers, Inc.

Chapter 28

OUTDOOR NAVIGATION SYSTEM FOR VISUALLY IMPAIRED PERSONS

Babar Chaudary[*], *MSc, Petri Pulli, PhD* and *Iikka Paajala, BSc*

Department of Information Processing Science,
University of Oulu, Oulu, Finland

ABSTRACT

One of the most challenging limitations for visually impaired persons (VIPs) is the inability of independent navigation. The purpose of this study is to build and test an outdoor navigation system to assist VIP navigation independently in urban areas. The proposed system assists VIPs to walk independently on sidewalks with the help of an augmented cane following magnetic or continuous metallic trails installed on sidewalks. They will be informed about points of interest (POI) such as turns and other decision points through serialized Braille vibrational guidance messages. Pre-test qualitative interviews and system usability testing was performed in Finland, Pakistan, and Sweden with total of 31 VIPs. In practical navigation tests, 15 out of 17 VI subjects were able to navigate the test track successfully with the prototype system. Based on the results, this kind of system would aid their navigation. The study also collected usability suggestions for further development of the system and factors affecting the acceptance of technological navigation aid by VIPs.

Keywords: visually impaired; outdoor navigation; Braille code; qualitative study, Quality Function Deployment (QFD), usability testing

---

[*] Correspondence: Babar Shahzad Chaudary, Doctoral Researcher Department of Information Processing Science, Faculty of Information Technology and Electrical Engineering, University of Oulu, Pentti Kaiteran katu 1, 90014 Oulu, Finland. E-mail: babar.chaudary@oulu.fi.

INTRODUCTION

Navigating complex routes and finding objects of interest are challenging tasks for VIPs. Outdoor navigation is termed as macro navigation or orientation in literature (1). It involves processing the remote environment, beyond the immediate perceptible ones. In the case of visual impairment, the main cues (e.g., landmarks and paths) for sensing the environment are degraded. This results in difficulties relating to orientation (2). A system that assists VIPs' orientation in real time will be of great benefit.

Despite over a decade of intensive research and development, the problem of delivering an effective navigation assistance to VIPs is largely unsolved (3). Navigation support for VIPs span the use of textured paving blocks, guide dogs, GPS based navigation systems, different sensors and wireless based systems among others (4). Other technologies include Radio Frequency Identification (RFID), using radio waves emitted from wireless LAN access points, infrared (IR), Bluetooth, and ultrasound based identification (USID) (5). Compared to public spaces and transport facilities, no progress is being made in providing commercial facilities with textured paving blocks. Guide dogs are effective for obstacle-free safe walkways but they cannot locate the intended destination of a person (6). As for GPS, the perceived accuracy is not always sufficient for blind navigation in urban areas. The urbanization phenomenon slows down GPS start up time. Most GPS systems use speech to convey directions to the user, but this approach is not valid for real-time tasks (7). RFID technology suffers from fluctuating signals accuracy, signals disruption, reader and/or tag collision, and slow read rates (8). The wireless LAN access point method has encountered issues with fluctuating positional accuracy due to reflected signals from the wireless LAN, obstacles, or the surrounding environment (8). The drawback of IR based systems is that natural and artificial light can interfere with it (9). IR based systems are costly to install due to large number of tags required to be installed and maintenance (10). For Bluetooth beacons based systems, the user has to walk slower than with other techniques because of the device delay (11). Bluetooth beacons suffer from heavy installation cost, maintenance, and line of site problems (12). Ultrasound based systems have the problem that walls may reflect or block ultrasound signals (13). It takes time to understand tactile maps by touch, and therefore, they are difficult to use when on the move (14).

To address these kinds of issues, our study aims to develop an effective navigation system that enables VIPs' independent navigation in urban areas and informs them about POIs.

SERIALIZED BRAILLE CODE

Braille is a tactile writing and reading system for VIPs (15). It employs group of dots to represent letters and numbers, in a domino-arrangement of two vertical columns of three dots each (see Figure 1). For convenience, a standard numbering system has been established for it (16).

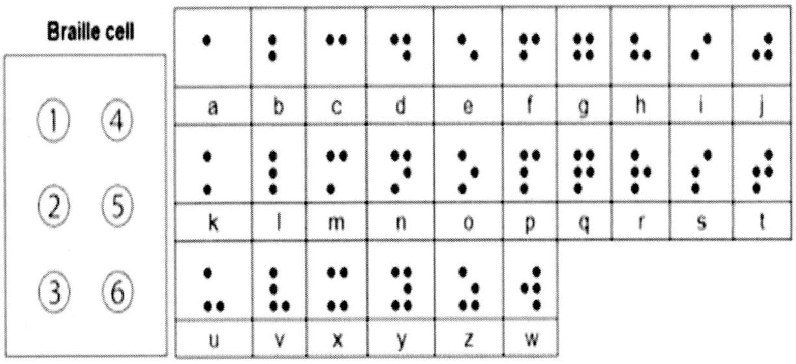

Outdoor navigation 247

Figure 1. Braille cell and Braille alphabet (17).

Braille was chosen as a communication mechanism for the system to guide VIPs. Though literature reports that reading Braille is more difficult than writing, making it difficult to use as a communication method in such navigation systems. For that reason, a serialized Braille version compliant with the traditional Braille was developed to be used as communication medium. A message encoded into it can be sent and read in the form of vibration.

The numbering system that is assigned to Braille cell dots is the basis for conversion of conventional Braille into serialized Braille. The serialized Braille was devised by positioning two columns serially rather than parallel and get numeral values for each Braille character.

SYSTEM DESIGN

The proposed navigation system comprises of four components: (i) an *Augmented Cane*, a regular white cane used by VIPs augmented with a small powerful ring shaped NdFeB magnet (17) reader at its bottom (see Figure 2); (ii) a *Stationary Magnet Point Trail*, comprising powerful disc type Neodymium magnets buried beneath the sidewalk forming a magnetic trail (see Figure 3). The VIPs can sense and follow the trail through augmented cane's magnetic reader; (iii) a *Metallic Trail*, comprising a tubular pure iron metallic pipe buried underneath the sidewalk (Figure 3), accessed in the same way; and (iv) the *Pulsing Magnet Apparatus*, installed at POIs on the sidewalks, this relays serialized Braille vibrational message about a POI (see Figure 4) to the augmented cane by vibrating it. Either of the stationary magnet point trail or metallic trail will be selected as component of the system after user testing.

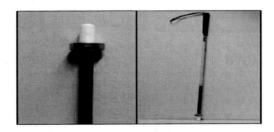

Figure 2. Augmented guidance cane.

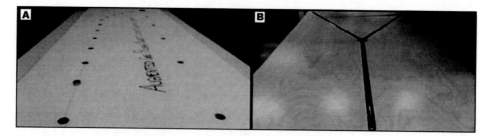

Figure 3. (A)Magnet points trail test bed, (B) Metallic trail test bed.

Architecture of the pulsing magnet apparatus

The pulsing magnet apparatus comprises of: (i) *Micro Controller Unit (MCU)* (18), which executes the serialized Braille transformation logic; (ii) an *Electromagnetic coil*, used to emit the serialized Braille guidance messages in the form of vibration through pulsing electromagnetism (Figure 4B). The polarity of electromagnetism is reversed with each successive pulse, causing the magnetic reader to be pushed/pulled by electromagnetic coil effecting a vibration in the cane; (iii) an *H-Bridge*, used to change the polarity of the electrometric coil, it is an electronic circuit that enables a voltage to be applied across a load in either direction (19); and (iv) a *Reed-Switch*, an electrical switch which conducts in the presence of a magnetic field and turns it off in absence (20). The pulsing magnet apparatus is activated when a VIP approaches it with the cane.

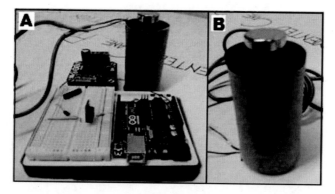

Figure 4. (A) Pulsing magnet apparatus, (B) electromagnet coil.

TEST PERSONS

Qualitative interviews

The first sessions of qualitative interviews were conducted in three countries:

- In *Finland*, 6 VIPs (3 females and 3 males, aged 21-55) were recruited, the recruitment being through personal communication; all interviews were conducted through email in the (non-native) language English.

- In *Pakistan*, 15 VIPs (4 females and 11 males, aged 19-58) were recruited through two third sector organisations (21, 22); all interviews were conducted in person, in the native language of subjects.
- In *Sweden*, 10 VIPs (6 female and 4 male, aged 34-70) were recruited through a research scientist at a University in Sweden; all interviews were conducted through email in the native language of subjects.

Study for the acceptance of technological navigation assistance by VIPs and blind persons

- In *Finland*, 19 VIPs (10 female and 9 male, aged 21-82) were recruited. Test subjects were recruited via Northern Ostrobothnia Association for the Visually Impaired and the Oulu Region Lutheran Parish. All interviews were conducted in person, in the native language of subjects.

Usability tests

- In *Finland*, two female VIPs who participated in the qualitative study also participated in the usability testing.
- In *Pakistan*, all VIPs and blind subjects who participated in the qualitative study also participated in the usability test.

End user consent and privacy protection

All VIP were given information on the study, that their participation was voluntarily and they had right to abort their participation at any point without any consequence. A signed consent was obtained. Permission of the interviewee was asked for audio recording of interviews and video recording of usability tests.

QUALITATIVE INTERVIEWS

A semi structured interview was used to collect qualitative data from VIPs. The first session of the interviews collected white cane usage specification data. The interviews were guided by a dramaturgical model (23). Quality Function Deployment (QFD) is a method for satisfying customers by translating their demands into design targets and quality assurance points (24). This framework will be utilized to convert VIPs' demands collected through interviews into design quality of the proposed navigation system.

Findings

The navigation specifications by VIPs collected through qualitative interviews are summed up as follows:

Finland

For outdoor navigation, VIPs use the white cane by left-right swiping on the ground or flat surface, as normal on trails, although it is slower on bricked surfaces, and normally in the rainy season. Soft snow makes navigation difficult for swiping and hides landmarks. Hard snow is identifiable and is easy to navigate though it also hides landmarks.

Big halls are difficult to navigate, as walls are the reference for navigation. In corridors, VIPs walk in the middle of corridor swiping cane on floor. On rising steps, the cane is held upright in front of the subject; the tip of the cane locates the step riser giving position and height of next stair. Navigating down steps, the cane is held as walking on a flat surface, without waving and touching next stair. On an escalator, the bumped surface at start is located; the end is identified by striking the escalator-floor interface. For lift usage, the cane is used to locate the door and to discern height difference of the lift floor (if any). Travelling by bus or car, the white cane helps in boarding or alighting from the bus by sensing the stairs and foothold of bus and surface of sidewalk, folding the cane within taxis or cars.

Sweden

On a flat surface, VIPs roll the cane from side to side for navigation. On bricks, they tap the cane instead of rolling. On a trail, they swipe cane with care so as to not tangle with foliage. The cane helps identify the presence of the slippery snow. In corridors, they use walls as reference for navigation by striking cane to it. In all other examples the operation is similar to Finland.

Pakistan

For outdoor navigation, they use cane by left right tapping on a flat surface, walk more slowly on bricks, and more carefully on trails. In all other examples the operation is similar to Finland. In a sub question, all users ranked the role of hearing for navigation above 80%.

STUDY FOR THE ACCEPTANCE OF TECHNOLOGICAL NAVIGATION ASSISTANCE BY VIPs

A complementary qualitative study is being conducted to acquire knowledge of factors affecting the acceptance of navigation assistance tools by VIPs. The project plans to design various solutions in addition to the system proposed in this article. The scope of this study includes aspects outside the scope of a smart cane system.

Acceptance issues with assistive tools

Previous studies have shown that assistive tools may have acceptance issues by some VIPs. There are several reasons for VIPs not accepting assistive tools (25). Tool-related reasons include availability and usability. User-related reasons include attitude to technology and perceived need for the tool (26).

Qualitative Interviews

The study is two-phased, with an interview and test sessions. The interview is designed to collect data on general technological acceptance issues. The field test session is still in a planning phase.

Using Unified Theory of Acceptance and Use of Technology (UTAUT2) model for finding out acceptance issues

The question set of the first round of interviews includes modified questions of the extended version of UTAUT2 model (27). The UTAUT2 model constructs are performance expectancy (PE), effort expectancy (EE), social influence (SI), facilitating conditions (FC), hedonic motivation (HM), price value (PM), and habit (HA).

'PE' is defined as the degree to which a user believes that the system will help him to attain gains in job performance. At the test sessions the goal is to find out whether the smart cane comes with enough extra performance so that it would be accepted as assistive tool. 'EE' is defined as the degree of ease of using the tool. The white cane is already familiar to most VIPs, the effort to learn to use the smart cane is low and therefore it should be accepted. 'SI' is defined as the degree of user's belief how family and friends view the usage of assistive tool. 'FC' is defined as the degree of user's belief of existing organizational support available for the system; the augmented cane system is heavily dependent on the infrastructure of magnetic trails. 'HM' is the aspect of fun or pleasure derived from using a technology. 'PV' is defined on user's perceived benefits from using a system compared to the monetary cost of using it (28); the cost of smart cane is negligible. 'HA' is defined as self-perceived habit or continual use of a system (27). After the future test session new data will be found on how the participants perceive if the habit of using a white cane would change if a smart cane is in use.

Preliminary results and future plans

The results are not analyzed yet, as the data collection continues. However, some preliminary results are presented here. Three of the interviewees (19 in total) did not use a white cane or any other tool for navigation, 14 used a white cane, and three a guide dog. Two of the dog owners preferred the dog to white cane. Eight of the participants used smartphones or tablet computers, but these devices were not used for navigation.

Considering reasons (tool- and user-related) behind assistive tool acceptance (29), our study indicates that white cane availability in Finland is very high. Usability of the cane is high as only two of the participants thought using was uncomfortable. Not every participant saw it as necessary. Attitudes for using the white cane was positive, as only three of the participants thought it was unpleasant to use.

In the future, the study continues to add the number of test subjects. Also, outdoor field tests are being planned with VIPs. The question of whether the extra benefits of the magnetic smart cane would increase the use of the white cane altogether will be studied.

Usability testing

The main objective of conducting the usability experiment is to remove problematic issues from the system which cause failure in achieving maximum desired system's usability (30). The usability experiment setting is defined as a specific number of participants, a moderator, and a set of tasks to test the system. It identifies problems which have remained hidden through the development process from developer's point of view (30).

Test scenarios

There are three phases of learnability for the proposed navigation system:

- 1st phase: User follows a walking trail successfully.
- 2nd phase: User senses the serialized vibration successfully at a given POI.
- 3rd phase: User reads the serialized Braille message successfully.

Test setting for the 1st phase usability testing

In the 1st phase, the users followed a straight line trail (100 cm) followed by a 45 degree bending curve (50 cm). Ability to follow the straight line and to turn was evaluated separately. Only the tests with stationary magnet points' trail were performed at this point.

Each VIP was given an oral briefing before the test about how the system works and how to use it. VIPs familiarized themselves with it by walking over the test trail. After familiarization, the real test walk was observed. The performance was evaluated as successful if the person was able to complete the track from start to end point. The subjects were then asked feedback questions.

Usability test results

Pakistan
13 out of 15 VI subjects were able to navigate the test trail successfully. They found proposed navigation system assistive for their navigation.

Finland
2 VI subjects participated in the usability test, both were able to navigate the test trail. They found proposed navigation system useful for the VIPs' navigation.

Discussion

The improvement of the autonomy and functional capabilities of people with special needs is often achieved through the use of assistive technologies. These technologies ensure an improvement of the general welfare of the people by enhancing their capabilities. However, their design will be limited if real end user requirements are not gathered through interaction with them. In this article, the prototype of a navigation system to assist VIPs in outdoor navigation was presented. A qualitative study as a part of the development was presented that collected accounts of VIPs' navigation specifications and acceptance of technological navigation tools. Usability tests to evaluate usability factor of the system were described and results of first phase testing were presented. Based on the results, it could be said that the proposed system has potential for navigational assistance to VIPs. Usability tests done so far have provided with actionable suggestions to increase usability of the proposed navigation system. Phases two and three of usability testing will be performed and reported in the future.

ACKNOWLEDGMENTS

This paper has been written as part of ASTS Project funded by Academy of Finland, Japan Science technology Agency (JST), and Faculty of Information Technology and Electrical Engineering (ITEE). We want to thank Timo Jämsä, Maarit Kangas, Niina Keränen, Eeva Leinonen, Pekka Räsänen, and Zeeshan Asghar for contribution and co-operation. We would like to expand our thanks to Doc. Intzar Hussain Butt (POB Trust), Sadia Butt (MID) for helping in tests and interviews in Pakistan, and Parivash Ranjbar in Sweden.

REFERENCES

[1] Katz BF, Kammoun S, Parseihian G, Gutierrez O, Brilhault A, Auvray M, et al. NAVIG: augmented reality guidance system for the visually impaired. Virtual Reality 2012;16(4):253-69.

[2] Downs RM, Stea D. Maps in minds: Reflections on cognitive mapping. New York: Harper Row, 1977:264-72.

[3] Kamiński Ł, Bruniecki K. Mobile navigation system for visually impaired users in the urban environment. Metrology Measurement Systems 2012;19(2): 245-56.

[4] Hersh M, Johnson MA. Assistive technology for visually impaired and blind people. Dordrecht: Springer, 2010.

[5] Yelamarthi K, Haas D, Nielsen D, Mothersell S. RFID and GPS integrated navigation system for the visually impaired. In: Circuits and Systems (MWSCAS), 2010 53rd IEEE International Midwest Symposium on. IEEE, 2010:1149-52.

[6] Letham L. GPS made easy: Using global positioning systems in the outdoors. Victoria, BC: Rocky Mountain Books, 2011.

[7] Kolodziej KW, Hjelm J. Local positioning systems: LBS applications and services. Boca Ratoin, FL: CRC press, 2010.

[8] Moreira A, Valadas R, Oliveira Duarte A. Reducing the effects of artificial light interference in wireless infrared transmission systems. In: IEEE Colloquium on Optical Free Space Communication Links, London: IEEE, 1996:510.

[9] Bulusu N, Heidemann J, Estrin D. Gps-less low-cost outdoor localization for very small devices. IEEE Pers Commun Magazine 2000;7:28-34.

[10] Chawathe SS. Low-latency indoor localization using bluetooth beacons. In: Intelligent Transportation Systems, 2009. ITSC '09. 12th International IEEE Conference, 2009:1-7.

[11] Hightower J, Borriello G. Location systems for ubiquitous computing. IEEE Computer 2001;34:57-66.

[12] Ran L, Helal S, Moore S. Drishti: An integrated indoor/ outdoor blind navigation system and service. In: Pervasive Computing and Communications, IEEE International Conference, 2004:23-30.

[13] Lorincz K, Welsh M. A robust, decentralized approach to rfibased location tracking. In: Location- and Context-Awareness 3479, 2004:49-62.
[14] Nakajima M, Haruyama S. Indoor navigation system for visually impaired people using visible light communication and compensated geomagnetic sensing. In: Communications in China (ICCC), 2012 1st IEEE International Conference, IEEE 2012:524-9).
[15] Braille L. Procedure for writing words, music and plain-song using dots for the use of the blind and made available to them. Paris: Institut National des Jeunes Aveugles, 1829.
[16] Wormsley DP, D'Andrea FM, eds.. Instructional strategies for Braille literacy. New York: American Foundation for the Blind, 1997.
[17] Neodymium magnet. URL: http://en.wikipedia.org/wiki /Neodymium_magnet.
[18] Arduino board. URL: http://www.arduino.cc/en/Main/ ArduinoBoardUno.
[19] H_bridge. URL: https://en.wikipedia.org/wiki/H_bridge
[20] Reed switch. URL: http://en.wikipedia.org/wiki/Reed_ switch.
[21] Pobtrust. URL: http://pobtrust.org/.
[22] Midpakistan. URL: http://www.midpakistan.com/
[23] Myers MD, Newman M. The qualitative interview in IS research: Examining the craft. Inform Organ 2007; 17(1):2-26.
[24] Akao Y. Quality function deployment: integrating customer requirements into product design. Cambridge, MA: Productivity Press, 2004.
[25] Nordqvist B. Nähdä. In Apuvälinekirja Salminen, A-L. (toim.) Helsinki: Kehitysvammaliitto, Oppimateriaal ikeskus, 2003. [Finnish]
[26] Salminen A-L. Apuväline toimintaa edistämässä. In: Apuvälinekirja Salminen, A-L. (toim.) Helsinki: Kehitysvammaliitto, Oppimateriaalikeskus, 2003. [Finnish].
[27] Venkatesh V, Morris MG, Davis GB, Davis FD. User acceptance of information technology: Toward a unified view. MIS Quart 2003;27(3):425-78.
[28] Venkatesh V, Thong JYL, Xu X. Consumer acceptance and use of information technology: Extending the unified theory of acceptance and use of technology. MIS Quart 2012;36(1):157-78.
[29] Donahue GM, Weinschenk S, Nowicki J. Usability is good business. URL: http://www.yucentrik.ca /usability .pdf.
[30] Nielsen J. Usability inspection methods. Conference Companion on Human factors in computing systems, ACM. 1994:423-4.

Submitted: July 15, 2015. Revised: August 15, 2015. Accepted: August 26, 2015.

In: Alternative Medicine Research Yearbook 2017
Editor: Joav Merrick
ISBN: 978-1-53613-726-2
© 2018 Nova Science Publishers, Inc.

Chapter 29

EXPLORING HAPTIC FEEDBACK FOR ROBOT-TO-HUMAN COMMUNICATION

Ayan Ghosh[1],*, MSc, Jacques Penders[1], PhD, Peter Jones[2], PhD, Heath Reed[3] and Alessandro Sorranzo[4], PhD

[1]Materials and Engineering Research Institute, Sheffield Hallam University, Sheffield, United Kingdom
[2]The Department of Humanities, Sheffield Hallam University, Sheffield, United Kingdom
[3]Art and Design Research Group, Sheffield Hallam University, Sheffield, United Kingdom
[4]The Department of Psychology, Sociology and Politics, Sheffield Hallam University, Sheffield, United Kingdom

ABSTRACT

Search and rescue operations are often undertaken in low-visibility smoky environments in which rescue teams must rely on haptic feedback for navigation and exploration. The overall aim of our research is to enable a human being to explore such environments using a robot. In this article we focus on creating feedback from a robot to a human. We describe our first designs and trials with vibration motors. The focus is on determining the potential use of vibration motors for message transfer and our trials reflect whether different messages can be discriminated. We describe the testing procedure and the results of our first tests. Based on these results, we conclude that close spatial arrangement of the motors blurs individual signals.

Keywords: exploration, navigation, haptic feedback, remote sensing

---

* Correspondence: Ayan Ghosh, Materials and Engineering Research Institute, Sheffield Hallam University, Sheffield, United Kingdom. E-mail: ayan.ghosh@student.shu.ac.uk.

Introduction

Search and rescue operations in fire incidents, are undertaken only when the ground is relatively passable (1); the major problem however is that the environment is smoke-filled and noisy. Lack of visual and auditory feedback make rescue teams rely on haptic feedback for navigation and exploration. Navigation concerns finding the way, while exploration involves exploring the environment and finding possible victims. Robots with a range of sensors on board might be helpful for such conditions. In addition, there are also everyday situations where vision and audibility are low, for instance, a visually impaired person trying to walk along a street.

An early work on robotic navigation assistance to the visual impaired is described in Tachi et al. (2) where they developed a guide-dog robot for the visually impaired. The robot tracks the handler using active sonar, and the handler wears a stereo headset, which provides coded aural feedback to notify whether the handler is straying from the path. There are no means to communicate with the robot, and the handler must learn the new aural-feedback code, the robot serving as a mobile beacon that communicates with the headset. More recently, Allan Melvin et al. (3, 4) developed a robot guide to replace a guide dog and also described a robotic guide where the emphasis is on how well a person follows the robot; however, the human does not have any control over the robot and thus cannot explore.

There is quite a difference between guidance and exploration. Guidance is limited to the robot leading the person or handler. This setting presupposes that the robot does the way-finding and the person just follows. Exploration concerns investigating the direct but yet unknown environment. As there is no-visibility, exploration has to rely on active haptic sensing. A widely used device for haptic exploration is a white cane as intended for the visually impaired. Inspired by this, Ulrich and Borenstein developed the GuideCane (5), a cane like device running on unpowered wheels which uses Ultra Sound to detect obstacles. The handler has to push the GuideCane – it has no powered wheels – however, it has a steering mechanism that can be operated by the handler or operate autonomously. In autonomous mode, when detecting an obstacle the wheels are steered away to avoid the obstacle. Obviously the feedback to the human remains implicit: the handle is the medium.

Our project aim is to build a robotic device for exploration purposes. We previously reported on our initial haptic mode experiments in which a person uses a simple passive device (a metal disk fixed with a rigid handle, as shown in figure 1) to explore the immediate environment (6). The feedback from the disk to the handler remains implicit: it is restricted to what the handler feels when holding the stick. Experiments demonstrated the extreme sensitivity and trainability of the haptic channel and the speed with which users develop and refine their haptic proficiencies, permitting reliable and accurate discrimination between objects of different weights. The disc with rigid handle provided implicit feedback to the handler while the handler was operating it. The final aim is to use a powered robotic device. However, a major issue with a powered robotic device is that there is no room for active haptic sensing by the human and the feedback to the handler has to be made explicit. Here we focus on creating feedback from a powered robot to the handler. We describe our first designs and trials with vibrating motors. At this stage the focus is on determining the potential of a set of vibration motors for message transfer; the trials investigate whether different messages can be discriminated.

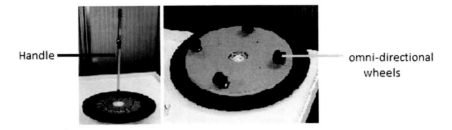

Figure 1. Metal disc fixed with a fixed handle.

Feedback device

Our design incorporates a robot with an impedance filter, which is connected with a handle to the handler. Figure 2 shows the impedance filter – a skirt-like structure – which sits on top of the robot (7). The figure also shows the handle, the physical interface between robot and the handler. Our previous work (4) has reflected on various aspects of the handle design. While encountering an obstacle, the skirt is displaced. The displacement is measured (using Cable Reel Transducers); these measurements need to be transformed into some sort of a haptic input to the handler. Defining and designing the input signal for the human handler is our current objective.

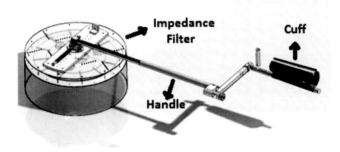

Figure 2. The handle (with feedback cuff) and the impedance filter.

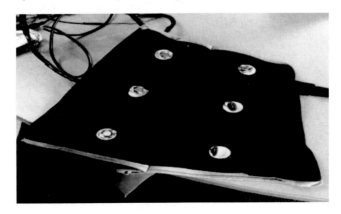

Figure 3. Feedback cuff.

We apply six vibrating motors, which are fixed on a wearable cuff (as shown in Figure 3) attached to the crutch-like part of the handle (as shown in Figure 2). The motors vibrate for short periods (3-5 seconds) on the lower arm of the handler. The motors are individually controlled; however, all motors operate at the same frequency and intensity. They are connected through a microcontroller and operated using a software interface developed in Labview.

Testing protocol

Figure 4 shows a person wearing the cuff on the lower arm. Our first question is whether subjects are able to distinguish which individual motors are activated; in addition our aim is to study whether different combinations of concurrent vibrating motors are recognisable. After one or more vibration motors were turned on for 3-5 seconds, the subjects were asked to report on the positions of the motors, by pointing out the options shown in the picture (see figure 4 right). To make it easier to understand, we named the positions as following: motors close to the wrist, Under Arm Bottom (UB) and Over Arm Bottom (OB), in the Middle as Under Arm middle (UM) and Over Arm Middle (OM) and close to the Elbow as Under Arm Top (UT) and Over Arm Top (OT), refer to Figure 5. Every subject was given noise cancelling ear protectors to neutralise all possible auditory cues.

Six subjects, aging between 22 and 55 without any medical conditions, took part in our experimental study. Each subject was asked to undergo four sessions with twelve trials in each session. Before the commencement of the trials, the subjects were briefed about the experiment and went through a pre-trial in order to make them accustomed with testing environment and the apparatus. In the first trial set any of the six vibration motors is activated, but only one at the time. In the second trial set two motors are activated concurrently but in varying patterns and in the third set three motors are activated in varying patterns. The final session consists of a mix of single, double or triple motor activations in a random order.

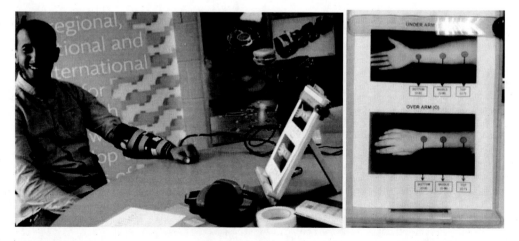

Figure 4. (Left) The cuff on trial and the trial's feedback display. (Right) The picture placed in front of the subjects for pointing out the positions.

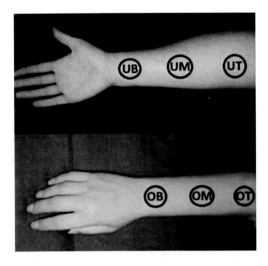

Figure 5. Position of the vibration Motors.

RESULTS

Figure 6 shows the errors subjects made in identifying the specific motors for the first three trial sets. The figures show motor positions on the horizontal axis; the vertical axis shows the proportion of errors (0-1) made when the respective motors were activated. Figure 6 left, shows the error proportions with single vibrating motors; the middle graph shows error proportions with two vibrating motors; and the right graph shows error proportions with three vibrating motors. We notice that there is an increase in the number of errors as the number of vibrating motors increases. It is evident that the subjects were most accurate in determining the positions of vibrations when only a single vibration motor was turned on.

Average proportions of errors for the 3 different trial sets were as follows:

- Set 1 (single vibrating motor; 6 trials): 0.125 (0-1)
- Set 2 (2 motors vibrating concurrently; 12 trials): 0.22 (0-1)
- Set 3 (3 motors vibrating concurrently; 12 trials): 0.40 (0-1)

These results indicate the increasing difficulty in accurate identification of vibrating motor(s) over the three sets.

For the first set of trials involving single vibration motors, error rates were low. A repeated one-way ANOVA measure on the arc sin transformation of the proportion of errors showed no significant difference across the six motor positions ($F(5,5) = .87$; p. = 0.51).

For the second set of trials, error rates were higher than for the first set but still rather low. A repeated one-way ANOVA measure on the arc sin transformation showed no significant difference in proportion of errors across the twelve trial conditions ($F(5,11) = .73$; p. = 0.7) involving pairs of concurrently vibrating motors.

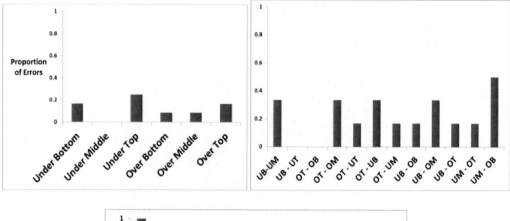
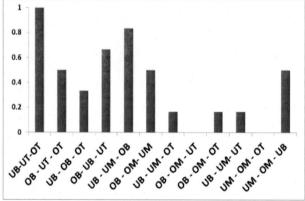

Figure 6. Proportion of errors, single (left); double (middle); triple (right).

In the third set of trials in which three motors were activated concurrently, the error rates are high. Furthermore, the one-way ANOVA ($F(5,11) = 3.89$; $p < 0.01$) showed a significant difference in proportion of errors across the twelve trials. It would appear, then, that the task becomes much more challenging with three vibration motors switched on and also that some of the triple-combinations are more readily identifiable than others, although the precise reasons for this extra level of difficulty are not clear. Anecdotal evidence suggests that identification difficulties may be associated with distribution or proximity of the motors on the arm but we were unable to establish this from our present data.

Conclusion

The findings of the experimental trials raise a number of issues that need to be taken into account for future re-design of the cuff and the message-sending configurations of vibrating motors. The trial data show that subjects were easily able to distinguish when individual vibration motors were activated but that the difficulty of the task increased when motors were combined. Combinations of three motors, in particular, were especially difficult to identify accurately.

For these reasons, present work is focussed on the use of a cuff with only four vibration motors (two on each side) which will be used either singly or in pairs to transmit messages.

Future experiments will also investigate whether specific signatures in vibration frequency and intensity for each motor may improve recognition. A next step is to define and design feedback signals (a sort of haptic alphabet) that correspond with displacements of the impedance filter.

REFERENCES

[1] Penders J, Alboul L, Witkowski U, Naghsh A, Saez-Pons J, Herrechtsmeier S, et al. A robot swarm assisting a human firefighter. Adv Robotics 2011;25:93-117.

[2] Tachi S, Mann RM, Rowell D. Quantitative comparison of alternative sensory displays for mobility aids for the blind. IEEE Trans Biomed Engineering 1983;30(9): 571–7.

[3] Allan Melvin A, Prabu B, Nagarajan R, and Bukhari I. ROVI: a robot for visually impaired for collision-free navigation, Proceed International Conference on Man-Machine Systems (ICoMMS), 2009.

[4] Ghosh A, Penders J, Jones P, Reed H. Experience of following a Robot using a Haptic Interface without Visual Feedback. IEEE Ro-Man, Edinburgh, 2014.

[5] Ulrich I and Borenstein J. The GuideCane-applying mobile robot technologies to assist the visually impaired. Systems, Man and Cybernetics, Part A: Systems and Humans, IEEE Transactions on Issue Date: Mar 2001;31(2):131-136.

[6] Jones P, Ghosh A, Penders J, Read H. Towards human technology symbiosis in the haptic mode. *International Conference on Communication, Media, Technology and Design,* Famagusta, North Cyprus, 2013 May 2-4:307-12.

[7] Janani A, Holloway A, Reed H, Penders J. Design of a mechanical impedance filter for remote haptic feedback in low-visibility environment. Oxford: TAROS, 2013.

Submitted: July 15, 2015. *Revised:* August 17, 2015. *Accepted:* August 26, 2015.

In: Alternative Medicine Research Yearbook 2017
Editor: Joav Merrick
ISBN: 978-1-53613-726-2
© 2018 Nova Science Publishers, Inc.

Chapter 30

RAISED-DOT SLIPPAGE PERCEPTION ON A FINGERPAD USING AN ACTIVE WHEEL DEVICE

Yoshihiko Nomura*, DrEng and Hirotsugu Kato, BEng

Department of Mechanical Engineering, Mie University, Japan

ABSTRACT

To improve the slippage perceptual characteristics with the fingertip cutaneous sensation, raised dots were introduced on the surface of a rotating wheel. As a result of psychophysical experiments, we obtained factor effects on the perception; statistical tests showed a significant difference among the three surfaces: the 3.2 mm and 12.8 mm periods of raised dot surfaces, and the without-raised-dot surface.

Keywords: raised-dot, slippage perception, fingerpad, active wheel device

INTRODUCTION

A prototype of a slippage-displaying device that embodied a wheel rotating on an index fingerpad was studied in this paper. Perceiving velocities for some periods, subjects can continuously move their hand; concatenating the motions, they can further perceive line drawings such as the multi-stroke characters. It would be helpful for visually impaired persons to perceive line drawing in such the way. To improve the slippage perceptual characteristics via cutaneous sensation, we have introduced raised dots on the sliding surfaces of the wheel. The raised dots give subjects distinct stimuli of concave deformations moving on the fingerpad skin surface; the distinctiveness is expected to enhance the slippage perceptual characteristics (1).

---

* Correspondence: Professor Yoshihiko Nomura, Dr Eng, Department of Mechanical Engineering, Mie University, Kurimamachiyacho, Tsu, 514-8507, Japan. E-mail: nomura@mach.mie-u.ac.jp.

Sarada et al. also reported some perceptual characteristics with slip velocities and directions (2). Together with a sandblasted homogeneous rough surfaces, they employed a specific dot surface made of small circular bulging edges: the Weber fraction with the slip-speed perception was improved from 0.25 to 0.04, and the difference thresholds between slip-directions were also improved from 11.7 to 3.6 degrees. Taking notice of not only the velocity, but also the perceptual time period, the authors extended perceptual tasks from the velocity to the length (3). Iit was also found that a speed perception scheme worked for the high-speed condition or the multiple dot contact condition, while a dot counting scheme did so for the low-speed and single dot contact condition (3). In this work, the mechanical configuration was extended from the linear actuator-based translation to servomotor-based rotation towards the development of mouse type tactile devices (3).

As with the mouse type fingertip tactile devices, Kyung et al. (4) proposed a multi-functional mouse providing 1-D grabbing force and 2-D translational force together with pin array tactile patterns. Gleeso et al. (5) proposed a device providing a 2-D tangential skin displacement. Tsagarakis et al. (6) used a V-configuration of frustum cones to provide the 2-D tangential slip/stretch as the velocity vector by the form of producing a vector sum: the discrimination angle was 15 degrees with about 70% correct answer rate. Webster et al. (7) produced the sliding contact through the rotation of a ball: values relating to just noticeable differences (JNDs) with directional differences were given as 20–25°. Contrasting to these with non-bumpy surfaces, the authors introduce raised dots to enhance the slippage perceptual performance in this work.

METHODS

Three kinds of films were introduced: (i) a surface with a dot spacing interval of 3.2 mm, see Figure 1(a), referred as the "3.2mm-dot surface"; (ii) a surface with a dot spacing interval of 12.8 mm, referred as the "12.8mm-dot surface"; and (iii) a non-bumpy flat surface, referred to as the "flat surface." The flat surface was introduced to clarify the advantages of the raised dots. Considering Japanese Standard with raised dots for tactile graphics, the raised dot size were 1.5 mm in diameter, and 0.4 mm in height. In addition, all the three films were made of a film that is commercially available (#2000, grain size of 9μm, 3M Corp.) to make the experimental results general. The films were affixed to the cylindrical surface of a wheel. The wheel was 65 mm in diameter, and was rotated with respect to orthogonal two axes by a couple of servomotors. One servomotor was connected to the other base-fixed servomotor via a swivel joint. This mechanism made the wheel possible to rotate in 2-DOF (see Figure 1(b), (c)).

Experimental procedure

Six right-handed male subjects, aged 22 to 59 years, voluntarily participated in the experiment. Twisting neither their body at the waist nor their head at the neck, subjects were seated on a chair, facing to the front (see Figure 1(d)). Setting their elbow flexion angle at about 90°, their forearm was set parallel to the table base, and was also set parallel to the direction in the sagittal plane. A white noise sound was applied to the subjects via headphones for avoiding any side effects on the slippage perception. Subjects touched the wheel surface using their fingerpad through a hole (12.8 mm diameter) made in a polyester film (100μ thick); the wheel was activated after arbitrary waiting times: the wheel was swivelled to a direction, and rotated by a specific angle where the servomotors drove the wheel in rectangular velocity patterns. The presented line lengths were 25, 50, 75, 100, 125, and 150 mm. The line directions were 0° (right) to 330° with an interval of 30° in the counterclockwise direction. The speed was set at 60 mm/s because the speed of 60 mm/s is considered to be natural in ordinary active touches. The 6 lengths and 12 directions made a combination of 72 line segments which were ordered in a pseudo random way, and were presented twice for each of the three surface types. Consequently, the total number of 432 (6 × 12 × 2 × 3) runs of line segment were presented for each subject. The experiment took about 2 hours per subject. During experiments, the subjects were instructed to relax, and to focus on perceiving the presented linear sliding lengths via their index fingerpad. They answered the perceived lengths and directions in the following way: just after the wheel stopped, they opened their eyes, looked at the answer board (see Figure 1(d)), and phonated a code number that represents the length and the direction.

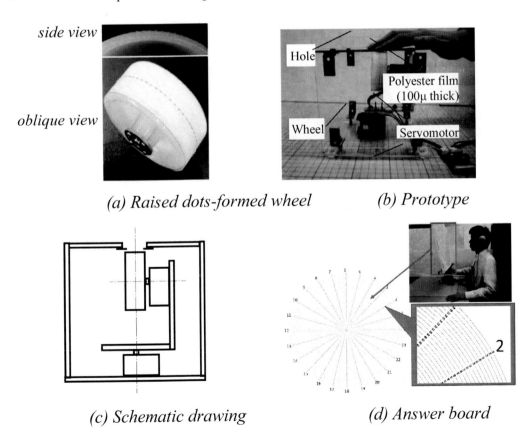

Figure 1. Experimental device.

RESULTS

The relationships between the perceptual and actual lengths are shown in Figure 2 for each of the three surfaces: (i) 3.2mm-dot; (ii) 12.8mm-dot; and (iii) flat. Although a length-related nonlinearity occurred for all the three surfaces, the nonlinearity in both the dot surfaces seemed to be much smaller than that in the non-bumpy flat surface.

The relationships between the perceptual angle errors and the actual angles are shown in Figure 3 for each of the three surfaces. There can be seen a trigonometric function patterns with approximately the same amount of biases of several degrees in the counterclockwise direction.

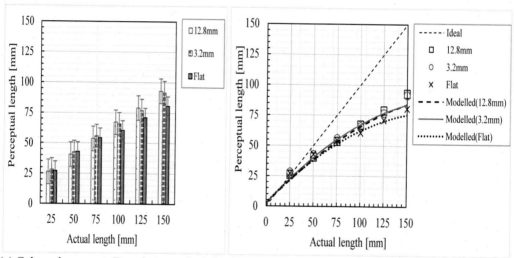

(a) Column bar; mean. Error bar; standard deviation.   (b) Symbol; mean. Line; modelled.

Figure 2. Perceptual length characteristics for the 12.8mm-dot, 3.2 mm-dot, and flat surfaces.

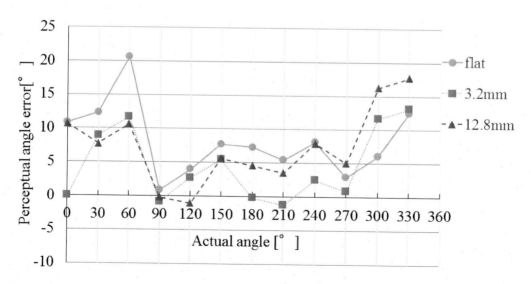

Figure 3. Mean deviation of the perceptual direction for the three surfaces with respect to the directions.

Table 1. ANOVA tables

(a) ln α (α, proportional coefficient wrt perceived lengths)

Factor	Level	Mean	Factor effect	Stand. dev.	DOF	Test stats. F-value	Dicision
Surface	12.8mm	0.94	-0.18	0.76			
	3.2mm	1.16	0.03	0.96			
	Flat	1.28	0.15	0.86			
					2	4.1	*
Direction					11	0.79	NS
Interaction					22	0.49	NS
Error				1.01	396		
Global		1.12		1.11	431		

(b) β (exponential coefficient wrt perceived lengths)

Factor	Level	Mean	Factor effect	Stand. dev.	DOF	Test stats.	Dicision
Surface	12.8mm	0.7	0.044	0.18			
	3.2mm	0.657	0.001	0.21			
	Flat	0.612	0.044	0.17			
					2	4.68	**
Direction					11	1.14	NS
Interaction					22	0.76	NS
Error				0.19	396		
Global		0.656		0.21	431		

(c) Perceived directional errors

Factor	Level	Mean	Factor effect	Stand. dev.	DOF	Test stats. F-value	Dicision
Surface	12.8mm	7.36	0.53	16.05			
	3.2mm	5.12	-1.71	13.28			
	Flat	8.00	1.17	20.52			
					2	7.75	***
Length					5	0.18	NS
Direction	0°	9.44	2.62	16.7			
	30°	9.65	2.82	18.29			
	60°	13.47	6.64	16.3			
	90°	-0.07	-6.9	12.4			
	120°	1.88	-4.95	19.4			
	150°	6.25	-0.58	18.37			
	180°	3.89	-2.94	13.63			
	210°	2.57	-4.26	17.56			
	240°	6.18	-0.65	16.57			
	270°	2.92	-3.91	10.72			
	300°	11.32	4.49	16.68			
	330°	14.44	7.62	16.99			
					11	19.39	***
Interaction					10	1.93	***
Error				15.98	2579		
Global		6.9		16.92	2591		

* $P<0.05$, ** $P<0.01$, *** $P<0.001$

Discussion on perceptual lengths

After fitting a curve to the above explained data, a statistical ANOVA test was applied. A model value, l_{model}, for the perceived length, l_{perc}, was assumed to be given by a power function relation with the actual length, L, as in

$$l_{model} = \alpha\, L^{\beta} \qquad (1)$$

The length-related nonlinearity can be expressed by parameters β: the further away from the ideal value of 1 the value of β is, the larger the nonlinearity effect is. After taking logarithms of Eq. (1)

$$\ln l_{model} = \ln \alpha + \beta \ln L, \qquad (2)$$

a linear least squares method was applied to the data for each of the combinations of the 3 surfaces, 12 directions, 6 subjects and 2 iterations. Then, the 432 pieces of the coefficient pairs, $\ln \alpha$ and β, were estimated. Averages of the estimated $\ln \alpha$ and β for each of the three surfaces were shown in Figure 2 together with the modelled values.

Next, an ANOVA test was applied to the estimated coefficients (see Table 1(a), (b)). It was concluded that there were significant differences among the three surface levels for each of the coefficients, ln α and β, with the significant level of 0.1%, and that the 12.8mm dot showed a bit better performance than the others, while there was no significant difference with respect to the direction factor and the interaction factor.

ANOVA was also applied to the perceived angle errors (see Figure 3). We can conclude from Table 1(c) that there were significant differences of a 0.1% level among the three surface levels and that the 3.2 mm dot showed much better performance than the others from the viewpoints of both the mean error and the random error (standard deviation). Although there were also significant differences with respect to the direction factor and the interaction factor besides the surface factor, the direction factor effect was the largest among them.

Conclusion

Introducing raised-dots for enhancing slide-length perceptual characteristics, the authors made a prototype of wheel-type slippage presentation device which was able to display velocity vectors via tactile sensation on a human fingerpad. By integrating the perceived velocities over duration times, line segments can be perceived. The sample size was not enough to conclude definitely, and further examinations are necessary. The followings were tentatively obtained as a pilot study.

- Based on the Steven's power law, the perceived lengths were modelled.
- Perception of length: the 12.8 mm dot surface showed a bit better performance than the other 3.2 mm dot surface and the flat one.
- Perception of angle: the 3.2 mm dot surface showed much better performance than the other 12.8 mm dot surface and the flat one.

The experimental equipment used in this study was not compact enough to make use of mouse-interface, and further development of miniaturization would also be needed in the future studies. In addition, since the experiments were conducted by sighted persons, the results should be applied to acquired blindness, and further studies shall be necessary for congenital blindnesses.

In the future, embedding the much smaller size of the wheel into a mouse, the authors would like to construct a prototype of active wheel mouses.

Acknowledgments

This work was supported by KAKENHI (Grant-in-Aid for Challenging Exploratory Research 25560112 from Japan Society for the Promotion of Science (JSPS)).

References

[1] Dépeault A, Meftah EM, Chapman CE. Tactile speed scaling: contributions of time and space. J Neuro-physiology 2008;99:1422–34.

[2] Salada M, Colgate JE, Vishton P, Frankel E. Two experiments on the perception of slip at the fingertip. Proceed 12th International Symposium on Haptic Interfaces for Virtual Environment and Teleoperator Systems (HAPTICS'04), 2004:146–53.

[3] Nomura Y, Yusoh SMNS, Iwabu K, Sakamoto R. Sliding raised-dots perceptual characteristics: Speed perception or dot count, Proceed ACHI 2013: The Sixth International Conference on Advances in Computer-Human Interactions, 2013:303–8.

[4] Kyung KU, Choi H, Kwon DS, Son SW. Interactive mouse systems providing haptic feedback during the exploration in virtual environment. Dordrecht: Springer. 2004:136–46.

[5] Gleeso BT, Horschel SK, Provancher WR. Design of a fingertip-mounted tactile display with tangential skin displacement feedback. IEEE Transactions Haptics 2010;3(4):297–301.

[6] Tsagarakis NG, Horne T, Caldwell DG. SLIP AESTHEASIS: a portable 2D slip/skin stretch display for the fingertip. First Joint Eurohaptics Conference and Symposium on Haptic Interfaces for Virtual Environment and Teleoperator Systems, 2005:214–9.

[7] Webster III RJ, Murphy TE, Lawton NV, Okamura AM. A novel two-dimensional tactile slip display: Design, kinematics and perceptual experiments. ACM Transactions Appl Percept 2005;2(2):150–6.

Submitted: July 16, 2015. *Revised:* August 19, 2015. *Accepted:* August 26, 2015.

Section three - Children, disability and abuse

In: Alternative Medicine Research Yearbook 2017
Editor: Joav Merrick

ISBN: 978-1-53613-726-2
© 2018 Nova Science Publishers, Inc.

Chapter 31

PHYSICAL ABUSE AND NEGLECT IN CHILDREN WITH DISABILITIES: MEDICAL EVALUATION

Dena Nazer[*], *MD*
Wayne State University School of Medicine,
Children's Hospital of Michigan,
Kids-TALK Children's Advocacy Center, Detroit, Michigan, US

ABSTRACT

Children with disabilities are at a much higher risk for physical abuse and neglect, as compared to those with no disabilities. Both these forms of child maltreatment may result in severe injury and ultimately in death with neglect being more associated with maltreatment deaths than any other kind of maltreatment. Not only should severe cases of physical abuse and neglect be recognized, but subtler indicators of abuse and sentinel injuries need to be identified by the different professionals caring for the child to identify children at risk and prevent further abuse. In addition, recognition of the child's needs and the multiple contributors to neglect at the level of the child, parents, family, community, and society is essential to address the child's needs and increase collaboration between the families and the different professionals caring for the child to prevent neglect. This article focuses on the medical evaluation of children who are suspected of being physically abused or neglected.

Keywords: children, disability, abuse, neglect, medical evaluation

INTRODUCTION

In the United States alone, child protective services (CPS) agencies received an estimated 3.6 million referrals involving approximately 6.6 million children in 2014 (1). The highest rate of victimization was in children less than 1 year of age with the most common type of

---

[*] Correspondence: Dena Nazer, MD, Kids-TALK Children's Advocacy Center Medical Clinic, 40 East Ferry St, Detroit, Michigan 48202, United States. E-mail: dnazer@med.wayne.edu.

maltreatment overall being neglect (75%) followed by physical abuse (17%). A nationally estimated number of 1580 children died as a result of maltreatment in 2014, mostly as a result of neglect and most of whom were younger than 3 years of age. When looking at these numbers, one realizes the increased vulnerability of children especially those that are younger than 3 years of age, and especially when coupled with disability and the increased demands placed on caregivers.

Reporting an accurate number of children with disability who are victims of child maltreatment is challenging due to disability not always being reported. In addition, not all children who are maltreated are assessed for the presence of a developmental disability. Further adding to the complexity are the diverse definitions of disability, the diverse definitions of child neglect, and what constitutes physical abuse. According to the American Association on Intellectual and Developmental Disabilities (AAIDD), developmental disabilities are severe chronic disabilities that can be cognitive (intellectual) or physical or both. The disabilities appear in childhood and are likely to be lifelong. Intellectual disability is a disability characterized by three essential elements: limitations in intellectual functioning (such as learning and reasoning), limitations in adaptive behavior, which covers many everyday social and practical skills, and onset originating before the age of 18 years. The term intellectual disability has replaced the previously used "mental retardation" term. Intellectual disability affects about one percent of the population, and of those about 85% have mild intellectual disability. Some disorders include both physical and intellectual disability such as fetal alcohol syndrome while others are mainly physical like cerebral palsy.

Children with disabilities are at a higher risk of child maltreatment as compared to children with no disability and providers need to be aware of this risk (2). The health care provider should be able to recognize injuries suspicious for physical abuse and differentiate abusive injuries from accidental injuries and those that result from conditions that mimic child abuse. Neglect also should be addressed with a focus on the needs of the child especially when the needs of children with disabilities are increased compared to other children. The health care provider is also tasked with the responsibility of coordinating the medical services needed to treat the underlying disability, consequences of the maltreatment, and collaborate with community agencies. In addition, the health care provider is mandated to report cases of physical abuse and neglect to the appropriate authorities to prevent the detrimental lifelong consequences including death resulting from these types of maltreatment..

PHYSICAL ABUSE

The World Health Organization (WHO) defines Child maltreatment as the abuse and neglect that occurs in children under 18 years of age. It includes all types of physical and/or emotional ill-treatment, sexual abuse, neglect, negligence and commercial or other exploitation, which results in actual or potential harm to the child's health, survival, development or dignity in the context of a relationship of responsibility, trust or power. Exposure to intimate partner violence is also sometimes included as a form of child maltreatment and may result in physical injuries to the child.

Although the exact definition of physical abuse may vary from one country to another and even in between States in the US, it commonly includes the presence of a non-accidental or inflicted injury that the child sustains by a caregiver. The definition of what constitutes physical abuse is influenced by one's professional experience and personal and cultural background (3).

Physical abuse results in both physical and mental health problems in children that may exacerbate the child's underlying medical condition and disability. It is also considered one of the adverse childhood experiences that leads to long term health consequences, chronic diseases and early death (4).

NEGLECT

Neglect is the most common reported form of child maltreatment in the US. Neglect is commonly defined in state law as the failure of a parent or other person with responsibility for the child to provide needed food, shelter, clothing, medical care, or supervision to the degree that the child's safety, health, and well-being are threatened with harm. Some states specifically mention types of neglect in their statutes such as medical neglect, educational neglect, and abandonment; in addition, some States include exceptions for determining neglect, such as financial considerations for physical neglect and religious exemptions for medical neglect. However, a more child focused definition of neglect as a condition when the child's needs are not met draws attention to the child's basic needs and allows a more collaborative approach between health providers and parents (5).

RISK FACTORS FOR PHYSICAL ABUSE AND NEGLECT

It is essential to identify the risk factors of child abuse when evaluating children with disabilities. Identifying the risk factors assists in identifying and creating prevention programs for families especially those that are identified as high risk. However, one has to remember that child abuse affects all children of different socioeconomic, religious, and ethnic backgrounds and the mere presence of these risk factors is not diagnostic. Infants and toddlers are at greatest risk for abuse, proving age of the child as the most significant risk factor for abuse. Children with disabilities--whether intellectual or physical--are at higher risk for physical abuse.

Risk factors for abuse and neglect include those that are parent-related (mental health disease, substance abuse, and interpersonal violence) and those that are child related (disability, prematurity, and low birth weight). Families who live in poverty, are socially isolated, and have lower level of education are at further risk for abuse. There are certain types of abusive injuries associated with specific developmental stages which may vary depending on the developmental abilities of the child. For example, abusive head trauma is associated with excessive crying and scald burns are associated with toilet training.

In addition, children with disabilities may place additional financial, social, physical, and emotional demands on their caregivers (6). A child may require closer supervision and assistance with performing daily routines such as hygiene which may overwhelm a caregiver who has limited support. Poverty and the lack of available services in the area the child resides in may further contribute to neglect and the child's needs not being met such as the lack of mental health services, affordable dental care, and the lack of a medical home which ensures comprehensive care is provided for a child.

CORPORAL PUNISHMENT

Parents of children with disability may struggle with discipline as children may not cognitively understand recommended methods of behavioral modification such as loss of privileges and time out. The American Academy of Pediatrics strongly opposes the use of physical punishment in children. Spanking, especially in infants, may be harmful and result in physical injuries especially when on sensitive areas such as the face (7). Laws differ in relation to what is acceptable and what constitutes acceptable physical discipline so one should be familiar with the laws and sensitive to the cultural norms and perspectives.

Appropriate discipline is a main concern for families with children especially for those who have children with disabilities. It is much harder to discipline a child with disability as the child may not comprehend loss of privileges or the reason for the discipline. However, parents of all children including those with disabilities need more guidance on acceptable and effective modes of discipline that do not result in injuries, physical or mental.

PRESENTATION OF PHYSICAL ABUSE AND NEGLECT

Children who are victims of physical abuse have various presentations depending on their age, developmental ability, type of injury and severity. The child may be brought in for routine care when a provider notices the presence of an injury, for example, a bruise or a burn on the child's body or the parent may bring the child in for care due to an injury for example pain and decreased mobility in an extremity. The child may also present with severe life-threatening manifestations. Making the diagnosis of physical abuse is difficult as one has to accept that the child's caregivers, who in many cases have a long standing relationship with the medical provider, injured the child (8). In addition, the highest risk of physical abuse is in the younger children who are nonverbal because of their age, disability, or as a complication of the physical injury. Caregivers may also not provide an accurate history and the presentation may be similar to other medical problems diverting the physician from making a diagnosis of physical abuse.

When evaluating a child for neglect, the provider needs to be sensitive, avoid blame, and engage the family in an active treatment plan (9). Proper communication is essential when evaluating any child especially when maltreatment is suspected. Families need to understand the concerns, the proposed plan of evaluation and the necessity to report certain cases to the appropriate organizations. The medical evaluation is a part of the multidisciplinary evaluation needed in cases of abuse and neglect and compliments the additional assessments done by other services.

There are several elements in the history and physical examination that prompt the physician to initiate a child abuse physical assessment. Concerning factors include injury in a nonmobile or nonverbal child, inconsistent or changing history, unexplained delay in seeking medical care and a disclosure of physical abuse by a verbal child (8). As in other medical conditions, an evaluation consists of a medical history, physical examination, imaging and laboratory testing when needed.

MEDICAL HISTORY

Medical history is an important component of assessment of injuries and one should answer the question of whether a particular injury is consistent with the history provided.

Injuries may be different due to developmental abilities, verbal skills and how pain is felt and expressed. One should attempt to obtain a history from the child alone and from each caregiver separately. However, for nonverbal children, a history from the child of how the injury occurred would be lacking. Questions that may help include asking about the events that lead to the injury, details of the fall or injury, supervision, when was the child last well, and development and progression of symptoms.

All assessments of children with disabilities should include a developmental assessment in order to better understand the abilities of the child and whether the history is consistent with the injury. For example, while a healthy 1-year-old child may pull to stand and fall resulting in a bruise on his forehead, a developmentally delayed 4-year-old may not be able to do that, making a bruise suspicious in the latter case. Intellectual disability also needs to be considered; for example, a 16-year-old with intellectual disability may still need supervision around electric outlets, stoves and other potentially dangerous house hold objects.

Additional important elements in the history include information regarding the child's past medical history (hospitalizations, surgeries, and medical conditions), child's birth, and dietary history. An assessment of the child's needs as a result of these medical illnesses and disabilities helps determine the needs of the child and the challenges facing the family in securing these needs. It also provides a child's needs approach to child neglect vs. a parental omission approach which is less blaming, offers a broader response to contributing factors to the child's condition and is more constructive (5, 9).

A complete social history is crucial as it is the child's social environment that is a key determinant of the child's current and future health (10). A social history serves to identify both strengths to reinforce and weaknesses to address specifically in cases where neglect is suspected and a treatment plan is being formulated with the family. Adverse childhood experiences are directly linked to risky health behaviors, chronic health conditions, and early death. A comprehensive social history may help in prevention of these adverse experiences and thus decreasing their negative outcome (4).

Due to the significant overlap of child maltreatment and intimate partner violence (IPV), the medical provider should also screen for and detect IPV in the family when evaluating the child (11). As mentioned above, IPV is sometimes included in the definition of child maltreatment. Not only do children who live in violent environments have a higher risk for child maltreatment, but children who witness IPV are at a higher risk of behavioral, psychological and adverse health problems. Victimization resulting from IPV starts even prior to the child's birth with several poor health outcomes related to abuse during pregnancy such as preterm labor and low birth weight. IPV may also result in physical injuries to the child, whether from a direct hit when being held by the parent or in older children when trying to intervene in the fight (12). Thus, identifying IPV in the clinical setting has a role in both preventing child maltreatment and better detection of high-risk families where abuse may be occurring. The American Academy of Pediatrics recognized the unique role of the pediatrician in identifying and addressing IPV and how this identification may be one of the most effective means of preventing child maltreatment (13). When IPV is recognized, the health care provider should be able to address the various health needs and refer to appropriate services for assessment and intervention.

PHYSICAL EXAMINATION

Children who are suspected of being physically abused or neglected need a complete thorough physical examination. The medical provider needs to be attentive to the general hygiene of the child, the bonding between the child and the parent, and the appropriateness of the clothing to the season during the examination.

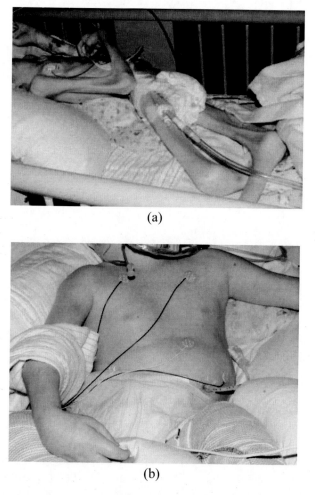

Figures 1a, 1b. Sixteen-year-old with cerebral palsy who presented with failure to thrive.

The medical provider also needs to measure and plot the growth parameters (height, weight, and head circumference) to assess for proper growth and detect any concerns of failure to thrive (lack of appropriate growth and weight gain) whether due to neglect, an underlying medical condition or food insecurity (14). Children with certain medical conditions are also at risk for being overweight as a result of excessive food intake relative to the expenditure of energy (lower metabolic rates and lack of ambulation and exercise). Neglect needs to be considered in cases of obesity when it results in increased risk of harm and medical complications and there is noncompliance with the medical weight management plan (15). Although the measurement may be difficult especially if the child is unable to stand, has contractures, or scoliosis, these measurements need to be accurate and done regularly and plotted over time.

Case 1

16-year-old child with a medical diagnosis of cerebral palsy presented with severe failure to thrive and weight loss (1a). On admission to the hospital, he weighed 9 kg (the average weight of a 9 month old infant). He was not receiving the full amount of the nutritional supplement prescribed by his pediatrician resulting in weight loss. Other elements of neglect were assessed and he had not attended school or followed up with physical therapy resulting in severe contractures. After 6 months of appropriate nutrition and corrective surgeries, he doubled his weight and the contractures had improved dramatically (1b).

Growth in children is influenced by several factors including nutrient intake, environmental circumstances, and genetics. In children with special health care needs, additional factors may impact growth such as congenital abnormalities, the medical condition, medications, and the degree of developmental disability. There are conditions that alter the growth of the child for example chromosomal disorders (e.g., trisomy 21) and genetic disorders. In addition, some conditions have the potential to alter growth such as conditions with feeding problems and those that impair ambulation.

Any problem with feeding that results in insufficient nutrient intake may affect the child's growth. Children with disabilities may have structural abnormalities of the oral area, oral-motor dysfunction, swallowing difficulties, or gastroesophageal reflux. They may also have feeding problems as a result of emotional or behavioral issues. Other than feeding difficulties, children who are non-ambulatory as a result of their medical condition lack the weight bearing which provides physical stress on the long bones of the leg required to stimulate bone growth.

Depending on the medical cause of the developmental disability, the child may need to be plotted on a special growth chart such as for children with trisomy 21, Prader-Willi syndrome, Williams syndrome, Turner syndrome, and Achondroplasia. For example, children with trisomy 21 (also called Down syndrome) have a different pattern of growth and generally have a shorter stature and a smaller head circumference. Thus, these children need to be plotted on an alternate growth chart for this patient population (16). It is not recommended to use these charts however for those children with neurologic disorders without known underlying genetic or medical conditions.

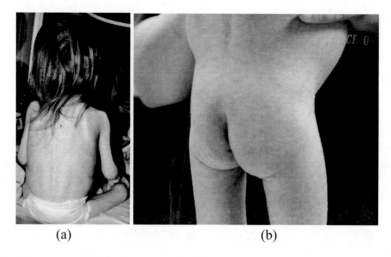

Figures 2a, 2b. Three-year-old girl who presented with failure to thrive. Notice the thin extremities, the protruding ribs, and the loss of subcutaneous fat in the buttocks.

Case 2

A 3-year-old child presents to the emergency department after her sister died from complications of pneumonia and failure to thrive. She had lost weight and upon reviewing her records weighed less at 3 years of age than she did when she was 9 months old. She was noted to be weak and unable to walk which resolved with optimal nutrition. An extensive medical workup was done and no medical cause was found to explain the failure to thrive other than neglect. She had missed follow up appointments with her pediatrician.

CUTANEOUS INJURIES

A thorough skin exam is required when evaluating children for suspected child maltreatment. It is also necessary when examining children for other health care needs as well. The skin needs to be examined from head to toe and bruises, and injuries found need to be documented. The child needs to be undressed when evaluated and areas that may be overlooked need to be examined for example the ears and inside the oral cavity. The genitals, and anus should also be examined (8).

Case 3

The scar on her forehead would have been easily missed with her hair style and without conducting a full medical exam and looking under her hair. Figure 3a shows the child with her hair covering her forehead. Figure 3b shows the child exposing the forehead to show the burn.

The presence and location of bruises are linked to the developmental stage and ability of the child. As children become more mobile, they bruise more often as the number of accidental injuries increases with ambulation. However, these bruises are typically on bony prominences. In Sugar's study, those "who do not cruise rarely bruise" (17), and any bruise in a nonambulatory child needs a full evaluation as to the etiology and whether there is an explainable mechanism of injury consistent with the development of the child (see Figures 4 and 5). Physicians need to be more aware of sentinel injuries when present. The presence of a bruise or an intra-oral injury in a nonmobile infant without a history even when minor needs to prompt an evaluation for physical abuse. Even when the remainder of the evaluation is negative, one should still report these injuries to the appropriate authorities to prevent future more severe abuse in the infant.

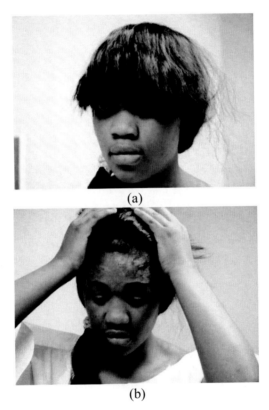

Figures 3a, 3b: A child who has a history of an old burn on her forehead.

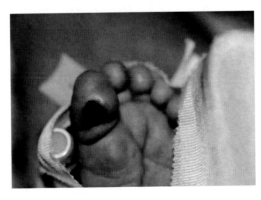

Figure 4. Two-month-old who presented with an abrasion on his big toe with an inconsistent history.

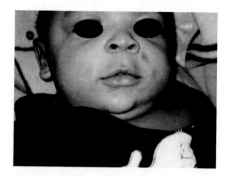

Figure 5. Infant with sentinel injury.

Case 4

This 2-month old baby who was born prematurely and has a history of developmental delay presented with an abrasion to his big toe with a history of the infant self-inflicting the abrasion by friction resulting from trying to move his foot on a carpeted floor he was placed on. The infant developmentally was barely able to move his extremities let alone move his foot with enough force to create a carpet friction burn on his toe. This injury was not consistent with the history provided because it is an injury in a pre-mobile infant which is inconsistent with his developmental age. This injury despite being small and heals with little medical treatment should alert professionals to perform a full medical assessment looking for other signs of physical abuse and identifying this family as a high risk family which needs further assessment and follow up.

Case 5

Infants may present with sentinel injuries such as this bruise on the face of a 3-month old infant. These injuries need to prompt an evaluation to prevent further abuse. In this infant, a skeletal survey was performed and showed multiple rib fractures.

Bruises as a result of abuse have certain discriminating factors that distinguish them from accidental bruises (18, 19). The mnemonic 'TEN 4' is an easy way to identify bruises that are of concern for abuse: T-torso; E-ear; N-neck; and 4-in children less than 4 years of age and any bruise in an infant under 4 months of age (see Figures 6a and 6b). There are also certain patterns of injuries that may identify the inflicting agent for example loop marks from extension cords, ropes or strings and small double bruises from pinch marks.

Case 6

This 1-year-old child presented with multiple bruises with no history of how the injury happened. Multiple concerns in this child included the age of the child (less than 4), the location of the bruises (torso, ear, and neck) and the absence of a history to explain the in injury.

Physical abuse and neglect in children with disabilities 283

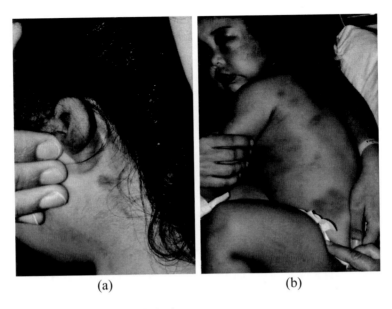

Figures 6a, 6b. One-year-old with multiple bruises.

Burn injuries make up about 10% of all child abuse cases, and about 10% of hospital admissions of children to burn units are the result of child abuse. It is crucial to identify abusive burns to protect the child from further injury as well as other children in the home. Children with abusive burns may also have other associated abusive injuries, have a higher mortality, and have longer hospitalizations as compared to those children with accidental burns.

Children presenting with burns require a thorough and complete medical evaluation (see Figure 7). The evaluation includes a history from the child if the child is verbal as well as a history from the parent and any other witnesses who were present when the burn occurred (20). Specific questions in cases of burns include:

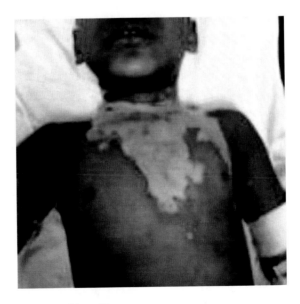

Figure 7. Two-year-old with an accidental burn.

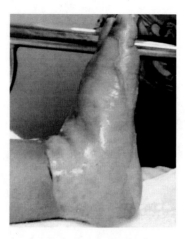

Figure 8. Two-year-old boy with an immersion burn to his left foot.

1. What was the child wearing when the burn occurred?
2. How long was the child in contact with the hot water or the hot object?
3. Does the child have any medical condition that impairs consciousness or the child's ability to move or sense pain or?
4. What are the child's developmental capabilities and motor skills?

Case 7

This 2-year-old child who presented with a burn after running in the kitchen and bumping into his mother who was holding a pot of hot water. The burn is consistent with the mechanism; however parental education was conducted regarding safety and supervision. The case was not reported to child protective services as no further concerns of abuse were present.

As with other injuries resulting from physical abuse, abusive burns are more frequent in younger children. Most are less than 10 years of age with the majority younger than 2 years of age. They are also associated with certain developmental stages. For example, abusive immersion burns are more commonly associated with toilet training as a form of punishment and immersion in hot pots is associated with children playing near a stove. Abusive burns may result from hot liquid, grease, chemicals, hot objects, microwave ovens, or electricity. Concerning characteristics of burns include children who reported inflicted injury, absent or inadequate explanation, hot water as agent, immersion scald, a bilateral/symmetric burn pattern, total body surface area >/=10%, full thickness burns, and co-existent injuries (21).

Scald burns are the most common type of abusive burns in childhood with immersion being the most frequent reported mechanism. Immersion scald burns are characterized by the presence of well-demarcated areas and the absence of splash or flow marks (see Figure 8). The depth and the pattern of immersion burns reflect the position that the child was held in, with "glove" and "stocking" distributions occurring when the burns are circumferential and involve the hands and/or feet respectively. After completing the medical history, the medical physician should perform a thorough head to toe examination documenting the burns and looking for any other associated injuries.

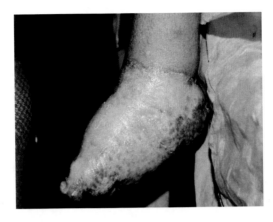

Figure 9. Six-year-old with meningomyelocele who presented with a burn to her right foot.

Case 8

2-year-old boy was left with the mother's boyfriend during the time the mother was at work. When the mother of the child came back home, she noticed the child to be in extreme pain and was crying. She then noticed the burns and was not provided with any history of how the burns occurred. The child was not able to provide a history of how the burn occurred. This burn is concerning not only because of the absence of a history but also because of the clear line of demarcation separating the burned skin from the normal skin and is consistent with an immersion burn.

Developmental disability and paralysis may contribute to the extent of the injury. For example, a child with paralysis in the lower extremities may not withdraw from the pain of hot water. Thus may have more significant burns and may also have an absence of splash marks. Children may not feel the pain or express it as other children may with no disabilities (see Figure 9). However, these children would need closer supervision and more attention when bathing especially with burns being preventable.

Case 9

6-year-old child with a medical history of meningomyelocele and paralysis and absent sensation in both her lower extremities presents with a burn to her right foot. Her father was helping her bathe. He seated her in her bathtub seat and had heated up the water in a bucket then placed her foot in the bucket not realizing how hot the water was. The child did not withdraw from pain due to her paralysis and she did not perceive pain. The burn appears to be an immersion burn and has the characteristics of an immersion burn with the clear line of demarcation. In this case the child was not able to provide a history due to her developmental delay making the diagnosis rather difficult considering her medical condition. However, neglect is a serious consideration in this case as the father should have been more careful when warming the water and placing her foot in the bucket of water to wash it. This case was reported to child protective services with concerns of neglect resulting in serious injury. Abuse could not be ruled out in this case.

SKELETAL INJURIES, FRACTURES, AND IMAGING

As with other injuries, child abuse is suspected when a child presents with a fracture with no underlying bone fragility and no mechanism to explain the fracture especially in non-ambulatory children (19). Physical abuse is also suspected when the child presents with multiple fractures, or with fractures that have a high specificity for child abuse such as fractures of the ribs, scapulae, classic metaphyseal lesions of the long bones, vertebrae, and sternum. The most important risk factor for skeletal injuries is age, with younger children and infants at a higher risk for abusive fractures as compared to older children. The radiologist plays a critical role in the evaluation and diagnosis of fractures (22).

Imaging in cases of suspected physical abuse is used to identify injuries present, including those that may be clinically silent and to demonstrate other radiological evidence of an associated or an alternative diagnosis as to the causation of injury (22). The American College of Radiology currently recommends a 21 dedicated view skeletal survey in children when physical abuse is suspected in children less than 2 years of age. A follow up skeletal survey is also indicated in 2 weeks when the abuse is suspected clinically or the initial findings are equivocal or abnormal. Abusive head trauma is the leading cause of death from physical abuse and results in significant mortality and morbidity. Professionals caring for children need to consider the diagnosis of abusive head trauma in children who present with nonspecific symptoms such as vomiting, lethargy, apnea or seizures so that cases are not missed (23). Head imaging (CT or MRI) would be indicated in these cases as well as a funduscopic exam for detection of retinal hemorrhages.

FURTHER INVESTIGATIONS

After comprehensive history and detailed physical examination, certain investigations are needed to further evaluate for the presence of injuries in children suspected of being victims of physical abuse. Some injuries may be subtle and may not be detected on physical examination, necessitating further work up to identify the injuries and assist in reaching a diagnosis of abuse or another medical condition that explains the presentation. The investigations depend on the initial injury, its severity, and the age of the child. These investigations include laboratory tests: a complete blood count and liver function tests. Imaging is indicated in certain cases includes imaging of the head and a skeletal survey. An ophthalmologic examination in cases of head trauma is needed. It is best to consult a child abuse pediatrician and a trauma specialist when evaluating these injuries to ensure a full evaluation is conducted and injuries are managed appropriately.

CONCLUSION

Child maltreatment in general including physical abuse and neglect is more common in children with disabilities as compared to those with no disabilities. However, evaluation is more difficult in non-verbal children due to the absence of a history of how the injury occurred. In addition, children with paralysis or loss of sensation, development disabilities may react differently to pain from physical injuries and hot liquids or objects. The evaluation requires a multidisciplinary approach including a scene investigation in certain cases of suspected abuse. The evaluation also requires a comprehensive assessment of the child's needs and the family's risk factors to prevent abuse and neglect prior to its occurrence. Professionals should also be aware of certain injuries and subtle warning signs of abuse and initiate a medical evaluation when necessary. The medical provider needs to initiate an evaluation for siblings, especially for those less than 2 years of age and twins, which are at higher risk. Medical care providers are also mandated reporters and are obligated by law to report cases of suspected child maltreatment.

REFERENCES

[1] US Department of Health and Human Services, Administration for Children and Families, Administration on Children, Youth and Families, Children's Bureau. Child maltreatment 2014. Washington, DC: Author, 2016. URL: http://www.acf.hhs.gov/sites/default/files/cb/cm2014.pdf.

[2] Hibbard RA, Desch LW, American Academy of Pediatrics Committee on Child Abuse and Neglect, American Academy of Pediatrics Council on Children with Disabilities. Maltreatment of children with disabilities. Pediatrics 2007;119(5):1018-25.

[3] Ferrari AM. The impact of culture upon child rearing practices and definitions of maltreatment. Child Abuse Negl 2002;26(8):793-813.

[4] Felitti VJ, Anda RF, Nordenberg D, Williamson DF, Spitz AM, Edwards V, et al. Relationship of childhood abuse and household dysfunction to many of the leading causes of death in adults. The Adverse Childhood Experiences (ACE) Study. Am J Prev Med 1998;14(4): 245-58.

[5] Dubowitz H, Newton RR, Litrownik AJ, Lewis T, Briggs EC, Thompson R, et al. Examination of a conceptual model of child neglect. Child Maltreat 2005;10(2):173-89.

[6] American Academy of Pediatrics Committee on Child Abuse and Neglect and Committee on Children With Disabilities. Assessment of maltreatment of children with disabilities. Pediatrics 2001;108(2):508-12.

[7] American Academy of Pediatrics Committee on Psychosocial Aspects of Child and Family Health. Guidance for effective discipline. Pediatrics 1998;101(4 Pt 1):723-8.

[8] Glick JC, Lorand MA, and Bilka KR. Physical abuse of children. Pediatr Rev 2016;37(4):146-56;quiz 157.

[9] Dubowitz H. Neglect in children. Pediatr Ann 2013;42(4):73-7.

[10] Pierce MC, Kaczor K, and Thompson R. Bringing back the social history. Pediatr Clin North Am 2014;61(5): 889-905.

[11] American Academy of Pediatrics Committee on Child Abuse and Neglect. The role of the pediatrician in recognizing and intervening on behalf of abused women. Pediatrics 1998;101(6):1091-2.

[12] Christian CW, Scribano P, Seidl T, Pinto-Martin JA. Pediatric injury resulting from family violence. Pediatrics 1997;99(2):e8.

[13] Thackeray JD, Hibbard R, Dowd MD, Committee on Child Abuse and Neglect, Committee on Injury, Violence and Poison Prevention. Intimate partner violence: The role of the pediatrician. Pediatrics 2010; 125(5):1094-100.

[14] Homan GJ. Failure to thrive: A practical guide. Am Fam Physician 2016;94(4):295-9.

[15] Harper NS. Neglect: failure to thrive and obesity. Pediatr Clin North Am 2014;61(5):937-57.

[16] Cronk C, Crocker AC, Pueschel SM, Shea AM, Zackai E, Pickens G, et al. Growth charts for children with Down syndrome: 1 month to 18 years of age. Pediatrics 1988;81(1):102-10.

[17] Sugar NF, Taylor JA, and Feldman KW. Bruises in infants and toddlers: Those who don't cruise rarely bruise. Puget Sound Pediatric Research Network. Arch Pediatr Adolesc Med 1999;153(4):399-403.

[18] Pierce MC, Kaczor K, Aldridge S, O'Flynn J, Lorenz DJ. Bruising characteristics discriminating physical child abuse from accidental trauma. Pediatrics 2010;125(1):67-74.

[19] Christian CW, American Academy of Pediatrics Committee on Child Abuse and Neglect. The evaluation of suspected child physical abuse. Pediatrics 2015; 135(5):e1337-54.

[20] Toon MH, Maybauer DM, Arceneaux LL, Fraser JF, Meyer W, Runge A, et al. Children with burn injuries--assessment of trauma, neglect, violence and abuse. J Inj Violence Res 2011;3(2):98-110.

[21] Pawlik MC, Kemp A, Maguire, S, Nuttall D, Feldman KW, Lindberg, DM, et al. Children with burns referred for child abuse evaluation: Burn characteristics and co-existent injuries. Child Abuse Negl 2016;55:52-61.

[22] American Academy of Pediatrics Section on Radiology. Diagnostic imaging of child abuse. Pediatrics 2009; 123(5):1430-5.

[23] Jenny C, Hymel KP, Ritzen A, Reinert SE, Hay TC. Analysis of missed cases of abusive head trauma. JAMA 1999;281(7):621–6.

Submitted: August 03, 2016. *Revised:* August 15, 2016. *Accepted:* August 31, 2016.

In: Alternative Medicine Research Yearbook 2017
Editor: Joav Merrick

ISBN: 978-1-53613-726-2
© 2018 Nova Science Publishers, Inc.

Chapter 32

MEDICAL EVALUATION AND MANAGEMENT OF SEXUAL ABUSE IN CHILDREN WITH DISABILITIES

Dena Nazer[*], *MD*

Wayne State University School of Medicine, Children's Hospital of Michigan, Kids TALK Children's Advocacy Center, Detroit, Michigan, US

ABSTRACT

Child sexual abuse is a public health problem with grave consequences affecting the child and the community. Children are vulnerable merely because of their age; furthermore, the presence of disability increases their vulnerability making children with disabilities at a greater risk for abuse as compared to children with no disabilities. This article will focus on child sexual abuse and its medical evaluation and management in children with disabilities.

Keywords: children, disability, sexual abuse, evaluation, public health

INTRODUCTION

When discussing the issues surrounding children with disabilities and their risk for child abuse, the absence of a universally accepted definition of disabilities adds to the complexity of accurately assessing the problem. Disability has variable definitions making it hard to identify its true incidence and characteristics in maltreated children. The Centers for Disease Controls and Prevention (CDC) describes developmental disabilities as a group of conditions due to an impairment in physical, language, learning, or behavior areas which begins during the developmental period, usually lasts throughout the person's life time and may impact the daily life.

---

[*] Correspondence: Dena Nazer, MD, Kids TALK Children's Advocacy Center Medical Clinic, 40 East Ferry St, Detroit, Michigan, 48202, United States. E-mail: dnazer@med.wayne.edu.

Intellectual disability, according to the American Association on Intellectual and Developmental Disabilities AAIDD), is a disability characterized by three essential elements: limitations in intellectual functioning (such as learning and reasoning), limitations in adaptive behavior, which covers many everyday social and practical skills, and an onset originating before the age of 18 years. The term intellectual disability has replaced the previously used "mental retardation" term.

In the United States, about one in six, or about 15%, of children aged 3 through 17 years have a one or more developmental disability. Intellectual disability affects about one percent of the population, and of those about 85 percent have mild intellectual disability. Diagnosis and identification of these children is essential as they are more vulnerable and subsequently at higher risk to be victims of abuse and neglect. Not only do medical providers need to be aware of the increased risk of maltreatment in this patient population but they also need to evaluate any child who is maltreated for the presence of developmental disabilities (1).

Child maltreatment includes all forms of physical and emotional ill-treatment, sexual abuse, neglect, and exploitation that results in actual or potential harm to the child's health, development or dignity. Within this broad definition, five subtypes can be distinguished– physical abuse; sexual abuse; neglect and negligent treatment; emotional abuse; and exploitation.

Sexual abuse occurs when a child is engaged in sexual activities that he or she cannot comprehend, for which he or she is developmentally unprepared and cannot give consent, and/or that violate the law or social taboos of society (2). The sexual activities may include all forms of oral, genital, or anal contact by or to the child or abuse that does not involve contact, such as exhibitionism, voyeurism, or using the child in the production of pornography. Thus the spectrum of sexual abuse includes activities ranging from physically less intrusive sexual abuse to rape.

Risk factors for sexual abuse in general include gender with girls reporting more sexual abuse than boys. Age is also a factor with teenagers having the highest rates of sexual assault as compared to other age groups. Other potential risk factors include absence of protective parent, prior sexual victimization, and physical disability.

There are many factors that increase the risk of sexual abuse in a child with disability in addition to the condition itself. Children with disabilities may be viewed as unable to comprehend sexual education thus they miss out on learning opportunities at schools and from parents on how to protect themselves from sexual abuse.

There is a lack of awareness from parents and society that children with disabilities are potential victims of sexual abuse at even higher rates than other children, and they are less diligent with safety measures around these children. Depending on the severity of the disability, these children may become increasingly isolated from the general community and more dependent on the caregiver to provide assistance in daily activities that may include intimate care. This makes the child accustomed to certain activities and less likely to differentiate intrusive behaviors from those of routine daily care. As the child becomes more dependent on the caregiver, the child becomes more compliant with adults who assume an authoritative role in the child's life and becomes less likely to resist and less likely to report sexual abuse. Even when children try to communicate and disclose, their disability may prevent them communicating or describing effectively with a clear credible statement the sequence of events and care givers may explain what happened as part of the child's routine.

PRESENTATION OF CHILD SEXUAL ABUSE

Children who are victims of sexual abuse present in a multitude of ways depending on their age, developmental level, and the nature of the sexual abuse. They may present after making a disclosure of sexual abuse to a parent, teacher, social worker or another trusted individual. These disclosures and the circumstances and questions that lead to the disclosures need to be documented. Children may also present with physical or behavioral symptoms which necessitate further evaluation for sexual abuse.

Physical signs and symptoms include nonspecific complaints such as abdominal pain, headaches, and fatigue. Children may also complain of genital pain, itching, discharge or other genitourinary symptoms related to the sexual abuse.

Behavioral changes include aggression, withdrawal, problems in school, regression (e.g., return to thumb sucking), sleep disturbances, fear of people or certain locations, depression and eating disturbances. The problem with these behaviors is that although they may indicate sexual abuse, they are nonspecific and may be a result of the child acting out to other stressors. In addition, the behavior may be attributed to the child's disability or underlying condition.

SEXUAL BEHAVIORS

Most children engage in sexual behaviors at a certain time in their childhood that is mostly age appropriate, transient and only requires guidance and monitoring. Some children however may exhibit sexual behavior which may initiate a sexual abuse evaluation or be both concerning to caregivers and distressing at school.

A broad range of sexual behaviors are exhibited by both children who have a history of sexual abuse and those where there is no concern of sexual abuse. This behavior is related to the child's age, maternal education, family sexuality, family stress, and family violence (3, 4). These behaviors are exhibited at a varying level of frequency with the most frequent including self-stimulating behaviors, exhibitionism, and behaviors related to personal boundaries. Self-stimulating behaviors include the child masturbating, or touching or rubbing different parts of the body to induce pleasure. Examples for behavior related to personal boundaries may include children standing too close, rubbing against people, or casually touching their mother's breasts or father's genitals. This behavior is mostly seen in the younger children who are still learning the culturally acceptable interpersonal distance between people. The less frequent behaviors are the more intrusive behaviors. This may pose a challenge for children with disabilities as they may not fully comprehend personal boundaries or understand what is hurtful for others and not accepted socially.

Children with disabilities may exhibit behaviors that correspond to their development vs. their chronological age. When assessing these behaviors, one should consider the developmental age vs. the chronological age. For example, a 16-year-old boy who functions at a developmental level of a 2-year-old may display sexualized behavior that is considered normal for a 2-year-old but not a developmentally normal 16-year-old.

Sexual behavior appeared to be inversely related to age with a peak frequency at age 5 for both boys and girls followed by a decrease in frequency over the next 7 years. Sexually abused children exhibit sexual behavior at a greater rate when compared to children who were not abused (5). However there is not a single sexual behavior that is indicative of sexual abuse.

EVALUATION OF CHILD SEXUAL ABUSE

The evaluation all children who are suspected of being sexually abused requires a multidisciplinary team approach, and this requirement is no different in children with disabilities. Each team member has a unique perspective and an area of expertise that is essential in the full comprehensive evaluation of children. Depending on the community, a child advocacy center or a sexual abuse response team may take the lead in addressing and evaluating the child's special needs in these cases. These teams include law enforcement, a child protective services worker, a medical provider, a forensic interviewer and other personnel for example a child advocate depending on the community where the child is being evaluated.

All victims of sexual abuse should be offered a medical examination by a medical professional trained in sexual abuse evaluations. The medical exam is necessary and helpful for all survivors of violence, regardless of the level of abuse disclosed. The role of the physician also includes the assessment of the physical, emotional, and behavioral consequences of sexual abuse, and coordination with other professionals to provide comprehensive treatment and follow-up of victims (6). In the US, the physician is also mandated to report cases of child maltreatment including cases of suspected sexual abuse to the appropriate authorities. The medical evaluation includes as in the assessment of other conditions obtaining a medical history, conducting a physical examination, collecting appropriate laboratory data, and in some cases forensic evidence depending on the nature of disclosure and the time since the last incidence of suspected sexual abuse.

The timing of the medical evaluation requires consideration of multiple factors including the medical, therapeutic and evidentiary purpose of such an evaluation (7). It also requires the consideration of where the best location for the assessment is as well as who is the most qualified provider who is able to evaluate children who are suspected of being sexually abused and is experienced in evaluating children with disabilities.

There are cases when the medical examination may be an emergency and needs to be performed without delay, or the need may be less urgent. These are cases where emergency contraception or post exposure prophylaxis for sexually transmitted infections (STIs) including human immunodeficiency virus (HIV) is needed. It is also emergent when there are medical, psychological, or safety concerns such as acute pain or bleeding, suicidal ideation, or suspected human trafficking. The need for forensic evidence collection may require the medical evaluation to be done emergently if the sexual assault may have occurred within the previous 72 hours (or other state-mandated time interval). This collection needs to consider the timing of when the sexual abuse took place and not depend on the presence of physical findings. The medical provider needs to become familiar with the laws as some jurisdictions have expanded the time frame of when the evidence collection is recommended (7).

A medical evaluation is urgent but not emergent in cases where the suspected sexual abuse occurred within the previous two weeks, without immediate medical, psychological, or safety needs identified. In cases where the suspected sexual abuse occurred more than two weeks prior without urgent medical, psychological, or safety needs and in cases where sexual abuse is suspected because of other symptoms, the medical examination is non-urgent (8).

MEDICAL HISTORY

The medical history is a key component of the evaluation of sexually abused children and is in many cases the strongest evidence of abuse (9). The medical history focuses on the health and well-being of the child and complements the forensic interview and other interviews conducted by other professionals. It serves the purposes of collecting information relevant to the health of the child and also serves to help address the effects the abuse has on the family and the child's perceptions of the problem.

To effectively obtain a history, the medical provider must be familiar with communicating with children and those with developmental delay and impaired communication skills and seek the help of an interpreter when needed. Children of different ages interact and express themselves differently and that needs to be taken into account when obtaining the medical history. The medical provider also needs to be compassionate, objective, and nonjudgmental. The disclosure needs to be preserved and documented along with the circumstances of how and why the child disclosed.

It is best to obtain the history with the child alone without the parent or caretaker. This would make the child more comfortable to talk and would decrease the influence the caretaker may have on what the child says and the caretaker's reaction to the disclosure. Questions need to be mostly open ended and non-leading so that a detailed accurate history may be obtained and documented.

Medical information and details also need to be obtained from the caregiver. The medical provider needs to ask about the details of the disclosure and circumstances around it. These details may assist in the differential diagnosis of the presenting symptoms. Elements of the medical history also include asking about the past medical and surgical history, medications the child is taking, developmental history, and social history. Further information about the genitourinary and gastrointestinal history may also help in assessing children for other conditions that may mimic the presenting symptoms of abuse. The medical provider needs to ask about urinary symptoms, change in bowel habits, and genital bleeding or discharge.

One aspect when obtaining the history that the provider needs to be aware of is the age of consent in the jurisdiction, which is the age a person is considered to be competent to consent to sexual acts under the law. Children may provide a history that they consented for the sexual activity and that there was no coercion or force used. The medical provider, however, must be aware that the developmental disability may compromise the capacity of a child to consent for sexual activity even if the child has attained the legal age of consent. It is thus important not only to consider the age when evaluating cases of sexual assault but also the developmental abilities of the child and his/her understanding and ability to provide consent.

Table 1. Normal genital anatomy to be examined in cases of suspected sexual abuse

Gender	Examination
Girls	The examination should include inspection and assessment for any signs of injury or trauma of the medial aspects of the thighs, labia majora and minora, clitoris, urethra, periurethral tissue, hymen, hymenal opening, fossa navicularis, posterior fourchette, perineum, and perianal tissues.
Boys	The exam should include inspection and assessment for any signs of injury or trauma. of the thighs, penis, scrotum, perineum, and perianal tissues

PHYSICAL EXAMINATION

Children who disclose sexual abuse or are suspected of being sexually abused require a complete comprehensive head-to-toe medical examination including an examination of the anogenital area. The physical examination findings or laboratory testing are rarely sufficient in making the diagnosis and it is the disclosure and history from the child that is of immense importance. However, the physical examination has several objectives making it a crucial part of the evaluation despite the low rate of positive findings (6, 10). The objectives include:

- Recognition of injuries and other medical needs that require immediate medical attention
- Comprehensive anogenital examination (see Table 1) and identification of abnormalities and interpreting findings or normal exams appropriately
- Identification of injuries outside of the anogenital region whether as a result of abuse or self-inflicted
- Detection and testing for sexually transmitted infections (see Table 2)
- Collection of forensic evidence
- Addressing patient and family concerns about physical health that may arise subsequent to abuse

The medical evaluation in this high risk population is also important because it may identify other health care needs that need evaluation and medical care such as decreased visual acuity and dental caries (11). These medical needs may be higher in children with disabilities who may lack a medical home and have concurrent concerns of neglect.

The health care provider performing the examination must effectively communicate and explain the nature and the purpose of the examination to the child and to the parent or guardian as well. The child may choose for the parent to be present during the exam to relief anxiety and give a sense of security. The time of the examination is also a good opportunity to educate the child on body safety and why it is acceptable for the examiner to examine the anogenital area. Every effort should be made to preserve privacy including the use of drapes and gowns. As these examinations involve the evaluation of the anogenital area, the presence of a chaperone is recommended, and medical policy needs to be established and communicated to the family (12).

Parents and in some cases children may be highly anxious prior to the exam, and explaining that the medical evaluation is noninvasive and not painful may alleviate that stress. In addition, the health care provider needs to explain to the parents that the most important evidence in these cases is the child's disclosure of abuse and that physical findings are absent in most cases. It is also the role of the medical provider to further explain to the family and members of the multidisciplinary team why the examination is normal in most cases.

There have been a number of research studies that concluded that most child victims of sexual abuse and even those who disclose repetitive penile-genital contact that involved some degree of perceived penetration had no definitive evidence of penetration on examination of the hymen (13-15). Even when exams of pregnant teenagers were reviewed, most did not have observable evidence of penetration on examination of the genital area (16).

Table 2. Testing for sexually transmitted infections and their implications in children evaluated for sexual abuse

STI	Testing	Implication
Chlamydia trachomatis*	Girls: Anal and vaginal cultures. NAATs can be used for detection in vaginal specimens or urine in girls. Boys: Anal cultures and a meatal specimen if urethral discharge is present.	Diagnostic for sexual abuse if not likely to be perinatally acquired and rare vertical transmission is excluded.
Neisseria gonorrhea*	Girls: Pharyngeal, vaginal and anal cultures. NAAT can be used for detection in vaginal specimens or urine from girls; however, culture remains the preferred method for testing urethral specimens or urine from boys and extragenital specimens (pharynx and rectum) from all children. Boys: Phayngeal, urethral, and anal cultures	Diagnostic for sexual abuse if not likely to be perinatally acquired and rare vertical transmission is excluded.
Trichomonas vaginalis*	Culture for *T. vaginalis* infection and wet mount of a vaginal swab	Highly suspicious for sexual abuse if not likely to be perinatally acquired and rare vertical transmission is excluded.
Human papillomavirus	Diagnosis is usually clinical, made by visual inspection. Biopsy is indicated only in specific cases	Suspicious and needs to be reported if evidence exists to suspect abuse, including history, physical examination, or other identified infections.
Syphilis	Serology for antibodies to *T. pallidum*	Diagnostic for sexual abuse if not likely to be perinatally acquired and rare vertical transmission is excluded.
HIV	When indicated, HIV antibody testing needs to be done during the original assessment, at 6 weeks, 3 months, and 6 months after the assault.	Diagnostic for sexual abuse if not likely to be perinatally acquired and rare vertical transmission is excluded.

NAAT: Nucleic acid amplification tests.
* Reports of suspected sexual abuse need to be made in these cases to the appropriate authority.

There are many reasons why the physical examination may not show any signs of trauma and these reasons should be taken into context when the medical provider explains the diagnosis in the medical report. Depending on the child's statement, the child may have disclosed forms of sexual abuse, such as being photographed or watching pornography, that do not involve contact and are not expected to leave any findings on physical examination. The sexual abuse may have involved only touching or fondling and would not result in injury or exam findings. In children who disclose penetration, the medical provider should note that penetration perceived by the child may only be penetration in-between the labia and not into the vagina, which is not expected to cause any medical findings.

In addition, most children do not disclose immediately and the disclosure may be delayed for days, weeks or even months after the sexual abuse took place. This period of time depending on the severity of the initial injury and location would have given enough time for the genital injuries to heal completely. Some genital injuries have been shown to heal as quick as a few days (17, 18). The hymenal and anal tissues also have the ability to stretch without injury, which is also a factor when explaining the absence of findings in children who disclosed penetration. Both the hymen and the anus may stretch without being injured. It is the medical provider's role to explain these reasons to the family and also to other members of the multidisciplinary team who may share misconceptions about the nature of the exam and expected medical findings.

One of the important roles of the medical evaluation is testing for STIs. However, each case should be evaluated individually for the need for testing and the rate of the STIs in the community where the child resides should be considered (19). Factors that should lead to testing children for STIs include the child being abused by a stranger or by a perpetrator known to be infected or at high risk for STIs. In addition, if the child has symptoms or signs of a STI such as genital discharge, or has experienced penetration or had evidence of healed penetrative injury to the genitals, anus, or oropharynx, the child should be tested. The physician also needs to test if a sibling, or relative of person in the house hold has an STI and in cases where the parent or the child is concerned and requests the testing (6, 19, 20). For the commonly tested STIs, please refer to Table 2.

In most cases, only one medical examination of the anogenital areas by an experienced medical provider is needed and documented. However, follow-up medical evaluation may be indicated in certain cases, especially when the findings on the initial examination are unclear or questionable or when there is a need for further STI testing that was not identified or treated during the initial examination. Follow up may also assist in confirmation of the initial examination findings, when initial examination was performed by an examiner who had conducted fewer than 100 of such evaluations, and for documentation of healing or resolution of acute findings present on the initial examination (8).

COMMERCIAL SEXUAL EXPLOITATION OF CHILDREN WITH DISABILITIES

Similar to sexual abuse, child commercial sexual exploitation (CSEC) and sex trafficking are global health problems requiring a multidisciplinary approach (21). Children in general are vulnerable to sexual exploitation; however, those with learning disabilities or a history of sexual abuse, physical abuse, or neglect are at a higher risk. In addition, other factors such as runaway youths and those with substance abuse problems, history of juvenile justice or child protective services involvement and those from dysfunctional families increase the risk for exploitation.

Although there is currently no validated clinical tool to identify CSEC, there are certain indicators that may help identify victims. When children give a history of someone asking them to have sex in exchange for money or other items such as food or shelter, if they were asked to have sex with someone else of if sexual pictures were taken of them and posted on the internet, sexual exploitation arises as a main concern and should be addressed and reported.

Identifying patients that are at victims of sexual exploitation may be hard though as these victims often do not self-identify as such and depending on the level of their intellectual disability, may lack an understanding of exploitation and its dangers (22). A screening tool has been proposed to better identify these children and differentiate them from other sexual abuse victims in the adolescent population (23). The American Academy of Pediatrics suggests that pediatricians should become more aware of potential victims of human trafficking and gives guidance on how to provide for the medical needs of these victims (21). The medical professional's role is vital since most victims of human trafficking seek medical care at a certain point. In addition, the medical professional can serve as a link to initiate the multidisciplinary collaboration for evaluation these children.

CONCLUSION

Child sexual abuse is a public health problem affecting children with disabilities at higher rates compared to children with no disabilities. The evaluation needs to be completed by a multidisciplinary team specialized in evaluating victims of sexual abuse. The medical evaluation is an integral part of this evaluation. Specifically, the medical evaluation and assessment follows a similar approach with various modifications in the communication and examination techniques to address the child's special needs. Most children who are victims of sexual abuse have a normal exam, making the child's disclosure the strongest evidence that abuse has occurred. The medical provider needs to be trained on the appropriate evaluation, management and interpretation of findings or lack of thereof in children who were sexually abused. The medical provider also needs to be aware of resources in the community that ensure the child's safety and wellbeing and prevents further abuse from taking place. Future efforts need to focus on the training of health care providers and professionals on how to detect, evaluate, and respond to child sexual abuse in general and more specifically for this increasingly vulnerable group.

REFERENCES

[1] American Academy of Pediatrics Committee on Child Abuse and Neglect and Committee on Children with Disabilities. Assessment of maltreatment of children with disabilities. Pediatrics 2001;108(2):508-12.
[2] Kempe CH. Sexual abuse--another hidden pediatric problem: The 1977 C Anderson Aldrich lecture. Pediatrics 1978;62(3):382-9.

[3] Friedrich WN, Fisher J, Broughton D, Houston M, Shafran CR. Normative sexual behavior in children: A contemporary sample. Pediatrics 1998;101(4):e9.
[4] Kellogg ND. Sexual behaviors in children: Evaluation and management. Am Fam Physician 2010;82(10): 1233-8.
[5] Friedrich WN, Fisher JL, Dittner CA, Acton R, Berliner L, Butler J, et al. Child Sexual Behavior Inventory: Normative, psychiatric, and sexual abuse comparisons. Child Maltreat 2001;6(1):37-49.
[6] Kellogg N, American Academy of Pediatrics Committee on Child Abuse and Neglect. The evaluation of sexual abuse in children. Pediatrics 2005;116(2):506-12.
[7] Christian CW. Timing of the medical examination. J Child Sex Abuse 2011;20(5):505-20.
[8] Adams JA, Kellogg ND, Farst KJ, Harper NS, Palusci VJ, Frasier LD, et al. Updated guidelines for the medical assessment and care of children who may have been sexually abused. J Pediatr Adolesc Gynecol 2016; 29(2):81-7.
[9] Finkel MA, Alexander RA. Conducting the medical history. J Child Sex Abuse 2011;20(5):486-504.
[10] Fortin K, Jenny C. Sexual abuse. Pediatr Rev 2012; 33(1):19-32.
[11] Girardet R, Giacobbe L, Bolton K, Lahoti S, McNeese M. Unmet health care needs among children evaluated for sexual assault. Arch Pediatr Adolesc Med 2006; 160(1):70-3.
[12] Committee on Pediatric Ambulatory Medicine. Use of chaperones during the physical examination of the pediatric patient. Pediatrics 2011;127(5):991-3.
[13] Adams JA, Harper K, Knudson S, Revilla J. Examination findings in legally confirmed child sexual abuse: It's normal to be normal. Pediatrics 1994;94(3): 310-7.
[14] Anderst J, Kellogg N, Jung I. Reports of repetitive penile-genital penetration often have no definitive evidence of penetration. Pediatrics 2009;124(3):e403-9.
[15] Berenson AB, Chacko MR, Wiemann CM, Mishaw CO, Friedrich WN, Grady JJ. A case-control study of anatomic changes resulting from sexual abuse. Am J Obstet Gynecol 2000;182(4):820-31; discussion:831-4.
[16] Kellogg ND, Menard SW, Santos A. Genital anatomy in pregnant adolescents: "Normal" does not mean "nothing happened". Pediatrics 2004;113(1 Pt 1):e67-9.
[17] McCann J, Miyamoto S, Boyle C, Rogers K. Healing of nonhymenal genital injuries in prepubertal and adolescent girls: A descriptive study. Pediatrics 2007; 120(5):1000-11.
[18] McCann J, Miyamoto S, Boyle C, Rogers K. Healing of hymenal injuries in prepubertal and adolescent girls: A descriptive study. Pediatrics 2007;119(5):e1094-106.
[19] Jenny C, Crawford-Jakubiak JE, Committee on Child Abuse and Neglect, American Academy of Pediatrics. The evaluation of children in the primary care setting when sexual abuse is suspected. Pediatrics 2013; 132:e558–67.
[20] Workowski KA, Bolan GA, Centers for Disease Control and Prevention (CDC). Sexually transmitted diseases treatment guidelines, 2015. MMWR Recomm Rep 2015;59(RR-03):1–137.
[21] Greenbaum J, Crawford-Jakubiak JE, Committee on Child Abuse and Neglect, American Academy of Pediatrics. Child sex trafficking and commercial sexual exploitation: Health care needs of victims. Pediatrics 2015;135(3):566-74.
[22] Reid JA. Sex trafficking of girls with intellectual disabilities: An exploratory mixed methods study. Sex Abuse 2016. Published online Feb 17, 2016.
[23] Greenbaum VJ, Dodd M, McCracken C. A short screening tool to identify victims of child sex trafficking in the health care setting. Pediatr Emerg Care 2015; 12:856-9.

Submitted: August 06, 2016. *Revised:* August 17, 2016. *Accepted:* September 02, 2016.

In: Alternative Medicine Research Yearbook 2017
Editor: Joav Merrick
ISBN: 978-1-53613-726-2
© 2018 Nova Science Publishers, Inc.

Chapter 33

SEXUAL BEHAVIORS IN CHILDREN WITH DEVELOPMENTAL DISABILITIES

Alyse Mandel, MS, LCSW and Ellen Datner, PsyD*

Bellevue Hospital Frances L Loeb Child Protection and Development Center,
New York City Health and Hospitals, New York, New York, US

ABSTRACT

Humans are sexual beings. Like all aspects of development, sexual development begins in infancy and continues throughout the human lifecycle. Children develop across many domains: emotional, social and physical, and at different rates and developmental stages. The topic of sexual development is often overlooked as an expected area of development. This could be due to societal beliefs and/or parental, cultural or religious differences. The normative progression of sexual development may not apply within a clear framework if a child has a developmental disability or delay. This topic has not been frequently studied historically, but more clinicians and researchers are now looking at how young people with disabilities experience sexual feelings or behaviors, whether at a normative rate, as a result of trauma or abuse, or the possibility of another explanation. Unfortunately, children with intellectual disabilities and developmental delays experience sexual abuse at a higher rate than peers who are not developmentally delayed. These children are especially at risk for abuse due to cognitive, social and emotional deficits. As with typically developing peers, problematic sexual behavior (PSB) can occur in children with developmental delays as a result of sexual abuse, but there may also be other factors at play. In this review, we will first present a brief overview of normative and PSB in youth and then explore some of the reasons PSBs are prevalent in developmentally delayed populations, focusing on children and adolescents diagnosed with higher functioning autism spectrum disorder (ASD) formerly known as Asperger's Disorder (AD). We will also discuss various methods to assess sexual behaviors and treatment options for this population.

Keywords: children, disability, sexuality, sexual behavior

---

[*] Correspondence: Alyse Mandel, MS, LCSW, Bellevue Hospital, Child Protection and Development Center, 462 First Avenue, New York, NY 10016, United States. E-mail: Alyse.Mandel@bellevue.nychhc.org.

INTRODUCTION

Research from several disciplines has contributed to our understanding of sexual identity, attitudes and behaviors. Sexual development is influenced by a variety of factors including biological, social and environmental contexts which can result in a diversity of sexual behaviors at different developmental stages (1). Sexuality is a multifaceted part of human development that evolves in the context of interactions with one's environment (2). "Sexuality is influenced by the interaction of biological, psychological, social, economic, political, cultural, legal, historical, religious and spiritual factors" (3). It can be expressed in numerous ways such as through thoughts or fantasies, attitudes, behaviors, identity, relationships, beliefs and values, for example. However, each individual may not experience or express all these aspects of sexuality (3).

Sexual development falls across all developmental stages from birth through adolescence into adulthood (1). Youth experience different sexual feelings and engage in a variety of sexual behaviors depending on their developmental age. Children and adolescents' understanding of sexuality is influenced by their exposure to sexual material as well as their ability to understand the experience (4). They are influenced by their parents, media, technology and peers. Problems arise when sexual behavior becomes aggressive, persistent and/or falls outside society's norms. The Association for the Treatment of Sexual Abusers' (ATSA) Task Force on Children with Sexual Behavior Problems (5) defined PSB in children 12 years old or younger who initiate these behaviors as "behaviors involving sexual body parts (i.e., genitals, anus, buttock or breasts) that are developmentally inappropriate or potentially harmful to themselves or others" (5). In terms of causation, throughout the literature there appears to be a significant amount of research on the correlation between sexual abuse and sexual behaviors. However, few studies address this association among children with disabilities (6). Sexual behaviors can also result from other experiences and recent literature discusses these possibilities (2, 7, 8).

Despite sexuality being an integral part of child development and public concerns about atypical sexual behaviors and child maltreatment, there is a paucity of research on the complexities of both normative and PSB. Even fewer studies address these behaviors in young populations with intellectual and developmental disabilities. A lack of knowledge regarding childhood sexual behavior can have potential negative consequences for children and their families in the home, school and social environments as well as in health care and child welfare and legal systems. The aim of several current studies is not only to improve our understanding of sexual behaviors in youth but also to contribute to the development of guidelines that can assist professionals in the assessment and treatment of these behaviors (8).

The "Diagnostic and statistical manual of mental disorders, fifth edition (DSM-5)" has made autistic spectrum disorder (ASD) the umbrella term for three previously separate diagnoses: Asperger's disorder (AD), childhood disintegrative disorder and pervasive developmental disorder, not otherwise specified (9). For the purpose of this review, we will use Asperger's disorder as a way to distinguish high functioning from low functioning autism, although the DSM-5 no longer recognizes this label.

NORMATIVE CHILDHOOD SEXUAL BEHAVIOR

In the beginning of the 20th Century, Freud introduced concepts that included sexuality as part of child development (10). At that time, ideas about childhood sexuality were primarily theoretical (11). Increased awareness of sexual abuse in the second half of the century, and more recent awareness of children engaging in sexually aggressive behaviors, have led to attempts to define typical sexual development in youth and sparked an increase in studies on the sexual behaviors of children. However, more research is needed, and a clear understanding of normative child sexual development including children's sexual knowledge, interests, experiences (10) and sexual behaviors is still lacking (8, 12).

Much of the existing research on childhood sexual behaviors is focused on PSB in children who have been sexually abused. Accurately differentiating typical sexual behavior in children from those resulting from maltreatment or other factors is of great importance. Such knowledge could aid in the proper assessment and identification of the presenting behavior (13) and inform developmentally-tailored treatment interventions (5, 13). For example, in cases of childhood sexual abuse (CSA), misdiagnosis of sexual behaviors can lead to negative and harmful outcomes for the child, family and/or accused perpetrator (13).

Different research methods have been used to obtain baseline information regarding typical childhood sexual behaviors (14) and the designs of the available studies appear to impact the measured prevalence rates of these behaviors (8). The majority of studies have gathered information from parents' and teachers' observations of their children's and students' sexual behaviors. Common measures used with caregiver and teacher informants to gather information on child sexual behavior include the sexual behavior items on the Child Behavior Check List (CBCL) (15) and the Child Sexual Behavior Inventory (CSBI) (16). The CSBI has been utilized in several studies on typical and atypical sexual behaviors and allows for comparison of studies (8). Additional studies have utilized adults' retrospective reports about their childhood sexual experiences or data gathered from populations of children seeking treatment for sexual behavior difficulties. Although more research is needed, what has been gathered so far has demonstrated some consistencies about childhood sexual behavior (17-19). For example, young children commonly engage in sexual behaviors such as genital touching, viewing others' genitals, showing their genitals to others, attempting to touch a woman's breasts, masturbation and playing "doctor" (14, 18, 20).

A wide range of sexual behaviors have been observed in typically developing child populations at varying frequencies. However, potential mediators of normative behaviors as well as problem behaviors is less known (21). Children learn about themselves, their bodies and their roles through their environment (2). Young children's curiosity about their body, including their genitalia, and those of others is a developmentally expected occurrence (18, 20). Sexual knowledge and behavior in children is influenced by a variety of factors including, but not limited to, the child's age and developmental level, family environment, exposure to sexual material, culture and societal norms (5, 10, 18). In addition, the expression and interpretation of sexual behaviors in children can also vary across contexts (8). Therefore, defining what is "normal" childhood sexual behavior is an arduous task (4).

In addition to the complexities of defining normative sexual behavior in young children, defining norms for older children is even more complicated as this population is often socialized to hide their sexual activities. As youth mature, they tend to seek privacy and engaging in sexual behaviors in public may be viewed as "taboo." Defining sexual behavior or interactions between children presents difficulties as well. Characteristics such as age, size and status used to determine if an encounter is typical or abusive may be difficult guides to assess child sexual play (10).

Very few studies exist on the impact of culture on childhood sexual behaviors and on behavioral differences between cultures. To address cultural influences, studies have compared rates of sexual behaviors in American and European populations. Consistencies were found in rates of less frequent sexual behaviors while more inconsistencies were discovered with more common sexual behaviors (8). One study (8) looked at American ethnic minority populations. Results showed that African American parents reported decreased solitary sexual behaviors compared to Caucasian parents. More research on diverse populations is greatly needed to further our understanding of the impact of culture on childhood sexual behaviors (8).

Children's knowledge and attitudes about sexuality and sexual behaviors are also influenced by the level of adult support and responses to their behaviors (10) and the beliefs of their families and communities (4). Western society tends to view children as "innocent," asexual beings who do not possess sexual thoughts or interests (10). Many adults and families hesitate to discuss or educate children about sexual development and behavior. In contrast, frequent images and themes of sexual behavior exist in our society. Children are often exposed to sexual images in the media and adults may delay discussing or explaining these images to children. They may also believe that children are not interested in or have the ability to understand mature sexual images (13). One researcher (10) suggested that the diversity of sexual attitudes and beliefs in society, and lack of guidance for parents to address sexuality with their children, leave youth to try to interpret and understand what acceptable sexual behavior is. Others (10) have suggested that the lack of comprehensive sex education programs that include not only responsible sexuality but also positive and pleasurable aspects of sexuality reflects a cultural belief that denies the data showing sexuality being a vital part of child development (10).

Sexual development includes physical changes, information learned about sexuality and demonstrated behaviors (22). Sexual behaviors in children can cause concern for caregivers and professionals due to the association between sexual abuse and sexualized behaviors. However, it has been demonstrated that children of all ages engage in a variety of sexual behaviors. Understanding of normative sexual behavior can help to minimize alarm, to assess the potential source of the behavior and to manage the behavior (17). Given the important decisions, policies and interventions made for many children and families, it is also imperative for professionals, child protective services (CPS) and court systems to be knowledgeable about typical and PSBs in youth and those that may be indicative of maltreatment (5).

Despite increasing knowledge, more research is needed to determine typical sexual behaviors in children. Defining normative sexual behavior is not only important to the understanding of child development but also to the assessment and diagnosis of atypical childhood sexual behaviors (18). Lack of baseline data can lead to the minimization of problematic sexual behaviors or over-reaction to expected and developmentally appropriate behaviors. For example, normative sexual behaviors can be pathologized, seen as unusual and/or misinterpreted as indicators of child maltreatment. Whereas, oversight of such

YOUNG CHILDREN

Gil (23) describes sexual curiosity and behavior as progressive over time. Children from birth to 4 years old commonly have limited peer contact. Their behavior focuses on self-exploration and stimulation and has a tendency to be disinhibited. They discover that touching certain body parts is pleasurable and may repeat this behavior. Sexual behaviors are mediated by caregivers' reactions and limit setting. If their reactions are punitive, the behavior may decrease or cease (e.g., touching self during a diaper change). Imitative play can be influenced by behaviors children are exposed to or have seen. For example, they may role play adult sexual activities seen in the home. Toddlers and preschoolers experiment through play and may for example, stick objects into body orifices. However, if this behavior is repetitive and does not appear to cause pain to the child, further assessment of the behavior may be needed. According to Gil (23) school aged children interact more with their peers of both sexes, experience periods of inhibition and experiment with their interactions. They may also be exposed to new sexual behaviors by peers and experiment with these behaviors. Latency aged children continue to interact with school, may explore sexual interests and have periods of inhibition and disinhibition. Physical development and puberty at this stage impacts physical and emotional reactions, feelings and behaviors (23).

By their nature, typically developing young children are very curious and inquisitive (18). Early childhood is a time of discovery and exploration (13). There is a natural exploration of all body parts (2) and young children engage in genitally-oriented behavior (14). Sexual behaviors are observed starting in infancy (24). Infants engage in a variety of self-stimulating behaviors such as finger sucking, rocking and cuddling (1) and an explicit interest and play involving genitalia is most frequently observed in 2-6 year old children (17, 18, 21, 25). This overt interest declines as children age, become more involved outside the home and are subjected to societal norms (17, 18, 24). The preschool years are a time of rapid and sizable change (26). Curiosity about sexuality including sexual feelings, exploring body parts and stimulation is expected and has been commonly observed in youth (18). Some studies have shown that certain normative and PSBs have an inverse relationship with age (17, 28). Examples of proposed explanations for this relationship include the immaturity of younger children (17) and decreased opportunities for adults to observe older children engaging in sexual behaviors (18). Sexual behaviors that have been found to decrease as a child ages include exhibitionism (e.g., showing genitals), voyeurism (e.g., looking at others' naked bodies), behaviors related to personal boundaries (e.g., standing too close to others) and self-stimulating behaviors (e.g., genital touching), the most frequent behavior observed in young children. However, interest in the opposite sex, asking questions about sexuality, viewing nude pictures or drawing genitalia for example, have been observed as more frequent in older children (28).

Parents and daycare providers have reported a variety of child sexual behaviors that are distinguished by their occurrence rates and specificity (8). Behaviors that are reported as occurring less frequently include behaviors that reflect adult sexual behaviors or that are more aggressive or intrusive (e.g., attempted intercourse, oral-genital contact, inserting objects into the vagina or rectum and masturbation with objects). Though such behaviors are shown to occur in approximately less than 3% of children in community samples, they are reported in all investigations using the CSBI (16, 19, 28).

Sexual behaviors are common in children, but the frequency of specific behaviors can vary (13). One European study (13) found that behaviors such as touching self and touching a mother's breasts for example, were widespread in children 0-11 years old. However, uncommon behaviors in this population included imitating sexual behavior with dolls, making sexual sounds and asking to watch explicit adult sexual behavior on television. The researchers of this study also found that 1 in 4 of a group of 670 children showed their genitals to adults or peers. Some behaviors decreased in frequency with age (undressing others, touching mother's breasts, hugging strangers) while others were more frequent among older children. Older children tended to demonstrate interest in the opposite sex, play doctor, ask questions about sexuality, look at pictures of nude bodies, draw genitalia, talk about sexual acts and ask to view sexually explicit television (13).

Larsson and Svedin (18) conducted a cross-sectional study comparing the frequency and range of sexual behaviors observed in the home environment and in daycare centers among 185 Swedish children aged 3-6 years. In addition, researchers asked caregivers and teachers about the children's general behaviors and their personal views of child sexual behavior. In this study, parents reported observing more sexual behaviors and daycare providers reported encountering more general behavior problems. A significant difference was found between the two setting where children tended to engage more in specific sexual behaviors (e.g., masturbation, showing own genitalia, trying to touch other children's genitals and talking about sex) in the home. A significant difference in sexual behaviors among boys and girls was found in the daycare setting only. Girls were observed by parents using sexual words, showing genitals to other children and role playing male roles significantly more (20-30%) at home than in daycare (4-5%). Boys at home were observed engaging more in four behaviors including rubbing genitals, masturbation with an object, touching genitals in public and talking about being female. However, these behaviors did not occur as frequently as others. On average, boys in the daycare centers engaged in more sexual behaviors. Children sought body contact with all adults but more so with their parents. The number of "advanced sex-play" behaviors was not significant in either setting. Larrson and Svedin's (18) research is consistent with other studies reporting more severe sexual behaviors as uncommon (14). Results of this and other studies indicate that non-maltreated children engage in a wide variety of sexual behaviors and highlights the difficulty of categorizing specific sexual behaviors that are indicative of sexual abuse in children (17, 24).

Sandnabba et al.'s (19) research looked at sexual behaviors in 364 Finnish 2-7 year olds attending day care. The children were not assessed for developmental or psychiatric difficulties or histories of CSA. School staff served as observers/informants. The researchers looked at frequency of behaviors as well as age and gender differences. Information on the frequency of sexual behaviors in children can provide a framework for understanding these behaviors in children and distinguishing typical from atypical sexual behaviors (10). Compared to earlier studies with normative samples and larger age ranges of subjects, the frequency of sexual behaviors in this population was lower. However, other studies have shown lower frequencies of sexual behaviors reported in day care settings compared to home settings (18). Proposed limitations of this study included but were not limited to the focus on preschool-aged subjects and the pre-school setting where there may be less opportunity to observe sexual behaviors and where behaviors may not be acceptable, the influence of the teachers' biases regarding behaviors and the direct nature of questions presented to informants. The authors highlighted that their study reflects an exploratory survey about students' childhood sexual behaviors and does not reflect the actual occurrence rates of these behaviors in the general population. Consistencies with other studies (14, 18, 20) were seen in the most frequently occurring sexual behaviors including, but not limited to, sexual interest and self-exploration, genital play, toilet behavior, engaging in behaviors with other children and voyeuristic behavior. Also consistent with other studies, was the absence of behaviors not expected in this age group including oral and genital penetration and intrusive and odd behaviors (19).

Davies et al. (14) interviewed a small, non-randomized but diverse group of 58 English preschool staff who reported commonly observing children's interests in genitalia through touching or showing genitalia, looking at peers' genitalia and touching women's breasts. Behaviors that infrequently occurred in this young population included insertion of an object into body orifices, oral contact with a peer's or doll's genitals and asking others to touch their genitals. Teachers reported less concern about common behaviors unless specific factors related to the behavior (e.g., frequency) or the child (e.g., child's age, demeanor and comments made while engaged in the behavior) were taken into account. Open and direct questions presented to the teachers appeared to influence their responses. Direct questions yielded responses describing the more rarely observed behaviors. Half of the subjects reported observing some children drawing or modeling genitalia occasionally, as a one-time occurrence or in a phase. Drawings identified as sexual in nature have been viewed by some professionals as an indicator of CSA and it is important to note that this may be a typical childhood sexual behavior. Despite some methodological differences, this study's results regarding the occurrence of common and rare sexual behaviors are consistent with similar studies conducted in different cultures.

OLDER CHILDREN

Friedrich et al. (28) conducted a community-based survey of 880 preadolescent children to assess the frequency of sexual behaviors in a normative population and their association to age, gender, family variables and socioeconomic status (SES). Mothers were questioned about their 2-12 year old children's sexual behaviors as well as demographic information. Youth with histories of CSA were excluded. Subjects reported a wide range of observed behaviors that varied in frequency and that peaked between the ages of 3-5 and decreased in frequency as the children matured. Aggressive and adult-like behaviors were rare. Older children were observed to engage in less sexual behaviors. Sexuality was related to general behavior problems and family nudity but not to SES.

In a later study, Friedrich et al. (17) studied the incidents of sexual behaviors in a somewhat diverse group of 1,114 children aged 2-12 years. Attempts were made to study children who did not have a history of CSA in order to identify other variables associated with childhood sexual behaviors. Questionnaires were used to gather data from the children's primary female caregivers. Examples of information gathered included demographic information, hours spent in daycare, occurrence of children's sexual behaviors, children's internalizing and externalizing problem behaviors, peer relationships, family sexuality, mother's views of childhood sexual behavior and children's exposure to family violence, illness and death. Results were consistent with previous studies and indicated that children display a wide range of sexual behaviors at varying frequencies. The most common behaviors found were self-stimulating behaviors, exhibitionism, and behaviors related to personal boundaries. Intrusive sexual behaviors were the least frequent in this population. As the children aged, the frequency of behaviors observed declined. Twenty percent of mothers of male and female children aged 2-5 years endorsed observing a wide range of sexual behaviors. Frequency of sexual behaviors peaked at age 5 years and continuously decreased until age 12. However, an increase in behaviors in 10 year old girls and 12 year old boys was observed and appeared to be related to a reported increased interest in the opposite sex. These results are consistent with Kendall-Tackett et al.'s (25) study that found sexual behaviors to be common in preschool children, to decrease with age and then reemerge in adolescence.

In the above study (17), researchers found that mothers with a higher level of education, and who viewed childhood sexual behavior as normal, reported more sexual behaviors in their children. The study's authors hypothesized that these mothers may have more open attitudes about sexuality and more opportunities to observe their children's behavior. A direct relationship between family sexuality and children's sexual behaviors was also found and may be due to more openness around sexuality or more ease of reporting behaviors. Ethnicity in this study was correlated to income but not to differences in sexual behaviors. Significant relationships were also found between observed sexual behaviors and hours spent in daycare. Reasons for this association are unclear but the researchers hypothesized that these relationships may reflect youths' exposure to other children with different levels of sexuality. Family violence and total life stress were associated with sexual behavior as well. These experiences have also been associated with other behavioral problems. The authors postulated that family stress may lead to inconsistent parenting, and that family violence, which often includes poor interpersonal boundaries and intrusiveness, could have impacted the children's behavior. The youths' sexual behavior was also related to the mothers' reports of their children's overall behavioral difficulties. Sexual behaviors as well as other childhood behaviors are viewed on a continuum and can overlap at the extremes of the continuum. Limitations to this study included the possibility that some of the children may have had a history of abuse which therefore could have increased the incidence of sexual behaviors. In addition, fewer behaviors observed in older children may reflect decreased opportunities for parents to observe their children engaging in such behaviors (17).

Pithers et al. (28) proposed that there are both common and rare behaviors associated with specific age groups. In their study, Sandnabba et al. (19) found that age had more of an impact on the extent of boys' behaviors especially as they matured. Their behaviors became more expressive while girls' sexual behaviors became more social with age. Girls engaged in more stereotypic gender role behaviors and boys were more explorative and engaged in information-seeking behaviors. In addition, these researchers found no gender differences in a group of behaviors that included for example, talking negatively about children of the opposite sex, games that had romantic or sexual characteristics and that tended to increase with age. However, older girls demonstrated less involvement in behaviors related to development and expressed interest in the characteristics of the opposite sex.

Based on the results of several studies, a summary of typical childhood sexual behaviors is presented in Table 1.

Table 1. Typical childhood sexual behaviors

Preschool children	Young children	School-aged children
– Exploring, touching, rubbing (with hand or object) and/or exposing genitals – Removing clothes – Peeking at others undressing or naked – Taking about "poop" and "pee" with same age peers	– Public or private masturbation – Mimicking adult social behaviors (e.g., kissing) – Playing "doctor" – Stating "naughty" words that they may or may not know the significance of	– Asking for more privacy – Privately masturbating – Engaging in sexual play (e.g., "truth or dare," "girlfriend/boyfriend") – Viewing nude pictures – Viewing sexual material through media – Experiencing sexual attraction towards peers

*Adapted from NCTSN (4) and NCSBY (26).

Data on observations of childhood sexual behavior may not be a true indicator of the prevalence and frequency of these behaviors given factors such as privacy or secrecy. Such factors may prevent observations of children engaging in sexual behaviors (14). Retrospective studies have been used to address the limitations of informant reports. In these studies, adults are asked about their early experiences engaging in sexual behavior. These studies have used different methodologies to define sexual behavior. Despite differences, the research indicates that broadly defined sexual experiences between children are common. A significant number of young adults across studies reported engaging in sexual behavior with their peers. Frequency of experiences in the younger ages were lower, however and may reflect the participants' ability to recall such early experiences (8).

SEXUAL PLAY

Compared to the small number of studies on typical sexual behavior in children, there is even less research on childhood sexual play. Sexual play is also common in childhood (30), but becomes more covert as children mature. Overt sexual behaviors appear to decline with age in part due to the influence of social norms or expectations for such behaviors (17, 19). Children engage in play to re-experience past events as well as practice future (adult) roles and behaviors (10). Play activities can include sexual play with peers (18). Children between the ages of 3-7 years practice and explore gender roles and become aware of genital differences between males and females. Play activities may include "house" and "doctor" (10).

In a review of various retrospective studies using adults' recollections of their child sexual play, Elcovitch et al. (8) noted that various sexual experiences between children are common and that 42-94% of subjects across these studies reported engaging in sexual play. Based on a retrospective study with adult subjects, Lamb and Coakley (11) identified categories of typical childhood sexual play. In their study, a group of United States female college students were asked to recall their childhood sexual play experiences. Researchers found that 85% of their population remembered engaging in a sexual game during their childhood and 76% engaged in this activity with their primary friends. Activities described by the subjects were categorized and included "playing doctor" (examining body parts, genitals), which was the most frequently reported game; exposing body parts to peers; exploring physical contact that included arousal; kissing games; exploring adult roles through fantasy sexual play; and others (e.g., mimicking sexual activity with dolls). The average age the subjects reported engaging in sexual play was 7.5 years. The adults (majority being parents) in the subjects' lives reportedly found out about these activities in half of the cases. Limitations of this study included the subjects' ability to accurately recall their past experiences, their choice of experiences to discuss, underreporting, and generalizability of subjects' experiences to other populations. Games reported as played by this population were experienced as a source of sexual excitement. Subjects were more likely to have been persuaded or manipulated into the play by boys. The researchers suggested that the play may have reflected enactments of socially defined gender roles. The researchers also found that bullying and manipulation were a part of "normal" sexual play activities. Girls were more likely to feel coerced or manipulated into an activity that made them feel uncomfortable. It was suggested that girls may be less likely to stop or report abuse if coercive experiences are interpreted as play and if they initially and willingly participated in the play. Recommendations for assertiveness training for children who may be confronted by another child to engage in sexual play were also discussed (11).

In a later retrospective study, Larsson and Svedin (30) found that more than 80% of a group Swedish students in their late teens reported engaging in solitary and mutual sexual experiences with a peer prior to the age of 13. Sexual experimentation and exploration appeared to be most prominent in the years before puberty. While solitary, exploratory behaviors increased prior to puberty, exploratory play with a peer decreased after age 10. The majority of mutual play occurred with a peer of a similar age, while 5% reported engaging in sexual play with a sibling. This is consistent with another study (10) where 9% of college age subjects reported engaging in sexual behavior with a sibling. Larsson and Svedin (30) also found that male and female subjects reported positive reactions to their sexual experiences, however, girls experienced more feelings of guilt. Boys engaged in slightly more play with peers and girls engaged in more same sex mutual play. The majority of subjects described their sexual activities as typical. Thirteen percent reported being tricked, bribed, threatened or physically forced into sexual activity. Girls reported more experiences that involved coercion and 10% of girls and 2% of boys reported engaging in sexual behaviors with someone 5 years older. In most cases, the older person was a relative (non-sibling) or a friend under 19 years old. This group also reported more mutual experiences in general and more experiences involving coercion. A small percentage (8.2%) of the subjects reported coercing others into sexual activity. Limitations of this study include the subjects' ability to remember details of their experiences and their interpretation of their experiences. The study authors suggested future research further address the impact of socialization on childhood sexual behaviors as well as differences between subjective and objective experiences of mutual and coercive sexual activities (30).

The ATSA report (5) differentiates problematic from typical childhood sexual play and curiosity. Normative sexual play is described as unprompted and sporadic. When the behavior involves other children, it is mutual and non-coercive and does not cause emotional distress. It also does not include adult sexual behaviors such as intercourse and oral sex. Typical child sexual development includes curiosity about sexual behavior and body parts and interest in sexual stimulation (5). How these behaviors are expressed is influenced by a child's developmental stage and culture (10, 28). Tolerance of behaviors in one culture may be prohibited in another (5). Children's relationships with caregivers and attachment experiences, which include positive physical contact, can influence future sexual and emotional relationships. In early childhood, children learn about gender roles and expectations through socialization experiences. Parents' restrictions on sexual behaviors can lead children to hide their behaviors and/or seek information from other sources such as peers and the media. Preadolescents may experience sexual attraction and sexual fantasies and as they get older may participate in dating and group activities with peers. Such activities provide them with social experiences to explore intimate relationships (1).

ADOLESCENTS

Adolescents are faced with changes associated with puberty including biological changes and an increase in sexual interests. These changes reflect sexual maturing. Social influences can have an impact on adolescent sexual involvement and behavior. Rates of engaging in heterosexual intercourse increase as adolescents age. In 1999, 48% of females and 52% of males in grades 9-12 reported engaging in sexual intercourse (31). Age of first sexual intercourse experience varies across cultures. For example, one study (32) found African Americans first sexual experience occurs on average at age 15.5 while Mexican Americans have sex for the first time on average at 17 years old. Boys in these groups tend to have sex at younger ages than girls. Differences between these groups may reflect differences in the adolescents' family structure, church attendance and socioeconomic opportunities such as employment rates and parent education level. Another study (1) found that 5 to 10% of adolescent boys and 6% of adolescent girls report having a sexual experience with someone, usually another adolescent, of the same gender. A portion of these adolescents engage in very few of these experiences out of curiosity (1). One of the psychosocial tasks of adolescence is defining one's identity and role in society in an environment that provides contradictory or inconsistent information. Gender identity is an important part of one's overall identity. In addition, adolescents are faced with learning how to navigate relationships including emotional and physical intimacy. According to the Kaiser Family Foundation (1), youth aged 10-15 most frequently identified media (movies, television, magazines, etc.) as their source of information about sex and intimacy, while fewer identified their parents, peers, sex education programs and professionals.

Brown and Cantor (33) proposed that media has a dominant influence on adolescents and has become a significant part of modern western society. Latency and teen aged youth use different forms of media up to several hours a day. Media has become more interactive and multisensory and is interpreted by youth in multiple ways. Youth can gather a lot of information about sexuality through the media though less is known about the effects of media exposure on youth. Exposure to media is also mediated by factors such as the child's age, sex, ethnicity and reasons for viewing the material (13). Brown and Witherspoon (34) reported a significant increase in sexual incidents portrayed in television since the mid-1970s. Sexual behavior on television is primarily verbal but physical portrayals occur in movies.

Cable television and videos are means for youth to view adult sexual behavior at home. In addition, music which historically focuses on love and sex has increasingly portrayed sexual images. According to Brown and Witherspoon (34), half of adolescents learn about pregnancy and birth control through the media and half of females report learning about sex through magazines. Research has also demonstrated that children have learned the meaning of words such as prostitution and homosexuality from television and that television and music portray premarital sex as acceptable. Media exposure can influence youths' sexual knowledge and development. However, less is known about the influence of media exposure compared to the incidents of young populations viewing sexual behavior through the media (13).

PROBLEMATIC SEXUAL BEHAVIOR (PSB)

Atypical and developmentally inappropriate sexual behaviors in children below the age of 13 have been gaining attention in the child welfare and mental health fields (5). Increased interest in these behaviors began with earlier research demonstrating a significant association between PSB and CSA (24, 25). Children presenting with PSBs are a heterogeneous group, engage in a variety of these behaviors and may require varied treatment approaches (29, 35). Both girls and boys exhibit sexual behavior problems (36). Children with PSB range in age and socioeconomic levels and come from a variety of cultural, social and familial environments and structures. Some have a history of traumatic experiences, maltreatment or mental health difficulties while others do not. Children with PSB can involve other children, siblings or peers in their behavior and their behaviors are not related to their sexual orientation (37).

Research and clinical experience have demonstrated that children and adolescents engage in a variety of typical and developmentally expected sexual behaviors. Despite the common occurrence of these behaviors, some sexual behaviors in youth are atypical and potentially problematic (25). When a child's behavior or awareness of sexual behavior is not commensurate with his/her age and developmental level, there is cause for concern (13). Studies have looked at a variety of factors that are related, contribute to and maintain problematic sexual behavior in children. These include biological, familial, economic and cultural factors (21). Research has also attempted to categorize subtypes of children with PSB but these categories greatly overlap (29) and suggest that PSBs differ in severity and intensity (5). PSBs have often been viewed on a continuum and the most aggressive behaviors are deemed the most pathological on the spectrum. In a retrospective study, Hall et al. (38) attempted to develop a typology of sexual behavior problems. They obtained data from the clinical records of a group of 3-7 year old children with a history of CSA. Characteristics related to the child and family functioning were included. The five types of sexual behavior problems derived from the study differed in terms of the behaviors as well as child and family functioning and treatment outcomes. Characteristics that differentiated the types of PSB most included aspects of the child's sexual abuse experience, opportunities for social modeling and practice with problematic behavior, and features of the family that impacted the occurrence of the behaviors. These factors also influenced treatment compliance and outcome. Implications for treatment interventions were discussed and highlighted the importance of tailoring treatment to the needs of the child and family (38).

Kendall-Tackett et al. (25) and others have identified several problematic sexual behaviors such as insertion of objects into the anal-genital regions of the body, excessive and/or public masturbation, asking adults or other children to engage in sexual stimulation, drawing genitalia, and knowledge of adult sexual behavior beyond the developmental level of the child. The types of PSBs that involve more than one child can differ as well, and the level of mutuality and potential for harm can vary. The most alarming PSBs involve children with significant differences in age and developmental functioning, aggressive or coercive acts that cause or have the potential to cause harm and advanced sexual behaviors (5).

The meta-analyses conducted by Kendall-Tackett et al. (25) identified sexual behavior problems in 34% of 351 sexually abused children up to the age of 12. Sexual behavior problems as well as symptoms of PTSD were the only sequelae that occurred significantly more in a population of sexual abused children compared to non-abused children from a clinical setting. Results suggest that assessment of children presenting with sexual behavior problems should consider several psychosocial risks including CSA as contributing to the behavior (25). More research on the variety of PSBs and associated treatment outcomes is needed (8).

Problematic sexual behaviors can have a variety of origins (39) and can occur independently and concurrently with other behavior problems. Children with the most problematic sexual behaviors tend to have co-morbid mental health, familial and social difficulties (5). Efforts to understand and treat PSB is complicated by the various definitions of the behavior used in research studies (40). Chaffin et al. (5) suggested that younger children with PSB may be more diverse than adolescents with PSB and adult sex offenders, who are predominantly male. Given their immature developmental and cognitive abilities, including a lack of verbal skills, preschool children are prone to engage in sexualized behavior when faced with stressful and confusing situations (26). There are considerable amounts of young boys and girls with PSB (41) and they do not appear to have a unique group of characteristics that distinguish them from other groups of children. The number of children referred for CPS, juvenile justice systems or treatment for PSBs has recently increased. The cause of this increase is unknown and could be the result of increasing PSBs in children, increased awareness and identification of PSBs and/or changing definitions (5).

The antecedents to PSBs are still unclear. Early research implicated CSA as the primary source of PSB in children (24). However, more recent research has demonstrated that many children with PSBs do not have a history of CSA (41) and several factors have been identified as potential causes of PSBs. Studies (5) have identified family, social, economic and developmental factors, child maltreatment, poor parenting practices, media exposure to sexually explicit material, living in a sexualized environment and exposure to family violence as precipitants to sexual behavior difficulties. PSBs have also been shown to result from exposure to adult sexual material or behavior in and outside of the home, inclusion in sexual activities with an older child or adult and/or lack of boundaries, guidance and nurturance in the home (23). Additional precipitating factors include family sexuality patterns, non-sexual behavior problems and physical abuse (36). Pithers et al. (29) described PSBs as one piece of a configuration of disruptive behaviors and Langstrom et al. (42) suggested that heredity may influence the presence of PSB. Childhood neurological and psychiatric disorders that include impulse control difficulties or obsessive–compulsive personality traits may contribute to an increased tendency for a child to engage in PSBs. Studies on such etiological factors and their development into adult maladaptive or offending sexual behaviors have received less attention in the literature (42).

Research has consistently identified several risk factors for the development of PSB in preadolescence. These include both severe sexual and physical abuse, families highly distressed by factors such as poverty, perpetration of sexual abuse in the extended family, incarceration for criminal behavior, domestic violence, poor parent-child attachment and familial obstacles to recovery from maltreatment (27). Hall, Mathews and Pearce (38) also identified four predictors of problematic sexual behaviors in children with a history of sexual abuse, including sexual arousal or sadism during the child's own abuse, history of physical and/or emotional abuse, and who the child blames for the abuse.

PSB is not diagnosed as a medical or psychological disorder. Behaviors can present in a variety of combinations and are perceived as beyond society's view of acceptable behavior (5). Based on an analysis of several evaluations of sexual behaviors in developmentally appropriate children below the age of 12 years, Johnson (43) found groups of behaviors falling on a continuum. These groups comprised children with healthy sexual behaviors to sexually reactive children, children who mutually engage in adult-like sexual behaviors and children who sexually abuse other children. Proposed criteria to differentiate typical and problematic sexual behaviors between children include, but are not limited to, differences in the children's age, developmental level, size and status; type of sexual behavior; dynamics and affective quality of the sexual activity or play; frequency, intensity and impulsivity of the behavior; and the use of threats, coercion and dominance (5). Gil and Cavanaugh-Johnson (23) define "sexualized children" as children who engage in problematic sexual behaviors through language, behavior, and excessive thoughts. These children include those who force, bribe, coerce or trick other children to engage in sexual behaviors. Davies et al. (14) identified characteristics of sexual behavior in youth that pose concern including frequency and the child's demeanor or statements while engaged in the behavior. The purpose of PSBs may or may not be used to achieve sexual gratification or stimulation and may be associated with a variety of other factors such as anxiety, attention-seeking and self-soothing behaviors (5). Sexual behavior can become problematic when it is repetitive, interferes with a child's cognitive or social functioning, involves coercion, force or intimidation, occurs under emotional distress, occurs between children of significantly different ages and/or developmental levels, continues to occur in secret despite adult intervention and has the potential to be harmful (36).

ASSOCIATION WITH SEXUAL ABUSE

Atypical sexual behavior can be a red flag for child maltreatment (13). Given the significant incidence of CSA and increased attention in the media to CSA, it is no surprise caregivers and childcare providers become concerned when they observe children engage in sexual behaviors (22). Unfortunately, children around the globe are negatively affected by sexual abuse, and many exhibit PSB. In addition, a significant percentage of sexual abuse offenders are adolescents (44). CPS agencies suggest that a large percentage of sexual abuse is performed by youth below the age of 20 (27). In a sample of 66 children, Gray et al. (27) found that subjects with PSBs had a significant history of child maltreatment (sexual, physical and emotional abuse, and neglect) were abused by an average of 2.5 perpetrators and the perpetrator was under the age of 18 in 40% of the cases.

Sexual behaviors are more often reported by parents with children who have experienced CSA. Therefore, sexual behavior in children can raise concerns of possible abuse (14). However, sexual behaviors in all categories have been reported by parents who had no concerns of abuse (39) and research has demonstrated that although PSB difficulties can be one consequence of CSA, they can occur absent of an abuse history (7, 41). Therefore, the association between CSA and sexual behavior problems is not seen in all children with PSB and most children who are sexually abused do not demonstrate these behaviors. Those who are abused however, tend to exhibit more frequent and intrusive sexual behaviors (8).

Historically, research on the impact of CSA has focused on adult populations. However, this has changed in the last 2-3 decades. Studies on CSA in young populations have focused on specific types of child victimization and their outcomes, and used different methodologies, leading to more child-friendly interventions. This literature has also allowed for the consideration of a developmental framework, the influence of mediating factors and potential outcomes of CSA (25). Several studies have documented a relationship between CSA and sexual behavior problems (19, 24, 25, 44, 45). Many of these studies have looked primarily at clinical populations with a history of CSA and compared them with non-clinical, non-abused populations. Therefore, focus is on problematic sexual behaviors in a population of sexually abused individuals. Rates of sexualized behavior in populations of sexually abused children were found to be higher compared to children who are not abused and children diagnosed with a psychiatric disorder (29).

Recent concerns about sexual abuse between children and between children and adolescents have identified a need to increase our understanding of normative sexual play. Distinguishing typical play from abusive behaviors is often complicated for caregivers, professionals and the court system. A better understanding of normative play may help in the assessment and intervention of problematic behaviors among children and adolescents. There is evidence (11) that a substantial number of CSA involves children or adolescents abusing other children. Abuse has been seen among siblings and cousins as well. In a pilot study (11), whether force or threats were used, the disclosure of abuse was less likely when it occurred with another child or adolescent. Authors hypothesized that children may not disclose the abuse because they may be unclear as to whether the behavior is abusive and may see themselves a responsible for choosing to engage in something that began as play but became exploitative (11).

A consequence of sexual abuse is traumatic sexualization, which can lead to a variety of psychological sequelae including but not limited to sexual aggression and preoccupation, and confusion of sex with love. Studies using parent and self-report psychological assessments and behavioral observations have differentiated sexually abused children, non-abused children and non-abused children with psychiatric diagnoses. Most of the research uses clinical samples. However, several studies comparing clinical populations, including neglected and physically abused children and children with a psychiatric history demonstrate differences in rates of sexualized behaviors. Assessment measures used appear to influence the observation of sexual behaviors (29). More research is needed to further clarify rate of PSB in child population (46).

Meta-analyses have demonstrated that CSA can lead to a variety of traumatizing outcomes. Sexualization and symptoms of PTSD are frequent but not universal outcomes of

CSA. The range of outcomes for children who have been sexually abused including lack of symptoms makes assessment and diagnosis difficult. Lack of a single pattern of responses calls for a comprehensive assessment of CSA and has implications for forensic assessments. Symptoms alone or the lack thereof cannot confirm or disconfirm abuse. In addition, few research studies address what leads to symptoms, if present, subsequent to CSA (23). Data on the occurrence rates of sexual behavior in children is important to the diagnosis, treatment and investigation of child abuse cases (25).

Childhood sexual behaviors present and change in frequency and at different ages (28). Gil (23) reported that inserting objects in the anal-genital areas of the body occurs with greater frequency in populations of sexually abused children. Kendall-Tackett et al. (25) showed that sexualized behaviors and PTSD are the most reliably associated outcomes of CSA. However, a majority of these studies focused on the most problematic behaviors in clinical populations of sexually abused individuals as compared to non-clinical, non-abused samples (12) Although research has shown an increased frequency of sexual behaviors in populations of children with a history of sexual abuse, the abuse histories of subjects were not proven, results of the studies are mixed and the type and methods of research limits generalizability.

Research methods used to identify subjects who were sexually abused also complicates conclusions about the relationship between sexual abuse and sexual behavior problems. Using the CSBI, Drach et al. (39) studied a group of 247 children referred for CSA assessment by a multidisciplinary team in a forensic setting. Results did not indicate a significant association between sexual behavior problems and a diagnosis of CSA or a significant association between a diagnosis of CSA and behavior problems as assessed by the CBCL. Sexual behaviors were variable within and between each group of subjects. Variability has been shown in abused and non-abused populations. There is little consensus in the literature as to what defines healthy, typical sexual behaviors in youth. However, behaviors that imitate adult sexual activity are observed more in populations of sexually abused children (10, 18, 20, 24). This increase in behaviors may not persist over time compared to non-abused children, and a variety of hypotheses have been made to try and explain PSBs in this population (27).

OTHER POTENTIAL CAUSES FOR PROBLEMATIC SEXUAL BEHAVIOR

Given our current understanding, and the research findings and limitations regarding the correlation between CSA and PSBs, it is important to consider multiple contextual variables and other child maltreatment experiences when evaluating sexual behaviors in children; and assessment and future research should consider variables other than CSA as potential antecedents (18, 21). The National Research Council (12) suggested that to better understand the antecedents and outcomes of child maltreatment and specifically the relationship between sexualized behaviors and child maltreatment, consideration should be given to several characteristics of the maltreatment including but not limited to severity, age of onset, resulting injury, chronicity, substantiation and exposure to maltreatment. Merrick et al. (12) looked at characteristics of maltreatment (timing and type) other than CSA that contribute to sexualized behaviors. A large sample of primary caregivers was interviewed about their 8 year old children's behaviors. Participants were obtained from the LONGSCAN Consortium.

The children in the study had a history of maltreatment other than CSA or were at risk for maltreatment. Results indicated that early and late reports of physical abuse and late reports of emotional abuse increased the probability of the child engaging in sexualized behaviors. Whereas early reports of emotional abuse were associated with decreased probability of sexualized behaviors, a history of physical abuse was predictive of sexualized behaviors and predicted more sexualized behavior for boys (e.g., exposing private parts, sexual intrusiveness) compared to girls (e.g., boundary difficulties). Although effect sizes were small, they demonstrated that experiences other than CSA can influence the probability of a child engaging in PSB.

It has been theorized that children with PSBs have emotion and behavior regulation difficulties (5) externalizing behavior problems (40) and poor social skills (24). The authors of the above study (12) suggested several hypotheses for the association between PSB and maltreatment other than CSA. For example, maltreatment such as physical abuse can create anxiety and difficulties regulating emotions for children. Subsequently, children may engage in sexual behaviors to manage these emotions and/or seek intimacy to cope with traumatic experiences. Difficulties regulating emotions and behavior can result in externalizing behavior problems. Sexual behavior is an externalizing behavior and may respond to effective self-regulation skills (21). However, maladaptive coping, including aggressive sexual behaviors (12) and contributing factors may lead to negative outcomes such as juvenile delinquency (29). In addition, child maltreatment is associated with family characteristics that may increase a child's exposure to sexual material and poor socialization skills (12). Rates of developmental and mental health difficulties in children who have a history of maltreatment and exposure to risk factors range from 50-80%. These statistics highlight the importance of effective coping skills to buffer the negative effects of maltreatment (12).

Additional studies have explored antecedents, other than CSA, to PSB. For example, Silovsky and Niec (41) found rates of physical abuse and witnessing family violence higher than CSA in a population of preschool children with problematic sexual behaviors. In addition, research by Friedrich and Trane (21) demonstrated that physical abuse and domestic violence have been associated with sexual and other behavior problems in children. As mentioned above, Langstrom et al. (42) looked at the influence of genetic and environmental factors influencing child sexual behavior problems. They focused on masturbatory behaviors in a group of Swedish 7-9 year old same-sex twins. Data was collected from over 1,000 parents/caregivers using items on the CBCL that address sexual behavior problems. Results indicated that the presence of problematic masturbatory behavior could be influenced by genetically determines "personality traits" (e.g., impulse control) and/or a genetically determined vulnerability to engage in problematic sexual behavior subsequent to environmental stress. They suggest that stressful life events as well as genetic factors should be considered in the evaluation of pre-pubertal children presenting with atypical masturbatory behavior.

A history of CSA is a risk factor for offending behavior, however, the majority of CSA victims do not subsequently offend. Furthermore, compared to experiences of CSA and neglect, a larger majority of physically abused kids have been shown to engaged in sexual offending (44). Scant research has been conducted on the sexual behaviors of young children and the influence of family variables and other child behaviors. More research has drawn general conclusions about specific child sexual behaviors and when they occur (17).

CHILDREN WITH ASD AND PSBs

Autism spectrum disorder (ASD) is a disorder of development that affects psychological and behavioral functioning. Both ASD and Asperger's disorder (AD) fall on a spectrum of severity but are characterized by deficits in reading social cues and social communication, by limited interests and perseverative or repetitive behaviors. AD differs from other disorders, however, in its relatively normal language and cognitive abilities (9, 47). Similar to typically developing peers, children with AD experience different sexual development stages. A common fallacy is that children with AD or other developmental disorders either do not experience sexual feelings or are extremely delayed. This can create problems for children with AD because they are not being adequately educated on sexual development and behaviors, such as appropriate touching of their own bodies as well as others. Children with disabilities need the same sex education and guidance as their typically developing peers in order to develop a sexual identity and have a framework for what is sexually appropriate and what is not. Without this information, coupled with an inability to understand social norms, social reciprocity, and likelihood of engagement in repetitive or self-stimulating behaviors, children with ASDs may be at risk for victimization, re-victimization or for victimizing others (35).

Sullivan and Caterino (48) suggested that individuals with ASD experience a large number of sexual behaviors which can be perceived as problematic due to societal norms. Social norms are difficult for individuals with ASD to recognize. These social deficits are fundamental characteristics of the disorder, complicating forming appropriate relationships. Specific impairments include: difficulty respecting personal boundaries, differentiating public vs. private behaviors, obsessional interests which may not correlate with the developmental stage of peers and which may include sexualized behavior, challenges in accurately reading or interpreting social cues, lack of empathy or not considering the viewpoint of another and difficulties handling anxiety. Youth with ASD may also receive negative reinforcement from peers or caregivers for sexualized behaviors. For adolescents, premature sexual development or puberty can lead to changes in hormones which can affect or change behavior. If norms do not apply, specifically the core impairments of AD listed above, PSBs can emerge (48). Frequently reported inappropriate sexualized behaviors in individuals with ASD include, touching self, touching others, masturbation (excessive or in public), and sexual talk.

EFFECTS OF DISABILITY AND OTHER CO-MORBID FACTORS

Children and adolescents with ASD may present with comorbid psychiatric, medical and behavioral difficulties such as attention deficit hyperactivity disorder (ADHD) and oppositional defiant disorder (ODD). Comorbid conditions can increase the likelihood that youth with ASD engage in sexualized behaviors. (41,47). For example, a study comparing individuals with ASD and those with obsessive compulsive disorder (OCD) found that people with both of these diagnoses reported more sexual obsessions than people with OCD without ASD (47). These two disabilities have overlapping features--ritualistic behavior and obsessional qualities--which may be influencing the unwanted behaviors. Consider the following case example:

A 10-year-old child with a complicated birth history has been diagnosed with multiple neurological and behavioral conditions, including AD and ADHD. This child has struggled with social, behavioral and attentional issues including impulsivity and poor decision making. It has been difficult to tease out the primary diagnosis due to the array of issues presented which have also complicated overall assessment and treatment planning. For several years, this child has exhibited problematic and perseverative behaviors but the primary treatment goal has focused on decreasing PSBs. As the child has gotten older, there is an increased desire to be with peers, but his behavioral issues, repetitive thoughts and difficulty accurately reading social cues have interfered with achieving success.

For individuals with ASD, anxiety is a primary affective experience and is commonly due to the desire to control their environment (49). Their anxiety can be manifested in self-stimulating behaviors and other behavioral issues. Individuals with AD struggle with social, attentional and behavioral issues including impulsivity, inattention, executive functioning difficulties and poor decision making (49). The 10 year old child referred to above has had some success in decreasing several behavioral difficulties, but less success in permanently decreasing or eradicating the sexualized behavior. There may be several reasons for this, including the consequences given for the sexualized behavior having the opposite intended effect. Instead of decreasing the sexualized behaviors, negative consequences could be providing reinforcement in terms of giving attention. For many parents, not providing consistent consequences but providing an abundance of attention (although negative) may inadvertently encourage behavior. Educating parents about appropriate sexualized behavior, behavior management, accepting their child's limitations, understanding the reasons why the sexualized behaviors are manifested and the neurological component are necessary.

Ray and Marks (49) discussed the possibility of PSB becoming a "pattern of behavior." Children with AD cognitively understand right from wrong, but lack insight into their own behavior, misinterpret societal rules, and view what others may think in a secondary light. They can also perceive other children's lack of verbal refusal (e.g., saying 'no') or compliance as agreement to take part in behaviors. One 7-year-old client of average cognitive ability diagnosed with AD, for example, demonstrated her knowledge of rules regarding appropriate and inappropriate sexual behaviors but this knowledge did not deter her from engaging in PSB. In fact, lying and purposefully finding opportune moments where she can be alone with another child have manifested. A major concern for this child's future is that her sexual preoccupation and various other contributing factors become increasingly severe and problematic despite treatment efforts.

ADOLESCENTS WITH ASD AND SEXUALIZED BEHAVIORS

The challenges faced by children with autism continue into adolescence but can be further complicated by puberty and the desire for intimate relationships. Navigating adolescent relationships is challenging for all teenagers, but adolescents with ASD display more inappropriate sexualized behaviors due to significant problems with social skills, identifying their own feelings, experiencing empathy and a failure to accurately understand another person's intended message (47, 50, 51). The difficulty they have expressing their feelings should not be mistaken for not having feelings (47). Although adolescents with ASD experience sexual urges like their typically developing peers, problems arise because they have difficulty processing nonverbal interactions, such as body language, facial expressions and tone of voice, and they do not understand the social norms necessary to figure out the nuances of intimate relationships.

Adolescents with ASD or other developmental disabilities therefore are at increased risk for exhibiting inappropriate sexual behaviors as well as for being physically, emotionally and sexually abused. Chan and John (47) discussed several factors that may contribute to these risks. Depending on the severity of the ASD or other developmental disability, adolescents may need adult assistance or supervision with daily living skills. This assistance may include helping with physical needs (e.g., toileting, dressing). This population is also less likely to receive sex education from their parents or school personnel. Parents may not have the skills needed to provide their adolescents information about changes in physical development and/or appropriate and inappropriate touching or inappropriate sexualized behaviors. This lack of information can increase the adolescent's vulnerability and risks of being taken advantage of or victimized by others. Given that many adolescents with ASD experience social awkwardness and difficulty recognizing proper social cues, some parents may be fearful of providing their children information that they think could be misunderstood by their child or others as permission to engage in these behaviors. This can lead adolescents with AD to feel frustrated and angry as they try to seek out relationships and intimacy, and their behaviors may be misinterpreted as PSBs (46, 52).

Typical adolescents develop a sense of self and sexuality from many sources, including day to day interaction with peers. This can be difficult for a teenager with ASD who, as mentioned earlier, may not understand subtle social innuendos or have the opportunity to experience intimate relations. They may also not learn as well through observation of others and misinterpret what they see and/or hear. This can lead youth with ASD to copy behaviors that may be out of context or inappropriate for a given situation. For example, a 12-year-old female diagnosed with ASD observed her older sister kissing her boyfriend which she misinterpreted as permission to kiss others. Her subsequent kissing behaviors led her family to believe she could have been sexually abused. It is not uncommon for inappropriate sexual behaviors to be misconstrued as signs of sexual abuse (53). Peers also may not serve as the best role models for this population because they can purposefully provide inappropriate information in order to cause embarrassment or humiliation. For these reasons and others, it is essential for parents to provide information about sexuality and puberty.

The literature (46, 50, 51) has discussed the frequency of sexualized behaviors and masturbation amongst adolescents with AD/ASD. It is normal for all teenagers to have sexual urges and masturbate. Those without developmental difficulties, however, have enough insight and impulse control to do this in private, as appropriate (54). According to Henault (51), public masturbation is the most frequently reported form of inappropriate sexual behavior for male adolescents with ASD. Many people with ASD are impulsive and hyperactive, and may use masturbation as a self-soothing behavior when they have a sexual urge, are feeling anxious, or are in a stressful situation. These feelings can especially be brought on in a new environment, with new routines or when there is uncertainty about when future events will occur. Like other ASD behaviors, masturbation can become compulsive and/or a distraction and can lead to exposure of genitals. Connor (46) defined inappropriate masturbation as "that which is constant, is maintained regularly but associated with feelings of shame, or is carried out in front of people."

It is necessary for youth with ASD to understand that masturbation is a normal and expected behavior, but that boundaries are needed. Depending on the reactions of others to this behavior, adolescents may not understand these boundaries or feel they are doing something 'bad,' which can create feelings of guilt. Concrete examples and supportive interventions need to be provided to help individuals distinguish between conducting this behavior in private vs. public places. It may also be beneficial to review multiple topics, including public exposure or masturbation, at an earlier age before behaviors become problematic (46, 51).

ISSUES FOR ASSESSMENT

For the assessment of childhood sexual behaviors, it is important to consider a variety of factors that could have precipitated or influenced the behavior. For example, does the behavior ordinarily occur among children of the same developmental stage or culture? Is the behavior repetitive? How preoccupied is the child with the behavior or sex? And can the behavior be corrected with adult intervention? When more than one child is involved in the behavior, assessment should consider for example, the difference in the children's ages and developmental stages, elements of force, coercion or intimidation, emotional distress in one or more of the children, potential for injury from the behavior and the possible negative impact on a child's social development from engaging in the behavior (55). Behavioral assessment of sexual behaviors should also include a chronology of behaviors and corresponding events using multiple informants (5).

Stress can have an impact on a child's behavior including exacerbating already existing behaviors. When a child is engaging in repetitive, stimulating sexual behaviors, it is important to assess if the behavior can be easily redirected, if the child performs the behavior in public and if the child's behavior is negatively affecting his/her overall functioning. Assessment of any sudden changes in behavior should also be considered. When gathering information about a child who engages in sexual behaviors, it is essential to assess if there is any history of child maltreatment, exposure to adult sexual material, such as pornography, and exposure to adult sexual activity. Assessment of sexual behaviors in children can yield different outcomes. For example, assessment results could lead to a referral to a child advocacy center to rule out child abuse, a report to CPS and/or a referral for treatment (13).

Adult's knowledge, beliefs and personal experiences can influence their interpretation of observed sexual behaviors in children (14). Professionals should especially be aware of their personal biases and values when assessing child sexual behaviors and follow accepted guidelines. Assessment of sexual behaviors informs subsequent recommendations and interventions and accuracy of the assessment can potentially lead to a positive or negative outcome for the child. Lack of available information on typical and atypical sexual behaviors in youth can lead to the possibility of personal standards influencing assessment practices. Few studies have addressed professionals' interpretations of typical child sexual behaviors. Given the potential influence of their work and professional roles on their perceptions, Heiman et al. (10) chose to compare the perspectives of professionals working with sexually abused children with professionals and medical students working and training in the area of human sexuality. These researchers found that sexual behaviors involving oral, anal or vaginal penetration were consistently viewed as abnormal in children under 12 years old. A lack of consensus among subjects was found when self-directed behaviors were assessed. Interactive sexual play was assessed as more atypical than self-directed sexual behavior, even among similar behaviors. Consistent with other research, female subjects perceived sexual behaviors as more atypical than male subjects. The authors hypothesized that socialization and gender role responsibilities may have an influence on the interpretation of sexual behaviors. Professional roles had a significant impact on interpretation of behaviors. Professionals working directly with sexually abused children assessed certain sexual behavior as more "abnormal." However, results did not indicate that the CSA experts over-pathologized behaviors. Agreement was found among subjects regarding their assessment of a young child inserting her fingers into an anatomically detailed doll's vagina as typical. This finding is inconsistent with previous concerns about the misdiagnosis of abuse when dolls are used in child abuse investigations, and supports the observation that young children's exploration of dolls' body parts is typical. Significant disagreement was found on 6 of 20 scenarios presented between subjects with the most diverse professional backgrounds. The majority of these items represented interactive, adult-like, sexual behaviors and were similar to behaviors assessed in previous (e.g., 19) studies as low frequency behaviors. CSA experts and medical students demonstrated the most disagreement. Compared to medical students and CSA trainees, CSA experts tended to view behaviors as more "normal" and differentiated types of behaviors vs. assessing individual behaviors as "normal" or "abnormal." Trainees and facilitators of human sexuality groups demonstrated directional (towards abnormal or normal) bias (10). Sexual behaviors are one part of a child's overall functioning (43) and there is not one way to determine typical sexual behavior. However, lack of knowledge regarding typical and atypical sexual behaviors in youth may create a risk for professionals using personal standards to assess these children (56). In the investigation of suspected child sexual abuse, knowledge of age-appropriate sexual behaviors is imperative for the professionals assessing if abuse occurred (10).

As discussed in the ATSA report (5), a good assessment should attempt to identify the situation(s) in which the sexualized behaviors are occurring. An assessment should look at environmental, contextual and genetic factors and whether the sexualized behaviors are self-focused or directed at other children. Clinicians should try to determine if the behaviors are occurring when a child is feeling stressed or anxious, is responding to environmental triggers, or during moments of opportunity, such as during play dates or sleepovers. The frequency and duration of the behaviors as well as the presence of other behavioral issues should also be determined. Multiple sources can be used to gather this information. Sources may include parents, teachers, therapists and possibly other children in order to obtain a more accurate and complete picture (5).

In addition to assessment of sexual behaviors, children's general behavioral and psychological functioning, co-morbid conditions and history of traumatic experiences should be assessed. PSB can be a primary or secondary concern. Children with PSB may have co-morbid disruptive behavior difficulties, anxiety and depression, developmental and cognitive difficulties and a history of maltreatment and/or exposure to violence (5).

For research and clinical purposes, two standardized instruments have been used by professionals to assess sexualized behaviors. The Child Sexual Behavior Checklist (CSBCL–

II) (5, 56) lists 150 behaviors related to sex and sexuality in children, and the Child Sexual Behavior Inventory (CSBI) (5, 16) measures the frequency of common and atypical behaviors and sexual knowledge. In 2002, Friedrich (57) developed the third edition, CSBI–III, which added four additional items that assess aggressive sexual behaviors. The outcome of these measures in conjunction with information obtained through other channels previously described can help guide professionals toward the most effective and best treatment options for each individual case.

If there is concern that a child has been sexually abused and the sexualized behaviors are seemingly secondary to the potential trauma, it is important to first conduct a forensic interview to help determine if in fact the abuse occurred. Forensic interviews are used as an initial assessment to rule out sexual abuse as the cause of inappropriate sexualized behaviors and protocols are put into place to conduct these interviews. There are special considerations that need to be taken into account when interviewing children or adolescents with ASD or any population with developmental disabilities (58, 59). Difficulties with communication, length of the interview, likelihood of a single interview and introduction to a new environment are some of the obstacles professionals may encounter when attempting to conduct a valid and reliable interview with these populations (49).

Prior to the first interview appointment, the forensic team should gather comprehensive information on the extent of the youth's developmental disability, including any psychiatric, psychological and educational evaluations and individualized education plans (IEP). An example of additional information to gather prior to the forensic interview includes, information regarding the child's emotional and behavior reactions to new situations. This data can be useful when preparing for the interview and support the forensic team's efforts to address the child's individual needs. During the initial stage of the forensic evaluation process, building rapport with the child and conducting an informal developmental assessment is especially important as the child's level of comfort and functioning can influence possible accommodations needed to conduct a reliable interview (58).

With all forensic interviews, the goal is to obtain the most valid and accurate information. This is typically achieved through open-ended questions in order to decrease suggestibility. For children or adolescents with developmental disabilities, there are several factors that may complicate the interview process For example, language difficulties, impaired memory, and problems with free recall may make using open-ended questions with this population difficult. However, youth with developmental disabilities can provide accurate and reliable information if they are interviewed properly (59, 60). The developmental and mental age of the child must be strongly considered, not just the chronological age. Questions should be asked at a slow pace, using simple language and correct pronouns. In addition, more open-ended questions should be introduced first, followed by cued invitations and more direct yet non-leading questions (61). Nonverbal interview aids should be available, such as crayons, dollhouses, visual aids or drawings to aid verbal disclosures. Other possible interview accommodations could include shortening the length of each session, eliminating noise or distractions and/or utilizing an extended forensic interview model which allows for multiple sessions over time (59, 61)

After the forensic evaluation is completed, a comprehensive functional assessment can take place to help determine if the sexualized behaviors are the primary issue or secondary, and whether non-sexual behaviors could be impacting the sexualized behaviors. Sexual development in children with ASD or developmental delays is complicated by the increased likelihood of sexual abuse, comorbidities and various other factors related to their developmental delays such as anxiety and a decreased ability to read social cues and conform to social norms. There are a number of assessment tools and methods available to practitioners to help determine the drivers of sexualized behaviors in this population as well as various treatment options. The outcome of a comprehensive evaluation and/or functional assessment should help guide the clinician in formulating a treatment plan or to make appropriate referrals.

In contrast to forensic investigations that seek to determine if a behavior occurred or to rule out CSA, clinical evaluations of children with PSBs can aid in the development of interventions and treatment plans and provide recommendations to child welfare and juvenile justice agencies who are engaged in case planning and decision making (e.g., placement decisions). ATSA (5) recommends that assessments should be conducted by licensed mental health professionals with expertise in a variety of areas related to child development, childhood mental health and behavioral difficulties and who are familiar with the current research in these areas. It is also suggested that these professionals have knowledge of factors related to children with PSB such as contextual factors impacting children's behaviors, and the influence of culture on parenting and child sexual behaviors. In addition, assessments should be tailored to individual cases and include an assessment of the environments (e.g., family and school environments) in which the behaviors occurred. Individual characteristics of a child may be less potent than the child's environment in influencing behavior. Changes in the environment are frequently necessary to change an individual child's behavior. Environmental factors both in and outside a child's home recommended to be assessed include, but are not limited to, the quality of the parent-child relationship and parenting skills, presence of positive role models, cultural influences, areas of resilience, history of traumatic experiences and child maltreatment, and exposure to sexual and/or violent material from adults, peers or through the media (5).

ISSUES FOR TREATMENT

PSBs can be resolved for most children with outpatient treatment and supervision. More severe and aggressive sexual behavior that may co-occur with a psychiatric or other behavioral disorder and that has not responded to other interventions may require a higher level of care (e.g., inpatient treatment). Children who are supervised and receive appropriate interventions for sexual behavior problems can live with other children. However, children who engage in ongoing intrusive and aggressive sexual behaviors and do not respond to close monitoring or treatment should be separated from other children until the behavior is resolved (36). For children in placement, assessment and intervention should occur in the current and future placements, including during reunification with the family of origin (5).

For children with AD, a change in environment may exacerbate or decrease sexualized behaviors. Prior to formulating a treatment plan, it may be helpful to determine if there are any triggers for the behavior or whether environmental changes can be made in order to decrease sexual behaviors. This may include removing objects that are associated with the behavior or changing attire on the child, for example, by adding a belt (62). Placing children in a setting that is very structured may decrease feelings of anxiety and their need to control their surroundings. This type of predictable environment, coupled with consistent supervision, may also lead to a decrease in sexualized behaviors.

Given the multiple antecedents to and expressions of sexual behavior difficulties in youth, a variety of interventions may be needed (63). ATSA (5) describes PSBs as diverse and that vary in severity and potential for harm to other children. There is no specific set of characteristics that identifies youth with PSB or rules that dictate decisions regarding, for example, placement. Legal adjudication issues should be made on a case by case basis. In addition, interventions should be revisited regularly given the possible changes that can occur with the individual child and their environments. Treatment should include modifications to the environments surrounding the child to help eliminate factors that can trigger or maintain the PSBs as well as identification of resources that can help address the problem behaviors (5).

Much concern has been expressed regarding children who have sexual behavior difficulties and their potential for future sex offending behavior. Current research indicates that when proper treatment is provided, the risk for re-offending is low and no greater than with other clinical populations. In addition, the risk for future offences may equal the risk for victimization. Children with PSBs generally respond well to cognitive behavioral and psychoeducational interventions that involve their caregivers. Few cases of children with PSBs require more intensive and restrictive interventions. Children with PSB are quite different from adult sex offenders and are not seen as their child counterparts. Interventions for adults are not applicable to children with PSBs. In addition, actions that attempt to protect society by isolating and criminalizing children with PSB may only lead to more difficulties and shame for these children (5).

Treating children or adolescents with sexualized behaviors can be challenging. Specific treatment modifications need to be considered for youth with ASD, AD and other developmental disabilities due to their limited insight, impulsivity, concrete understanding of concepts, possible cognitive limitations, linguistic issues and difficulty generalizing acquired knowledge to real life scenarios. There are several treatment options depending on whether the sexualized behaviors are considered internalizing or externalizing behaviors. The focus of the interventions should be determined on a case to case basis after a careful analysis is completed and the primary problematic behavior is identified. Treatments such as trauma focused-cognitive behavioral therapy (TF-CBT) target trauma symptoms (i.e., posttraumatic stress disorder) and may be indicated for children or adolescents with internalizing behaviors. However, if a child presents with externalizing or disruptive behaviors, the primary focus of this chapter, other behavioral interventions may be more effective (64).

Concrete behavioral strategies that use behavior charts and reward systems with immediate consequences can be effective in shaping target behaviors in children and adolescents with ASD. When formulating a chart, it is useful to isolate the primary problematic behavior and focus on decreasing the frequency of its occurrence prior to moving on to other issues. Other possible interventions for any child with behavioral difficulties, but specifically for individuals with ASD, include role playing, "social stories" and video modeling to help assist with social skills development, emotion regulation, linking feelings of anxiety to social situations, and helping children understand the impact of their behavior on other people's feelings (47,65,67). Often children and adolescents with ASD present behaviors that are more impulsive than compulsive, so strategies such as cognitive restructuring, or understanding the abuse cycle may not be as effective with this population.

Consistent use of effective interventions is an important element to ensure permanent eradication of an undesirable behavior. Short-term success and intermittent reduction in sexualized behaviors can often occur during periods of consistent supervision in a predictable environment. Therefore, interventions need to continue even if the sexualized behaviors decrease, or they will not likely have a lasting effect (68).

Several researchers (65, 67) have discussed the use of "social stories" to help children and adolescents manage problematic behaviors. The stories provide information youth may need to achieve success in a social situation. Using a step-wise approach, the stories address specific issues or situations by teaching the child or adolescent the appropriate expected behavior. The stories are individually tailored to the child's needs and developmental abilities. For individuals diagnosed with AD and language difficulties, the use of a social story can combine verbal directions with pictures or prompts. Self-monitoring strategies may also assist in decreasing sexualized behaviors, and the techniques used are dependent on the age or developmental level of the child. A self-regulation chart, such as an emotions thermometer, measuring levels of excitability, may be used to help a child with developmental disabilities recognize when he/she is overstimulated and how to respond accordingly. For example, a child may be directed to use self-calming strategies or take a break from the source of excitement. Other strategies may use visual aids or prompts, such as cards with red and green lights and stop signs. These can be placed around the home to indicate where certain behaviors are or are not acceptable. Pictures can also be placed on the child as reminders or to help them generalize appropriate behaviors to other settings. Another behavioral intervention includes providing a replacement behavior that can help comfort or redirect a child from the undesired sexual behavior. For example, when working with a 10-year-old male who would frequently grab his genitals in public, a squeeze ball was introduced in order to redirect his attention.

Regardless of whether treatment is focused on young children or adolescents or which treatment option is employed, parental or primary caregiver support and consistency needs to be maintained to achieve any success (69). Communication between the clinician and the parent is important to ensure continuity and consistency of information given and techniques used, and to assist the parent in determining appropriate language to be used with their child and that corresponds with the age and abilities of their child. There are several treatment modalities that can be used to accomplish this including, dyadic treatment, parent collateral sessions and/or family therapy. Caregivers need to be educated about normal sexual development in order to recognize inappropriate sexual behaviors if they arise, and to respond promptly and effectively. They should provide their child information on appropriate and inappropriate touch, boundaries and privacy rules, model appropriate attire and affection with others, and encourage and demonstrate positive and appropriate peer interactions (5).

Professionals need to consider a variety of factors that may impact families' reactions and receptivity to interventions that address sexuality and sexual behaviors. These include, but are not limited to, racial identity, ethnicity, religion, socioeconomic status, cultural beliefs and norms, and the social environments within which the child interacts. It is important to assess the family's beliefs, values and practices in regards to sexuality and sexual behavior. These include the family's implicit and explicit rules about sexual behavior, relationships and intimacy, and their comfort in addressing these issues. Openness, respect and understanding of a family's culture may strengthen the working relationship and make the family more receptive to the professional's interventions. Professionals should also be aware of the knowledge, beliefs and values about sexuality and sexual behavior they possess that coincide or conflict with their family clients, and that could have the potential to negatively impact the provision of services and/or the professional relationship. Information provided by the professional about sexuality and sexual behaviors should be consistent with their family clients' beliefs (4).

When incidents of sexual behavior or CSA, and subsequent concerns about a child's safety warrant discussions with families whose practices (e.g., cultural or religious) do not include an openness about sexuality or sexual behavior, it is important for professionals to respect the family's values, explain the reasons for their interventions and work with the family to identify options for discussing the presenting concerns and for making recommendations and initiating interventions. This requires flexibility on the part of the professional. Subsequent treatment interventions should not only consider the child's social and cultural context, developmental abilities and family beliefs and values, but also the parents' acceptance of information provided to their child during the treatment (4).

THE IMPACT OF CAREGIVERS

The development of children's or adolescents' sexual knowledge is influenced by the information they receive from a variety of sources including their family, culture, school, peers, community, the media and by the developmental abilities they possess to understand and interpret this information. This information can be implicit, explicit and conflicting. As children mature, they develop knowledge and attitudes that are also influenced by the presence or absence of support and reactions from adults (e.g., caregivers and teachers). Studies have shown that parents can help to reduce youth engagement in some risky sexual behaviors and mediate sexual information obtained through the media through close supervision and effective communication with their child (4).

Several theories explain the impact of context or environment on a child's emerging sexual development (2). Socialization has an early influence on an individual's development. Children are taught rules, norms and values about their culture, relationships, and behavior. These norms and values are learned through observation and imitation, the responses of others to their behaviors and direct instruction. This socialization process includes acquiring rules about sexuality. Gil (23) states that parent reactions to children's sexual behavior can mediate the child's sexual development. Parents who are inflexible and punish typical sexual behaviors may produce feelings of guilt and shame in their children and possibly lead them to hide subsequent behaviors or concerns about sexuality. In contrast, parents who do not limit exposure to sexual content may trigger their children to act out sexually. Children may learn that certain sexual behaviors are prohibited while others only occur in a private setting (21). Parents' decisions to provide information to their children can be influenced by the child's age and developmental level, concerns about safety and cultural beliefs, for example. Information about sexuality can be provided formally or informally to children (4). Sex education requirements across school systems vary and may be different from the information children receive in their home. Despite the shock and disbelief caregivers often experience when they observe their children engage in sexual behavior, the assumption that their children possess a sophisticated or mature understanding of sexuality and/or their sexual behaviors is often inaccurate and can add to the caregivers' concerns.

Home environments tend to be less structured and provide opportunities for children to not only see family members undress, but also to show curiosity about nudity, have conversations with their caregivers about body functions and display sexual behaviors. The school environment is often a more structured and monitored group setting. Early in life, children are socialized to keep sexual behaviors private (10). Schools may place demands on children to conform to social norms and provide less opportunities for children to engage in sexual behavior.

Larsson and Svedin (18) found that 67% of the parents and 41% of the teachers in their study never spoke to their children and students about sexual behaviors but their attitudes about sexuality were found to be quite open. Discussions more commonly occurred when the children initiated the conversation. More than half of the teachers spoke to parents about children's sexual behaviors while the majority (92%) of parents did not speak with the teachers. Teachers were viewed as slightly more liberal than parents regarding child sexual behavior. One fifth of all of the adult informants did not have names for the children's genitals. More adults referred to boys genitalia with accurate labels while girls were more likely given inaccurate or colloquial names for their genitals. Researchers also found that the majority of their adult informants believed that it is normal for children to be curious about sexuality, engage in sexual play and experience sexual feelings but less frequently believed that children engage in sexual behavior. Studies such as Larrson and Svedin's (18) support the importance of context when evaluating sexual behaviors in children.

Parents often have the unexpected experience of encountering their child exploring their bodies or engaging in sexual play. Many parents may feel uncomfortable or uncertain in these often spontaneous events and can react in a number of ways. They may react with shock, anger, anxiety and/or embarrassment and have concerns about their child's safety and development (22). The increase in information and attention on sexual abuse may also produce confusion for parents addressing issues of sexuality with their children. Parents' responses or management of sexualized and non-sexualized behaviors can influence a child's sexual development (13). Adult expectations for gender specific behaviors or "gender role stereotypes" can also influence a child's socialization and behaviors (19). It is important for clinicians to normalize sexual behaviors in children for parents (13) and to address the distress they may experience when witnessing their children engage in sexual behaviors.

Educating children about sex and sexuality is often a difficult task for parents. It is suggested that they provide accurate and developmentally appropriate information to their children in order to enhance safety, healthy habits and self-confidence with their bodies (4). It is also suggested that parents talk with their children about sexuality and development, privacy and safety. Parents' awareness and guidance can help address information the child is exposed to outside the home, clarify questions and define what is acceptable. In addition, supervising the child's media use can help to protect, prevent and address exposure to inappropriate sexual material (13).

Children learn rules of physical interactions through the reactions of others to their behavior. Boundaries for such behavior can promote privacy for self and others and identity protection in future sexual interactions. The reactions of adults and peers to young children who break such boundaries can produce feelings of shame for the child that can be long-lasting and internalized. Parents are often surprised and anxious when they encounter their child engaging in sexual behavior. Their alarm may result in a variety of questions and concerns. They may fear that their child has been exposed to adult sexual material or been abused. They may also question if their child's behavior is developmentally inappropriate or typical. Parents' reactions can vary and are influenced by their familial and cultural backgrounds and belief systems. When appropriate, validating the child's behavior as typical can often ease parents' fears of sexual abuse and influence their reactions and management of the behavior. They often need support and education regarding developmentally expected child behaviors. Intervention includes the family and it is important to assess the parents' backgrounds and beliefs about sexual development and behavior as well as their past experiences including trauma history and current stressors (13).

Parenting a child with sexualized behaviors and developmental disabilities (DDs) can be very stressful, have negative implications for the family unit and lead to feelings of isolation from friends or family. It may be helpful for parents to join a support group for families with children exhibiting similar problematic behaviors. With additional support, families have an opportunity to understand and accept the deficits surrounding their child's diagnosis and how DDs may contribute to sexualized behaviors. Depending on the origin of the sexualized behaviors, the parents' understanding that their child may be unable as compared to unwilling to stop these behaviors could help them possibly empathize with the child's inability to stop. The possibility of a neurological component in individuals with multiple diagnoses (e.g., ADHD, AS, OCD) may affect the client's ability to control their sexual impulses. Understanding the implication of a neurological origin may help reduce the parent's self-blame and reinforce the need for supervision, highlight the necessity for behavioral interventions and the formation of a safety plan, and guide treatment decisions (70, 71).

SEX EDUCATION

In order to help decrease PSBs and risks for sexual abuse as well as support positive feelings of sexuality and the formation of healthy relationships, individuals with DDs and ASD should be involved in an age and developmentally-appropriate sex education program and/or receive information about sexuality and sexual development from an early age through adolescence. Possible topics to be addressed include information about their bodies and how they work, basic hygiene, personal safety, inappropriate and appropriate touching and saying 'no' followed by individualized instructions that are brief, concrete, concise and repetitive (53, 72, 73). The amount of information offered, and to what extent, will depend on the individual child or adolescent's cognitive and linguistic abilities. Within any program, youth should be taught how to identify a potentially abusive situation, increasing the likelihood they can avoid one. This is especially important in populations diagnosed with a DD where individuals may be more likely to trust others and be easily manipulated. Lumley and Miltenberger (69) discussed the importance of assessing an individual's knowledge following the completion of a specific sex education program using role-play and in situ assessment. This would allow clinicians to see how much information is retained and if newly learned skills have been generalized to real life scenarios.

Although there has been attention on the importance of providing sex education to individuals with developmental delays and AS, there has been less discussion in the literature about formal sex education curricula. The few programs reviewed focus on sex education for individuals with ASD or AD are centered on social and communication issues, but elements of these programs can and should be modified to each individual depending on their cognitive, developmental, linguistic, social and emotional abilities. The overall goal of these programs is to provide information, protect against victimization, increase self-esteem and promote age-appropriate sexual habits. Three established programs specifically mentioned in the literature are TEACCH, which focuses on 4 levels of curriculum depending on the child's cognitive ability, the Devoreaux Centers, which attempt to use parents as teachers as much as possible to communicate a wide array of topics, and the Benhaven program, for more severely impaired individuals focusing on self-care and appropriate behavior (48, 73). For adolescents with AS, Stokes and Kaur (54) discussed the need for a 'specialized' sex education program with an emphasis on social interactions integrated into the program.

Conclusion

The topic of sexual development is often overlooked as an expected area of development, especially among children with disabilities. However, more clinicians and researchers are now looking at how young people with disabilities experience sexual feelings or behaviors normatively, as a function of their disability and/or comorbidities, as a result of trauma or abuse, or as the result of other risk factors. Unfortunately, children with intellectual disabilities and developmental delays experience sexual abuse at a higher rate than peers who are not developmentally delayed due to cognitive, social and emotional deficits. As with typically developing peers, problematic sexual behaviors can occur in children with developmental delays as a result of sexual abuse, but there are often other factors at play. In this chapter, we first presented a brief overview of normative and problematic sexual behaviors and then explored some of the reasons they are more prevalent in developmentally delayed populations, focusing on children and adolescents diagnosed with higher functioning Autism Spectrum Disorder. We then discussed various methods to assess sexualized behavior and treatment options for this population with a focus on working with their families in their cultural context and providing appropriate sex education.

Chaffin (74) provided commentary regarding misconceptions placed on children and adolescents who display PSB and recent scientific data which may alter policies involving treatment, practice and perceptions of these behaviors. Knowledge and effectiveness of utilizing evidence-based treatment for children with PSBs has grown over the last decade and has shown a positive outcome with less likelihood of sexual behaviors reoccurring. He points out that "reeducation" of professionals and policy makers is necessary to prevent every adolescent and child with a history of PSB from being labeled a perpetrator. An incorrect label could change the direction of the most effective treatment options (74).

Children and adolescents with developmental delays exhibiting PSB's can be especially difficult to interview and assess, therefore, compromising the formulation of an effective treatment plan and placing the child at risk for incorrect and damaging labels. At an administration level, staff must receive proper training regarding normative sexual development, PSBs, and developmental disabilities in order to provide effective, comprehensive and sensitive services. Lack of expertise amongst clinicians, high turnover rates, and poor communication and collaboration between agencies and providers are ongoing issues that need to be addressed. At an institutional level, future research could assist in determining efficacy of different treatment modalities specific to this population. Future research needs to look beyond developmentally appropriate individuals and focus efforts on evidence-based practice that is developmentally sensitive and considers cognitive, emotional and behavioral characteristics which are often overlooked in this vulnerable population. (68). Based on current research and our clinical experience in a hospital based children's advocacy center that specializes in the evaluation of child maltreatment of children with disabilities, we believe that there is a core set of skills and competencies which can be developed to optimally assess and treat children with disabilities who may have been abused. However, many professionals currently doing this work have expertise in either the evaluation and treatment of child maltreatment or of children with disabilities, but not both. These children require an integrated approach with additional professional time, services and expertise, as well as sex education and preparation tailored to their specific abilities and needs. This is particularly true when they have entered the child protection system which, unfortunately, often does not have the resources available for these often complex evaluations. With additional training and research into normal sexual development and how cultural context and maltreatment affects sexual behavior in children with disabilities, we believe we can improve lives and mitigate harm among this very special, but very vulnerable, population.

REFERENCES

[1] DeLamater J. Human sexual development. J Sex Res 2002;39:110-4.
[2] Balter AS, Van Rhijn TM, Davies AWJ. The development of sexuality in childhood in early learning settings: An exploration of early childhood educators' perceptions. Can J Hum Sex 2016;25(1):30-40.
[3] World Health Organization. Report of a technical consultation on sexual health, 28–31 January 2002, Geneva: WHO, 2006.
[4] National Child Traumatic Stress Network (NCTSN). Cultural and family differences in children's sexual education and knowledge. Culture and Trauma Brief 2008;3:1. URL: http://www.NCTSN.org.
[5] Chaffin M, Berlinger, L, Block, R, Cavanaugh Johnson, T, Friedrich, W Garza Louis, D. Report of the ATSA Task Force on Children with Sexual Behavior Problems. Child Maltreat 2008;13:2:199-218.
[6] Mandell D, Walrath C, Manteuffe B, Sgro G, Pinto-Martin J. The prevalence and correlates of abuse among children with autism served in comprehensive community-based mental health settings. Child Abuse Negl 2005;29:1359-72.
[7] Bonner BL, Walker CE, Berliner L. Children with sexual behavior problems: assessment and treatment – final report. Washington DC: US Department of Health and Human Services, National Clearinghouse on Child Abuse and Neglect, 1999.
[8] Elkovitch N, Latzman RD, Hansen DJ, Flood MF. Understanding child sexual behavior problems: A developmental psychopathology framework. Clin Psychol Rev 2009;29:586-98.
[9] American Psychiatric Association. Diagnostic criteria for autism spectrum disorder. Washington, DC: APA, 2013. URL: http://www.dsm5.org.
[10] Heiman ML, Leiblum S, Cohen ES, Malendez PM. A comparative survey of beliefs about "normal" childhood sexual behaviors. Child Abuse Negl 1998;22:289-304.
[11] Lamb S, Coakley M. "Normal" childhood sexual play and games: Differentiating play from abuse. Child Abuse Negl 1993;17:515-26.
[12] Merrick MT, Litrownik AJ, Everson MD, Cox CE. Beyond sexual abuse: The impact of other maltreatment experiences on sexualized behavior. Child Maltreat 2008;13(2):122-32.
[13] Hornor G. Sexual behavior in children: Normal or not? J Pediatr Health 2004;18(2):57-64.

[14] Davies, SL, Glaser, D, Kossoff, R. Children's sexual play and behavior in pre-school settings: Staff's perceptions, reports, and responses. Child Abuse Negl 2000;24(10):1329-43.
[15] Achenbach T, Edelbrook C. Manual for the child behavior checklist and revised child behavior profile. Burlington VT: University of Vermont, Department of Psychiatry, 1983.
[16] Friedrich WN. Child sexual behavior inventory: professional manual. Odessa, FL: Psychological Assessment Resources, 1997.
[17] Friedrich WN, Fisher J, Broughton D, Houston M, Shafran CR. Normative sexual behavior in children: A contemporary sample. Pediatrics 1998;101(4):E9.
[18] Larsson I, Svedin CG. Teacher's and parent's reports on 3 to 6 year old children's sexual behavior--A comparison. Child Abuse Negl 2002;26:247-66.
[19] Sandnabba NK, Santtila P, Wannas M, Krook K. Age and gender specific sexual behaviors in children. Child Abuse Negl 2003;27:579-605.
[20] Lindblad F, Gustafsson PA, Larsson, I, Lundin B. Preschooler's sexual behavior at daycare centers: An epidemiological study. Child Abuse Negl 1995;19:569-77.
[21] Friedrich WN, Trane ST. Sexual behavior problems across multiple settings. Child Abuse Negl 2002;26: 243-5.
[22] National Child Traumatic Stress Network (NCTSN). Sexual development and behavior in children: Information for parents and caregivers 2009. URL: http://nctsn.org/nctsn_assets/pdfs/caring/sexualdevelopmentandbehavior.pdf.
[23] Gil E, Johnson TC. Sexualized children: Assessment and treatment of sexualized children and children who molest. Rockville, MD: Launch Press, 1993.
[24] Friedrich WN. Sexual victimization and sexual behavior in children: A review of recent literature. Child Abuse Negl 1993;17:59-66.
[25] Kendall-Tackett KA, Meyer Williams L, Finkelhor D. Impact of sexual abuse on children: A review and synthesis of recent empirical studies. Psychol Bull 1993;113:164-80.
[26] Hewitt SK. Assessing allegations of sexual abuse in preschool children: Understanding small voices. Thousand Oaks, CA: Sage, 1999.
[27] Gray A, Pithers WD, Busconi A, Houchens, P. Developmental and etiological characteristics of children with sexual behavior problems: Treatment implications. Child Abuse Negl 1999;23(6):601-21.
[28] Friedrich WN, Grambsch P, Broughton D, Kuiper J, Bielke RL. Normative sexual behavior in children. Pediatrics 1991;88:456-464.
[29] Pithers WD, Gray A, Busconi A, Houchens P. Children with sexual behavior problems: Identification of five distinct types and related treatment considerations. Child Maltreat 1998;3:384-406.
[30] Larsson I, Svedin CG. Sexual experiences in childhood: Young adult's recollections. Archives of Sexual Behavior 2002;31:3:263-273.
[31] Center for Disease Control (CDC). National survey of family growth. URL: http://www.cdc.gov/nchs/nsfg/key_statistics/s.htm#.
[32] Day RD. The transition to first intercourse among racially and culturally diverse youth. J Marriage Fam 1992;54:749-62.
[33] Brown JD, Cantor J. An agenda for research on youth and the media: Conference proceedings. J Adolesc Health 2000;27:2-7.
[34] Brown JD, Witherspoon EM. The mass media and American adolescent health: Supplemental article. J Adolesc Health 2002;31:154-70.
[35] Greydanus DE, Pratt HD. Childhood and adolescent sexuality. In: Greydanus DE, Patel DR, Pratt HDS, Calles Jr JL, Nazeer A, Merrick J, eds. Behavioral pediatrics, 4th ed. New York: Nova Science, 2015:413-38.
[36] National Center on the Sexual Behavior of Youth (NCSBY) Fact sheet: Adolescent sex offenders: Common misconceptions vs. Current evidence. Oklahoma, OK: University of Oklahoma, 2003.
[37] Child Traumatic Stress Network (NCTSN). Understanding and coping with sexual behavior problems in children: Information for parents and caregivers, 2009. URL: http://nctsn.org/nctsn_assets/pdfs/caring/sexualbehaviorproblems.pdf.

[38] Hall DK, Mathews F, Pearce J. Sexual behavior problems in sexually abused children: A preliminary typology. Child Abuse Negl 2002;26:289-312.
[39] Drach KM, Wientzen J, Ricci LR. The diagnostic utility of sexual behavior problems in diagnosing sexual abuse in a forensic child abuse evaluation clinic. Child Abuse Negl 2001;25:489-503.
[40] Allen B. Children with sexual behavior problems: Clinical characteristics and relationship to child maltreatment. Child Psychiatr Hum Dev 2016 Feb 29.
[41] Silovsky JF, Niec L. Characteristics of young children with sexual behavior problems: A pilot study. Child Maltreat 2002;7:187-97.
[42] Langstrom N, Grann M, Lichtenstein P. Genetic and environmental influences on problematic behavior in children: A study of same sex twins. Arch Sex Behav 2002;31:343-50.
[43] Johnson TC. Understanding the sexual behavior of young children. Washington, DC: SIECUS Report, 1991:8-15.
[44] Pratt HD, Patel DR, Greydanus DE, Dannison L, Walcott D, Sloane MA. Adolescent sex offenders. Int Pediatr 2001;16:1-8.
[45] Palusci VJ, Cox EO, Cyrus TA, Heartwell SW, Vandervort FE, Pott ES. Medical assessment and legal outcome in child sexual abuse. Arch Pediatr Adol Med 1999;153(4):388-92.
[46] Connor MJ. ASD and inappropriate (as perceived) sexualized behavior. OAASIS 2007. URL: http://www.mugsy.org/connor90.htm.
[47] Chan J, John RM. Sexuality and sexual health in children and adolescents with autism. J Nurse Pract 2012; 8:306-15.
[48] Sullivan A, Caterino L. Addressing the sexuality and sex education of individuals with autism spectrum disorders. Educ Treat Child 2008;31:381-94.
[49] Ray F, Marks C, Bray-Garretson H. Challenges to treating adolescents with Asperger's syndrome who are sexually abusive. Sex Addict Comp 2004;11:265-85.
[50] Realmuto GM, Ruble LA. Sexual behaviors in autism: Problems of definition and management. J Autism Dev Disord 1999;29:121-7.
[51] Henault I. Asperger syndrome and sexuality. London: Kingsley, 2006.
[52] Hellemans H, Deboutte D. Autism spectrum disorders and sexuality. Presentation to the World Autism Congress, Melbourne, 2002.
[53] Greydanus DE, Omar HA. Sexuality issues and gynecologic care of adolescents with developmental disabilities. Pediatr Clin North Am 2008;55:1315-35.
[54] Stokes MA, Kaur A. High functioning autism and sexuality. Autism 2005;9:266-89.
[55] Hall DK, Mathews F, Pearce, J. Factors associated with sexual behavior problems in young sexually abused children. Child Abuse Negl 1998;22:10:1045-1063.
[56] Johnson TC, Friend C. Assessing young children's sexual behaviors in the context of child sexual abuse evaluations. In: Ney T, ed. True and false allegations of child sexual abuse: Assessment and case management. Philadelphia, PA: Brunner/Mazel, 1995:49-72.
[57] Friedrich WN. Psychological assessment of sexually abused children and their families. Thousand Oaks, CA: Sage, 2002.
[58] Ballard MB, Austin S. Forensic interviewing: special considerations for children and adolescents with mental retardation and developmental disabilities. Educ Train Dev Disabil 1999;34:521-5.
[59] Edelson-Goldberg M. Sexual abuse of children with autism: factors that increase risk and interfere with recognition of abuse. Disabil Stud Q 2010;30(1). URL: http://www.dsq-sds.org/article/view/1058/1228.htm.
[60] Dent H. The effects of age and intelligence on eyewitnessing ability. In: Dent H, Flin R, eds. Children as witnesses. Chichester: John Wiley, 1992:1-13.
[61] Cronch LE, Viljoen JL, Hansen DJ. Forensic interviewing in child sexual abuse cases: current techniques and future directions. Aggress Violent Behav 2006;11:195-207.
[62] Pithers WD, Gray A, Busconi A, Houchens P. Caregivers of children with sexual behavior problems: Psychological and familial functioning. Child Abuse Negl 1998;22:129-41.
[63] Tuzikow J. Responding to inappropriate sexual behaviors displayed by adolescents with autism spectrum disorders. URL: http://www.opwdd.ny.gov/ node/118.

[64] Allen J, Berliner L. Evidence-informed, individual treatment of a child with sexual behavior problems: a case study. Arch Sex Behav 2015;44:2323-2331.
[65] Gray CA, Garand J. Social Stories: improving responses of students with autism with accurate social information. Focus Autistic Behav 1993;8:1-10.
[66] Reynhout G, Carter M. Social stories for children with disabilities. J Autism Dev Disord 2006;36:445-69.
[67] Ali S, Frederickson N. Investigating the evidence base of social stories. Educ Psychol Pract 2006;22:355-77.
[68] McLay L, Carnett A, Tyler-Merrick G, Van der Meer L. A systematic review of interventions for inappropriate sexual behavior of children with adolescents with developmental disabilities. Rev J Autism Dev Disord 2015;2:357-73.
[69] Lumley VA, Miltenberger RG. Sexual abuse prevention for persons with mental retardation. Am J Ment Retard 1997;101:459-72.
[70] Children with sexual behavior problems. TDMHSAS best practice duidelines, 2007. URL: https://tn.gov/ assets/entities/behavioralhealth/attachments/.
[71] O'Malley K, Rich S. Clinical implications of a link between fetal alcohol spectrum disorders (FASD) and autism or Asperger's disorder. A neurodevelopmental frame for helping understand and management. In: Fitzgerald M, ed. Recent advances in autism spectrum disorders, vol 1. Rijeka, Croatia: INTECH, 2013. URL: http://dx.doi.org/10.5772/54924.
[72] Balazs T. Review of effective interventions for socially inappropriate masturbation in persons with cognitive disabilities. Sex Disabil 2006;24:151-68.
[73] Koller Rebecca. Sexuality and adolescents with autism. Sex Disabil 2000;18:125-35.
[74] Chaffin M. Our minds are made up-don't confuse us with the facts: commentary on policies concerning children with sexual behavior problems and juvenile sex offenders. Child Maltreat 2008;1:110-121.

Submitted: August 10, 2016. *Revised:* September 01, 2016. *Accepted:* September 05, 2016.

In: Alternative Medicine Research Yearbook 2017
Editor: Joav Merrick
ISBN: 978-1-53613-726-2
© 2018 Nova Science Publishers, Inc.

Chapter 34

CHILDREN WITH MEDICAL COMPLEXITY: NEGLECT, ABUSE, AND CHALLENGES

Alex Okun[*], *MD*

New Alternatives for Children, New York, New York, US

ABSTRACT

This review on recognizing and responding to suspected maltreatment of children with medical complexity is organized around several questions: 1) What is meant by the term, "children with medical complexity?" Does this term represent something distinct from "children with special health care needs," or "children who are medically fragile?" 2) What constitutes medical neglect of children with medical complexity? How can it be distinguished from expected and reasonable shortcomings in the care that can realistically be provided to a child? 3) How can health care providers recognize instances of "medical child abuse" in which the harm results from interventions that health care providers undertake in response to exaggerated or fabricated reports from parents or other family caregivers? 4) What are some of the challenges facing mandated reporters and members of the health care and case planning teams in recognizing and responding to suspected medical neglect or abuse of children with medical complexity?

Keywords: children, disability, special needs, abuse, neglect, medical neglect

INTRODUCTION

In this review our knowledge about recognizing and responding to suspected maltreatment of children with medical complexity is discussed. There are many challenges facing mandated reporters and members of the health care and case planning teams in recognizing and responding to suspected medical neglect or abuse in this population, beginning with its definition. The term "children with medical complexity" has been variously defined and

---

[*] Correspondence: Alex Okun, MD, Medical Director, New Alternatives for Children, 37 West 26th Street, New York, NY 10010, United States. E-mail: aokun@nackidscan.org.

refers to a subset of "children with special health care needs," many of whom are also considered to be "medically fragile." What constitutes medical neglect of children with medical complexity is also poorly defined, as it can be difficult to distinguish from expected and reasonable shortcomings in the care that can realistically be provided to a child. It can be especially challenging for health care providers to recognize instances of "medical child abuse" in which the harm results from interventions that health care providers undertake in response to exaggerated or fabricated reports from parents or other family caregiver.

Fictional case histories of two children ("Angel" and "Robin") are presented to illustrate issues that arise when maltreatment is suspected in children with medical complexity. These three-part vignettes are complicated and lengthy, in keeping with the nature of biomedical, psychosocial and care coordination needs of children with medical complexity, but they highlight the important issues for this especially vulnerable population.

The case of Angel, part I of III

Angel was a 34 month old born at 24 weeks' gestation, weighing 650 gm (1 lb., 7 oz.). The mother's early pregnancy was complicated by alcohol and cocaine use before she became aware that she was pregnant. Several years prior, her two oldest children, now adults, had been placed in foster care following police reports of domestic violence and allegations against the mother that she was engaging in commercial sex work. Angel's mother and father lived together with their healthy 3 year-old.

Angel required respiratory support for the first six months of life. Most of the intestines had to be surgically removed due to necrotizing enterocolitis (a severe inflammatory or infectious condition affecting the GI tract), resulting in a gastrostomy, jejunostomy and colostomy (in which the intestinal contents drain through holes, or ostomies, created in the abdominal wall) and dependence on parenteral (intravenous) nutrition.

Shortly after the first birthday, Angel was discharged from the neonatal intensive care unit with the diagnoses of short bowel syndrome (in which too little of the intestines remain to meet a person's overall nutritional needs), liver disease associated with parenteral nutrition, and chronic lung disease of prematurity (also known as broncho-pulmonary dysplasia). Prior to discharge, the mother demonstrated what were judged to be good skills meeting Angel's special needs. The home care regimen included supplemental oxygen, parenteral nutrition, trophic enteral feeds (a slow trickle of formula fed continuously into the stomach in order to promote intestinal growth), and nine medications, each given once to four times daily. State Medicaid authorized 40 hours per week of private duty nursing services to be provided in the home.

What is meant by the term "children with medical complexity?"

The literature on classification of "children with special health care needs" includes a vast body of work in the fields of policy, advocacy and research. A long list of terms, such as "children with chronic conditions," "children who are medically fragile" and "children with medical complexity," has been used to describe and classify children that are the focus of this chapter. Some of these terms are listed in Table 1.

Most early research on psychological and social outcomes of children with chronic health conditions was conducted on groups of children with identical or similar disorders (e.g., reports of depressive symptoms among adolescents with cystic fibrosis or of body image among children with inflammatory bowel disease). From the research of Stein (1, 2) and others (3) the needs of families and children living with chronic health conditions were shown to be quite similar across a broad range of diagnoses (e.g., service gaps in common among children with diabetes, hemophilia, severe asthma, or cerebral palsy and their families, or psychological and financial impact on caregivers and children living with these conditions) (1-3).

"Children with special health care needs" are defined as those who are at "increased risk for chronic physical, developmental, behavioral or emotional condition(s)" and "require health and related services of a type or amount beyond those required of children generally" (4). This conceptualization, referred to as a "non-categorical definition," led to transformation of the processes used to determine eligibility for Social Security/Disability benefits, based previously on whether the conditions of children applying for coverage could be found on lists of qualifying diagnoses.

Table 1. Terms used to refer to children with special health care needs, or the chronic conditions with which they live, over the past five decades

Time	Term
Pre 1970s	Crippled (or handicapped) children Chronic illness or disease Disabled children
1970s	Chronically ill children
1980s	Chronic conditions Technology-dependent (later, technology-assisted) children Children with chronic physical, developmental, behavioral or emotional conditions Children with special needs Children (or children and youth) with special health care needs Medically complex children
1990s	Children with significant disabilities Condition (proposed to replace the terms, "illness," "disease," "disorder," "disability," "impairment," "handicap") Children/persons with developmental disabilities/intellectual disabilities Complex medical needs
2000s	Medically fragile children Functional limitations Children with medical complexity Complex chronic conditions Complex needs Complex health conditions Significant chronic conditions

Increased attention has been directed more recently to the needs of "children with medical complexity," those with the most complicated chronic conditions, and to those of their families. Inquiry has been focused on ways to improve the care they receive, enhance the quality of their lives and reduce health care costs. Some of this research, conducted using administrative datasets drawn from large population groups, has given rise to new terms and conceptualizations such as, "significant chronic conditions," and subgroups of "chronic conditions" classified as "dominant," "moderate," "minor," "catastrophic" and "malignant" (5-7). Definitions of terms used most commonly in reference to children with special health care needs appear in Table 2.

Table 2. Definitions of a sample of terms used to refer to children with a variety of special health care needs and their conditions

Chronic health condition: Any medical condition that can be reasonably expected to last at least 12 months (unless death intervenes) and to involve either several different organ systems or 1 organ system severely enough to require specialty pediatric care and probably some period of hospitalization in a tertiary care center (3).

Children with special health care needs: Those who have or are at increased risk for a chronic physical, developmental, behavioral, or emotional condition and who also require health and related services of a type or amount beyond that required by children generally (4).

Technology-dependent: Refers to need for support by technology for basic life function (e.g., a feeding tube, tracheostomy, ventilator, dialysis unit).

Technology-assisted: Refers to support by technology that provides compensation for lost function but is not essential for survival (e.g., power wheelchair chair or assistive communication device).

Children who are medically fragile: High morbidity and mortality, require extensive nursing care in the home in order to prevent death or worsening disability, and depend on skilled supportive services, often technology-based, to support fundamental organ function (24).

Functional status differences, per the ICF Classification scheme (25):
- *impairment:* When specific body system or body part's functioning are impacted
- *activity limitation:* When a whole individual's function is impacted, resulting in difficulty doing basic tasks
- *participation restriction*: When an individual is unable to fully engage in life events

Children with medical complexity (12): Those who have chronic conditions, functional limitations, high health care use and medical fragility and intensive care needs that are not easily met by existing health care models. This definition incorporates:
- characteristic chronic and severe conditions;
- substantial family-identified service needs;
- functional limitations; and
- high health care resource use, involving:
  - intensive hospital and or community based service need;
  - reliance on technology, polypharmacy and or home or congregate care to maintain basic quality of life;
  - risk of frequent or prolonged hospitalizations; and/or elevated need for care coordination

While children with medical complexity make up less than 1% of the pediatric population, their health care needs have been estimated to consume up to one third of the costs of health care for children in the United States (8). They are considered to be at extremely high risk for complications and challenges in the domains of physical, developmental and psychosocial well-being. Families of children with medical complexity report spending substantial time each week on care coordination and direct home care (9). Most experience significant financial difficulties, find that a family member must leave their job in order to care for the child, and report challenges accessing non-medical services for their children (10).

A consensus definition for "children with medical complexity" is still evolving. Several tools have been developed and validated to identify individual children with special health care needs (11), but no valid and reliable instrument has been published to classify children as having medical complexity.

The case of Angel, part II of III

During the first year and a half at home, Angel was hospitalized over a dozen times and made many more emergency department visits for suspected bloodstream infections; skin breakdown around the ostomies; diarrhea and weight loss; catheter obstruction, fracture or dislodgement; and exacerbations of chronic lung disease. Members of the health care teams involved recognized that these episodes of illness compromised Angel's nutritional status and overall well-being were but were not surprised by their frequent occurrence, given the degree of medical complexity. They were primarily concerned that liver disease associated with long-term use of parenteral nutrition was worsening and would lead to liver failure.

Staff at the hospital also wondered whether Angel's poor weight gain and some of the complications involving the central venous catheter could have been averted had more skilled care been provided in the home. They were aware that the family experienced poverty and other psychosocial stressors but did not understand them in depth, as Angel's mother preferred not to discuss them. They were reassured by evidence of the mother's bond to Angel and her attendance at most outpatient appointments. Some described the status of Angel's care as situated chronically in a "grey zone," in which reports of medical neglect could have been justified on any of a number of occasions but were strongly indicated on none of them.

Emerging neurodevelopmental problems included expressive language delays, spastic diplegia (a common type of cerebral palsy, predominantly affecting the legs) and myopia (nearsightedness). Angel was prescribed corrective lenses to prevent the development of amblyopia (permanent vision impairment). After the second birthday, Angel was referred to a special preschool with capacity to serve children with complex medical needs, where a variety of therapies could be provided.

After a few months, staff at the school became concerned when they noticed that Angel was arriving at school in diapers and clothes that appeared not to have been changed recently, and without glasses. Some days, Angel arrived over an hour late. The school sent home supplies of diapers and donated clothes and asked that the mother bring the glasses to school, where they could be stored in the classroom for Angel to wear there. The school social worker attempted to ensure that Angel's mother could access federal, state and community based entitlements (such as SSI/Disability, WIC, food stamps and public assistance) and other supportive services, as had social workers at the hospital.

Two months later, Angel came to school one day without a sufficient supply of parenteral nutrition or formula. The following week, the central venous catheter dressing was discovered detached and soiled when Angel arrived. At a meeting held at the school, the mother was noted to have facial bruises and injury to the front teeth. She acknowledged suffering with depression and having had a physical altercation with Angel's father. She asked that the school keep this confidential, lest her family face eviction from a landlord to whom she owed back rent and who did not want law enforcement officials visiting the home.

The first in a series of reports to state child protective services was made by the school. Angel eventually stopped attending the school altogether. When local child protective service workers visiting the home noted Angel to be malodorous and dehydrated, Angel was admitted to the hospital for stabilization. From the hospital, Angel was discharged to foster care.

Angel's case meets all the criteria for medical complexity proposed by Cohen et al. (12). Several chronic and severe conditions existed, the most significant of which were consequences of short bowel syndrome: progressive liver disease, nutritional compromise and poor wound healing, among others. Substantial family-identified service needs included extreme poverty; threats to safety, housing and permanency; maternal depression and possible substance use disorder; and support from home care services that fell short of meeting Angel's needs. Angel had functional limitations, which though significant, were far less severe than they are for many children with medical complexity. A large proportion of children with medical complexity have severe neurological impairment resulting in intellectual disability, irritability, chronic pain, epilepsy, feeding difficulties, progressive lung disease and musculoskeletal disorders. Angel's care consumed extensive health care resources, the final criterion proposed by Cohen et al. (12).

Health care professionals and staff at the school were concerned that Angel's medical needs were not being met consistently. At many junctures in Angel's life at home, the failure to provide needed medical care could have been considered medical neglect.

What constitutes medical neglect of children with medical complexity?

Medical maltreatment or neglect was first defined in the US in a revision of the Child Abuse Prevention and Treatment Act of 1974 (CAPTA) simply as, "failure to provide adequate medical care." It was considered reportable to state child protective service agencies when it was associated with "harm or significant risk of harm" to the child (13). Specific definitions and processes for responding to reports of medical neglect were left to the states to develop. Through 2011, eleven of the fifty states had done so, most choosing broad descriptions such as "failure to provide needed medical or mental health care" (14).

Children with medical complexity experience elevated risk of maltreatment and medical neglect, as do children with disabilities generally. This can occur in the form of omission of or inconsistent adherence with important regimens of medications, feeds, therapies or use of technologies; a level of supervision at home that is unreliable or inadequate to assure safety; lack of regular follow up with primary or subspecialty medical care; dental neglect; and excessive school absences.

When Angel was brought to school with soiled clothes and diapers, it posed no significant harm or threat to health, although it was recognized as a sign of stressors in the household or the mother's life. School staff appreciated that Angel's mother experienced numerous barriers to meeting Angel's care needs more consistently and felt that she tried as hard as she could to do so. The proposal to store Angel's glasses in the classroom was thought to be a good compromise solution to one unmet need.

When Angel arrived with inadequate supplies of parenteral nutrition or formula, or with the entrance site of the central venous catheter exposed and vulnerable to infection, staff at the school felt that there was significant risk of harm. As mandated reporters, they acted accordingly to notify child protective services of suspected medical neglect.

In the year before preschool enrollment, Angel and the mother had extensive contact with a number of health professionals and teams providing outpatient, emergency and inpatient care. These individuals and groups regarded the consequences of Angel's short bowel syndrome as substantial. They felt, as did staff at the school, that Angel's mother was trying as hard as she could to care for her child.

The remainder of this chapter is devoted to challenges faced by health care providers, families and social service workers when medical neglect of children with medical complexity is suspected. First, we will look at a special subtype of medical complexity in which numerous serious disorders are believed to exist in a child but the truth is more complicated.

The case of Robin, part I of III

Robin was a 5 year old who, as an infant, had been admitted frequently to "Children's Hospital" for suspected intestinal dysmotility (slowed intestinal peristalsis), weight loss, and accounts of irregular breathing observed in the home during sleep. The mother had reported episodes at home, none witnessed by emergency responders, when she had found Robin pale or blue, and either limp or posturing. Physicians were concerned that these might represent manifestations of epilepsy, metabolic or mitochondrial disease (dysfunctions at the level of the body's cells or systems of energy production) or a central disorder of the control of respiration (a functional deficit, originating in the brain, leading to inadequate breathing). Work-ups included extensive imaging studies and analyses of blood, urine and spinal fluid; numerous EEGs; invasive procedures involving the GI tract; and biopsies of skin, muscle and rectum.

At the time, Robin's mother was regarded by hospital staff as an educated and reliable reporter, usually to be found at the bedside. They empathized with her frustration at not having found an answer to Robin's instability at home. Despite negative studies, Robin was treated with antacids, pro-motility agents (drugs to promote peristalsis), anti-epileptic drugs and an array of special formulas. Eventually these were fed by nasogastric tube, followed by the creation of a gastrostomy to assure adequate nutrition.

The family moved out of state when Robin was 16 months old and returned when Robin was 5. The mother reported that in the interim, the diagnosis of intestinal dysmotility had been confirmed, and that severe constipation had developed. Robin had also been found to have a low-lying brainstem (known as Chiari malformation) and possible hydrocephalus (accumulation of excess spinal fluid in and around the brain). Two surgical procedures were performed urgently in which portions of bone were removed from the base of the skull to alleviate any impact this could be having respiration (which is driven by a center in the brainstem), followed by placement of a ventriculoperitoneal shunt (a catheter tunneled underneath the skin that allows excess cerebrospinal fluid to drain into the abdomen). The shunt had been revised or replaced emergently several times in response to complaints of recurrent headache that were accompanied, on occasion, by breathing pauses observed at home.

At the time of return to Children's Hospital, Robin was being given two anti-epileptic medications, two antacids, continuous feeds of an elemental (non-allergenic) formula 20 hours per day through a gastrojejunostomy tube (a long, thin tube threaded through a gastrostomy, ending in the small intestine), two medications to alleviate constipation, and a low dose of corticosteroids for possible adrenal insufficiency (an endocrine disorder that, unrecognized, can lead to dehydration and shock). The mother reported that Robin had developed allergies to wheat, soy, eggs, cow's milk protein, acetaminophen, morphine, diphenhydramine, hydroxizine (both antihistamines), senna, docusate (both treatments for constipation) and several brands of adhesive tape and dressings.

The mother expressed frustration that the constipation remained refractory to medical treatment, because she felt that this worsened the dysmotility. She was worried that Robin would eventually require parenteral nutrition. She inquired about the creation of a colostomy to permit irrigation of the colon as another means to address the constipation. She asked that once the state-based insurance was active, Robin be prescribed a pulse oximeter so that in the event that Robin's breathing slowed during sleep (and the blood oxygen level dropped), an alarm would sound and awaken her. The team learned that she had moved out of state years before to escape a relationship with Robin's father that was characterized by violence and controlling behaviors, and that each time he learned of their new whereabouts, she and Robin would move to a different address.

How can health care providers recognize instances of "medical child abuse?"

Now 40 years since the classic case reports by Meadow (15), what was then labeled "Munchausen Syndrome by Proxy" has come to be re-conceptualized in ways that emphasize recognizing and acting on suspicions that the child is a victim of "medical child abuse" (16-18). The terms "factitious disorder" and "caregiver fabricated illness" have been proposed in recent years to replace, "Munchausen syndrome by proxy" but the original label remains in common use.

In cases of "medical child abuse," the "instruments" or "vehicles" of the abuse are the health care providers. Based on reports of serious concerns that, unbeknownst to them, are invented or exaggerated by a parent or one or more family caregivers, they feel compelled to order invasive studies and treatments, often repeatedly (16). Why do providers find themselves colluding, unintentionally, in this abuse?

Routine medical care for children is based in the assumption that reports provided by parents or other family caregivers are honest and as accurate as possible. This is particularly important when the information provided has critical implications for the child's well-being. This assumption is part of an unspoken "contract" between provider and parent or other family caregiver, more of which will be explored in the next section of this chapter. As in other forms of child maltreatment, when medical child abuse is occurring, this contract has in effect been broken, something that is often hard to recognize.

Medical child abuse is among the most covert forms of child maltreatment. The concerns expressed by parents or family caregivers are typically believable and deeply concerning. In Robin's case, each of the neurosurgical interventions performed during the time away from Children's Hospital took place in an atmosphere of crisis following reports by the mother of portentous signs and symptoms that were not documented or observed by medical personnel.

Health care providers may be astonished when parents or other family caregivers who have been regarded as loyal, persistent, courageous, even heroic advocates for their very sick children are revealed to have been deceitful and, in effect, seduced providers into enacting the abuse in the form of medical procedures. At interdisciplinary team conferences convened to discuss the possibility that medical child abuse is taking place in the care of a particular patient, it is not uncommon for one member of the care team to object vehemently to the proposed explanation, being offended by the suggestion by other members of the team that the reports of deeply concerning signs and symptoms did not require intervention.

Medical providers are trained to be vigilant for potentially serious signs and symptoms and act expeditiously to assure that important diagnoses or complications are not missed. Invasive tests or procedures may be recommended, "just to be on the safe side." Physicians may also be worried about the consequences of a missed diagnosis and their liability in the event that the family brings legal action against them. The irony in these situations is that many decisions made in the care of children experiencing medical child abuse serve to perpetuate the abuse, rather than ensuring their safety.

The performance of procedures and studies continues to be rewarded in most settings today on a fee-for-service basis. No empiric study has been published into the extent to which this may influence physicians' decision making in the care of children with medical complexity and promote further invasive interventions.

When providers are asked to investigate worrisome complaints about a childlike Robin but feel it would be better to avoid intervening further, they may worry that saying "no" to the family will provoke confrontation or lead the family to transfer the child's care elsewhere (16). When the possibility of medical child abuse is being considered, providers are urged to follow many of the same steps, listed in Table 3, that are indicated in caring for other children who are suspected as having been maltreated. Hospitalization may be required. Restricting access the family or certain caregivers are permitted to have to the child can generate conflict. There is a role for covert video surveillance in the diagnostic investigation of some cases of suspected medical child abuse. Hospitals should have established policies and procedures in place whenever this is considered. Despite the most careful and fair implementation processes, covert video surveillance, if exposed, can lead to backlash on the family's part and even create additional risk to the child (19).

Table 3. Medical child abuse: Steps needed (16)

- Identify that the abuse has occurred
- Stop the abuse from occurring
- Provide for ongoing safety of the child
- Treat the physical consequences of the abuse
- Treat the psychological consequences of the abuse
- Try to maintain integrity of the family

The case of Robin, part II of III

At age 5, Robin appeared thin but otherwise well, with surgical scars and the shunt and tube described. Robin preferred not to leave the mother's side and did not speak to members of the team at Children's Hospital. After a series of requests for medical records from the medical center where Robin was treated out of state, the team found chart notes indicating that Robin was believed to have severe constipation, but likely not intestinal dysmotility. They saw that extensive assessments of brain anatomy and intracranial pressure had never been definitively abnormal, even though the neurosurgical procedures had in fact been performed. The mother had expressed concerns for multiple allergies and adrenal insufficiency, but testing had been performed and the disorders "ruled out." Because Robin's mother had continued to request that investigations and treatment be pursued for what she maintained were multiple disorders in spite of repeated reviews of study results and attempts at reassurance, she was suspected of "Munchausen Syndrome by Proxy." The providers at that medical center made a state child protective services report.

The care team at Children's Hospital was now faced with arriving at consensus as to whether some or all of the concerns for Robin's health had been invented by the mother, leading to invasive and burdensome interventions by medical providers, including members of their own team some 4 years previously. It sought to decide what actions to recommend now that would help Robin avoid a potentially unnecessary procedure like the requested colostomy or intensification of monitoring at home, and still promote the opportunity to re-establish a therapeutic relationship with Robin's mother.

What are some of the challenges facing mandated reporters and members of the health care and case planning teams in recognizing and responding to suspected medical neglect or abuse of children with medical complexity?

Investigating cases of suspected medical child abuse or medical neglect is threatening to families and challenging for all professionals involved. Health care professionals and other mandated reporters face significant moral, ethical and practical challenges throughout the process of child welfare involvement for children with medical complexity and their families. These challenges may arise long before a state child protective service report is called in, during an extended period, like the "grey zone" described by some of Angel's providers, when reports of medical neglect would be justified but there are other interventions that seem preferable to try first.

Amidst the many uncertainties that characterize decision-making in the care of children with medical complexity, health professionals and other mandated reporters may question whether their suspicions of neglect are justified. The ways that these doubts can lead to repeated, potentially harmful interventions by health care providers are described in the previous section of this chapter on medical child abuse.

Children with medical complexity and their families often have long-lasting, close relationships with members of the health care team that are characterized by mutual loyalty, honesty, commitment and respect. Health professionals may feel that making a child protective services report represents a betrayal of that relationship, particularly when there are feelings of affection for the parent or other family caregivers.

Removal from the family household is among the most painful consequences for any child and family involved in investigation of suspected maltreatment. Parents and other family caregivers may feel unjustly accused by the very care team on which they relied for their child's life-sustaining care; vulnerable by virtue of the limited capacity of some child protective service workers to appreciate the complexities of their child's needs and family stressors; helpless in court systems in which decisions can seem arbitrary and inconsistent; and susceptible to prejudice and discrimination by systems of medical care, child protective services, law enforcement and the courts.

Providers are aware of these foreseeable harms to the child and family. Based on past experience, they may anticipate that child protective service involvement is unlikely to lead to positive change or benefit to the child. They feel committed first to find ways to address unmet needs and improve care for the child and may defer or postpone making child protective service reports.

The time and effort required of health care providers to be involved in child protection work for children with medical complexity can be enormous, generally unreimbursed, and characterized by redundancy, uncertainty, and frustration. Many physicians are reluctant to give deposition or testify in court proceedings, given the challenges recalling precise details of remote events and facing hostile cross-examination. Child protective service workers and legal professionals often struggle to comprehend the concerns for medical neglect or medical child abuse in children with disorders of which they understand little. They carry large and challenging caseloads and experience pressure for casework to come to closure quickly. They typically work with children and families with needs that are far more common and easily understood than the nuances of suspected medical neglect of children with rare and complex conditions. They commonly experience difficulty reaching involved physicians, obtaining their full participation in the investigatory process, deciphering confusing accounts of diagnoses and treatments, and retaining physicians' ongoing involvement in case planning activities.

Families with stronger socioeconomic, social and family support systems are best equipped to handle the overwhelming needs of care at home for children with medical complexity. They are more likely than families living in poverty to have the resources to afford the needed time off from work; enlist the help of family and other members of their social network; overcome barriers to transportation and care for their other children that would otherwise impede availability to attend numerous outpatient appointments; and advocate effectively with health care organizations, suppliers, insurers, education systems and other agencies and programs charged with supporting care at home for their children with medical complexity.

Other families may not have such assets to call on in times of need. Disparities persist in access to care and quality of care provided to children living in poverty and those who are members of racial and ethnic minority groups. Children identified as African-American or multiracial made up 25% of those in foster care in 2014, a significant overrepresentation relative to the population distribution of the United States (20). Aware of these inequities, providers must be mindful of any component of implicit bias that may be operant during the decision making process around initiating child protective service involvement.

Taken together, these experiences, disincentives and sensitivities may discourage some health care professionals from reporting suspected medical neglect of children with medical complexity. Independent of their legal obligation, physicians have ethical and professional commitments to report suspected medical neglect. These include minimizing the risk of harm, present and future, and doing all that is feasible to maximize the chances of best outcomes in the child's health, quality of life and, in some instances, survival.

Sensitive, respectful and responsible work with families requires that health care professionals take steps to interpret caregivers' actions in the context of culturally based health beliefs and practices. They need to take into account the impact that poverty, family chaos, limited health-related knowledge and distrust of the health care system can have on care that the family is able to provide (21). Beyond recognizing and treating the biomedical complexities of their patients, they have an obligation to address problems related to violence, substance use disorders, mental health problems and other life stressors that impair the capacity of families to care optimally for their children with medical complexity (22, 23).

In some settings, state and local child protective service systems have developed collaborations with groups of committed and qualified pediatric medical providers in children's hospitals or across communities, or with private, non-profit child welfare organizations that have expertise in work with children with a range of special health care needs and their families. At one such organization based in New York City, master's level social workers serve as case planners for children with special health care needs and families who are involved in foster care, prevention, aftercare programs and other initiatives. Restricted caseloads permit intensive, community-based work with each child's medical, educational and other service providers, and with the parent's, family caregivers' and other children's providers of medical and mental health and community based services. Casework is conducted in collaboration with agency-based team professionals who have expertise in pediatric complex care, pediatric nursing, child and adult psychiatry, psychotherapy, psycho-educational and developmental evaluation, educational advocacy, recreation and creative arts. Contracted payments for casework and reimbursement for the pediatric medical and mental health services provided fall far short of supporting such resource-intensive services. Long-term sustainability remains dependent on private and government grant provision and charitable support.

The case of Robin, part III of III

The team at Children's Hospital came to consensus not to grant Robin's mother's request to create a colostomy for irrigation. It offered to hospitalize Robin electively for the purposes of an extensive multispecialty work up involving possible sleep study, video EEG recording, motility studies, allergy testing, definitive relief of constipation and potential food challenges. Contact with the mother was subsequently lost. A state child protective service report was made, but the family could not be located at their address and other means of contact on record.

The case of Angel, part III of III

Angel was placed in care with a foster parent who had retired from work as a nurse in a pediatric intensive care unit and had cared in her home for several children who were assisted by technology. Formula feedings were advanced. Angel gained weight well, the abdominal wounds healed, and parenteral nutrition was weaned over the course of the next six months. The liver disease resolved.

Angel's mother engaged in mental health services, renewed an order of protection against Angel's father and was assisted in securing affordable housing. She made consistent and reassuring visits with Angel, supervised at first, then progressing to overnight visits in her new home. She cared effectively and safely for Angel during these stays and met all other goals of the service plan. Angel was returned to her care after 16 months in foster care and continued to gain weight, even after skilled nursing services were curtailed. Angel was not readmitted to the hospital.

CONCLUSION

Children with medical complexity comprise a small proportion of the population of children in the United States yet require immense expenditures to provide ongoing, costly, specialized multidisciplinary care to ensure their survival and optimal health outcomes and quality of life. When they are suspected as being subject to medical neglect or medical child abuse, the level of involvement required of members of health care, educational and social service teams is extensive, complex, largely unreimbursed and fraught with challenges for the professionals involved. The development of innovative, collaborative interventions demands a support, expertise, creativity and teamwork to an extent that exceeds what has generally been available in order to address successfully the profound medical and social complexities involved.

REFERENCES

[1] Stein RE. To be or not to be noncategorical. J Dev Behav Pediatr 1996;17:36-7.
[2] Stein RE, Bauman LJ, Westbrook LE, Coupey SM, Ireys HT. Framework for identifying children who have chronic conditions: The case for a new definition. J Pediatr 1993;122:342-7.
[3] Perrin EC, Newacheck P, Pless IB, et al. Issues involved in the definition and classification of chronic health conditions. Pediatrics 1993;91:787-93.
[4] McPherson M, Arango P, Fox H, Lauver C, McManus M et al. A new definition of children with special health care needs. Pediatrics 1998;102:137-40.
[5] Neff JN, Sharp VL, Muldoon J, Graham J, Popalisky J, Gay JC. Identifying and classifying children with chronic conditions using administrative data with the clinical risk group classification system. Amb Pediatr 2002;2:71-9.
[6] Feudtner CF, Feinstein JA, Zhong W, Hall M, Dai D. Pediatric complex chronic conditions classification system version 2: Updated for ICD-10 and complex medical technology dependence and transplantation. BMC Pediatr 2014;14:199-205.
[7] Simon T, Cawthon ML, Stanford S, Popalisky J, Lyons D, Woodcox B, et al. Pediatric Medical complexity Algorith: A new method to stratify children by medical complexity. Pediatrics 2014;113:e1647-54.

[8] Berry JG, Hall M, Neff J, et al. Children with medical complexity and Medicaid: Spending and cost savings. Health Aff (Millwood) 2014;33(12):2199-206.

[9] Feudtner CF, Christakis DA, Connell FA. Pediatric deaths attributable to complex chronic conditions: A population-based study of Washington State, 1980-1997. Pediatrics 2000;106:205-9.

[10] Kuo DZ, Cohen E, Agarwar R, Berry JG, Casey PH. A national profile of caregiver challenges among more medically complex children with special health care needs. Arch Pediatr Adolesc Med 2011;165(11):1020-6.

[11] Van der Lee JH, Mokkink LB, Grootenhuis MA, Heymans HS, Offringa M. Definitions and measurement of chronic health conditions in childhood: A systematic review. JAMA 2007;297(24):2741-51.

[12] Cohen E, Kuo DZ, Agrawal R, Berry JG, Bhagat SKM, et al. Children with medical complexity: An emerging population for clinical and research initiatives. Pediatrics 2011;127:529-38.

[13] American Academy of Pediatrics (AAP) Committee on Bioethics. Conflicts between religious or spiritual beliefs and pediatric care: Informed refusal, exemptions and public funding. Pediatrics 2013;132:962-5.

[14] Casey Family Programs State Welfare Policy Database. Medical Neglect specifically defined in statute. URL: http://www.childwelfarepolicy.org/maps/single?id=144.

[15] Meadow R. Munchausen Syndrome by Proxy: The hinterland of child abuse. Lancet 1977;310:343-5.

[16] Roesler TA, Jenny C. Medical child abuse: Beyond Munchausen syndrome by proxy. Elk Grove Village, IL: American Academy of Pediatrics, 2009.

[17] Flaherty EG, Macmillan HL, AAP Committee on Child Abuse and Neglect. Caregiver-fabricated illness in a child: A manifestation of child maltreatment. Pediatrics 2013;132(7):590-7.

[18] Bass C, Glaser D. Early recognition and management of fabricated or induced illness in children. Lancet 2014; 383:1412-21.

[19] Fisher MA. Caring for abused children. Pediatr Rev 2011;32(7):e73-8.

[20] US Department of Health & Human Services, Administration for Children and Families, Administration on Children, Youth and Families, Children's Bureau. Child maltreatment 2014. Washington, DC: Author, 2016. URL: http://www.acf. hhs.gov/programs/cb/research-data-technology/statistics-research/child-maltreatment.

[21] Jenny C, Committee on Child Abuse and Neglect. Recognizing and responding to medical neglect. Pediatrics 2007;120(6):1385-9.

[22] Palusci VJ, Haney ML. Strategies to prevent child maltreatment and integration into practice. APSAC Advisor 2010 (Winter):8-17.

[23] American Professional Society on the Abuse of Children. Practice Guidelines: Integrating prevention into the work of child maltreatment professionals. Columbus, OH: Author, 2010.

[24] Law M, Rosenbaum P. Service coordination for children and youth with complex needs. Hamilton, ON, Canada: Can Child Centre for Childhood Disability Research, McMaster University, 2004.

[25] World Health Organization. International classification of functioning, disability and health (ICF). URL: URL:http://www.who.int/classifications/icf/en/.

Submitted: August 15, 2016. *Revised:* September 05, 2016. *Accepted:* September 08, 2016.

Chapter 35

CHILDREN WITH DISABILITIES: LEGAL ISSUES IN CHILD WELFARE CASES

Frank E Vandervort, JD and Joshua B Kay, PhD, JD*
University of Michigan Law School, Ann Arbor, Michigan, US

ABSTRACT

In this review we examine the legal framework applicable when child maltreatment and disability intersect. It begins with a brief description of the constitutional foundation for parent-child-state relations. It provides an overview of relevant federal child welfare laws, which today shape each state's child protection system. It then considers the application of various federal laws governing work with children and families when a child has a disability. In doing so, we consider the Americans with Disabilities Act, the Individuals with Disabilities Education Act, and Section 504 of the Rehabilitation Act, and we touch upon Social Security benefits for children. This review does not examine child well-being legislation that establishes and funds programs such as Temporary Assistance to Needy Families (TANF), Supplemental Nutrition Assistance Program (SNAP), or publicly funded health care for children such as the State Children's Health Insurance Program.

Keywords: children, disability, welfare, legal

INTRODUCTION

According to the Census Bureau in the United States (US), approximately 2.8 million school-aged children (ages 5–17 years) have a disability (1). These disabilities range from physical to cognitive, sensory to emotional. Having a disability may place a child at higher risk for maltreatment. In turn, maltreatment may cause a child to have a disability, such as when a child suffers from an inflicted head injury. Inevitably, children with disabilities will come into

---

* Correspondence: Professor Frank Vandervort, University of Michigan Law School, 701 S. State Street, Ann Arbor, Michigan 48109, United States. E-mail: vort@umich.edu.

contact with the child protective system. Nationally each year, the confirmed cases of child maltreatment approach 1,000,000, which involve some 3,000,000 children. Among these are hundreds of thousands of children with disabilities and maltreatment in the US who will be involved in disparate legal proceedings designed for one or the other, but not both.

UNITED STATES CONSTITUTIONAL FRAMEWORK

The Constitution of the United States does not explicitly mention parents, children or families. For nearly a century, though, the Supreme Court has interpreted the Constitution to protect the rights of parents to raise their children and the rights of children to benefit from familial attachment free from interference by governmental authorities. At the same time, the Court has recognized a compelling governmental interest in protecting children from maltreatment at the hands of their parents, guardians or custodian. The establishment of these rights is rooted in the xenophobia surrounding World War I (2).

Before the advent of World War I, most states in the country protected the right of parents to educate their children in the language of their choice. During that war, however, a number of states enacted legislation requiring that public school children be taught in English, and prohibited educational lessons taught in other languages. The State of Nebraska enacted one such law in April 1919, which "made it a misdemeanor to teach any subject in a foreign language, or any foreign language as a subject" (2).

A year after the statute was enacted, a county attorney entered the classroom in Hampton, Nebraska, where Robert Meyer was teaching in German. Meyer was charged with violating the statute prohibiting the use of any foreign language when teaching school children. He was convicted of the misdemeanor and given the minimum fine provided by the law, $25. He appealed his conviction on grounds that the law prohibiting him from teaching in German violated his right to liberty under the Fourteenth Amendment to the Constitution, which provides that "No state shall ...deprive any person of life, liberty, or property without due process of law" (3). The Nebraska Supreme Court upheld his conviction, and he appealed to the US Supreme Court.

In 1923, the Court issued its opinion in the case. The Court acknowledged that it had "not attempted to define with exactness the liberty thus guaranteed" (3). However, the court noted,

> "Without doubt, it denotes . . . the right of the individual . . . to marry, establish a home and bring up children . . . and generally to enjoy those privileges long recognized at common law as essential to the orderly pursuit of happiness by free men" (3). Thus, the court observed, "it is the natural duty of the parent to give his children education suitable to their station in life" (3). Because the parents of Mr. Meyer's students possessed this "natural duty," they had a right, protected by the liberty clause of the Fourteenth Amendment, to engage Mr. Meyer to fulfill this responsibility. Although the court recognized the State "may do much, go very far...in order to improve the quality of its citizens, physically, mentally and morally...the individual has certain fundamental rights which must be respected" (3).

Two years later, in *Pierce v. Society of Sisters* (1925), the Court held that the fundamental right established in *Meyer* extended to a parent's right to choose to educate his or her children in non-public, religious or military schools (4). In doing so, the Court observed that "The child is not the mere creature of the State; those who nurture him and direct his destiny have the right, coupled with the high duty, to recognize and prepare him for additional obligations" (4). Together, the *Meyer* and *Pierce* cases established the fundamental right of a parent to direct the upbringing of his or her child without undue interference from governmental authorities.

In both *Meyer* and *Pierce*, however, the Court made clear that State authorities are not entirely without power to regulate schools or, more broadly, parents' choices in directing their children's upbringing. The limitations on a parent's right to direct their children's upbringing were addressed in 1944. Massachusetts had enacted certain child labor laws, which prohibited children of certain ages from engaging in certain activities. Sarah Prince was charged with violating the law when she permitted her two children and a third child over whom she had legal guardianship to sell religious pamphlets for $.05 on the streets of Brockton, Massachusetts. She was convicted of violating the law and appealed.

The case *Prince v Massachusetts* raised two issues related to the Constitutional right to liberty: 1) the right of a parent to direct a child's religious development; and 2) the right of the children to observe and participate his or her family's religious activities. In *Prince*, the Court more squarely articulated the sometimes adverse positions of the parent and the state vis-à-vis the child. The Court acknowledged both the parent's interest in raising her or his child without governmental interference and the right of the State, as the ultimate guardian of the child, to act to protect the child's welfare. The Court noted, "It is cardinal with us that the custody, care, and nurture of the child reside first in the parents" (5). But the Court went on to state that "the family is not beyond regulation in the public interest...neither the rights of religion nor rights of parenthood are beyond limitation. Acting to guard the general interest in youth's wellbeing, the state...may restrict the parent's control" in a number of ways, including by mandating school attendance and prohibiting child labor (5). Thus, the Court ruled, "the state has a wide range of power for limiting parental freedom and authority in things affecting the child's welfare" (5).

What of the rights of children relative to the rights of the state and the parents in this mix? The rights of children in this triangle of rights are somewhat less defined. Courts have, however, recognized that, generally speaking, parents and children have reciprocal rights. Parents have the right to raise their children as they see fit and children have the right to benefit from the day-to-day nurturing provided by parents and to their benevolent decision-making (6). That is, parents have the right to care, custody and control in raising of their children and children have the right to benefit from that care and concern. However, "the power of the parent...may be subject to limitation under *Prince* if it appears that parental decisions will jeopardize the health or safety of the child, or have a potential for significant social burdens" (7).

In subsequent years, the Supreme Court has applied this basic doctrine balancing the rights of parents and the rights of state authorities to familial living arrangements (8), medical and mental health decision-making (6), and whether a grandparent has the right to visit a child over the objections of the custodial parent (9). The rule that pertains from the Court's cases, read together, is that a fit parent, one who has not been found to have maltreated his or her child, has the right in the first instance to raise his or her child as he or she sees fit. Parents' rights are weakest when they have been shown to have maltreated their child.

CHILD MALTREATMENT AND THE UNITED STATES CONSTITUTION

The law begins with the presumption that a parent is fit and will, therefore, make parenting decisions that are in the best interests of her or his child. The Supreme Court has articulated the rationale for this presumption: "The law's concept of the family rests on the presumption that parents possess what a child lacks in maturity, experience and capacity for judgment required for making life's difficult decisions...[H]istorically, it has recognized that natural bonds of affection lead parents to act in the best interests of their children" (6). While the state may have a legitimate interest in separating a child from an abusive or neglectful (i.e., unfit) parent, the state has no legitimate interest in separating a child from a fit parent (10).

When one wishes to invoke the law in order to protect a child from parental neglect or abuse, that individual must assume the burden of demonstrating parental unfitness. In asserting the unfitness of a parent to parent his or her child, the law will not rest on presumptions, and the actual unfitness of the parent must be demonstrated (10). Thus, for example, where the State of Illinois enacted a law that presumed that all unmarried fathers were unfit to provide care and custody for their children upon the death of the child's mother and automatically took the children into the foster care system, the Court held the law to be an unconstitutional violation of the father's right to both equal protection of the law due process of law (10). Under the state's statutory scheme, a mother, a married father or a divorced father had the right to have a hearing at which state authorities were required to demonstrate the parent's unfitness before their children could be removed. The statute, however, allowed the state to remove children from their father if he had never married their mother on the theory that because most unwed fathers were unfit, the children of all these fathers could be removed. The Supreme Court struck down this law, requiring that state authorities demonstrate that the particular father at issue is unfit to care for his children.

Cases involving the fathers of children present some unique legal challenges. While a child's mother is known, and her rights established, at the time of birth, the identity of a child's father may be more difficult to ascertain, and determination of his rights more complicated. In *Lehr v. Robertson*, the Supreme Court was required to define the rights of a father who was not married to the child's mother and who had never established a relationship with his child (11). Because the father did not grasp the opportunity to parent his child, he did not have the same rights as a father who had grasped that opportunity. In short, a father must actually exercise his parental rights and attend to his parental responsibilities or he may be deprived of his rights more easily than a father who has asserted them.

While parents and children possess reciprocal rights in their relationship with one another and share an interest in the preservation of their family free from governmental interference (12), there is no absolute constitutional right to remain together as a family, and state authorities, acting on the orders of a court, may remove a child from an abusive or neglectful parent's custody (13). Once a state trial court finds that a parent is unfit, the State's "urgent interest" in protecting the child from harm prevails over the parent's right to care, custody and control of the child.

While child protective services caseworkers may act to protect a child from harm by seeking to remove him from abusive or neglectful parents, the state is under no obligation to do so. Thus, where children's protective services were involved with a family but failed to remove the child from the parent's custody, the child could not successfully sue the state authorities after his father beat him causing extensive brain damage (13).

While the state may demonstrate parental unfitness by a preponderance of the evidence standard (i.e., that child maltreatment more likely than not occurred), it may not permanently terminate a parent's rights unless it can show by clear and convincing evidence that abuse or neglect has occurred (12). The Supreme Court has explained the need for this higher burden of proof:

> The fundamental liberty interest of natural parents in the care, custody, and management of their child does not evaporate simply because they have not been model parents or have lost temporary custody of their child to the State. Even when blood relationships are strained, parents retain a vital interest in preventing the irretrievable destruction of their family life. If anything, persons faced with forced dissolution of their parental rights have a more critical need for procedural protections than do those resisting state intervention into ongoing family affairs. When the State moves to destroy weakened familial bonds, it must provide the parents with fundamentally fair procedures (12).

Note that this standard applies only to non-Indian children. A higher standard, "beyond a reasonable doubt," applies to the termination of parental rights to an Indian child, as will be discussed more fully later in this chapter. While the Supreme Court has held that the Constitution does not require, as a matter of due process of law, that parents be appointed legal counsel in every case (15), most states, either in interpreting their constitutions (16) or by way of statutory enactment (17), provide for the appointment of a lawyer in every child protection proceeding at public expense if the parent is unable to afford one. Although appointment of legal counsel is not constitutionally required, the provision of a transcript of the trial court proceedings at public expense is mandatory if the parent is unable to afford to pay for the transcript to be produced (18). With this constitutional framework in mind, we will next consider the statutory schemes utilized by states to protect children from inadequate parenting.

THE FEDERAL STATUTORY FRAMEWORK OF CHILD WELFARE CASES

Every state has a statutory scheme for responding to alleged child maltreatment that occurs at the hands of a child's parents or legal custodians. (19) While these statutes differ in their particulars, they are substantially similar largely because of the federal government's involvement in funding child protection services since the mid-1970s. To understand how this came to be, it will be helpful to begin with a very brief history lesson.

The United States has always provided some mechanism by which the larger community can step in and assume the care of a child who is without parents or whose parents are unable or unwilling to provide an appropriate home. By the early 1800s, the doctrine of *parens patriae*—the notion that the sovereign was ultimately responsible for safeguarding the welfare of those who lacked legal capacity— was well-established in American law. Where children were placed when their parents were unable to provide and appropriate home has changed over time, from basically indenturing them to placing them in congregate care facilities, to foster family homes.

In the 1960s, in the wake of the publication of the Kempe et al. seminal paper "The battered child syndrome" in the Journal of the American Medical Association (20), states began to enact laws requiring physicians and other professionals to report cases of suspected child abuse to state authorities (21). Those laws were expanded over time to broaden both what was to be reported—e.g., child neglect and sexual abuse in addition to physical abuse— and categories of professionals who were mandated to report their concerns— initially only medical professionals were required to report, but that was expanded to social workers, teachers and others professionals who come into frequent contact with children. These laws resulted in substantial increases in the number of abused and neglected children coming to the attention of state child protection authorities.

By the mid-1970s, there were about half a million children in the foster care system nationwide. It was not unusual for children entering the foster care system to remain in the system for years with no effort being made either to reunify them with their families of origin or to move them into alternative permanent homes. This phenomenon came to be known as foster care "limbo" and was accompanied by another phenomenon, foster care "drift," in which children would often move from home to home. Children remained in foster homes for so many years that the United States Supreme Court was called on in *Smith v. Organization of Foster Families for Equality and Reform* to determine whether long-term foster families had the same or similar constitutional rights as biological families. Eventually, these concerns were brought to the attention of Congress, which enacted legislation intended to bring about reform of the nation's child protection systems. Space limitations do not permit a detailed discussion of federal child welfare law.

CHILD ABUSE PREVENTION AND TREATMENT ACT

The United States is a federal system, which means that some matters of public policy are handled by the federal government while others are handled by the individual states. Legal issues relating to families are regulated by the states. The federal government may influence state policy by enacting legislation pursuant to its spending authority and placing conditions on the receipt of federal money. In the child protection arena, the federal government has established a stream of funding that allows the states to draw down large amounts of federal money if they design their state child protection systems to meet federal standards.

The first such statute that Congress enacted was the Child Abuse Prevention and Treatment Act (CAPTA). Signed into law in 1974, and repeatedly amended and reauthorized since, CAPTA provides support for state systems of preventing and responding to reported cases of child maltreatment. CAPTA also provides funding to support research into all aspects of child maltreatment—causes, prevention, and consequences—as well as program evaluation and technical assistances to states, Indian tribes and non-profit organizations (22).

ADOPTION ASSISTANCE AND CHILD WELFARE ACT OF 1980

Concerned about the number of children in foster care, the length of time they remained in what was intended to be a temporary system, and placement instability, in 1980, Congress passed and the President signed into law the Adoption Assistance and Child Welfare Act of 1980. This statute added two sections to the Social Security Act to provide funding to states to address child protection. Broadly speaking, this statute, which, like CAPTA, has been amended and reauthorized repeatedly since its initial enactment, has three purposes: 1) reducing the number of children entering foster care; 2) shortening stays in foster care; and 3) moving children to permanent homes, either through return to their family of origin, or, when return home is not possible, moving children into adoptive homes. We will look at each of these goals in a bit more detail.

To reduce the number of children entering foster care, the law required that state child welfare authorities make "reasonable efforts" to prevent children from entering the system by developing programs to provide in-home services to children and their families aimed at maintaining the family. To accomplish this, Congress added Title IV-B to the Social Security Act, which funnels federal money to states to prevent the removal of maltreated children from their homes. In response, states developed intensive family preservation programs which seek to address the family's needs and problems in functioning in order that children may remain safely in their homes.

Next, the statute addressed those cases in which the child cannot be safely maintained in the home and must be removed. To accomplish this, Congress created Title IV-E of the Social Security Act. The law incentivizes states to make "reasonable efforts" to return children to their families. To accomplish this goal, states child protection authorities are required to develop individualized case plans aimed at addressing the needs of individual family members such as drug or mental health treatment for parents and medical and mental health care for the children. The aim of the service plan is to resolve the problems in functioning that lead to the child's removal and facilitate the safe return of the child to the custody of his or her parents.

The third requirement of the statute is that states consider "the child's sense of time." rather than adult's sense of time. Generally, Congress determined that children need decisions about returning home or being freed for adoption to be made much more quickly than was happening before the enactment of the stature. Thus, the law required that states hold permanency planning hearings (PPH) after a child had been in foster care for a designated period of time. Originally, the PPH was to be held 18 months after the child entered foster care. That requirement was subsequently shortened to one year.

Finally, the 1980 law provided a package of adoption incentives that were intended to move children from temporary foster care into permanent homes. These incentives include the state rather than the adoptive family paying for the costs of the adoption (e.g., court fees) and by providing both cash assistance and medical benefits for special needs children (e.g., children with disabilities and older children).

In the early 1980s, these statutes began to have their intended impact, the numbers of children entering foster care edged down slightly. But then two phenomena converged to increase the numbers of children entering care. First, a more conservative federal government began to cut public benefits available to families, increasing the risk of child maltreatment. Secondly, the combination of the crack cocaine epidemic and the advent of HIV/AIDS had devastating impacts on certain communities. The need for foster care increased.

A related problem also emerged. In the 1980 law, Congress never defined what it meant by "reasonable efforts," and many states, in part as a means of saving money, defined it to mean every conceivable effort had to be made before a child could be removed from the home. That is, states began to overuse intensive family preservation programs beyond their capacities, which resulted in a number of high profile child deaths and many lesser harms inflicted on children (23).

ADOPTION AND SAFE FAMILIES ACT

As a result, in 1997, Congress passed and President Clinton signed into law the Adoption and Safe Families Act (ASFA), which was intended to clarify the intent of Congress regarding the 1980 Act in general and the "reasonable efforts" requirement in particular. While it renewed the federal government's commitment to family preservation, it made clear that children's health and safety are to be the paramount concerns of the nation's child protection systems.

The ASFA maintained the basic framework of the 1980 Act but made a number of adjustments and clarifications. The new law tightened the timeline for permanency planning hearings from 18 months to one year. It also made clear that there is a set of cases involving very serious child maltreatment—e.g., death of a child, torture of a child—in which "reasonable efforts" shall not be made to preserve or reunify the family, and the state authorities are mandated to seek the termination of the parents' rights immediately.

Next, ASFA permitted each state to define for itself a category of "aggravated circumstances" cases in which state authorities may determine that "reasonable efforts" to either preserve or reunify a family are unnecessary, and thereby permit the child protection agency to pursue immediate termination of parental rights. While each state is free to define this group of cases for itself, the federal legislation suggests that appropriate circumstances for its use include abandonment, chronic abuse, and sexual abuse.

The final major change in the law under ASFA is that the state child welfare agency may seek, and the juvenile or family court may grant, termination of parental rights in any case without making "reasonable efforts" to preserve or reunify the family if the specific circumstances warrant such action. Illinois is one state that has codified this possibility. It statute provides that parental rights may be terminated "in those extreme cases in which the parent's incapacity to care for the child, combined with an extremely poor prognosis for treatment or rehabilitation, justifies expedited termination of parental rights" (24).

In the wake of ASFA's enactment a number of states have adopted definitions of "reasonable efforts" in order to guide state child welfare authorities and courts in making decisions about whether this requirement has been complied with. For instance, Missouri law provides as follows:

> "Reasonable efforts" means the exercise of reasonable diligence and care . . . to utilize all available services related to meeting the needs of the juvenile and the family. In determining reasonable efforts to be made and in making such reasonable efforts, the child's present and ongoing health and safety shall be the paramount consideration. In support of its determination of whether reasonable efforts have been made, the court shall enter findings, including a brief description of what preventive or reunification efforts were made and why further efforts could or could not have prevented or shortened the separation of the family. The [state child welfare authorities] shall have the burden of demonstrating reasonable efforts (25).

ASFA also permitted the use of concurrent planning, which allows state child protection authorities to simultaneously seek to reunify the family and develop an alternative plan in the event that reunification services are not successful. By engaging in the duel planning process, children's stays in foster care can be shortened and they can achieve permanency more quickly. The law also expanded permanency options to include both permanent legal guardianship and a designation called "another planned permanent living arrangement," which is typically used in cases of older foster children who can neither be returned to their families of origin nor placed for adoption, and includes alternatives such as independent living or, perhaps, discharge into the adult foster care system for incapacitated adults.

MULTIETHNIC PLACEMENT ACT AND THE INTERETHNIC ADOPTION PROVISIONS

Historically, minority children, particularly African Americans, were excluded from receiving public child welfare services. In more recent years, there has been concern not of underserving minority children but of the overrepresentation of minority — again, specifically African American — children in the child protection system. As a result, there has been debate about the availability of services to meet the needs of these children. One ongoing controversy is the placement of African American children across racial lines for adoption. One response to this concern was for state authorities to engage in conscious race matching. As a result, some African American children's placement from institutional care into foster family homes or for adoption in a suitable home was delayed or denied. Some jurisdictions had explicit waiting periods before a child could be placed into or adopted across racial lines.

In 1994, Congress enacted the Multiethnic Placement Act, which sought to eliminate (or, at least, dramatically reduce) the use of race, color or national origin as a basis on which foster or adoptive placement could be determined. The law's language, however, was easily interpreted as permitting some racial matching, so two years later, Congress passed clarifying language in the Interethnic Adoption Provisions, which were intended to ban outright the use of race, color or national origin in placement decision-making except in the rarest of circumstances.

If the placement of a child into either a foster home or adoptive home is delayed or denied on the basis of race, color or national origin, the law explicitly provides that the aggrieved person— the child or the foster parent/adoptive parent— may sue the state child welfare agency. This is a rare exception to the governmental immunity from lawsuits typically enjoyed by child welfare agencies.

THE FOSTER CARE INDEPENDENCE ACT

Each year, approximately 20,000 children age out of the foster care system. Many of these youth are ill-prepared to make a successful transition to young adulthood. Historically, most had not graduated from high school, many were ending up homeless, nearly half were themselves parents, and some 80% of them were unable to support themselves financially. To address the unique problems facing this sub-population of the foster care population, Congress enacted The Foster Care Independence Act in 1999, commonly known as the "Chafee Act," so named for its author, Senator John Chafee (1922-1999).

The Chafee Act provided a separate funding stream to states to allow them to develop programming for children who were in the foster care system on or after their 14th year birthday. In addition to providing Medicaid coverage for these youth until the age of 21 years, the Act required that foster parents of these youth be specially trained to meet their needs and that state agencies assist youth in developing independent living skills such as how to seek employment and how to manage a household budget. Agencies were also to provide assistance with completing high school and making the transition to job training or college. The law also provided additional adoption subsidies to encourage and support the adoption of these older children.

In 2008, the Congress amended Title IV-E to allow states to extend these youth in the foster care system until their 21st year birthday. It also mandated that state agencies develop a personalized, youth-directed plan for each youth in order to address the transition to adulthood, including educational, housing, health insurance, and other considerations.

INDIAN CHILD WELFARE ACT

In 1978, in an effort to respond to overzealous child welfare practices aimed at assimilating Indian children into the dominant culture through unnecessary removals, Congress enacted the Indian Child Welfare Act (ICWA). Unlike the other federal child welfare laws discussed in this chapter, which are funding statutes, the ICWA is substantive law. That is, unlike the funding statues, which the states may choose to follow or not (if they choose not to, of course, they will not be able to draw down some or all of the federal funding they would be able to draw down if they complied), the states are mandated to comply with the ICWA in every child protection case involving an "Indian child." This distinction results because the Constitution of the United States explicitly reserves to the Congress the authority to make laws relating to the Indian tribes.

Two threshold issues are important to keep in mind regarding the application of the ICWA. First, the law defines an "Indian child" as "any unmarried person who is under age eighteen and is either (a) a member of an Indian tribe or (b) is eligible for membership in an Indian tribe and is the biological child of a member of an Indian tribe." The federal government has given formal recognition to 567 "tribal entities" across the country. Of note, it is possible for a child to be of Native American ancestry but not qualify as an "Indian child" within the meaning of the law, because each tribe defines for itself its tribal eligibility requirements. Some, but not all, tribes have a blood quantum requirement. Secondly, unlike child protection proceedings involving non-Indian children, in a proceeding involving an "Indian child" the child's tribe is a party to the proceeding. Thus, the tribe or the parents may, generally speaking, elect to move the case from the state court to a tribal court. Alternatively, the tribe may intervene as a party to and participate in a state child protection proceeding.

When an "Indian child" resides on a reservation, state courts may make only emergency orders that are necessary to ensure a child's immediate safety. In situations such as this, the law provides that the case must be transferred the tribal court. Most tribes that have tribal courts have separate child welfare codes. However, these codes are substantially similar to state child welfare codes. As with state child protection systems, the various federal laws allow tribes to access federal funding to support their child protection efforts so long as the tribal system meets the federal requirements.

The ICWA provides a unique set of procedures applicable to cases of Indian children that are explicitly intended to make it more difficult to remove an Indian child from his or her home. The law accomplishes this goal in several ways. First, it increases the amount of evidence (i.e., the standard of proof) which state authorities must present to a court before an Indian child may be removed from the home. While a non-Indian child may typically be removed from the home based upon a showing of probable cause that a child has been harmed, before an Indian child may be removed, the state authorities must present clear and convincing evidence. This is the same standard by which the parental rights of a non-Indian child's parent may be permanently terminated. To terminate the rights of an Indian child's parents requires proof beyond a reasonable doubt, the highest standard of proof known to the law, which is typically used to convict a defendant of a criminal offense.

The ICWA also requires that at both the removal stage and the termination of parental rights stage in a child protection proceeding state authorities prove that "active efforts" have been made to maintain or reunify the Indian family. The Bureau of Indian Affairs within the Department of the Interior in 2015 issued updated guidance for state authorities in applying the ICWA. (26) It said that, "Active efforts are intended primarily to maintain and reunite an Indian child with his or her family or tribal community and constitute more than reasonable efforts" as required by other federal funding legislation. The BIA provides examples of "active efforts," including:

- "Identifying appropriate services and helping the parents to overcome barriers, including actively assisting the parents in obtaining such services."
- "Taking into account the Indian child's tribe's prevailing social and cultural conditions and way of life, and requesting the assistance of representatives designated by the Indian child's tribe with substantial knowledge of the prevailing social and cultural standards."
- "Offering and employing all available and culturally appropriate family preservation strategies."
- "Completing a comprehensive assessment of the circumstances of the Indian child's family, with a focus on safe reunification as the most desirable goal."

Some question the viability of the ICWA given that consideration of race in matters of public decision-making is restricted, and ask how the ICWA squares with the Multiethnic Placement Act and the Interethnic Adoption Provisions. The basic answer is that tribes are sovereign nations, and enrollment in a tribe constitutes a political designation rather than a racial or ethnic classification.

In response to the enactment of the ICWA, several states—e.g., Iowa, Michigan, Minnesota—have enacted comparable statutes at the state level. These statutes may be more expansive or protective than the federal law, and therefore may apply to children and families that would not be covered under the federal ICWA.

APPLICATION OF DISABILITY LAW TO CHILD WELFARE CASES: THE AMERICANS WITH DISABILITIES ACT AND SIMILAR LAWS

The services provided in child welfare cases to prevent the removal of a child from a parent's custody or to reunify a family often are designed to address parenting problems identified by the child welfare agency. These problems with parenting may be the ones that prompted agency involvement in the first place or may be ongoing or new concerns that contribute to continued foster care placement. In contrast, less attention may be paid to the social service and educational needs of children involved in the child protection system. Child welfare agencies need to carefully ascertain what kinds of assistance children may require, and special attention must be paid to ensuring that the needs of children with disabilities are met.

It is well-established that any services provided to parents by child welfare and associated agencies must reasonably accommodate a parent's disability under Title II of the Americans with Disabilities Act (ADA) (26). If these services do not reasonably accommodate a parent's disability, they may not be considered "reasonable efforts" by the courts, jeopardizing the state's access to federal funding in that case and potentially interfering with later efforts by the agency to terminate the parent's rights. Similarly, but perhaps considered less frequently by child welfare agencies and the service providers with whom they work, the ADA also protects children with disabilities. Therefore, any services provided to a child with a disability must accommodate that disability such that the child has an opportunity to benefit from the service as much as a non-disabled child might.

The ADA is a federal civil rights law that is designed "to provide clear, strong, consistent, enforceable standards addressing discrimination against individuals with disabilities" (27). It is not the only law to do so. For example, Section 504 of the Rehabilitation Act of 1973 also addresses disability discrimination, but only in entities that receive federal funding (28). Many organizations and agencies providing services to children in the child welfare system receive federal funds, so Section 504 would apply to them much as the ADA does. So too would analogous state disability rights statutes where they exist. Because the application is quite similar between these statutes, and the ADA is the more encompassing federal law, this chapter focuses on how the ADA applies in these cases. Readers should simply be mindful that other disability rights laws are likely to apply as well.

APPLICATION OF THE ADA

The threshold for whether the ADA applies to a child in a given child welfare case is whether the child has a disability. Disability is defined as "(A) a physical or mental impairment that substantially limits one or more major life activities of [the] individual; (B) a record of such an impairment; or (C) being regarded as having such an impairment" (29). Whether a person is disabled is to "be construed in favor of broad coverage" (30). The statute provides a non-exhaustive list of many "major life activities," both physical and cognitive, that may be limited and therefore fall under the Act (31). These include learning, reading, concentrating, thinking, and communicating, all tasks that are germane in educational and other contexts, such as psychotherapy and health care, in which children may engage. Impairments in these and other areas of functioning may interfere with a child's ability to benefit from services provided by child welfare and other agencies if reasonable accommodations are not made.

Unless the agency will stipulate to the fact that a child is disabled or has portrayed the child as disabled in its court pleadings or other documents or verbal statements, evidence of disability will be needed to trigger ADA protections. This evidence may include information from medical and mental health evaluation reports or other records, Social Security determinations, or educational evaluations and records. Although child welfare agencies frequently describe disabling impairments in parents, it is less common for them to note how the child functions in different domains. Therefore, practitioners should not rely on the agency to "tip them off" to a child's disability, and thorough evaluation of the child is a critical component of ensuring that any disabilities are identified and accommodated.

Sometimes, however, the agency does report that the child has a disability or describes the child's functional status in a way that implies that it regards the child as disabled. In these cases, the ADA applies. Under the ADA, disability may be inferred if a person is treated by a public entity as having an impairment that substantially limits a major life activity (32). In essence, this treatment by the agency amounts to the child being regarded as having an impairment, thereby triggering ADA protections.

In order to be eligible for ADA protection, the child must be a "qualified individual with a disability," which is defined as a person who, "with or without reasonable modifications," "meets the essential eligibility requirements for the receipt of services or the participation in programs or activities provided by a public entity" (33). There is no doubt that children with disabilities who are involved in child welfare proceedings are eligible to receive services from the agency and are therefore qualified individuals under the ADA. Finally, child welfare agencies are clearly public entities, including private agencies that enter into contracts with the state or county child welfare agency to do work that would otherwise fall to the public agency. Therefore, they are required to follow the requirements of the ADA. It is important to note that the ADA applies to child protection agencies regardless of whether the case is court-involved. Child welfare agencies take only a small fraction of cases to court, mostly when children must be removed from the custody of their parents. Many cases are handled by the agency directly with the families involved and never go to court, and in all of these matters, the agency must comply with the ADA. Therefore, the agency must accommodate the disabilities of the parents and children with whom they work, from ensuring accessibility to agency and other facilities to providing any educational materials in an accessible format and using training approaches tailored to the needs of the individual.

DEVELOPING REASONABLE ACCOMMODATIONS

When reasonable accommodations are required in order to meet the needs of a child with a disability who is receiving services, it is important to think carefully about exactly what kinds of accommodations might be in order. That determination may rely on having a thorough assessment, which may need to be a multidisciplinary assessment, of the child's needs. That assessment should take a "functional" view of disability. The functional view emphasizes the child's actual, functional abilities across whatever domains are relevant (34). Therefore, a functional evaluation may reveal how the child learns best or applies what he or she learns, or how the child navigates the word physically, or the child's behaviors in various circumstances, and the like. In addition, the functional perspective emphasizes the interaction of the individual and his or her environment, recognizing that the environment itself, including not only physical barriers but also policies, attitudes, and teaching styles, can be disabling or contribute to diminished functioning (35). A functional approach provides the most guidance in planning interventions, including how best to accommodate the disability.

In contrast, a "categorical" view of disability emphasizes the criteria for various categories of disability, such as a type of mental illness, intellectual disability, or a specific physical disability, much like a medical diagnosis. (34) The categorical approach reveals little about the person's actual functioning and thus provides scant information for the purpose of service planning and reasonable accommodations. Unfortunately, many professionals are tempted to approach disabilities categorically, because it is easier to diagnose and label than it is to do a deeper, more meaningful assessment. Over-reliance on the categorical approach contributes to service provision that is not tailored to the actual needs of the individual.

Given the complexities of disability coupled with the trauma history that is inherent to most child protection cases, the gold standard for an assessment that is likely to result in excellent service planning tailored to the child's needs is multidisciplinary, trauma-informed assessment completed by a team that has expertise in working with children with disabilities. These types of evaluation can yield rich data that effectively guide interventions across the medical, mental health, and educational spectra. When considering reasonable accommodations, there are no set approaches, and it is best to consult with the child if he or she is old enough, his or her parents, providers who may have worked with the child in the school, medical, and mental health contexts, and expert evaluators in order to determine what accommodations may be needed.

SPECIAL EDUCATION LAW

It is critical to consider the educational needs for every child in the child welfare system, and children with disabilities may encounter extra challenges in school. They also are supposed to receive specific protections. Children with disabilities are legally entitled to receive a "free, appropriate public education" (FAPE), and the special education system is intended to provide them with just that (36). The Individuals with Disabilities Education Act (IDEA) is the main federal law that governs the provision of special education services, though the ADA and Section 504 of the Rehabilitation Act of 1973 can be useful as well. A special education program is deemed appropriate if it was created through an Individualized Education Program (IEP) process and is reasonably calculated to confer educational benefit (37). Through special education, children with disabilities can receive specialized instruction, adapted transportation to and from school, various therapies, and a wide range of supplementary aids and services, including assistive technology devices, to the extent that any of these services are needed in order for the child to receive a FAPE (38).

Generally, education rights flow through the *parents* of children, not the children themselves. If a child with a disability remains with his or her parent during the pendency of a child welfare case, the parent can seek special education services for the child. Assistance from the child welfare agency in doing so may be necessary and appropriate, but the caseworker cannot sign an IEP. If a child is in foster care, a parent can still seek special education services, as can a foster parent (39). In addition, the court may designate a surrogate parent for the purposes of education planning if a child is a court ward (40).

A written referral indicating that a student may need special education services begins the process. School personnel may write these referrals, as can parents, guardians, or foster parents. The referral triggers an evaluation to determine the child's eligibility. Special education evaluations must be designed to assess both the student's eligibility and the student's educational needs in order to inform what services should be put into place (41). IDEA has numerous eligibility categories, such as cognitive impairment, specific learning disability, speech and language impairment, etc., but it is important to note that the category does not determine or limit what services the child might receive (42). Rather, the category simply makes the child eligible for all necessary services to benefit from his or her education. Therefore, advocates and caregivers should consider the eligibility category merely as a means of entry into the special education system. Once a parent or other caregiver consents to an evaluation, the school district has sixty calendar days or less to complete it (43).

Once an evaluation is completed, an Individualized Education Planning Team (IEPT) is convened to determine the student's eligibility for special education services based on the evaluation. As noted above, if a student is eligible for special education services, an Individualized Education Program (IEP) must be developed by the IEPT (44). The IEP must be reassessed at least yearly, and either the school or parent can request that an IEP meeting be held sooner if needed. The child must be educated in the least restrictive environment that is appropriate to meet his or her needs (45). The IEP should indicate the settings in which services will occur, exactly what services will be provided, how long and how often services will be provided, the student's current level of functioning, how progress will be measured, and any supplementary aids or services that are necessary for the student to receive a FAPE. The goals for what the student is expected to achieve in the following year should be clear, objective, and measurable. Special education students must be included in state educational testing, albeit with accommodations, or in alternate assessments if they cannot participate in state educational testing even with accommodations (46).

For children in foster care, all of this may be more difficult to accomplish, especially if the child has changed schools. If the parent is uninvolved, there may be a dearth of background knowledge about the child and his or her educational programming, even if the school has up to date records. Agency personnel and the child's lawyer should endeavor to bridge any gaps, which may include arranging for school personnel from the child's previous school to attend an IEP meeting and consult with the new school in an ongoing manner. Another option may be to advocate for a thorough re-evaluation.

Finally, caregivers and advocates should be aware that while IDEA is the primary legal scheme under which special education services are provided, some children with disabilities do not qualify under IDEA's eligibility categories. In such cases, the Americans with Disabilities Act or Section 504 of the Rehabilitation may still mandate that the school accommodate the child's disability. It is important to consult with a student advocacy center or with the state's Protection and Advocacy office for representation or advice about how to access special education services or other accommodations as appropriate. See www.ndrn.org for a list of state Protection and Advocacy offices.

SOCIAL SECURITY

Children with disabilities may be eligible for Supplemental Security Income (SSI) payments from the Social Security Administration. For SSI purposes, a child is considered disabled if he or she is under 18 years of age and "has a medically determinable physical or mental impairment, which results in marked and severe functional limitations, and which can be expected to result in death or which has lasted or can be expected to last for a continuous period of not less than 12 months" (47). If the child is in foster care, SSI payments will go to the child welfare agency to offset the cost of the child's care. Despite the fact that such payments might not appear to benefit the child directly, it is important to apply for SSI benefits if the child might be eligible. The child's disability may require ongoing financial support beyond the time that the child is in foster care, and either the child's family of origin or the child's adoptive family could benefit substantially from SSI payments, materially improving the child's standard of living. If a child is in foster care, the child welfare agency should apply for SSI benefits on the child's behalf.

To determine whether the child is disabled and therefore eligible for SSI benefits, Social Security requires detailed information about the child's condition and how it affects his or her functioning in daily life, including at home, in school, and in other contexts. Reports or other data from doctors, therapists, teachers, etc., also provide information for the eligibility determination. Unfortunately, it may be difficult to gather adequate medical and school records for children in foster care, especially if they have changed schools or providers and records have not transferred successfully, but it is important to try to do so. Also, the income and resources of the child's household will be considered in the SSI eligibility determination—if income and resources are more than the allowed amount, the child will not be eligible for SSI payments. However, this requirement should not affect children living in foster care.

CONCLUSION

It is inevitable that some children with disabilities will come to the attention of child protection authorities or that maltreated children will become disabled. This review has addressed the legal framework for addressing the needs of children when these two phenomena intersect. It has summarized the constitutional framework governing relationships between parents, child, and the state and provided an overview of important federal child protection and disability law. It is essential that child welfare agency caseworkers, lawyers, and other professionals consider a child's disability in the course of a child protection case and seek expert consultation as necessary so as to ensure that children's needs are met.

REFERENCES

[1] US Department of Commerce, Economic and Statistics Administration, U.S. Census Bureau. School—aged children with disabilities in the U.S. Metropolitan Statistical Areas: 2010. Washington, DC: US Census Bureau, 2011.

[2]   Cappozzola R. Uncle Same wants you: World War I and the making of the modern American citizen. London: Oxford University Press, 2008.
[3]   Meyer v. Nebraska, 262 U.S. 390 (1923).
[4]   Pierce v Society of Sisters, 268 U.S. 510 (1925).
[5]   Prince v. Massachusetts, 321 U.S. 158 (1944).
[6]   Parham v. J. R., 442 U.S. 584 (1979).
[7]   Wisconsin v Yoder, 406 U.S. 205 (1972).
[8]   Moore v. City of East Cleveland, Ohio, 431 U.S. 494 (1977).
[9]   Troxel v. Granville, 530 U.S. 57 (2000).
[10]   Stanley v. Illinois, 405 U.S. 645 (1972).
[11]   Lehr v. Robertson, 463 U.S. 248 (1983).
[12]   Santosky v. Kramer, 455 U.S. 745 (1982).
[13]   Doe v Oettle, 293 N.W. 2d 760 (Mich. 1980).
[14]   DeShaney v. Winnebago County Department of Social Services, 489 U.S. 189 (1989).
[15]   Lassiter v. Department of Social Services, 452 U.S. 18 (1981).
[16]   Reist v Bay Circuit Judge, 241 N.W.2d 55 (Mich. 1976).
[17]   Boyer BA. Justice, access to the courts, and the right to free counsel for indigent parents: The continuing scourge of Lassiter v. Department of Social Service of Durham. Loyola U Chicago Law J 2005;36:363-81.
[18]   M.L.B. v. S.L.J., 519 U.S. 102 (1996).
[19]   Mnookin RH, Weisberg, DK. Child, family, and state: Problems and materials on children and the law. New York: Aspen, 2009.
[20]   Kempe CH, Silverman FN, Steele BF, Droegemueller W, Silver HK. The battered child syndrome. JAMA 1962;181:17-24.
[21]   Vandervort FE. Mandated reporting of child maltreatment: Developments in the wake of recent scandals. APSAC Advisor 2012;24(4):3-9.
[22]   Child Welfare Information Gateway, About CAPTA: A legislative history, 2011. URL:https://www.childwelfare.gov/pubPDFs/about.pdf.
[23]   Gelles RJ. The book of David. How preserving families can cost children's lives. New York: Basic Books, 1996.
[24]   705 Ill Comp Stat Ann § 405/1-2(1)(c).
[25]   Mo Ann rev Stat § 211.183(2).
[26]   Kay JB. Representing parents with disabilities. In: Guggenheim M, Sankaran VS (eds). Representing parents in child welfare cases. Chicago, IL: American Bar Association Books, 2015:253-68.
[27]   42 U.S.C. § 12101(b)(2).
[28]   29 U.S.C. § 794.
[29]   42 U.S.C. § 12102(1).
[30]   42 U.S.C. § 12102(4)(A).
[31]   42 U.S.C. § 12102(2)(A)
[32]   28 C.F.R. § 35.104; 42 U.S.C. § 12102(3)(A).
[33]   42 U.S.C. § 12131(2).
[34]   Tymchuk AJ. The importance of matching educational interventions to parent needs in child maltreatment: Issues, methods, and recommendations. In: Lutzker JR, ed. Handbook of child abuse research and treatment. New York: Plenum Press, 1998:421-48.
[35]   Watkins C. Beyond status: The Americans with Disabilities Act and the parental rights of people labeled developmentally disabled or mentally retarded. Cal Law Rev 1999;83:1415-75.
[36]   20 U.S.C. § 1401(9).
[37]   Board of Education v. Rowley, 458 U.S. 176, 206 (1982).
[38]   See generally 20 U.S.C. § 1401 *et seq*.
[39]   20 U.S.C. § 1401(23)(A). State law may differ as to whether a foster parent can sign an IEP.
[40]   20 U.S.C. § 1401(23)(D).
[41]   20 U.S.C. § 1414(b).
[42]   34 C.F.R. § 300.304(c)(6).

[43] 34 C.F.R. § 300.301(c). State law or regulation may provide a shorter timeframe, which then overrides the federal rule.
[44] 20 U.S.C. § 1412(a)(4).
[45] 20 U.S.C. § 1412(5).
[46] 20 U.S.C. § 1412(16).
[47] 42 U.S.C.§ 1382c(a)(3)(C)(i).

Submitted: August 20, 2016. *Revised:* September 10, 2016. *Accepted:* September 20, 2016.

Chapter 36

CHILDREN WITH DISABILITIES: PREVENTION OF MALTREATMENT

*Vincent J Palusci**, MD, MS*

New York University School of Medicine and the Frances L Loeb Child Protection and Development Center, Bellevue Hospital, New York, New York, US

ABSTRACT

Those caring for children with disabilities have many reasons for wanting to prevent child abuse and neglect, not the least of which are to reduce pain and suffering and future health problems. These goals are particularly relevant for the weak and vulnerable in our population. However, the details of why, how, when, and where health care professionals can promote prevention may seem murky or ill-defined, especially as maltreatment and violence against children remains undercounted and under-addressed by many segments of society and by many of the systems designed to improve child welfare. This review provides both the rationale and strategies for prevention as well as some concrete ideas about how to professionals can integrate it into the day-to-day care of children with disabilities.

Keywords: children, disability, abuse, neglect, prevention

INTRODUCTION

Preventing child abuse and neglect spares children physical and psychological pain and suffering and improves their long-term health outcomes. Dubowitz (1) noted that prevention "is intuitively and morally preferable to intervening after the fact" and recent work from our

---

*Correspondence: Vincent J Palusci, MD, MS, Professor of Pediatrics, New York University School of Medicine, Bellevue Hospital Center, 462 First Avenue, New York, NY 10016, United States. E-mail: Vincent.palusci@nyumc.org.

understanding of the long-term physical and mental health effects from adverse childhood experiences calls us to action. Earlier intervention is more effective in preventing abuse and neglect, saves money for society, and improves peoples' overall health and well-being, perhaps the most important goals for civil society to accomplish.

The United States Advisory Board on Child Abuse and Neglect (2) reported that child maltreatment (CM) is an emergency requiring leadership through professional societies and research. Prevention is explicitly not the responsibility of any one agency, profession, or program, but is best framed as the responsibility of all to create a society less conducive to child maltreatment. In this paradigm, individual skill development, community and provider education, coalition building, organizational change, and policy innovations are all part of the prevention solution. Professionals who provide clinical or supportive services to victims of maltreatment or families facing serious challenges have a role and an obligation to be aware of and support the prevention efforts in their community and to be able to appropriately refer the families they see to these resources.

The American Academy of Pediatrics has made recommendations specifically for pediatricians as well (3). There is increasing evidence to demonstrate the elements of successful interventions, the populations and programs of most benefit, and the best implementation research to demonstrate that we have met our goals. In this paper, current strategies in child abuse prevention and guides for professionals in the integration of prevention activities into their daily work with children with disabilities (CWD) will be reviewed.

THE CASE FOR PREVENTION

Research has identified the physical and mental conditions increasingly being associated with adverse childhood experiences, such as physical abuse, sexual abuse, and neglect. Neurologic imaging and traumatology studies have delineated the chronic physiologic and structural changes that occur after chronic stress and abuse (4). Chronic stress and abuse are associated with specific disease processes and poor mental health outcomes in adults, and adverse childhood experiences (ACEs) have been associated with increased rates of teen pregnancy, promiscuity, depression, hallucinations, substance abuse, liver disease, chronic obstructive pulmonary disease, coronary artery disease, and identifiable permanent changes in brain structure and stress hormone function (5-8). Children with disabilities have been noted to have more ACEs than do children without disability, thereby increasing their risk even more (9). Emotional conditions associated with abuse and neglect, including depression, posttraumatic stress disorder, and conduct disorders, compound any direct physical injuries inflicted on individual children. As children mature, increased risk of low academic achievement, drug use, teen pregnancy, juvenile delinquency, and adult criminology add further burden. Although treatment after the fact can improve mental and physical health and prolong life and productivity, the direct and indirect costs of child maltreatment for both children and adults in poor health, pain, and suffering themselves warrant our taking action to prevent child abuse and neglect (10).

WHAT IS PREVENTION?

Child maltreatment prevention is endorsed by all those who are familiar with the problems associated with child maltreatment, and efforts aimed at preventing abuse are promoted by agencies, governmental officials, and individual practitioners. Unfortunately, beyond a blanket endorsement of the concept, there are many different ideas about what prevention actually means and what activities are considered effective. Definitions vary, yet three categories of prevention are generally described (11):

1. Primary: Efforts aimed at the general population for the purpose of keeping abuse from happening.
2. Secondary: Efforts aimed at a particular group with increased risk to keep abuse from happening.
3. Tertiary: Efforts aimed at preventing abuse from happening again to those who have already been victimized. This level includes treatment to reduce harm from the original abuse.

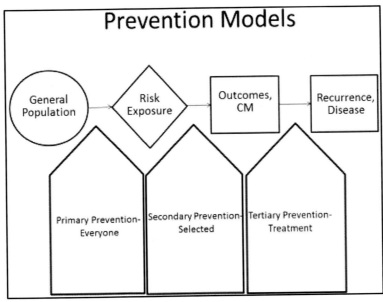

CM = Child Maltreatment.

Figure 1. Prevention levels and child maltreatment.

The Centers for Disease Control and Prevention (12) have emphasized that abuse operates in a societal context and requires an entire spectrum of necessary prevention strategies over time, thinking of prevention in terms of **when** it occurs (before or after abuse), **who** is the focus (everyone, those at greatest risk, or those who have already experienced abuse), and at **what** point to intervene (individual, relationship, community, or society level). A simplistic conceptual model is offered in Figure 1. These efforts are based on Bronfenbrenner's ecological model, which promotes intervening at the individual, relationship, community, and societal levels (13, 14). Approaches implied from these new labels emphasize a shift away from risk reduction as the predominant prevention approach and toward promotion of positive social change. Some argue that prior definitions limited prevention strategies by focusing primarily on potential individual targets of abuse and how to intervene rather than the environmental and societal context that supports and even condones abusive acts. Definitions of prevention based on timing which apply to all populations are:

1. Primary: taking action *before* CM has occurred to prevent it from happening.
2. Secondary: intervening *right after* CM has occurred.
3. Tertiary: taking the long view and working *overtime to change conditions* in the environment that promote or support CM.

CHILD MALTREATMENT PREVENTION STRATEGIES

Daro (15) has noted three important goals of CM prevention: (a) to reduce the incidence of abuse and neglect; (b) to minimize the chance that children who are maltreated will be re-victimized; and (c) to break the cycle of maltreatment by providing victims the help they need to improve how they parent children in the next generation. Systematic comparative effectiveness research is in its early infancy in this area, and the long-term effectiveness of most programs is still being studied (16). Most strategies, such as home visiting, are not uniformly effective in reducing all forms of CM but do appear to improve parenting or one or more risk factors. Some family programs are successful in reducing physical abuse but not neglect, for example, and sexual abuse educational programs have created controversy despite some promising improvements in mental health measures. Additional health and welfare outcomes, such as improved physical growth and development for infants, have also been noted, sometimes without measurable reductions in CM.

Few studies have looked specifically at children of intellectually or developmentally disabled parents. Many parents with intellectual disabilities lose custody of their children due to real or perceived parenting inadequacies, but it is not clear how parents who keep their children differ from parents who don't. In one study (17) comparing 30 mothers with an intellectual disability who still had custody of all their children to 17 mothers whose children were placed in care, mothers who still had custody of their children were more involved in their community, were more satisfied with the services they received, and had higher incomes with younger children than mothers who had lost their children. No significant differences were found concerning the behavior of their children, the mothers' health, adaptive behaviors, or the number of persons in their social network. The authors concluded that services should be offered to both mothers and children with IDDs and should be adapted as the children grow. Many available strategies tailor their programs to one or more levels of prevention while addressing different risk factors for intervention in different populations (see Table 1). This is appropriate given our understanding that child maltreatment occurs because of many factors acting simultaneously on the parent, child, family/relationship, community, and society levels (18). Some focus on children, others on parents, while still others address parent-child dyads or the environment in which parents raise children. Patno (19) has appropriately reminded us that "there is not, and never will be, one program that prevents all abuse and neglect" given the multifactorial causes. Thus, we will need multiple strategies which vary by method and approach to effectively address different forms of CM in different populations. While high standards must be set, there remains room for creativity and the use of feedback from diverse community settings to respond to shape strategies to meet their unique needs and situations. Some strategies may be hampered in their opportunity to be truly comprehensive, to reach broader audiences, and to use creative methods because of lack of funds, a problem that has been identified by many prevention program leaders. Demands for quality need to be combined with demands for adequate funding for prevention so that truly valuable programs can exist. Different forms of CM in distinctive communities and cultures will require unique types of prevention strategies.

Table 1. Examples of strategies by prevention level

Level	Strategy	Example(s)
Primary	Prepregnancy/Perinatal	"Safe haven" laws (38)
	Newborn AHT education	Dias (40), Period of Purple Crying (41)
	Homevisiting	Nurse Family Partnership (22), Healthy Families America (27)
	Medical services	Practicing Safety (46), No Hit Zone (42)
	Sexual abuse prevention	Personal Space & Privacy (68), Policies (50)
	Public health	Media campaigns (12)
	Social capital building	Triple P (48), subsidized child care (56)
Secondary	Family Wellness	Family Preservation (32), Family Connections (58), Parenting programs (34)
	Parent training	Parent-Child Interaction Therapy (60), Family Nurturing Program (35)
	Pediatric services	Anticipatory guidance (44), SEEK (43)
	Adolescent parents	Teen mother's groups (45)
	Substance abuse	Substance abuse treatment (51)
Tertiary	Mandated reporting	Universal mandated reporting laws (57)
	Mental Health Treatment	Counseling after psychologic maltreatment (66), Groups for children (52)
	Fatality review	Child death review programs (49)

Klevens and Whitaker (20) systematically reviewed the literature for 1980-2004 utilizing existing databases and found 188 primary prevention interventions that addressed a broad range of risk factors. However, few had been rigorously evaluated, and only a handful demonstrated impact on child maltreatment or its risk factors. From a public health perspective, they recommended that interventions that target prevalent and neglected risk factors such as poverty, partner violence, teenage pregnancy, and social norms tolerating violence toward children need to be developed and evaluated, and more attention should be given to low cost interventions delivered to the public, by society, or that require minimal effort from recipients.

The US Children's Bureau (21) has suggested that all prevention services need to embrace a commitment to a set of practice principles that have been found effective across diverse disciplines and service delivery systems. They have published a list of best practice standards that represent best practice elements that lie at the core of effective interventions. To the extent that direct service providers and prevention policy advocates hope to maximize the return on their investments, supporting service strategies that embrace the following principles will be essential:

- A strong theory of change that identifies specific outcomes and clear pathways for addressing these core outcomes, including specific strategies and curriculum content
- A recommended duration and dosage or clear guidelines for determining when to discontinue or extend services that is systematically applied to all those enrolled in services
- A clear, well-defined target population with identified eligibility criteria and strategy for reaching and engaging this target population
- A strategy for guiding staff in balancing the task of delivering program content while being responsive to a family's cultural beliefs and immediate circumstances
- A method to train staff on delivering the model with a supervisory system to support direct service staff and guide their ongoing practice
- Reasonable caseloads that are maintained and allow direct service staff to accomplish core program objectives
- The systematic collection of information on participant characteristics, staff characteristics, and participant service experiences to ensure services are being implemented with fidelity to the model, program intent, and structure

One should keep in mind other important principles as we discuss a number of strategies which have been used in an attempt to prevent or reduce child maltreatment. These include considering the conceptual model represented by the strategy, whether a risk factor or intermediate outcome is being addressed, whether there are co-morbidities or other factors such as disability which modify or moderate the effects, how things are being measured and paid for, whether a strategy is implemented with fidelity, and how it is disseminated and scaled to larger populations. It is also important to consider whether some analysis has been done looking at efficacy, effectiveness and cost-effectiveness.

HOME VISITING

Home visiting programs aim to prevent child abuse and neglect by influencing parenting factors linked to maltreatment. These are: (a) inadequate knowledge of child development, (b) belief in abusive parenting, (c) lack of empathy, (d) insensitive, unresponsive parenting, (e) parent stress and lack of social support, and (f) the inability to provide a safe and nurturing home environment. By changing these factors, home visiting programs also seek to improve child development and health outcomes associated with CM. There have been reductions noted of 40% in child maltreatment in certain models (22, 23). In a comprehensive review, Gomby (24) found home visitation programs were most effective when they targeted families with many risk factors and used highly trained professionals who carefully followed a research-based model of intervention. Long-term follow-up with low-income single mothers who received home visitation services suggests that these programs are also effective in reducing child abuse and neglect in families where domestic violence is not present, decreasing the number of subsequent pregnancies, arrest rates, and the amount of time on welfare (25). Home visiting by nurses has been consistently more effective at reducing preterm and low-weight birth, increasing well child care medical visits and reducing deaths and hospitalizations for injuries and ingestions (16, 26). The findings have been replicated in a population of medically at-risk infants where home visiting using paraprofessionals was associated with lower use of corporal punishment, greater safety maintenance in the home, and fewer reported child injuries (27).

Programs such as Healthy Families America (HFA) have used paraprofessionals to provide services. In a randomized trial of HFA in New York, mothers in the program committed only one-quarter as many acts of serious abuse and neglect as did control mothers in the first two years (28). An evaluation of Healthy Families Florida found that the program using paraprofessionals had a positive impact on preventing child maltreatment, showing that children in families who completed treatment or had long-term, intensive intervention experienced significantly less child maltreatment than did comparison groups who had received little or no service. This effect was accomplished in spite of the fact that, in general, participants were at significantly higher risk for child maltreatment than the overall population. According to Williams, Stern and Associates (29), participants in HFA in Florida had 20% less child maltreatment than all families in their target service areas. In addition, families who completed the program fared much better than their comparison group counterparts and were more likely to read to their children at early ages. Also, HFA positively affected self-sufficiency, defined as employment. The program met or exceeded its goals for preventing maltreatment after program completion, provision of immunizations and well-baby checkups, increasing time between pregnancies, and participant satisfaction with services.

The Nurse-Family Partnership (NFP) is an evidence-based nurse home visitation program that improves the health, well-being, and self-sufficiency of low-income, first-time parents and their children. NFP models have been evaluated longitudinally across sites using randomized trials (36) and have been replicated in more than 250 counties. One analysis showed that for every $1 spent on the NFP, there were $4 in savings for taxpayers (30). Other specific programs have been reviewed, but overall, it is difficult to show cost effectiveness in improving key outcomes such as child abuse and neglect because the programs have wide variability in the job description of the home visitor, program implementation, and costs (31).

FAMILY WELLNESS AND PARENTING PROGRAMS

Family wellness programs include a variety of parent and family interventions and have been demonstrated to have some positive effects. These programs range from short-term counseling to parenting classes, sometimes with home visiting and sometimes with intensive "wrap-around" services for families at high risk for maltreatment. Many of these have been grouped together, making assessment problematic, but meta-analyses show promising reductions in child maltreatment (32). Intensive family preservation programs with high levels of participant involvement, an empowerment/strengths-based approach, and social support were more effective. In one series of 1,601 inner-city clients with moderate risk, programs designed to meet families' basic concrete needs and to provide mentoring were more effective than parenting and child development programming, and center–based services were more effective than home-based ones (33). At-risk parents who do not receive parent coaching or education have higher rates of child maltreatment, parent arrest, and child hospitalization for violence (30).

Parenting programs delivered by heath visitors, have been found to improve child mental health and behavior, and reduce social dysfunction among parents in one randomized controlled trial (34). Parent training models often differ, however, which often precludes direct comparisons. Parent training can include reviewing child development, teaching and practicing specific skills, identifying and addressing maladaptive behaviors, and supporting parents in managing their own emotions and responding to stress. Effect sizes overall have been found to be moderate, with outcomes affected by how training was delivered and under what conditions. Finally, family socioeconomic status, relationship with the trainer, inclusion of fathers, the need for additional child therapy, inclusion of a home visitor, proper length, delivery mode, and delivery setting must also be addressed to maximize potential outcomes (34).

A CDC meta-analysis of parent training programs (35) looked at program components and delivery methods that had the greatest effect on child behavior and parent skills. It concluded that teaching parents emotional communication skills and positive child interaction skills, while requiring practice with their children during each session, was the most effective in helping them to acquire effective parenting skills and behaviors. Teaching parents about the correct use of time out, to respond consistently to their child, to interact positively with their child, and to require practice were all associated with decreases in children's externalizing behaviors (35). In another model, Palusci et al. (36) found that parents with a variety of problems, including incarceration, substance abuse, and stress, had improved empathy, understanding of child development, and other improved parenting skills after an 8-week program of interactive classes using a family nurturing program.

The family support needs of parents with an intellectual disability are relatively unknown. One study (37) reviewed two types of intervention for parents with ID: those designed to strengthen social relationships and those teaching parenting skills. Using a literature search of electronic databases, only a limited number of evaluative studies were found, and the authors concluded that the evidence for interventions aimed at strengthening social relationships was inconclusive. Although positive changes were observed, there were limitations in study design which restricted the generalizability of the results. The evidence for parental skills teaching suggested that behavioral based interventions are more effective than less intensive forms such as lesson booklets and the provision of normal services, although these studies also had limitations.

THE PRENATAL AND PERINATAL PERIODS

Ray Helfer (38) noted the "window of opportunity" that is present in the perinatal period to enhance parent-child interactions and prevent physical abuse. This period, which he defined as from one year before birth to 18–24 months of life, was determined to be a critical time to teach new parents skills of interaction with their newborns. Several program models have shown promise based upon key periods within this time frame, including pre-pregnancy planning, early conception, late pregnancy, pre-labor and labor, immediately following delivery, and at home with the child. Opportunities for prevention in the early months of life include teaching parents and caregivers to cope with infant crying and how to provide a safe sleep environment for their infant. A recent meta-analysis of several early childhood interventions concluded that the evidence for their preventing child maltreatment in the first year of life is weak, but longer-term studies may show reductions in child maltreatment similar to other programs such as home visiting when longer follow-up can be achieved (39).

Many US state legislatures have enacted legislation to address infant abandonment and infanticide in response to a reported increase in the abandonment of infants (40). Beginning in Texas in 1999, "Baby Moses laws" or infant safe haven laws have been enacted as an incentive for mothers in crisis to safely relinquish their babies to designated locations where the babies are protected and provided with medical care until a permanent home is found. These laws generally allow the parent, or an agent of the parent, to remain anonymous and to be shielded from prosecution for abandonment or neglect in exchange for surrendering the baby to a safe haven. As of 2013, all 50 states, the District of Columbia, and Puerto Rico have enacted safe haven legislation. While national statistics have not been published, several states have reported hundreds of infants protected in this manner. Michigan, for example, had 170 infants relinquished using their safe haven laws during 2001-2015 (41).

HEALTH-BASED SERVICES

Health services in early childhood have generally not been shown universally to result in reduced child abuse and neglect. In the newborn period, Dias et al. (42) implemented a program in nurseries in western New York designed to teach new parents about violent infant shaking and alternatives to use when infants cry. The incidence of abusive head injuries decreased by 47% during the first 5 years of the program. The *Period of PURPLE Crying* uses a brief video and written material to educate new parents about normal crying and how to cope with infant crying. This program has been shown to improve mothers' knowledge about crying and to improve their behavioral response (43). Although these programs represent promising models and have been required in more than 15 U.S. states, neither has yet demonstrated strong evidence of effectiveness in the primary prevention of abusive head trauma or child maltreatment. Another hospital program, "No Hit Zone" has also been attempted to reduce the use of physical discipline, but it has not been systematically evaluated for CM prevention on a national scale (44).

A randomized trial of pediatric primary care screening and anticipatory guidance has shown lower rates of maltreatment, fewer CPS reports, less harsh punishment, and improved health services (45). This office-based prevention model, the Safe Environment for Every Child (SEEK), used pediatric residents who were trained to recognize factors that place a family at risk for maltreatment and a team to address any identified risk factors. When tested in a resident continuity clinic over a 3-year period, families had fewer reports of child maltreatment to child protective services, fewer incidents of medical nonadherence and delayed immunizations, and less harsh punishment by parents when compared with a control group. Some of the differences between the control group and the intervention group were of modest significance, however, and the program has not been systematically evaluated in a large number of pediatric practices. There were several barriers (professional time, training, culture, ability to deal with nonmedical issues) to widespread implementation that can be addressed by identifying potential strategies, such as the use of handouts and local news stories, to begin a dialogue during routine pediatric visits (46). In addition, there are several high-risk groups that need focused attention by the health care system, such as adolescent parents, addicted mothers, and depressed or mentally ill parents (47).

The American Academy of Pediatrics (AAP) has developed *Connected Kids: Safe, Strong, Secure* as an office-based intervention (48). Originally known as the Violence Intervention and Prevention Program (VIPP), the program was modeled after the AAP's Injury Prevention Program (TIPP) and uses a resilience-based approach to anticipatory guidance designed to help primary care physicians use their therapeutic relationship to support families. The *Connected Kids* program includes a clinical guide, online training materials, and parent education materials to educate both pediatricians and parents about discipline, parenting, and other related issues. *Connected Kids* is appealing to pediatricians, feasible to implement, and sustainable over a period of 6 months. A related project, *Practicing Safety*, was conducted by the AAP and funded by the Doris Duke Charitable Foundation to develop expanded anticipatory guidance modules for use in primary care offices. The seven modules provide pediatricians with suggested assessment tools, guidance, and resources to help parents cope with crying, develop parenting skills, ensure their children's safety when they are in the care of others, improve the family environment, provide effective discipline, assist with sleeping and eating, and help with toilet-training. However, neither the *Practicing Safety* nor the *Connected Kids* interventions led to significant decreases in child maltreatment in national samples.

There are been promising developments in medical-based parenting programs that are worth mentioning. A program of parenting intervention with videotaping parents during primary care pediatrics visits was associated with less use of physical punishment by parents at 2 years of age (49) and was maintained through three years (50). This program reduced parenting stress and physical punishment. In another analysis, the program improved social/emotional development in that children with reduced externalizing behavior may be less likely to be abused. Mediation pathways indicate that enhanced positive parenting through reading and play result in improved parent-child relationships, potentially reducing the risk of abuse (51). When used with a foster care population, a program using similar reflective video feedback during home visits also improved externalizing behaviors among maltreated children (52).

COMMUNITY STRATEGIES

A large body of theory and empirical research suggests that intervention at the neighborhood level can prevent child maltreatment among children with disabilities. This represents a "fourth wave" in prevention activities, with emphasis on altering communities in ways on par with those aimed at the individual parenting level (53). The two components of intervention that appear to be most promising are social capital development and community coordination of individualized services. Social disorganization theory suggests that child abuse can be reduced by building social capital within communities—by creating an environment of mutual reciprocity in which residents are collectively engaged in supporting each other and in protecting children. This is particularly relevant for disabled children, some of whom are highly dependent on residential or other care provided by specialized institutions. Research regarding the capacity and quality of service delivery systems in these communities underscores the importance of strengthening a community's service infrastructure by expanding capacity, improving coordination, and streamlining service delivery. Community strategies to prevent child abuse and promote child protection have focused on creating supportive residential communities whose residents share a belief in collective responsibility to protect children from harm, and on expanding the range of services and instrumental supports directly available to parents. Both elements—individual responsibility and a strong formal service infrastructure—are important. The challenge, however, has been to develop a community strategy that strikes the appropriate balance between individual responsibility and public investment.

Daro and Dodge (53) have also noted that, in the short run, the case for community prevention is promising on both theoretical and empirical grounds. Community prevention efforts are well grounded in a strong theory of change and, in some cases, have strong outcomes. At least some of the models have reduced reported rates of child abuse and injury to young children, altered parent-child interactions at the community level, and reduced parental stress and improved parental efficacy. When focusing on community building, the models can mobilize volunteers and engage diverse sectors within the community such as first responders, the faith community, local businesses, and civic groups in preventing child abuse. This mobilization can exert synergistic impact on other desired community outcomes, such as economic development and better health care.

One such program, the "Triple P" system, was designed as a comprehensive, population-level system of parent and family support with five intervention levels of increasing intensity and narrowing population reach. This system combines various targeted interventions to ensure a safe environment, including promoting learning, using assertive discipline, maintaining reasonable expectations, and taking care of oneself as a parent. These principles translate into 35 specific strategies and parenting skills. A large-scale randomized trial of the system published in 2009 noted lesser increases in substantiated child maltreatment, child out-of-home placements, and child maltreatment injuries in the intervention counties. Recent additional analysis which made use of a 5-year baseline yielded large effect sizes for all three outcomes that converged with those from the original analyses. The authors concluded that the study underscored the potential for community-wide parenting and family support to produce population-level preventive impact on child maltreatment (54).

A public health model follows a common pattern of intervention and evaluation when addressing a variety of conditions. A problem is defined, risk and protective factors are identified, prevention strategies are developed and tested, and if successful, are widely adopted (12). A key operating assumption in such efforts is that change initiated in one sector will also have measurable spillover effects into other sectors and that the individuals who receive information or direct assistance will change in ways that begin to alter normative behavioral assumptions across the population. This gradual and evolutionary view of change is reflected in many public health initiatives that, over time, have produced dramatic improvement in such areas as smoking cessation, reduction in drunk driving, increased use of seat belts, and increased conservation efforts. CDC and the US Maternal Child Health Bureau, for example, have strengthened the public health role and funding for child maltreatment and violence prevention (12). A caution is that the public health model for reducing adverse outcomes through normative change may not be directly applicable to the problem of child maltreatment. In contrast to the "stop smoking," "don't drink and drive," and "use seat-belts" campaigns, child abuse prevention often lacks specific behavioral directions that the general public can embrace and feel empowered to impose on others in their community.

Child fatality review has been a promising public health strategy which uses tertiary prevention to identify preventable patterns of CM fatality and near-fatality. Exceptions may exist for specific forms of maltreatment, such as shaken baby syndrome, but much maltreatment is neglect, which is less amenable to identification by this type of state-level public health interventions (55). Also, unfortunately, as the US Commission to Eliminate Child Abuse and Neglect Fatalities has found, there are relatively few promising or evidence-based solutions with research evidence showing a reduction in fatalities—one being the Nurse- Family Partnership (26). Likewise, they found only a handful of communities that identified reduction of child abuse and neglect fatalities as a goal, implemented efforts to achieve that goal, and demonstrated progress.

All organizations can develop policies and procedures that acknowledge that child abuse occurs, in and outside of child-serving agencies. Youth-serving organizations have an implicit responsibility to their clientele. However, even organizations that do not solely or primarily focus on children can, and should, be involved in the same prevention process. For example, doctors' offices, clinics, hospitals, community mental health centers, and other health care facilities that serve children could also enhance children's safety and decrease their own liability by taking similar actions (56).

Two community risk factors, poverty and substance abuse, have been singled out as particularly important in terms of the strength of their association with physical abuse and neglect (57). Increased recognition and integration of substance abuse treatment into child welfare was found to be an important first step to reduce co-existing substance abuse and CM. A motivationally-based public health approach for potentially at-risk parents could be proactive, brief, and repetitive and would incorporate substance abuse prevention messages into routine public health approaches spread over the parenting years. There is growing evidence that such programs, when implemented in multiple settings without stigmatizing parents, can appreciably reduce substance abuse and its associated CM (57). When children are exposed to violence as a result, some programs of secondary prevention such as group counseling have showed promise (58).

SOCIAL POLICIES

Policies can be powerful tools for prevention given their potential to affect conditions that can improve population-level health. Factors in society that can contribute to child maltreatment include the social, economic, health and education policies that lead to poor living standards, socioeconomic instability, warfare, or hardship as well as social or cultural norms that promote or glorify violence, demand rigid gender roles, or diminish the status of the child with regard to the parent (59). On the global scale, the United Nations Convention on the Rights of the Child offers a framework as a legal instrument for integrating the principles of children's rights with professional ethics and for the policy changes needed to enhance public health responses to prevent maltreatment (60). Each of these rights has specific implications for practice, advocacy, and research that can assist in defining, measuring, legislating, monitoring, and preventing child maltreatment. Achieving appropriate investments in community child abuse prevention programs will require a research and policy agenda that recognizes the importance of linking learning with practice. It is not enough for scholars and program evaluators to learn how maltreatment develops and what interventions are effective, and for practitioners, separately, to implement innovative interventions in their work. Instead, initiatives must be implemented and assessed in a manner that maximizes both the ability of researchers to determine the effort's efficacy and the ability of program managers and policy makers to draw on these data to shape their practice and policy decisions, which can affect society as well as families and communities (52).

Although evaluating societal CM prevention programs has been discussed for some time, it is only recently that the practice field has begun to develop the necessary capacity to understand and use evidence in decision making. National organizations, such as the US Centers for Disease Control and Prevention, Prevent Child Abuse America, Parents Anonymous, and the National Alliance of Children's Trust and Prevention Funds, have begun to assess and disseminate information about the effectiveness of programs (61). The World Health Organization (18) has also assembled a guide to assist policy makers and program planners in using and developing evidence-based programs. The CDC has promoted evidence in the creation and implementation of family programs, for example, which integrate evidence and evaluation into the program model. Programs should ideally monitor their impact, create and enhance new approaches to prevention based on those results, apply and adapt effective practices, and build community readiness for additional activities (12).

Klevens et al. (62) identified 37 state policies that might have impacts on the social determinants of child maltreatment and used available data to explore effects of 11 policies on child maltreatment rates. These included two policies aimed at reducing poverty, two temporary assistance to needy families policies, two policies aimed at increasing access to child care, three policies aimed at increasing access to high quality pre-K, and three policies aimed at increasing access to health care. Multi-level regression analyses identified two that were significantly associated with decreased child maltreatment rates: (a) lack of waitlists to access subsidized child care, and (b) policies that facilitate continuity of child health care. The presence of waitlists to access child care had a statistically significant association with child maltreatment investigation rates, with an increase in maltreatment investigations of 3.13 per 1000 children. States' continuity of eligibility for Medicaid/SCHIP was significantly associated with child maltreatment investigation rates that were 2.55 per 1000 lower than states without continuous eligibility. Klevens et al. theorized that these strategies decrease child maltreatment because child care and medical assistance with enriched early experiences in high-quality care settings can reduce childhood and adolescent behavioral problems that may trigger abusive parenting. Furthermore, continuous health insurance coverage and continuity of the medical home directly affect child health and development by enhancing parents' ability to provide an improved home environment and by removing financial stresses associated with uninsured medical costs. These findings were limited by the quality and availability of the data, and future research might focus on a reduced number of states that have good quality administrative data or population-based survey data on child maltreatment or reasonable proxies for child maltreatment and where data on the actual implementation of specific policies of interest can be documented.

Pediatricians have long been familiar with therapeutic preschools and with parenting programs. Participation in school-based child-parent centers, which provide extensive family education and support, can reduce maltreatment by 50% in high-risk populations (39). Access to affordable health insurance and high-quality early childhood education and child-care programs are additional interventions on a community level that address the problem of toxic stress by creating a healthier environment for children. Policies related to state provision of children's health care insurance such as the State Children's Health Insurance Program (SCHIP) can also potentially reduce maltreatment because children without insurance are less likely to receive health services in a timely manner, which might lead to medical neglect. Continuous insurance eligibility policies have enabled states to ensure continuity of care by providing Medicaid and SCHIP enrollees with continuous coverage for longer periods of time rather than on a month-to-month basis and they enable states to provide temporary coverage to children and pregnant women until a formal eligibility determination can be made. Other policies with prevention potential include criminalizing fetal exposure to drugs, designating child exposure to partner violence as child neglect, increasing access to abortion, and evaluating the effects of housing policies on stability for children and availability of child care.

Mandated reporting of suspected child abuse and neglect is a societal policy which can result in earlier and better identification of maltreated children. Palusci and Vandervort (63) evaluated the effects of universal mandated reporting laws on child maltreatment reporting rates to determine whether requiring all adults improved CM identification. Using county-level data from the US National Child Abuse and Neglect Data System for the years 2000 and 2010, they evaluated reporting rates for total reports, confirmed reports, and confirmed maltreatment types in a cross-sectional, ecological analysis. Controlling for child and community demographic variables such as child population size, gender, race, ethnicity, school attendance, disability, poverty, housing, high school graduation, parental marriage, religiosity, unemployment and crime, they found that counties in states with laws mandating that all adults must report suspected child maltreatment had significantly higher rates of total and confirmed reports. When mandates for clergy to report were changed, the results were less clear. They concluded that it is unclear whether changing state law or policy will enhance case identification.

TARGETING SPECIFIC TYPES OF CHILD MALTREATMENT

Instead of addressing specific methods or populations, some programs have been devised to target specific forms of CM. Several parent education programs, for example, have been evaluated for their association with decreases in physical abuse and neglect. *Family Connections*, a multifaceted, home visiting community-based child neglect prevention program, showed "cost effective" improvements in risk and protective factors and behavioral outcomes (64). To address a specific form of physical abuse, a hospital-based parent education program implemented immediately after birth that has been shown to decrease the incidence of shaken baby syndrome (42). After a similar program delivered to over 15,000 new parents in West Michigan, the number of SBS cases admitted to the hospital dropped from 7 per year to 5.3, a 24% reduction (65). *Period of Purple Crying* was able to increase maternal knowledge scores, knowledge about the dangers of shaking, and sharing that information with other caretakers, but no significant differences were noted in maternal behavioral responses to crying (43). Counseling and other therapies have been used with families with increased risk for CM, and Parent-Child Interaction Therapy (PCIT) is one evidence-based model which has shown promise in reducing physical abuse and neglect in young children (66).

One area which has historically been targeted with community interventions is sexual abuse prevention. Not all children who have experienced sexual abuse will be clearly identified or perhaps even identified at all until well into adulthood. Although some cases of sexual abuse are immediately apparent owing to the presence of sexually transmitted infections or acute physical injury, the vast majority of child sexual abuse is discovered through a child's own accidental or purposeful disclosure of abuse. Children often grapple with whether to tell, who to tell, and when to disclose so as to minimize negative outcomes to themselves or their families. These children may be faced with adults who are unprepared to respond appropriately because of lack of information, fears, or adults' own emotional reaction. Even when adults listen, they may respond in ways that upset the child or contribute to a retraction of the report or they may misinterpret the message, either exaggerating or minimizing the situation (67). Parents will react differently than their children and one another, and are critical to healing after abuse. Assessment of and attention to parents may be a critical component of successful intervention. Children with physical disabilities, cognitive impairments, or developmental delays have elevated risk of being sexually abused, and their parents and caregivers need to be especially informed of the need for safety (68). Yet, there is very limited empirical research evaluating methods to teach abuse-protection skills to CWD, and the studies available have focused on female participants with mild to moderate IDDs (69).

The big questions of how best to prevent sexual abuse, how to reduce rates over time, and eventually, eliminate sexual abuse remain unanswered. Until recently, few studies actually showed that participation in a prevention program resulted in reduced rates of sexual abuse for participants, with only anecdotal reports on successes and actions taken to stay safe as evidence (70). One study showed that college women who had participated in a child sexual abuse prevention program as children were significantly less likely to experience subsequent sexual abuse than those who had not had such a program (71). Additionally, although some argue that sexual abuse has not decreased as a result of sexual abuse prevention efforts, actual rates of sexual abuse do seem to be decreasing, and one proposed explanation is that sexual abuse prevention efforts may be at least part of the reason. Finkelhor (72) has concluded that these decreased rates and other available evidence support providing high-quality sexual abuse prevention education programs because children are able to acquire the concepts, the programs promote disclosure, there are lower rates of victimization, and children have less self-blame after attending these programs. Despite this, communities should be wary of relying on children to be solely or primarily responsible for their own safety and protection. All communities must do more than simply educate children about sexuality or abuse.

Despite the prevalence and demonstrated long-term effects of psychological maltreatment, there is little evidence detailing specific programs and practices designed specifically for its primary prevention. Several interventions do promote attachment and enhanced parent-child interactions, which by their very nature should decrease psychological maltreatment. However, given the varying definitions of psychological maltreatment and our difficulty in its accurate identification and reporting, it will be inherently problematic to show its reduction after prevention activities. One study showed that providing counseling services after confirmed psychological maltreatment was associated with a marked reduction in further confirmed psychological maltreatment (73).

IMPORTANCE OF HEALTH PROFESSIONAL INVOLVEMENT

Ray Helfer, a pediatrician who spearheaded the creation of the Children's Trust Funds across the United States, suggested decades ago that health professionals should be an important part of a multifaceted approach to prevent violence (74). Historically, approaches used included community commitment, mass media messages, training for new parents, early childhood development programs, interpersonal skills programs, and adult education programs for those caring for children. For children with disabilities, there are several reasons that health professionals should be more involved with prevention efforts. Most health professionals already understand and appreciate the linkages among prevention, intervention, and treatment, and they have an invaluable understanding of the effects of disabilities on children and families. It is critical that health care professionals embrace the importance of their role in prevention beyond merely treating and reporting suspicious injuries.

However, health care professionals are sometimes reluctant to intervene in potential cases of abuse. There are several reasons for this: lack of knowledge, fear of offending the patient (or caregiver), time pressures, discomfort of the patient with questions, fear of loss of control of the provider/patient relationship, and attitudes about accountability. Examining barriers to optimal service provision is important for every health care professional. Because health professionals have unique relationships with families, they have special opportunities to intervene to prevent abuse. Dubowitz (1) has suggested that it is important that physicians be able to ask sensitive questions, gather information, and use astute observation and careful assessment skills if they are to be successful in these endeavors. Keys to effectiveness are professional comfort with hearing sensitive issues, an ability to teach children about sensitive issues their bodies and personal space and privacy, familiarity with normal genital anatomy and routine child and parent concerns, an ability to diagnose and treat suspected maltreatment, and knowledge of the child welfare system (75). Screening for family and community violence should be included in routine health visits, even though some pediatricians need skills to better identify and manage injuries caused by such violence (76).

In addition to good clinical practice, medical providers can use and support a variety of strategies in the office, hospital, and their community to prevent child maltreatment. These include good clinical skills in properly recognizing and reporting suspected maltreatment, educating parents, and advocating for community programs and resources that will address the underlying problems that contribute to child maltreatment, such as poverty, substance abuse, mental health issues, and poor parenting skills. Collecting information about possible abuse experiences on intake forms is one way to learn about and create opportunities to address certain problems. Some physicians may be skeptical that patients would reveal information about a history of abuse on health forms, though patients are more forthcoming if asked than if never asked at all (77). In addition, by mentioning "unmentionable" topics, those providing health care show that they are aware of these issues and probably are knowledgeable about how to be helpful. The American Academy of Pediatrics *Connected Kids: Safe, Strong, Secure* (48) includes a guide for office clinicians, provides 21 parent/patient information brochures and supporting training materials, and encourages implementing a strengths-based approach for clinicians to provide anticipatory guidance to help parents raise resilient children.

Physicians and other medical professionals have now been invited by child welfare and public health officials to become more active in prevention as we think of CM as a long-term, public health problem. Prevention is explicitly not the responsibility of any one agency, profession, or program but is framed as the responsibility of all to create a society less conducive to child maltreatment. In this paradigm, individual skill development, community and provider education, coalition building, organizational change, and policy innovations are all part of the prevention solution for everyone, including health professionals (3).

INTEGRATING PREVENTION INTO PROFESSIONAL PRACTICE

Variability in outcomes after past programming has resulted in efforts to find more effective prevention programs. A current trend is toward "best practices" for ensuring quality, especially for care provided by medical professionals. Several conceptual standards have been suggested to evaluate programs, such as the content and approaches to imparting information to the target group, practice standards, and administrative standards. Recommendations for strategies include being family centered, community-based, culturally competent, and using a strengths-based approach. Other suggestions include being easily accessible, being linked to informal and formal supports, and having a long-range plan and ongoing evaluations. These efforts are promising and may help to build the highest quality into prevention programs that vary greatly in their efficacy and level of comprehensiveness. As we develop our understanding, evidence-based interventions will be useful, but standardizing programs across settings and cultures may not always effectively prevent CM.

Other professionals can take several roles in violence prevention, including advocating for resources for effective programs, screening, recognizing and referring at-risk families for services, and promoting nurturing parenting and child-raising styles (78). Beyond this, Plummer and Palusci (11), the American Academy of Pediatrics (3), and the American Professional Society on the Abuse of Children (79) have suggested several opportunities for professionals to CM prevention into their practice.

Table 2. Summary of steps to take to integrate prevention in daily work (72)

- Parent education
- Community awareness about the problem
- Bystander involvement in identification and reporting
- Early behavior problem identification
- Policy and organizational prevention efforts
- Improved clinical care and education
- Treatment and referral to optimal, accessible services
- Advocacy for resources and evidence-based programs
- Keeping up to date with practice in the field

Parent education

Professionals need to give parents effective strategies for discipline and nurturing by providing materials, consultation and referral. Parents should know about Internet safety, supervision, selecting safe babysitters, and choosing quality day care programs. Posters in waiting rooms, take-home brochures, and lists of Web addresses should be readily available for referrals for parents' use. Additional resources on child abuse prevention programs that exist in and around the community and referrals of parents to area agencies for additional information or assistance are vital prevention interventions.

Community awareness

Professionals need to offer to provide radio or TV public service announcements to build awareness of child abuse as a societal and public health issue and an issue related to physical and mental health. Health care professionals have the credibility to promote awareness of the links between childhood trauma and future health problems.

Bystander involvement

In personal or professional capacities, professionals need to be become involved when they are concerned about a child's safety and to seek supervision or consultation when necessary. Despite great demands on their time, professionals must be willing to make referrals to child protective services based on reasonable suspicion rather than waiting until they are certain to report child maltreatment.

Early behavior problem identification

Caregivers often consult with professionals about behavior problems with their children, who may be exhibiting reactive symptoms of being abused or stress after trauma exposure. Behavioral problems are often nonspecific, but professionals can guide parents to seek additional assistance, while guarding against parental overreaction to self-exploration or developmentally appropriate behavior.

Policy and organizational prevention efforts

Professionals should be willing to make changes in policy, hiring, supervision, and training in their own office or organization to put proven risk-reduction procedures in place. This can include establishing clinical practice guidelines to address these issues in the office and clinic.

Improved clinical care and education

Professionals need to recognize risk factors for violence when providing clinical care and be able to identify, treat, and refer violence-related problems at all stages of child development. Professionals need to identify issues with mental illness, substance abuse, stress, inappropriate supervision, family violence and exposure to media violence, access to firearms, gang involvement and signs of poor self-esteem, school failure, and depression. Professionals need to support early bonding and attachment, educate parents on normal age-appropriate behaviors for children of all ages, and educate parents about parenting skills, limit setting, and protective factors to be nurtured in children to help prevent a variety of injuries. Consistent discipline practices and body safety techniques should be emphasized.

Treatment and referral

Professionals need to know what they can handle through office counseling and when they need to refer families for help. They must also be cognizant of the resources available in their community to address these risks. This will require knowledge of the child welfare, emergency shelter, and substance abuse treatment systems and how to make referrals to appropriate therapists and mental health professionals.

Advocacy

Professionals should use their given status in the community to advocate for the needs of individual families and for the broader needs of children in society. This includes working on public policy and can best be achieved working in conjunction with organizations that address the needs of children in different arenas. Professionals can endorse and support quality, comprehensive, child-focused education and can serve on advisory boards for a local child abuse prevention agency or home visiting program, thereby assisting in networking alliances between prevention programs and the treatment field. Professionals can also be role models and leaders in their communities by offering support for family and neighbors who might need encouragement, help, or referrals and being advocates to assure that their communities have resources and services for parents.

Keeping up to date with the field

Professionals can be more effective advocates if they are knowledgeable about the current prevention field and evidence-based strategies for prevention. In CPS, professionals can identify prevention opportunities within the population of families and children who come to their system, but who are unsubstantiated or do not require that the children be taken into protective custody. Professionals in 'more traditional' fields of practice can help by recognizing the importance of their prevention work, participating in training, and helping to bridge the gap between research and practice.

PAYING FOR PREVENTION

While there is increasing evidence supporting the effectiveness of many of these universal and selective prevention interventions, a comprehensive assessment should include an analysis of cost and potential financial benefits (80, 81). For example, every $1 spent on childhood vaccinations in the US, $10.20 in disease treatment costs are saved, an estimated $13.5 billion saved annually in the US (82). Those attempting to justify the cost of CM prevention have often made comparisons to its measurable harms in an effort to show how resources used today can save money later. Advocates have estimated that every $1 spent on early childhood programs saves $4-7 for victims and taxpayers (30). All estimations are just that, relying on a series of assumptions about the direct and indirect costs, the costs of programs, the effectiveness of their implementation, and the potential reductions in societal costs as a result of those strategies.

Cost estimation for CM has historically focused on immediate costs in the medical, child welfare and criminal justice systems, but more recent analyses have attempted to estimate costs over the lifespan. In 1988, Deborah Daro (83) estimated a national and direct cost of $14.9 million for juvenile delinquency based on its incidence and rate among adolescent victims. She also found that 1% of severely abused children suffer permanent disability. Her analysis projected that the national cost and future productivity loss of severely abused and neglected children were between $658 million and $1.3 billion each year in the US as of 1988, assuming that impairments would reduce future earnings by as little as from 5% to 10%. In 1992, Robert Caldwell (84) looked at a single state (Michigan) and laid out what he thought were total costs in a variety of social systems and the savings that could be had. He estimated that the costs of a home visitor program in Michigan would be 3.5% of the $823 million estimated cost of child abuse, and small reductions in the rate of child maltreatment were thought to make prevention cost-effective. For 2002, he estimated that the yearly loss of tax revenue and productivity due to child maltreatment rose to $1.8 billion (8). Drawing from Maxfield and Widom's work (86), *Fight Crime: Invest in Kids* (30) noted that child abuse and neglect cost Americans at least $80 billion annually and affected taxpayers as well as those being directly affected. Potential benefits of prevention included mitigating the direct costs of child maltreatment as well as improving all of our lives through increased productivity and decreased crime and need for social services. Prevent Child Abuse America (87) used "conservative" estimates to calculate direct and indirect costs as $103.8 billion for the US in 2007.

In a more recent analysis of direct and indirect costs in the US, Fang et al. (88) estimated the average lifetime cost per victim of nonfatal child maltreatment to be $210,012 in 2010 dollars, including $32,648 in childhood health care costs; $10,530 in adult medical costs; $144,360 in productivity losses; $7,728 in child welfare costs; $6,747 in criminal justice costs; and $7,999 in special education costs. The estimated average lifetime cost per death was $1,272,900, including $14,100 in medical costs and $1,258,800 in productivity losses. The total lifetime economic burden resulting from new cases of fatal and nonfatal child maltreatment in the United States in 2008 was calculated to be approximately $124 billion. In a sensitivity analysis, the total burden was estimated to be as large as $585 billion. Compared with other health problems, the burden of child maltreatment is substantial and indicates the importance of prevention to address the high prevalence of child maltreatment. Similar conclusions have been reached internationally (89). The potential savings are thought to be substantial if CM is prevented or reduced, yet these savings cross multiple societal systems and funding streams. This acts as a disincentive to investment by segments of the economy unless they can capture potential savings from CM prevention.

One potential source for prevention funding comes from the health care system. On March 23, 2010, President Obama signed into law the Patient Protection and Affordable Care Act of 2010 (Affordable Care Act, ACA, P.L. 111-148), legislation designed to make quality, affordable health care available to all Americans, reduce costs, improve health care quality, enhance disease prevention, and strengthen the health care workforce (90). Through a provision authorizing the creation of the Affordable Care Act Maternal, Infant, and Early Childhood Home Visiting Program, the ACA was designed to use a health insurance model to strengthen and improve the programs and activities carried out under Title V; to improve coordination of services for at-risk communities; and to identify and provide comprehensive services to improve outcomes for families who reside in at risk communities. Home visiting is viewed as one of several service strategies embedded in a comprehensive, high-quality early childhood system that promotes maternal, infant, and early childhood health, safety and development and strong parent-child relationships. The long-term effects of the ACA are still being assessed, and recent federal policy changes may eliminate prevention or rescind the act entirely.

Given recent knowledge about the long-term health effects associated with adverse childhood experiences such as CM, we looked at potential medical savings for the healthcare system associated with reduced adult chronic conditions. We estimated disease-specific savings over the lifetime related to reductions in adverse childhood experiences (ACEs) to assess whether significant expenditures by healthcare systems for children are justified. Using annual healthcare expenditures in a single state (NH) for 4 of the chronic conditions in adulthood which were analyzed in the original ACEs studies (diabetes mellitus, cancer, heart disease and pulmonary disorders), we derived direct annual medical costs for each disease from national studies and NH data (91). Risk for adult disease based on childhood ACE scores was derived from the original ACEs studies, which found that a score of 4 or more was significantly related to increases in the adult condition of interest (6, 7). Recent research has suggested that these "conventional" ACE scores are significantly related to adult physical disease in diverse populations, although there is variability in relative risk (92).

Assuming that a combination of prevention strategies would result in the decrease of at least one adverse childhood experience for each child across the population, we then calculated the resultant decreases in adult disease costs based on changes in the population attributable risk fraction (PARf) associated with ACE score changes from 4 to 3 (see Table 3). Using program costs calculated from national data and our prior work, we then estimated the costs for providing three widely-available prevention strategies: home-visiting, office based parent screening programs, and hospital based newborn head trauma interventions. In this example, child population and births were estimated for the state of New Hampshire (NH) using census data.

Table 3. Risk reductions, cost estimates, and savings for selected conditions and strategies

1. Chronic disease costs/savings estimates

Disease*	Cost(NH)**	RR(4 v 0)	RR(3 v 0)	RR(4 v 3)	PARf(4 v 3)	Savings (4 v 3)*
CA	$220,000,000	1.9	1.0	1.900	0.474	$104,210,526
DM	$90,000,000	1.6	1.2	1.333	0.250	$22,500,000
HD	$180,000,000	2.2	1.4	1.571	0.364	$65,454,545
PD	$170,000,000	3.9	2.2	1.773	0.436	$74,102,564
						$162,057,110

*CA=Total Cancers; DM=Diabetes Mellitus; HD=Heart Disease; PD=Pulmonary Disorders
**NH annual direct medical cost estimate
***Calculations:
RR(4 v 3) = RR(4 v 0) / RR(3 v 0)
PARf (4 v 3) = (RR (4 v 3) - 1) / RR (4 v 3)
Savings (4 v 3) = Total Cost x PARf (4 v 3)

2. Prevention strategy cost estimates

Strategy	Unit Cost	Target	Population	Total Cost		
NB Ed	$20	Newborns	13,000	$260,000		
Screening	$500	Families w/children <5y	143,741	$71,870,500		
Homevisit	$2,000	Children <2y	26,000	$52,000,000		
						$124,130,500

3. Annual direct medical savings: $37,926,610

PARf calculations use risk ratios from: http://www.cdc.gov/violenceprevention/acestudy/outcomes.html.

The results are impressive. Total medical savings achieved in one year in NH for reductions in healthcare costs associated with these four adult chronic conditions amounted to $162 million (see Table 3). The total costs estimated for the three strategies delivered to the eligible populations were estimated to be $124 million, yielding a savings of $38 million annually in direct healthcare costs alone. This is likely a large underestimate of cost savings because it only includes four chronic conditions and does not include mental health or other behavioral issues which result in additional direct medical costs. This analysis makes several grand assumptions about the accuracy of the ACEs data, the effectiveness of prevention programs, the interactions of other risk factors with health and disease, and the economies of scale and program implementation. It is likely that any prevention program would reduce an individual's ACE score by more than 1 point, resulting in a larger decrease in adult disease; however, the efficacy of prevention strategies in reducing ACE scores has not been systematically evaluated. Despite these reservations, we conclude that the costs for just these three CM prevention programs are justified if the healthcare system can capture the savings in the future. The return on investment could be substantial, despite the long time frame to recoup the costs. In addition, given that medical costs are generally estimated to be 10-20% of the total direct and indirect economic burden of CM, an additional $1 billion or more in savings would accrue beyond direct medical costs. Thus, societies which are able to share costs and benefits across systems will be able to reap substantial economic benefit by preventing CM.

CONCLUSION

There are a variety of strategies which have been shown to reduce child abuse and neglect, although few studies specifically address their use or outcomes in populations of children with disabilities. Several steps have been taken to improve our identification of maltreatment specifically among disabled children, and children with disabilities who are maltreated are hopefully more readily identified and services are initiated earlier. While research is sparse, it is clinically believed that these interventions reduce the risk of abuse and neglect because of the additional emotional support which benefits child physical and emotional development. Health professionals can confidently support home visits in their community with appropriate referrals and can work to improve funding and access to affordable child care and prekindergarten interventions as evidence-based strategies which reduce CM. While there are several other strategies available, the evidence supporting these methods is promising but less robust. Regardless of the strategy used, the costs of CM to society are too high, and calculations showing the long-term savings achieved by reducing adverse childhood experiences justify significant expenditures. The medical system can afford to pay for prevention strategies for children if medical savings can be captured during adulthood. Our current state of knowledge and the evidence make this plainly obvious.

Yet additional steps can be taken by professionals to reduce CM. Little or no training is currently available specifically addressing the needs of children with disabilities. Clinicians and advocates need to be able to identify and report patterns of maltreatment while excluding mimics and other confounders. Children with disabilities need "medical homes" with professionals who follow them on a consistent basis and are integrated with community services. These reduce the risk of abuse or neglect and permit proactive, preventative services to be put into place. Further analyses are needed to better understand and disrupt the relationships between disabilities and child maltreatment, to answer questions about whether we can prove the causal links between adverse childhood experiences, and whether medically-based prevention programs in hospitals or the community can prevent child maltreatment. With more attention and additional research, we will hopefully demonstrably improve the lives of all children and adults, including those with disabilities.

REFERENCES

[1] Dubowitz H. Preventing child neglect and physical abuse: A role for pediatricians. Pediatr Rev 2002; 23(6):191–6.
[2] Krugman SD. Multidisciplinary teams. In: Krugman RD, Korbin JE, eds. C Henry Kempe: A fifty year legacy to the field of child abuse and neglect New York: Springer, 2013:71-8.
[3] Flaherty EG, Stirling J, American Academy of Pediatrics Committee on Child Abuse and Neglect. Clinical report: The pediatrician's role in child maltreatment prevention. Pediatrics 2010;126;833-41.
[4] De Bellis MD. The psychobiology of neglect. Child Maltreat 2005;10(2):150-72.
[5] Shonkoff JP, Garner AS, the Committee on Psychosocial Aspects of Child and Family Health, Committee on Early Childhood, Adoption, and Dependent Care, and Section on Developmental and Behavioral Pediatrics. The lifelong effects of early childhood adversity and toxic stress. Pediatrics 2012;129(1):e232-46.

[6] Felitti VJ, Anda RF, Nordenberg D, Williamson DF, Spitz AM, Edwards V, et al. Relationship of childhood abuse and household dysfunction to many of the leading causes of death in adults: the adverse childhood experiences (ACE) study. Am J Prev Med 1998; 14:245–58.

[7] Anda RF, Brown DW, Dube SR, Bremner JD, Felitti VJ, Giles WH. Adverse childhood experiences and chronic obstructive pulmonary disease in adults. Am J Prev Med 2008;34(5):396-403.

[8] Middlebrooks S, Audage NC. The effects of childhood stress on health across the lifespan. Atlanta, GA: Centers for Disease Control and Prevention, National Center for Injury Prevention and Control, 2008.

[9] Austin A, Herrick H, Proescholdbell S, Simmons J. Disability and exposure to high levels of adverse childhood experiences: Effect on health and risk behavior. NC Med J 2016;77(1):30-6.

[10] Palusci VJ. Adverse childhood experiences and lifelong health. JAMA Pediatrics 2013;167(1):95-6.

[11] Plummer C, Palusci VJ. The path to prevention. In: Kaplan R, Adams JA, Starling SP, Giardino AP, eds. Medical response to child sexual abuse. St Louis, MO: STM Learning Inc, GW Medical Publishing, 2011:365-95.

[12] Centers for Disease Control and Prevention (CDC). Preventing maltreatment: Program activities guide. Atlanta, GA: Author, 2007. URL: http://www.cdc.gov /ncipc/dvp/pcmguide.htm.

[13] Bronfenbrenner U. Toward an experimental ecology of human development. Am Psychologist 1977;32:513–30.

[14] Zielinski D, Bradshaw C. Ecological influences on the sequelae of child maltreatment: A review of the literature. Child Maltreat 2006;11:49–62.

[15] Daro D. Prevention of child abuse and neglect. In: Myers JB, ed. The APSAC handbook on child maltreatment, 3rd edition. Thousand Oaks, CA: Sage, 2011.

[16] MacMillan HL, Wathen CN, Fergusson DM, Leventhal JM., Taussig HN. Interventions to prevent child maltreatment and associated impairment. Lancet 2009;373:250–66.

[17] Aunos M, Goupil G, Feldman M. Mothers with intellectual disabilities who do or do not have custody of their children J Dev Dis 2004;10(2):65-79.

[18] World Health Organization. Report of the consultation on child abuse prevention. World Health Organization, Geneva, Switzerland: WHO Press, 1999. URL: http:// whqlibdoc.who.int/hq/1999/WHO_HSC_PVI_99.1.pdf.

[19] Patno KM. The prevention of child abuse and neglect. In: Jenny C, ed. Child abuse and neglect: Diagnosis, treatment and evidence. Philadelphia, PA: Elsevier Saunders, 2010:605-9.

[20] Klevens J, Whitaker DJ. Primary prevention of child physical abuse and neglect: Gaps and promising directions. Child Maltreat 2007;12;364-77.

[21] Child Welfare Information Gateway. Child maltreatment prevention: Past, present, and future. Washington, DC: US Department Health Human Services, Children's Bureau, 2011.

[22] Sweet MA, Appelbaum MI. Is home visiting an effective strategy? A meta-analytic review of home visiting programs for families with young children. Child Dev 2004;75(5):1435–56.

[23] Olds DL. The nurse-family partnership: An evidence-based preventative intervention. Inf Ment Health J 2006;27(1):5–25.

[24] Gomby DS. The promise and limitations of home visiting: Implementing effective programs. Child Abuse Negl 2007;31(6):793–99.

[25] Eckenrode J, Ganzel B, Henderson CR, Smith EG, Olds DL, Powers J, et al. Preventing child abuse and neglect with a program of nurse home visitation: The limiting effects of domestic violence. JAMA 2000;284(11): 1385–91.

[26] Commission to Eliminate Child Abuse and Neglect Fatalities. Within our reach: A national strategy to eliminate child abuse and neglect fatalities. Washington, DC: Government Printing Office, 2016. URL: http:// www.acf.hhs.gov/programs/cb/resource/cecanf-final-report.

[27] Bugental DB, Schwartz A. A cognitive approach to child maltreatment prevention among medically at-risk infants. Dev Psychol 2009;45(1):284–8.

[28] Dumont K, Mitchell-Herzfeld S, Greene R, Lee E, Lowenfels A, Rodriguez M, et al. Healthy families New York (HFNY) randomized trial: Effects on early child abuse and neglect. Child Abuse Negl 2008;32(2):295–315.

[29] Williams S. Health families Florida evaluation report: January1, 1999–December 31, 2003. Miami, FL: Author, 2005.
[30] Kass D, Miller C, Rollin M, Evans P, Shah R. New hope for preventing child abuse and neglect: Proven solutions to save lives and prevent future crime. Washington, DC: Fight Crime: Invest in Kids, 2003.
[31] Rigney L, Brown EJ. The use of paraprofessionals in a prevention program for child maltreatment: History, practice, and the need for better research. The APSAC Advisor 2009;21(winter):13–20.
[32] MacLeod J, Nelson G. Programs for the promotion of family wellness and the prevention of child maltreatment: A meta-analytic review. Child Abuse Negl 2000;24(9):1127–49.
[33] Chaffin M, Bonner BL, Hill RF. Family preservation and family support programs: Child maltreatment outcomes across client risk levels and program types. Child Abuse Negl 2001;25(11):1269–89.
[34] Patterson J, Barlow J, Mockford C, Klimes I, Pyper C, Stewart-Brown S. Improving mental health through parenting programmes: Block randomized controlled trial. Arch Dis Child 2002;87:472–7.
[35] Centers for Disease Control and Prevention (CDC). Parent training programs: Insight for practitioners. Atlanta, GA: Author, 2009.
[36] Palusci VJ, Crum P, Bliss R, Bavolek SJ. Changes in parenting attitudes and knowledge among inmates and other at-risk populations after a family nurturing program. Child Youth Serv Rev 2008;30:79-89.
[37] Wilson S, McKenzie K, Quayle E, Murray G. A systematic review of interventions to promote social support and parenting skills in parents with an intellectual disability. Child Care Health Dev 2013; 40(1):7–19.
[38] Helfer RE The perinatal period, a window of opportunity for enhancing parent-infant communication: An approach to prevention. Child Abuse Negl 1987; 11(4):565–79.
[39] Reynolds AJ, Mathieson LC, Topitzes JW. Do early childhood interventions prevent child maltreatment? Child Maltreat 2009;14(5):182–206.
[40] Child Welfare Information Gateway. Infant safe haven laws. Washington, DC: US Department Health Human Services, Children's Bureau, 2013. URL: https://www. childwelfare.gov/systemwide/ laws_policies/statutes/safehaven.cfm.
[41] State of Michigan Department of Health and Human Services. Safe Delivery Factsheet, January, 2016. URL: http://www.michigan.gov./documents/dhs/SAFE_DELIVERY_STATISTICS_-__UPDATE__ REVISED_as_of_September_7_2011_doc_REV_1_362698_7.pdf.
[42] Dias MS, Smith K, deGuehery K, Mazur P, Li V, Shaffer ML. Preventing abusive head trauma among infant and young children: A hospital-based, parent education program. Pediatrics 2005;115(4):470–7.
[43] Barr RG, Rivara FP, Barr M, Cummings P, Taylor J, Lengua LJ, Meredith-Benitez E. Effectiveness of educational materials designed to change knowledge and behaviors regarding crying and shaken baby syndrome in mothers of newborns: A randomized, controlled trial. Pediatrics 2009;123(6):972–80.
[44] Frazier ER, Liu GC, Dauk KL. Creating a safe place for pediatric care: A no hit zone. Hospital Pediatrics 2014; 4:247-50.
[45] Dubowitz H, Feigelman S, Lane W, Kim J. Pediatric primary care to help prevent child maltreatment: The Safe Environment for Every Kid (SEEK) model. Pediatrics 2009;123(3):858–64.
[46] Sege RD, Hatmaker-Flanigan E, De Vos E, Levin-Goodman R, Spivak H. Anticipatory guidance and violence prevention: Results from family and pediatrician focus groups. Pediatrics 2006;117:455–63.
[47] McHugh MT, Kvernland A, Palusci VJ. An adolescent parents programme to reduce child abuse. Child Abuse Rev 2015 Dec 30. doi: 10.1002/car.2426.
[48] American Academy of Pediatrics. Connected Kids: Safe strong secure. A new violence prevention program from the American Academy of Pediatrics. Elk Grove Village, IL: Author, 2005.
[49] Canfield CF, Weisleder A, Cates CB, Huberma HS, Dreyer BP, Legano LA, et al. Primary care parenting intervention and its effects on the use of physical punishment among low-income parents of toddlers. J Dev Behav Pediatr 2015;36:586-93.
[50] Cates CB, Weisleder A, Dreyer BP, Johnson SB, Vlahovicova K, Ledsma J, et al. Leveraging healthcare to promote responsiva parenting: Impacts of the Video Interaction Project on parenting stress. J Child Fam Stud 2016. doi: 10.1007/s10826-015-0267-7.

[51] Weisleder A, Cates CB, Dreyer BP, Berkule Johnson S, Huberman HS, Seery AM, et al. Promotion of positive parenting and prevention of socioemotional disparities. Pediatrics 2016;137(2):e20153239. doi: 10.1542/peds. 2015-3239.

[52] Pasalich DS, Fleming CB, Oxford ML, Zheng Y, Spieker SJ. Can parenting intervention prevent cascading effects from placement instability to insecure attachment to extenalizing problems in maltreated toddlers? Child Maltreat 2016. doi: 10.1177/10775595 16656398.

[53] Daro D, Dodge DA. Creating community responsibility for child protection: Expanding partnerships, changing context. Future Child 2009;19(2):67–93.

[54] Prinz, RJ, Sanders MR, Shapiro CJ, Whitaker DJ, Lutzker JR. Addendum to population-based prevention of child maltreatment: The US Triple P System Population Trial. Prev Sci 2016;17:410–6.

[55] Schnitzer PG, Covington TM, Wirtz SJ, Verhoek-Oftedahl W, Palusci VJ. Public health surveillance of fatal child maltreatment: Analysis of three state programs. Am J Public Health 2008;98(2):296–303.

[56] Saul J, Audage NC. Preventing child sexual abuse within youth-serving organizations: Getting started on policies and procedures. Atlanta, GA: Centers for Disease Control and Prevention, National Center for Injury Prevention and Control, 2007.

[57] Ondersma SJ, Chase SK. Substance abuse and child maltreatment prevention. The APSAC Advisor 2003; 15(3):8–11.

[58] Palusci VJ, Bliss R, Crum P. Outcomes after groups for children exposed to violence with behavior problems. Trauma Loss 2007;7(1):27-38.

[59] World Health Organization and the International Society for the Prevention of Child Abuse and Neglect. Preventing child maltreatment: A guide to taking action and generating evidence. Geneva: WHO, 2006.

[60] Reading R, Bissell S, Harvin J, Masson J, Moynihan S, Pais MS, et al. Promotion of children's rights and prevention of child maltreatment. Lancet 2009; 373:332–43.

[61] Prevent Child Abuse America. BECAUSE kids count! Building and enhancing community alliances united for safety and empowerment. URL: http://member.prevent childabuse.org/site/Page Server?pagename=research_because_kids_count.

[62] Klevens J, Barnett SB, Florence C, Moore D. Exploring policies for the reduction of child physical abuse and neglect. Child Abuse Negl 2015;40:1-11.

[63] Palusci VJ, Vandervort FE, Lewis JM. Does changing mandated reporting laws improve child maltreatment reporting in large US counties? Child Youth Serv Rev 2016;55:170-9.

[64] DePanfilis D, Dubowitz H, Kunz J. Assessing the cost effectiveness of Family Connections. Child Abuse Negl 2008;32(3):335–51.

[65] Palusci VJ, Zeemering W, Bliss RC, Combs A, Stoiko MA. Preventing abusive head trauma using a directed parent education program. Presented at the Pediatric Academic Societies Meeting. Atlanta, GA, May, 2006.

[66] Funderburk BW, Eyberg S. Parent-child interaction therapy. In: Norcross JC, Vandenbos GR, Freedheim DK, eds. History of psychotherapy: Continuity and change Second edition. Washington, DC: American Psychological Association, 2011:415-20.

[67] Jensen TK, Gulbrandsen W, Mossige S, Reichelt S, Tjersland OA. Reporting possible sexual abuse: a qualitative study on children's perspectives and the context for disclosure. Child Abuse Negl 2005;29:1395-413.

[68] Andrews AB, Veronen LJ. Sexual assault and people with disabilities. Special issue: sexuality and disabilities: a guide for human service practitioners. J Soc Work Hum Sex 1993;8:137-59.

[69] Doughty AH, Kane LM. Teaching abuse-protection skills to people with intellectual disabilities: A review. Res Dev Dis 2010;31:331-7.

[70] Plummer CA. Prevention of child sexual abuse: A survey of 87 programs. Violence Victim 2001;16(5): 575–88.

[71] Gibson L, Leitenberg H. Child sexual abuse prevention programs: Do they decrease the occurrence of child sexual abuse? Child Abuse Negl 2000;24(9):1115–25.

[72] Finkelhor D. Prevention of sexual abuse through educational programs directed toward children. Pediatrics 2007;120:640-5.

[73] Palusci VJ, Ondersma SJ. Services and recurrence after psychological maltreatment confirmed by child protective services. Child Maltreat 2012;17(2):153-63.
[74] Helfer RE. A review of the literature on the prevention of child abuse and neglect. Child Abuse Negl 1982; 6:251-61.
[75] Finkel MA. Child Sexual abuse prevention: Addressing personal space and privacy in pediatric practice. AAP SCAN Newsletter 2014;25(1):2,10-2.
[76] Trowbridge MJ, Sege RD, Olson L, O'Connor K, Flaherty E, Spivak H. Intentional injury management and prevention in pediatric practice: results from 1998 and 2003 American Academy of Pediatrics Periodic Surveys. Pediatrics 2005;116:996-1000.
[77] Diaz A, Manigat M. The healthcare provider's role in the disclosure of sexual abuse: The medical interview as a gateway to disclosure. Child Health Care 2000; 28:141-9.
[78] American Academy of Pediatrics, Task Force on Violence (AAP). The role of the pediatrician in youth violence prevention in clinical practice and at the community level. Pediatrics 1999;103(1):173–81.
[79] APSAC Prevention Taskforce. Practice guideline: Integrating child maltreatment prevention into professional practice. Elmhurst, IL: American Professional Society on the Abuse of Children, 2010.
[80] Mikton C, Butchart A. Child maltreatment prevention: A systematic review of reviews. Bull World Health Org 2009;87:353–61.
[81] Plotnick RD, Deppman L. Using benefit-cost analysis to assess child abuse prevention and intervention programs. Child Welfare 1999;78(3):381–407.
[82] Shurney D. Immunizations, prevention and lifestyle. J Managed Care Med 2016;19(Suppl 1):5-10.
[83] Daro D. Confronting child abuse: Research for effective program design. Washington, DC: National Academy Press, 1988.
[84] Caldwell RA. The costs of child abuse vs. child abuse prevention: Michigan's experience, 1992. URL: https:// www.msu.edu/~bob/cost1992.pdf.
[85] Noor I, Caldwell RA. The costs of child abuse vs. child abuse prevention: A multi-year follow-up in Michigan, 2005. URL: https://www.msu.edu/~bob/cost2005.pdf.
[86] Maxfield MG, Widom CS. The cycle of violence: Revisited six years later. Arch Pediatr Adol Med 1996;150(4):390–5.
[87] Wang CT, Holton J. Total estimated cost of child abuse and neglect in the United States. Chicago, IL: Prevent Child Abuse America, 2008.
[88] Fang X, Brown DS, Florence CS, Mercy JA. The economic burden of child maltreatment in the United States and implications for prevention. Child Abuse Negl 2012;36:156–65.
[89] Ferrara P, Corsello G, Basile MC, Nigri L, Campanozzi A, Ehrich J, et al. The economic burden of child maltreatment in high income countries. J Pediatrics 2015;167(6):1457-9.
[90] Affordable Care Act Maternal, Infant and Early Childhood Home Visiting Program. URL: http://www.hrsa.gov/grants/apply/assistance/homevisiting/homevisitingsupplemental.pdf.
[91] DeVol R, Bedroussian A. An unhealthy America: The economic burden of chronic disease charting a new course to save lives and increase productivity and economic growth. Santa Monica, CA: Milken Institute, 2007.
[92] Wade R, Cronholm PF, Fein JA, Forke CM, Davis MB, Harkins-Schwarz M, et al. Household and community-level adverse childhood experiences and adult health outcomes in a diverse urban population. Child Abuse Negl 2016;52:135–45.

Submitted: August 25, 2016. *Revised:* September 20, 2016. *Accepted:* September 22, 2016.

Section four - Virtual rehabilitation system design

In: Alternative Medicine Research Yearbook 2017
Editor: Joav Merrick
ISBN: 978-1-53613-726-2
© 2018 Nova Science Publishers, Inc.

Chapter 37

CHOOSING VIRTUAL AND AUGMENTED REALITY HARDWARE FOR VIRTUAL REHABILITATION: PROCESS AND CONSIDERATIONS

Sebastian T Koenig[*]*, Dipl-Psych, PhD*
and Belinda S Lange, BSc, BPhysio(Hons), PhD

Katana Simulations Pty Ltd, Adelaide, Australia
School of Health Sciences (Physiotherapy), Flinders University, Adelaide, Australia

ABSTRACT

Virtual and Augmented Reality hardware has become more affordable in the past three years, largely due to the availability of affordable sensors and smartphone displays as well as financial investments and buy-in through the entertainment industry. Many new consumer devices are now available to researchers, clinicians and software developers. With so many options available, planning a Virtual Rehabilitation project and selecting appropriate hardware components can be a challenge. This paper presents a stepwise selection process for Virtual and Augmented Reality hardware. The process is described through an example project in which clinical and technical implications of each hardware choice are discussed.

Keywords: virtual reality, virtual rehabilitation, augmented reality, development

INTRODUCTION

Recent advances in virtual reality (VR) and augmented reality (AR) technologies have provided a tremendous boost to the field of virtual rehabilitation. Two main drivers have contributed to the recent surge in VR/AR popularity and increased awareness in these

---

[*] Correspondence: Sebastian Koenig, Dipl-Psych, PhD, CEO, Katana Simulations Pty Ltd, Henley Beach South 5022, South Australia, Australia. E-mail: koenig@katanasim.com.

technologies: availability of affordable VR/AR hardware and availability of software development tools. Both of these factors also have a large impact on Virtual Rehabilitation applications.

Availability of affordable VR/AR hardware

Largely driven by the entertainment industry, prices for VR/AR head-mounted displays (HMDs) and tracking devices have become more affordable and accessible for consumers. Instead of spending tens of thousands of dollars for sophisticated HMDs and motion platforms, researchers, clinicians and educators can now purchase immersive VR/AR systems for under USD2000. Tracking solutions such as motion platforms, head-, hand- and body-tracking as well as a wide range of display methods have become available since the first Oculus Rift Prototype was released in March 2013 (1).

Availability of software development tools

Game and simulation engines are a key component for VR/AR content development. These engines give developers the tools to create interactive software applications and integrate VR/AR hardware. The trend for game and simulation engines has gone from expensive, closed systems to free access for everyone. Unity Technologies was the first company to start giving its engine away for free to individuals and small companies in 2009 (2). Over the past year, CryEngine (3) and Unreal Engine (4) followed a similar path and are now providing free licenses to their game engines. Other companies like Amazon (5) are joining the market with new free game engines, giving developers even more choices for software development.

Moreover, all major game engine providers have started to work with VR/AR hardware manufacturers to seamlessly integrate HMD-support and VR/AR user input into their products. Similarly, many companies releasing VR/AR hardware have started to provide integrations and example projects for the most popular game engines. This completely negates one of the main barriers to VR/AR adoption: a lack of platform compatibility between hardware and software components (6).

As a consequence, researchers, students and hobbyists can more easily become proficient in game and simulation development and even develop applications for fully immersive VR/AR systems. Game development courses at schools, universities and online learning platforms are becoming increasingly popular. Companies and researchers wishing to join the Virtual Rehabilitation field have a growing pool of skilled developers at their disposal. Developing VR/AR systems has transitioned from an expensive, narrow field of work to a growing industry that is open for anyone to join and start developing for free.

Taken together, both driving forces have had a large impact on VR/AR in general and the Virtual Rehabilitation field specifically. Researchers, clinicians, educators and developers have more hardware and development options available to them than ever before. However, with many new products and paradigms entering the market, a lack of standards, guidelines or prior experience with choosing and applying these new technologies can negatively impact Virtual Rehabilitation projects.

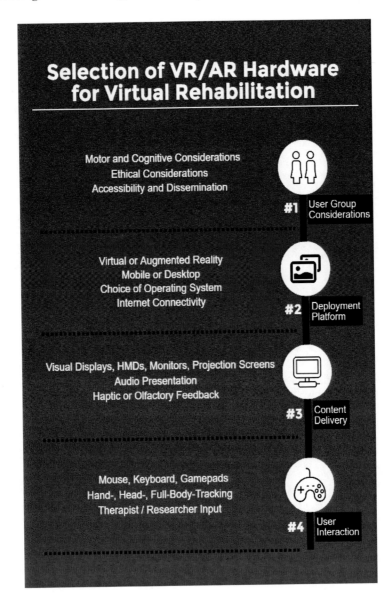

Figure 1. Selection process for VR/AR hardware.

This paper aims to provide guidance for selecting VR/AR hardware and software by describing a stepwise process (see Figure 1) that can be applied to Virtual Rehabilitation projects. The process includes 1) Considerations for User Groups; 2) Deployment Platforms; 3) Choice of Content Delivery; and 4) Choice of User Interaction. Each step of the process will be described through an example of a Virtual Rehabilitation project. The example project is a realistic simulation of a classroom which serves as an attention training and assessment. Available VR/AR hardware options and the implications of each option on clinical use and the end user are presented. The project used in this example has been ongoing for several years, however, this paper assumes the perspective of today's VR/AR market and discusses choices that are available as of Q1 2016.

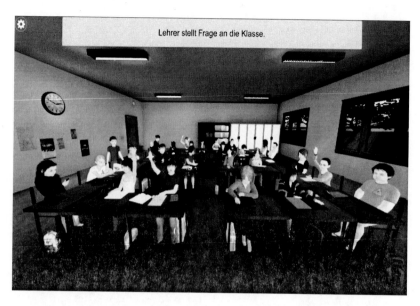

Figure 2. Virtual classroom scenario.

These steps are presented in an order that puts steps which are more selective at the start. However, it can be necessary to re-evaluate previous steps if a desired mode of content delivery or user interaction is not supported by the chosen platform. Such cases will be mentioned in the example project.

Decision process for selecting VR/AR hardware for virtual rehabilitation

The virtual classroom project (see Figure 2) aims to simulate an interactive classroom environment with students, teacher, distractions and learning content (7). The user is placed at a student's desk within the virtual environment and asked to monitor a task at the blackboard. Distractions are presented to challenge the user's sustained, focused and divided attention while the student has to respond to stimuli presented on the blackboard or by the teacher. The application is designed to be broadly used in research, education and clinical assessment and training. Depending on the intended use, the outlined decision process can vary considerably. The following stepwise process will focus on the training and assessment of attentional deficits in clinical use cases.

Considerations for user groups

Considering the needs of a user group or examining a clinical gap are fundamental steps in the planning and design of a virtual rehabilitation application. These considerations are essential for making any follow-up decision in steps two to four by choosing VR/AR technology that takes into account motor and cognitive deficits, accessibility and ethical principles when working with the relevant user groups.

Virtual rehabilitation applications are often designed for two user groups, patients and therapists/researchers/educators. This project targets school or university students and the therapists who are conducting the attention assessment or training. It seems reasonable to expect students to be at least familiar with computers, entertainment technology or occasionally even VR/AR hardware. Moreover, motor deficits, fatigue or other health conditions that limit the project's hardware selection seem unlikely unless comorbid conditions are expected. Ethical considerations are limited to a standard risk of simulator sickness when using immersive VR/AR systems. Consequently, no hardware or deployment options need to be ruled out based on the student user group.

No additional hardware has been excluded for this project as long as each device does not interfere with patient safety and allows the therapist/researcher/educator to directly interact with the virtual scenario in real-time. This aspect will be discussed when deciding on user interactions (step 4).

This first evaluation step ensures that projects and applications are not driven by the existence of exciting new technology, but rather with a focus on the clinical need. Eliminating hardware choices through user needs and limitations can involve very broad decisions that can be further refined in the upcoming steps. If, for example, the user group was a patient population with severe physical or cognitive limitations, and system use was limited to bedside treatment, the deployment platform, content delivery and user input would be vastly different from this described example application.

Choice of deployment platform

This decision influences most of the remaining choices in the process, as it determines which hardware, operating system and overall complexity the project will adopt. Deployment largely depends on where the system will be used. If the aim is to use the classroom in a lab setting, a Windows desktop PC is a viable choice. If the classroom focuses on clinical usage in private practices, a mobile solution with hardware such as the Samsung GearVR (8) and a smartphone are more appropriate options to provide portability and easy access. The availability of internet access in the target environment can also play a large role in choosing system components.

Most major game engines (e.g., Unity, Unreal Engine, CryEngine & Lumberyard) allow developers to deploy their software to multiple platforms without making major changes to the project. For most Virtual Rehabilitation projects and applications, the free license of CryEngine has to be excluded as a development option, as it excludes simulations and serious games. Further, CryEngine does not support deployment to mobile platforms. The remaining engines support deployment to Android, iOS and Windows, all of which seem valid choices for the Virtual Classroom project. Mac OS or Linux are not supported by most HMDs and have to be ruled out as target operating systems.

For this particular project, two additional factors play a deciding role for the deployment platform that is chosen. Firstly, attention assessments rely on highly accurate measurements of response timings. All available deployment options should undergo additional testing to guarantee that the latency between user input, response time measurement and a reaction on the system's display is within acceptable limits. Secondly, a simulation of over 20 animated characters requires substantial rendering capabilities. It has to be tested whether a modern smartphone can actually run an application with such complex graphics. Performance optimization and character rendering solutions are essential for deciding for or against mobile deployment, but these topics are beyond the scope of this paper.

This second decision step does provide several paths to follow for this project, but mobile and desktop deployment as well as VR and AR remain viable options. The following steps can narrow our choice of VR/AR hardware down further.

Choice of content delivery

Content delivery entails the presentation of visual, audio, tactile or even olfactory stimuli. Only visual and audio stimuli are relevant for this example project.

Visual stimuli presentation for the Virtual Classroom project can be achieved through monitors, HMDs or projection screens. It is essential for this project to allow the student user to freely look around the classroom. Distractions can occur in any part of the classroom and encourage the user to focus their attention on events away from the blackboard. The main goal of this application is to quantify attention and inattention. If the user looks at the blackboard and fails to respond to a relevant cue, an error is recorded. If the user is distracted and looks away from the blackboard while missing a cue, this event also captures inattention, but is a qualitatively different type of error.

Looking around the classroom can be achieved by three means: placing displays all around the user (e.g., CAVE environment), utilizing head-tracking or implementing virtual head movement. Multiple screens or CAVE environments require a complex hardware installation and are mostly prohibitive in cost and space requirements. Virtual head movement does not require actual movement by the user and is controlled via mouse, keyboard or other input devices. In light of affordable HMDs which include head-tracking, an HMD was chosen as the preferred option for head-tracking in this example project.

Mobile versus desktop deployment was already discussed in the previous section and the selection of HMD will obviously be impacted by the choice that was initially made with regard to the deployment platform. The main considerations for choosing mobile or Windows-based HMDs should be comfort, display quality, latency, integration in game engines, integrated tracking systems, price and availability of other compatible hardware such as handheld controllers. Market availability of existing HMDs may play an important role for products that have not been released as consumer versions yet and are only available as development kits. Development kits may change over time and new hardware and drivers may not be compatible with previous versions. This can negatively impact the development process and project timelines.

Comfort should be tested based on the intended maximum length of a session with the intended application. Features like padding material, total weight, weight distribution and cable-management should be considered. The weight and comfort of the newer HMDs such as the Oculus Rift or HTC Vive (9) was considered reasonable for use in the virtual classroom, because the scenarios run for no longer than one hour. Some smartphone-based HMDs require the user to hold the HMD with their hands or interact with the phone via buttons on the HMD. Such interactions were avoided for the Virtual Classroom as they interfere with the natural position of students sitting at a classroom desk.

An interesting potential option is the use of AR hardware to superimpose students, teacher and blackboard onto a real room. However, the use of this method is not suitable for a highly specific context such as the Virtual Classroom. An AR system would limit the use of the Virtual Classroom to real-world rooms that are spacious enough and contain believable furniture to support the simulation of a Virtual Classroom. In addition, the rendering of seated, fully-animated characters in unpredictable real-world spaces is a large technical challenge. Consequently, AR devices like the Microsoft HoloLens (10) and Meta2 (11) have not been chosen for the development of the application.

Consideration of the above criteria leave devices such as the Oculus Rift (1), HTC Vive (9), Razer OSVR Development Kit (12), Samsung GearVR (8), Google Cardboard (if used with plastic headmount) and Wearality Sky (when attached to hat and not handheld) (13) as potential hardware for displaying visual stimuli of the Virtual Classroom.

Auditory information is a key element of the virtual classroom for delivering distractions to the user. The spatial location of each audio cue is vital for systematically testing the user's spatial attention. Modern game engines usually support the spatial presentation of audio sources. Thus, auditory content delivery needs to support spatial audio. While some HMDs already have headphones included that support spatial audio, external headphones can usually be added to a VR/AR system without any problem.

Choice of user interaction

Recording user responses is vital for any cognitive assessment. The virtual classroom requires the user to respond to stimuli on the blackboard and to respond to input from the teacher.

If deployed as a mobile HMD, user input can be implemented through Bluetooth gamepads, keyboards or similar controllers. Speech recognition on Android or iOS are also valid options. In either case, latency variability needs to be taken into account when measuring response timings, as Bluetooth connections and voice recognition both add a slight delay to the response of the user. Desktop deployment provides more user input options, because many wired controllers, mice and keyboards with low input latencies are available. Desktop deployment also adds more options for writing, hand- and tool-tracking (i.e., pen) that can be used as a naturalistic response mechanism for the student user or as a detection method for fidgeting and motor activity. Such devices include writing tablets from companies like Wacom (14) and hand-tracking devices such as the Leap Motion (15).

Head-direction, as measured through head-tracking, can also be used as a means of user input. Facing other students can reliably be detected and used to start distracting animations. Head-direction is also an important variable for determining whether the user was looking at the blackboard when task-related stimuli were presented and potentially omitted by the user. The downside to using head-direction as an approximation for gaze-direction is that it is unknown what exactly the user was looking at or even whether the user's eyes were closed. Eye-trackers are not commonly integrated in HMDs yet, but several companies, for example Tobii (16) and Fove Inc (17), are working on advancing foveated rendering, which requires eye-tracking to adaptively change the resolution of the displayed image based on the user's gaze-target.

Lastly, the clinician's, researcher's or educator's interaction with the system needs to be considered. It is assumed that this user group requires a visual display of what the student user is experiencing in real-time. On a desktop VR system, the PC's monitor will usually display the point-of-view of the HMD. For mobile systems, the smartphone's display can be streamed to a TV via devices like Google Chromecast (18). Alternatively, Bluetooth or WifiDirect can be used to stream data from the smartphone to a second device that serves as the clinician's/researcher's/ educator's interface and live feed of the application. Further, it needs to be decided whether the clinician/ researcher/educator requires direct control over the application or whether the scenario is fully automated. For the Virtual Classroom these controls can include triggering distractions or changing the parameters of the primary task on the blackboard. It has to be noted that in some clinical or military environments the communication via Bluetooth or WifiDirect are prohibited and thus, mobile deployment or communication between multiple devices have to be ruled out as possible hardware choices. This limitation does not apply to the Virtual Classroom when used in a therapist's office or lab setting.

The choices presented in the previous steps are summarized in Figure 3.

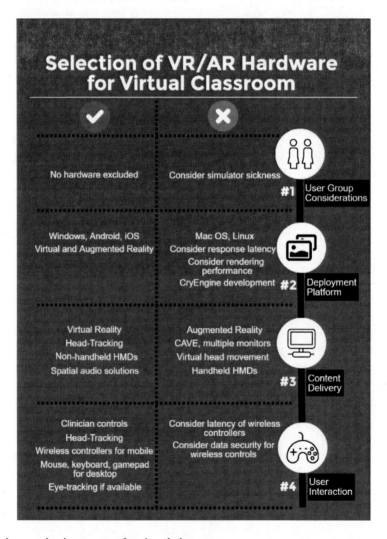

Figure 3. Hardware selection process for virtual classroom.

CONCLUSION

The example of the virtual classroom application can be applied successfully to different use cases with various user populations, even after excluding many technologies and VR/AR devices. Applying the selection process to this example project, two main configuration scenarios emerged for clinical and research use. When space and mobility are of less concern, a Windows desktop system with current HMDs such as the Oculus Rift and HTC Vive seems optimal. The clinician, researcher or educator can interact with the application through a normal PC monitor and use mouse and keyboard to change assessment and training scenarios. For improved mobility and flexibility, smartphone-based HMDs such as the Samsung GearVR are the preferred choice. The clinician, researcher or educator can monitor and interact with the application through a wireless connection of a separate tablet or laptop.

The virtual classroom is currently being used in three research trials. One trial investigates the influence of seating position during a simulated math class on student attention and retention of presented material. A second trial is testing the effect of a neurofeedback training in the virtual classroom on children diagnosed with ADHD. Lastly, the virtual classroom is utilized as a training tool for teacher trainees to provide hands-on scenarios for diagnosing disorders such as ADHD or dyslexia (7). The virtual classroom of the first two versions presents the user with a student's perspective and the third version puts the user in the perspective of a teacher who can observe the classroom and interact with students. The first two versions leverage the Oculus Rift and a Windows PC and the last version aims to make the virtual classroom accessible to a wide range of Windows-based laptops and desktop PCs.

The described selection is rehabilitation applications. Obviously, just as rehabilitation is not one size fits all, these solutions are not one size fits all. Virtual reality and AR applications have potential to improve rehabilitation by offering flexible, tailored tools that can provide multimodal feedback, quantitative measurement and user engagement. It is important to consider the technical aspects and how decisions about hardware and software will ultimately have an impact on the final product in this fast-paced market of VR and AR technologies.

ACKNOWLEDGMENTS

The authors have no affiliations with or financial investments in any of the mentioned companies or products and no endorsement of specific products is intended.

REFERENCES

[1] Oculus VR LLC. Oculus Kickstarter Campaign 2012 [Crowdfunding project description]. Accessed 2016 Feb 10. URL: https://www.kickstarter.com/projects/1523379 957/oculus-rift-step-into-the-game/description.

[2] Unity Technologies. Unity3D game engine product page [Product website]. Accessed 2016 Feb 10. URL: https://unity3d.com/.

[3] Crytek GmbH. CryEngine game engine product page [Product website]. Accessed 2016 Feb 10. URL: https://www.cryengine.com/.
[4] Epic Games Inc. Unreal game engine product page [Product website]. Accessed 2016 Feb 10. URL: https://www.unrealengine.com/.
[5] Amazon Web Services Inc. Amazon Lumberyard game engine product page [Product website]. Accessed 2016 Feb 10. URL: https://aws.amazon.com/lumberyard/.
[6] Rizzo AA, Kim GJ. A SWOT analysis of the field of virtual reality rehabilitation and therapy. Presence: Teleoper. Virtual Environ 2005;14(2):119-46.
[7] Klingsieck K, Al-Kabbani D, Bohndick C, Hilkenmeier J, Muesche H, Praetorius S, et al. Spielend eine diagnostisch kompetente Lehrkraft werden – mit der game- und e-learningbasierten, Problemorientierten und selbstgesteuerten Lernumgebung gePros. Konferenz der Deutschen Gesellschaft für Hochschuldidaktik, Paderborn, Germany, 2015. [German].
[8] Samsung Corporation. Samsung GearVR product page [Product website]. Accessed 2016 Feb 10. URL: http://www.samsung.com/global/galaxy/wearables/gear-vr/.
[9] HTC Corporation. HTC Vive Head-mounted display product page [Product website]. Accessed 2016 Feb 10. URL: http://www.htcvive.com/.
[10] Microsoft Corporation. Microsoft HoloLens product page [Product website]. Accessed 2016 Feb 10. URL: https://www.microsoft.com/microsoft-hololens/en-us/.
[11] Meta Company. Meta 2 Development Kit product page [Product website]. Accessed 2016 Feb 10. URL: https://www.metavision.com/.
[12] Razer Inc. Razer OSVR Development Kit product page [Product website]. Accessed 2016 Feb 10. URL: http://www.razerzone.com/osvr.
[13] Wearality Corporation. Wearlity Sky product page. [Product website]. Accessed 2016 Feb 10. URL: http://www.wearality.com/wearalitysky/.
[14] Wacom. Wacom digital writing tablets product page [Product website]. Accessed 2016 Feb 10. URL: http://www.wacom.com/.
[15] Leap Motion Inc. Leap Motion sensor product page [Product website]. Accessed 2016 Feb 10. URL: https://www.leapmotion.com/.
[16] Fove Inc. Fove Head-Mounted Display product page [Product website]. Accessed 2016 Feb 10. URL: http://www.getfove.com/.
[17] Tobii AB. Tobii Eye-Tracking for VR [Product website]. Accessed 2016 Feb 10. URL: http://www.tobii.com/tech/products/vr/.
[18] Google Inc. Google Chromecast product page [Product website]. Accessed 2016 Feb 10. URL: https://www. google.com/chromecast.

Submitted: December 20, 2016. *Revised:* February 10, 2017. *Accepted:* February 15, 2017.

In: Alternative Medicine Research Yearbook 2017
Editor: Joav Merrick

ISBN: 978-1-53613-726-2
© 2018 Nova Science Publishers, Inc.

Chapter 38

BAYESIAN MODELLING FOR INCLUSIVE DESIGN UNDER HEALTH AND SITUATIONAL-INDUCED IMPAIRMENTS: AN OVERVIEW

Bashar I Ahmad, PhD, BEng, Patrick M Langdon, PhD, BSc and Simon J Godsill, PhD, MA*

Signal Processing and Communications Laboratory (SigProC),
Engineering Department, University of Cambridge, Engineering Design Centre (EDC),
Engineering Department, University of Cambridge, UK

ABSTRACT

Predictive pointing enables smart interfaces, which are capable of inferring the user intent, early in the pointing task, and accordingly assisting on-display target acquisitions (pointing and selection). It adopts a Bayesian framework to effectively model the user pointing behaviour and incorporate the present perturbations induced by situational impairments as well as inaccuracies in the utilised sensing technology. The objective of the predictive pointing system is to minimise the cognitive, visual and physical effort associated with acquiring an interface component when the user input is perturbed due to a situational impairment, for example, to aid drivers select icons on a display in a moving car via free hand pointing gestures. In this paper, we discuss the ability of the predictive pointing solution to simplify and expedite human computer interaction when the user input is perturbed due to health induced impairments and disability, rather than a situational impairment. Examples include users with tremors, spasms, or other motor impairments. Given the flexibilities acceded by the Bayesian formulation, the applicability of the predictive pointing to inclusive design in general is addressed. Its intent prediction functionality can be adapted to the user's physical capabilities and pointing characteristics-style, thereby catering for wide ranges of health induced impairments, such as those arising from ageing. It is concluded that predictive displays can significantly facilitate and reduce the effort required to accomplish selection tasks on

---

* Correspondence: Bashar I Ahmad, PhD, BEng, Senior Research Associate, SigProC, Baker Building, Engineering Department, University of Cambridge, Trumpington Street, Cambridge, CB2 1PZ, United Kingdom.
E-mail: bia23@cam.ac.uk.

a display when the user input is perturbed due to health or physical impairments, especially when pointing in 3D via free hand pointing gestures.

Keywords: human machine interaction, health-induced impairment, situationally-induced impairment, Bayesian Inference

INTRODUCTION

Interactive displays, such as touchscreens, are becoming an integrated part of the car environment due to the additional design flexibilities they offer (e.g., combined display-interaction-platform-feedback module whose interface can be adapted to the context of use through a reconfigurable Graphical User Interface GUI) and their ability to present large quantities of information associated with In-Vehicle Infotainment Systems IVIS (1-4). The latter factor is particularly important since the complexity of IVIS has been steadily increasing to accommodate the growing additional services related to the proliferation of smart technologies in modern vehicles (5). Using an in-car display typically entails undertaking a free hand pointing gesture to select an on-screen GUI icon. Whilst this input modality is intuitive, especially for novice users, it requires dedicating a considerable amount of attention (visual, cognitive and physical) that can be otherwise available for driving (4). Additionally, the user pointing gesture and input on the display can be subject to in-vehicle accelerations and vibrations due to the road and driving conditions, which can lead to erroneous selections (6). This source of perturbations is dubbed Situationally Induced Impairment and Disability (SIID). Figure 1 depicts an example of free hand pointing gestures, in 3D, subjected to high levels of perturbations (i.e., SIID) in a moving car. The notable impact of the in-vehicle SIID originated perturbations is clearly visible in the pointing motion as jolts or jumps. Adapting to the present noise and/or rectifying incorrect selections will tie up more of the user's attention. This can render interacting with the touchscreen highly distracting, with potential safety consequences (4, 7).

Predictive interactive displays, proposed in (8, 9), utilise a gesture tracker to capture, in real-time, the pointing hand/finger locations in 3D in conjunction with appropriate probabilistic destination inference algorithm. It can establish the icon the user intends to select on the display, remarkably early in the free hand pointing gesture, and in the presence of perturbations due to road and driving conditions, i.e., SIID. The smart intent-aware display then accordingly simplifies and expedites the target acquisition by applying a *pointing facilitation scheme*. This can be in the form of, among other options, expanding or colouring the intended GUI icon(s) or even selecting the predicted item on behalf of the user, who then need not touch the display surface. Therefore, predictive displays can notably improve the usability of in-car interactive displays by reducing distractions and workload associated with using them. The Bayesian formulation of the fundamental problem of intent inference, see (8), enables the predictive displays to effectively handle varying levels and types of present SIID-originated perturbations and/or user pointing behaviour as well as incorporating additional sensory or contextual data when available. It is noted that several pointing gesture trackers, which can accurately track, in real-time, a pointing gesture in 3D, have emerged lately, e.g., Microsoft Kinect, leap motion and others. They are motivated by extending Human-Computer Interaction (HCI) beyond traditional keyboard input and mouse pointing.

On the other hand, using technological devices and the ubiquitous touchscreens becoming commonplace in everyday life, whether in work or domestic environments, led to the task of acquiring targets on a graphical user interface (e.g., to select buttons, menus, etc.) being a part of modern life and a frequent human-computer interaction undertaking. Hence, facilitating on-screen target acquisition (pointing and selection), reducing the effort incurred and improving its accuracy is critical for realising effective user interfaces. This is typically tackled by applying a pointing assistive strategies (e.g., expanding icon, altering its activation area, etc.), preceded by a mechanism to establish the intended GUI icon, i.e., to identify which icon to expand or alter, for example see (10-19). Whilst the user population is diverse and includes motion impaired, elderly and non-expert users, these HCI studies often consider able-bodied computer users and focus on pointing in 2D on a computer screen using a mouse or a mechanical device. However, similar to users experiencing SIID, the pointing-selection task can be challenging for users with a motion-visual impairment, i.e., Health Induced Impairment and Disability HIID (19-24), for example, Figure 2 shows 2D mouse cursor pointing tracks of a user suffering from cerebral palsy. The prediction approaches developed for mouse pointing are also in general unsuitable for pointing in 3D using free hand pointing gestures and/or have high computational-training requirements (8). Thereby, suitable prediction algorithms for pointing in 3D under situational impairment are proposed in (8), within a flexible Bayesian framework. Statistical techniques based on Kalman filtering and advanced state-space particle filter method are employed to smooth 2D pointing mouse cursor trajectories and 3D tracks of free hand pointing gestures (8, 19, 20). They compensate for (remove) HIID and SIID related perturbations, such that the resultant 2D or 3D pointing trajectories move only in the intended direction.

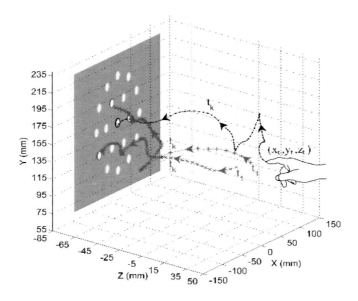

Figure 1. Full pointing finger-tip trajectories in 3D during three pointing gestures aimed at selecting a GUI item (circles) on the in-vehicle touchscreen surface (blue plane), whilst the car is driven over a harsh terrain with severe perturbations present. Arrows indicate the direction of travel over time, starting at $t_1 < t_k$.

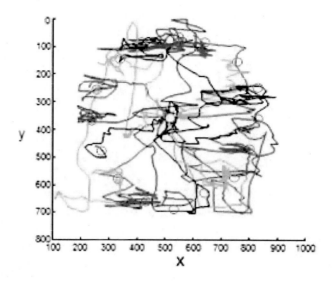

Figure 2. Several 2D mouse cursor tracks to acquire on-screen GUI icons (classical Fitt's law task, ISO 9241) for user with cerebral palsy (20).

In this paper, we highlight the potential of applying the predictive display solution, which was developed for perturbations due to SIID in automotive contexts and supports pointing gestures input modality in 3D, to facilitate HCI for users with a wide range of health induced impairment and disability. This includes HIID that arises from age, and not only severe forms of physical disability. Therefore, this HCI solution can be viewed as a means to promote inclusion. Inclusive design examines designed product features with particular attention to the functional demands they make on the perceptual, thinking and physical capabilities of diverse users. A predictive display can extend the usability of the interactive displays to a diverse population of users, for example, motion impaired or able-bodied users, elderly or young users, expert or non-expert users as well as those that are situationally impaired.

Here, we exploit the transferability of HCI solutions for HIID to SIID scenarios (and vice versa) (23, 26). This transferability assumes that any human user can be impaired (disabled) in their effectiveness by characteristics of their environment, the task and the design of the GUI. Such impairment may take the form of perceptual, cognitive and physical movement functional limitations, which translate into inability. For instance, attempting to enter text on an in-car touchscreen (e.g., for navigation) whilst driving in an off-road environment presents difficulties in perceiving the interface for multiple tasks (seeing on-screen icons, outside driving environment and vehicle controls), performing the attentional tasks necessary for safe driving (track/correct vehicle movement, maintaining car controls as well as monitor/correct the texting task), and carrying out the required physical movements (pointing, pressing, steering, braking, etc.). The Bayesian intent predictor applied within a predictive display system relies on defining a Hidden Markov Model (HMM) of the pointing motion in 3D, effectively capturing the influence of the intended endpoint on the pointing finger/hand movements (8). This is distinct from previous HCI research on endpoint prediction in 2D scenarios, e.g., (11-18), which often follow from Fitt's law type analysis and uses a static setting/model. The statistical modelling approach permits capturing the variability among users, motor capabilities and the noise of the motion tracking sensor via Stochastic

Differential Equations (SDE) that represent the destination-motivated pointing motion in 3D or even 2D.

Inclusive design from disability to HCI

Increasingly, mobile technology is proliferating, and due to the expected contribution of the Internet of Things (IoT), 5G and recent mobile communications technology, a plethora of possible applications integrating sensor networks, cloud based processing and storage and mobile contexts will present HCI challenges to interaction designers (24, 27). Challenges range from: network latencies, and lack of them; processing limitations; fusion of multiple sources of data, and the potential to overload the user's capabilities, both in terms of physical responses and also cognitive capacity. The field of inclusive design relates the capabilities of the population to the design of products by better characterising the user–product relationship. Inclusion refers to the quantitative relationship between the demand made by design features and the capability ranges of users who may be excluded from use of the product because of those features. By 2020, almost half the adult population in the UK will be over 50, with the over 80s being the most rapidly growing sector. These "inclusive" populations contain a great variation in sensory, cognitive and physical user capabilities, particularly when non-age-related impairments are taken into account. Establishing the requirement of end users is intrinsically linked to the user-centred design process. In particular, a requirements specification is an important part of defining and planning the variables to be tested and measured as well as the technology use cases to be addressed during the user trials.

In particular, inclusive design is a user-centred approach that examines designed product features with particular attention to the functional demands they make on the perceptual, thinking, and physical capabilities of diverse users, particularly those with reduced capabilities and ageing. It is known, for example, that cognitive capabilities such as verbal and visuospatial IQ show a gradually decreasing performance with aging. Attending to goal-relevant, task features and inhibiting irrelevant ones is important in interaction and this is known to be affected by ageing. Attentional resources may also be reduced by ageing, such that more mistakes are made during divided attention, dual task situations (28-30). Another perspective on inclusive design is that of ordinary and extraordinary design that aims to improve design for older, impaired users of low functionality while at the same time enhancing design for the mainstream and ordinary users in extreme environments. On this basis, design should focus on the *extraordinary* or impaired first, accommodating mainstream design in the process (31).

Not all functional disabilities result from ageing. Some common examples of non-age-related impairment include specific conditions such as stroke and head injury, which may affect any or all of perception, memory and movement. Other conditions are generally associated with movement impairment. For example, Parkinson's disease and cerebral palsy involve damage to the brain causing effects such as tremor, spasms, dynamic coordination difficulties, and language and speech production impairment. Of course, many other conditions such as Down's syndrome and multiple sclerosis may affect cognitive capability either directly, through language learning and use, or indirectly through its effects on hearing, speech production and writing. Of all the variations discussed, many differentially affect normal population ranges of capability. They may be rapidly changing and vary in intensity both within and between individuals, leading to a demanding design environment that requires close attention to conflicting user requirements and a better understanding of user capability. Again, this confirms that interaction design for future generations of products must be inclusive.

One area offering mitigation to these challenges is design of integrated multimodal display and control technologies for ease of input and task completion (20-23). Initially, in the domain of better design for elderly and impaired computer and TV users, this work is directly transferrable to the domain of the situationally impaired interface disability users as proposed by (26) and in the form of extraordinary user interfaces (32). This approach assumes that any human user can be impaired (disabled) in their effectiveness by characteristics of their environment, the task, and the design of the user interface they are presented with. Importantly, an inclusive design approach extends beyond the scope of conventional usability methods as it must accommodate extremes of capability range or situational contexts of task or stress, that are not normally accommodated by product design. For this reason, the predictive interactive display within a Bayesian framework is well suited to the human centred design of new information-rich and multimodal interfaces. It can effectively incorporate variabilities in physical-motor capabilities, interaction style, contextual information and additional sensory data (when available), within the stochastic pointing movement and measurement models as well as the modelling priors. In this paper, we start with a specific case, whereby the proposed statistical predictive techniques aim to facilitate the GUI icons acquisition on an in-vehicle touchscreen by a driver in a moving car, i.e., the pointing gestures can be heavily perturbed due to SIID. This has proven to be very effective in reducing the workload associated with using an interactive in-car display. Thus, the developed predictive displays framework is a promising approach to achieving substantial significant usability improvements to health impaired users, i.e., HIID, in similar pointing tasks. If so, this solution can significantly enhance the HCI capabilities of individuals with severe physical impairments such as tremor, spasm and athetosis.

Bayesian formulation and suitability

The free hand pointing gesture movements towards an on-screen interface item in 3D are not deterministic, but are rather governed by a complex motor system. They can also be subjected to external motion, vibrations, acceleration (e.g., in a moving platform), etc. Nonetheless, stochastic models can capture the variability in the pointing finger movements, albeit being driven by premeditated intent (33). Hence, predictions of the pointing object (e.g., finger) motion are not single fixed paths, but are rather probabilistic processes, such that the object position at a future time expressed as a probability distribution in space. By adequately incorporating this uncertainty, relatively simple models of the pointing finger motion can be used successfully to track finger movements and evaluate the corresponding *observation likelihoods* (8, 33). It is noted that the objective of a predictive pointing is not to accurately model the complex human motor system. It suffices to utilise approximate pointing motion models that facilitate establishing the on-display endpoint of a free hand pointing gesture, hence intent. Therefore, calculating the transition density of a stochastic model, for example, between two successive observation times is required to condition the tracked pointing finger state $\mathbf{X}_t$, (e.g., position, velocity, etc.) on a nominal endpoint on the display $\mathcal{D}_i$ (33).

Continuous-time motion models are a natural choice in such cases, where the tracked pointing object dynamics are captured by a continuous-time stochastic differential equation. This SDE can be integrated to obtain a transition density over any time interval (8, 33). Although numerous models exist, the class of Gaussian linear time invariant models for the evolution of $\mathbf{X}_t$ has proven to be effective to establishing the user intent and also lead to a low-complexity inference procedure (8, 33, 34). This class includes many models used in tracking applications, such as constant velocity and the linear destination reverting (LDR) models.

Intent inference
Predictive displays aim to estimate, in real-time, the probability of each of the selectable icons of the displayed GUI being the intended endpoint of the undertaken pointing task. At time instant t_k where the available pointing object (finger or mouse cursor) observations (e.g., positions) are $\mathbf{m}_{1:k} = \{\mathbf{m}_1, \mathbf{m}_2, \ldots, \mathbf{m}_k\}$, the system calculates

$$\mathcal{P}(t_k) = \{P(\mathcal{D}_I = \mathcal{D}_i | \mathbf{m}_{1:k}), i = 1, 2, \ldots, N\}. \qquad \text{Equation 1}$$

The intended destination, which is unknown *a priori*, is notated by $\mathcal{D}_I$ such that $\mathcal{D}_I \in \mathbb{D} = \{\mathcal{D}_1, \mathcal{D}_2, \ldots, \mathcal{D}_N\}$ and $\mathbb{D}$ is the set of selectable GUI items. It is noted that the locations of the interface components in $\mathbb{D}$ are known, however, no assumptions are made on their distribution or layout on the display. Following Bayes' rule, we can write: $P(\mathcal{D}_I = \mathcal{D}_i | \mathbf{m}_{1:k}) \propto P(\mathcal{D}_I = \mathcal{D}_i) P(\mathbf{m}_{1:k} | \mathcal{D}_I = \mathcal{D}_i)$, for each of the selectable GUI icons. This prior is independent of the current pointing task and can represent contextual information, user profile, frequency of use, etc. Sequentially determining the probabilities in Equation 1 demands only calculating the likelihoods $P(\mathbf{m}_{1:k} | \mathcal{D}_I = \mathcal{D}_i)$ at the arrival of a new observation (i.e., up-to-date position of the pointing finger or mouse cursor).

After evaluating $\mathcal{P}(t_k)$ in Equation 1, a simple intuitive approach to establish the intended destination at t_k is to select the most probable endpoint via

$$\hat{I}(t_k) = \arg\max_{\mathcal{D}_i \in \mathbb{D}} P(\mathcal{D}_I = \mathcal{D}_i | \mathbf{m}_{1:k}) \qquad \text{Equation 2}$$

Decision criterion other than Equation 2 can be applied within the Bayesian framework, see (8). For the linear destination reverting models, Kalman filters can be used (one per nominal destination) to calculate $P(\mathcal{D}_I = \mathcal{D}_i | \mathbf{m}_{1:k})$ in Equation 1 as per (8, 34). Adopting nonlinear motion or observation models can lead to advanced statistical inference methods such as sequential Monte Carlo or other related methods for online filtering.

Linear destination-reverting motion models
Since the pointing motion is intrinsically driven by the intended on-screen icon, destination-reverting models can be suitable for predictive pointing under health or situationally induced impairments. Following the integration of their respective SDEs and assuming that the intended endpoint is $\mathcal{D}_i$, LDR models can be expressed by

$$\mathbf{X}_{i,k} = \mathbf{F}_{i,k} \mathbf{X}_{i,k-1} + \boldsymbol{\kappa}_{i,k} + \mathbf{w}_k, i = 1, 2, \ldots, N, \qquad \text{Equation 3}$$

where $\mathbf{X}_{i,k-1}$ and $\mathbf{X}_{i,k}$ are the hidden model state vectors at two consecutive time instants t_{k-1} and t_k. For example, the state $\mathbf{X}_{i,k}$ can include the true pointing-finger location in 2D or 3D and other higher order motion dynamics such as velocity, acceleration, etc. Matrix $\mathbf{F}_{i,k}$ is the state transition and $\kappa_{i,k}$ is a time varying constant (both are with respect to $\mathcal{D}_i$), and the motion model dynamic noise is $\mathbf{w}_k$. For $\mathcal{D}_i \in \mathbb{D}$ possible endpoints on the display (i.e., selectable GUI icons), N such models can be constructed and their corresponding likelihoods are calculated with the appropriate statistical filtering algorithm where the (also) linear observation model is given by

$$\mathbf{m}_k = \mathbf{H}_k \mathbf{X}_{i,k} + \mathbf{n}_k. \quad\quad\quad \text{Equation 4}$$

The noise introduced by the sensor is represented by $\mathbf{n}_k$. For more details on the LDR models and their characteristics with and without the bridging distributions, the reader is referred to (8, 33, 34).

Bayesian inference with a hidden Markov model offers flexibility in terms of modelling the pointing motion with either HIID or SIID via the SDE and its integration in Equation 3. We recall that the variability in the pointing movement, e.g., due to the user behaviour and/or impairment, can be introduced through the noise element of the state $\mathbf{X}_k$ and the noise generated from the employed sensor (e.g., a particular gesture tracker) can be incorporated via the measurement noise in the observation model in Equation 4. Most importantly, the statistical filter utilised to determine the intent of the tracked object (e.g., mouse cursor in 2D or pointing finger for pointing gestures in 3D) can be applied to the same class of motion models, albeit altering the applied pointing motion model.

Smoothing noisy trajectories

The results of the N statistical filters applied to determine $\mathcal{P}(t_k)$ in Equation 1 can be employed to remove the unintentional perturbations-impairment-related movements as shown in (8, 34). However, in certain scenarios (e.g., severe perturbations) where it is desirable to maintain a simple linear motion model for the intent inference functionality, a pre-processing step/stage can be added such that the raw pointing data is filtered, e.g., using a particle filter (20, 25). The filtered track is subsequently used by the destination inference module. The effectiveness of the state-space-modelling for removing unintentional impairment-related pointing movement were demonstrated in (8, 19, 20, 25, 33, 34).

Examples: Situational and motor impairments

Figure 3 depicts results of utilising an in-vehicle predictive display under varying levels of SIID due to road/driving conditions when the predictive capability is off and on. In the former case, the experiment becomes a conventional task of interacting with an in-car touchscreen where the user has to physically touch the intended icon on the screen to select it. The benefits of the predictive display are assessed in terms of the system ability to reduce the workload of interacting with the in-car touchscreen and the pointing tasks durations T_p. NASA TLX forms, widely utilised in HCI studies, are used to evaluate the subject workload experienced by the users. In this study, a Leap Motion controller is employed to produce, in real-time, the locations of the pointing finger in 3D, i.e., $\mathbf{m}_k = [x_{t_k}\ y_{t_k}\ z_{t_k}]'$ at t_k. Pointing finger observations are then used by the probabilistic intent predictor to calculate the probabilities $\mathcal{P}(t_k)$ in Equation 1. The predictive display auto-selects the intended on-screen icon once a particular level of prediction certainty is achieved (the user need not touch the display surface to make a selection). This pointing facilitation scheme is dubbed *mid-air selection* (9). Figure 3 demonstrates that the predictive display system can reduce the subjective workload of interacting with an in-car display by nearly 50%. It can also be noticed that workload notably increases as more perturbations are experienced. Measured durations of pointing task also show that T_p can be reduced by over 35% under mild to severe accelerations-vibrations due to the road conditions (e.g., driving on a badly maintained road). Therefore, the predictive display system that uses a suitable Bayesian formulation can significantly simplify and expedite on-screen target acquisitions via free hand pointing gestures.

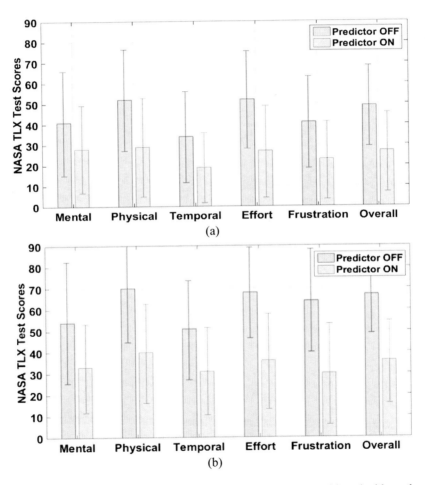

Figure 3. Workload scores for interacting with an in-vehicle touchscreen with and without the predictive capability for 20 participants under varying levels of experienced in-vehicle perturbations (9). (a) Minimum perturbations (motorway); (b) Mild-severe perturbations (badly maintained road).

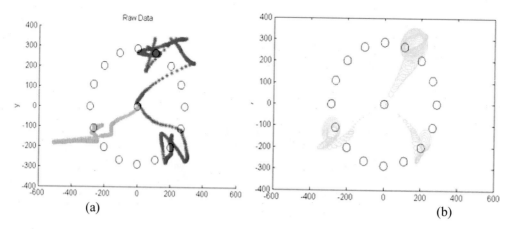

Figure 4. Filtering noisy mouse cursor trajectories due to HIID using a particle filter and showing the confidence ellipses (20). (a) Raw noisy 2D cursor trace data; (b) filtered traces. Units on the axes are pixels.

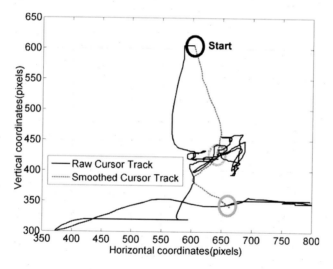

Figure 5. Smooth cursor track in 2D for a severe HIID-related perturbations (19). User is targeting two GUI icons (target 1 is the blue circle and then target 2 is the green circle). The start point is the black circle.

Figures 4 and 6 illustrate the ability of a sequential Monte Carlo method, namely the variable rate particle filter, to remove highly non-linear perturbation-related unintentional pointing movements when interacting with a touchscreen using pointing gestures in 3D and selecting icons of a GUI displayed on a computer screen via a mechanical mouse. Whereas, in Figure 5 Kalman filtering is applied. The raw cursor movement data in Figures 4 and 5 is for a user that suffers from cerebral palsy. Figure 4 exhibits the confidence ellipses obtained from the sequential Monte Carlo filter, which has visibly removed the health-induced-impairment jumping behaviour of the mouse cursor position and can assist identifying the user's intended destination (despite the ambiguity of the raw pointing data). On the other hand, unintentional situational-induced-impairment-related pointing finger movements in 3D are successfully removed in Figure 6.

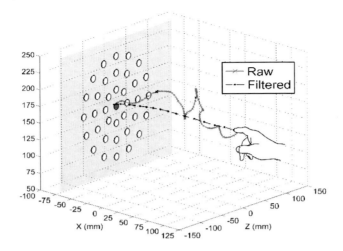

Figure 6. 3D pointing track before (blue) and after (dashed) applying a variable rate particle filter (25).

CONCLUSION

Using the Bayesian formulation developed for able-bodied touchscreen users in a perturbed environment has proved successful in improving performance and reducing workload. There is no reason to suppose these benefits may not be realised in the case of health-induced impairment and disability. We reported preliminary tests of this assumption, providing promising results. Spasm, weakness, tremor and athetosis can be mitigated or largely eliminated by the predictive approach based on the described Bayesian algorithms, original developed for automotive applications. In particular, motion impaired users, who may have difficulty pointing-selecting on interactive displays will benefit not only from prediction and automated selection (i.e., auto-selection), but also from the reduction of workload reported by the automotive trial participants, measured using NASA TLX scores.

Additionally, from an inclusive design perspective, the predictive display technology may greatly benefit those with age related or mild physical or perceptual impairments by enhancing performance in pointing-selection and reducing the associated workload. Mild functional impairments such as physical movement (reach and stretch, dexterity), visual acuity, and cognitive capacity could be improved. This predictive approach is also applicable to special purpose designs for specific cases, extreme impairment and disability. Experimental studies will be superseded by trials of the same algorithms and detection technologies with interfaces in mobile displays, walking scenarios, wheelchair use and on public transportation. Predictive displays are capable of incorporating and fusing additional sensory data or input modalities, e.g., eye-gaze or voice-based commands, via the Bayesian framework succinctly described in this paper. In conclusion, encouraging results suggest that these specific advanced predictive algorithms for pointing and selection have utility in a range of interfaces where performance is impaired, whether by situation or by health. The health based impairment is a rich area for future investigation.

REFERENCES

[1]   Burnett G, Porter JM. Ubiquitous computing within cars: designing controls for non-visual use. Int J Hum Comput Stud 2001;55:521–31.
[2]   Burnett G, Lawson G, Millen L, Pickering C. Designing touchpad user-interfaces for vehicles: which tasks are most suitable? Behav Inform Technol 2011;30:403-14.
[3]   Harvey C, Stanton NA. Usability evaluation for in-vehicle systems. London: CRC Press, 2014.
[4]   Jaeger MG, Skov MB, Thomassen NG. You can touch, but you can't look: interacting with in-vehicle systems. Proceedings of the SIGCHI Conf. on Human Factors in Computing Systems (CHI), 2008, Florence, Italy. ACM 2008:1139–48.
[5]   Bishop R. Intelligent vehicle technology and trends. Norwood, MA: Artech House, 2005.
[6]   Ahmad BI, Langdon PM, Godsill SJ, Hardy R, Skrypchuk L, Donkor, R. Touchscreen usability and input performance in vehicles under different road conditions: An evaluative study. Proceedings of the 7th International Conference on Automotive UI and Interactive Vehicular Applications (AutomotiveUI), 2015, Nottingham, UK, ACM, 2015:47-54.
[7]   Klauer SG, Dingus TA, Neale VL, Sudweeks JD, Ramsey DJ. The impact of driver inattention on near-crash/crash risk: An analysis using the 100-car naturalistic driving study data. National Highway Traffic Safety Administration, DOT HS 810 5942006, 2006.
[8]   Ahmad BI, Murphy JK, Langdon PM, Godsill SJ, Hardy R, Skrypchuk L. Intent inference for hand pointing gesture-based interactions in vehicles. IEEE Transactions on Cybernetics 2016;46:878-89.
[9]   Ahmad BI, Langdon PM, Godsill SJ, Donkor R, Wilde R, and Skrypchuk L. You do not have to touch to select: A study on predictive in-car touchscreen with mid-air selection. Proceedings of the 8th International Conference on Automotive UI and Interactive Vehicular Applications (AutomotiveUI), 2016, Ann Arbor, USA, ACM, 2016:1-8.
[10] MacKenzie IS. Fitts' law as a research and design tool in human-computer interaction. Hum Comput Interaction 1992;7:91-139.
[11] Meyer DE, Abrams RA, Kornblum S, Wright CE, Keith-Smith JE. Optimality in human motor perform-ance: ideal control of rapid aimed movements. Psychol Rev 1988;95:340–70.
[12] Murata A. Improvement of pointing time by predicting targets in pointing with a PC mouse. Int J Hum Comput Interaction 1998;10:23–32.
[13] Asano T, Sharlin E, Kitamura Y, Takashima K, Kishino F. Predictive interaction using the, 2005: 133-41.
[14] McGuffin MJ, Balakrishnan R. Fitts' law and expanding targets: Experimental studies and designs for user interfaces. ACM Transactions Comput Hum Interaction 2005;12:388–22.
[15] Wobbrock JO, Fogarty J, Liu SYS, Kimuro S, Harada S. The angle mouse: target-agnostic dynamic gain adjustment based on angular deviation. Proceedings of the SIGCHI Conf. on Human Factors in Computing Systems (CHI); 2009, NY, USA, ACM 2009:1401–410.
[16] Kopper R, Bowman DA, Silva MG, McMahan RP. A human motor behavior model for distal pointing tasks. Int J Hum Comput Stud 2010;68:603-15.
[17] Ziebart B, Dey A, and Bagnell JA. Probabilistic pointing target prediction via inverse optimal control. Proceedings of the 2012 ACM International Conference on Intelligent User Interfaces (IUI); 2012; Lisbon, Portugal. ACM; 2012. p. 1–10.
[18] Pasqual PT, Wobbrock JO. Mouse pointing endpoint prediction using kinematic template matching. Proceedings of the SIGCHI Conf. on Human Factors in Computing Systems (CHI), 2014, Toronto, Canada. ACM 2014:743–52.
[19] Ahmad BI, Langdon PM, Bunch P, Godsill SJ. Probabilistic Intentionality Prediction for Target Selection Based on Partial Cursor Tracks, Proceedings of the 8th International Conference on Universal Access in Human-Computer Interaction (UAHCI). Lecture Notes in Computer Science (8515), 2014. Crete, Greece: Springer, 2014:427-38.
[20] Langdon PM, Godsill SJ, Clarkson PJ. Statistical estimation of user's interactions from motion impaired cursor use data. Proceedings of the 6th Int. Conf. on Disability, Virtual Reality and Associated Technologies (ICDVRAT), 2006, Denmark, 2006.

[21] Keates S, Hwang F, Langdon PM, Clarkson PJ, Robinson P. Cursor measures for motion-impaired computer users. In: Proceedings of the Fifth Int. ACM Conference on Assistive Technologies (ASSETS), 2002, NY, USA, ACM 2002:135–42.

[22] Gajos KZ, Wobbrock JO, Weld DS. Automatically generating user interfaces adapted to users' motor and vision capabilities. Proceedings of ACM Symposium on User Interface Software and Technology, 2007, RI, USA, ACM 2007:231-40.

[23] Biswas P, Langdon PM. Developing multimodal adaptation algorithm for mobility impaired users by evaluating their hand strength. Int J Hum Comput Interaction 2012;28:576-96.

[24] Domingo MC. An overview of the internet of things for people with disabilities. J Network Comput Applications 2012;35:584-96.

[25] Ahmad BI, Murphy JK, Langdon PM, Godsill SJ. Filtering perturbed in-vehicle pointing gesture trajectories: Improving the reliability of intent inference. Proceedings of IEEE International Workshop on Machine Learning for Signal Processing (MLSP), 2014, Reims, France, IEEE 2014:1-6.

[26] Sears A, Lin M, Jacko J, Xiao Y. When computers fade. Pervasive computing and situationally induced impairments and disabilities. Proceedings of HCI International Conference, 2003. Crete, Greece: Springer, 2003:1298-302.

[27] Atzori L, Iera A, Morabito G. The internet of things: A survey. Comput Networks 2010;54:2787-805.

[28] Petrie H. Accessibility and usability requirements for ICTs for disabled and elderly people: A functional classification approach. In: Nicolle C, Abascal J, eds. Inclusive guidelines for human computer interaction. London: Taylor Francis, 2001.

[29] Schaie KW, Willis SL. Adult development and aging. New York: Prentice-Hall, 2003.

[30] Newell AF. Older people as a focus for Inclusive Design. Gerontechnol 2006;4:190-9.

[31] Newell AF, Gregor P, Morgan M, Pullin G, Macaulay C. User-sensitive inclusive design. Universal Access Inform Soc 2011;10:235-43.

[32] Newell AF, P. Gregor. Human computer interfaces for people with disabilities. In: Helander M, Landauer TK, Prabhu P, eds. Handbook of human computer interaction. Amsterdam: Elsevier Science BV, 1997 813-24.

[33] Ahmad BI, Murphy JK, Godsill SJ, Langdon PM, Hardy R. Intelligent interactive displays in vehicles with intent prediction: A Bayesian framework. IEEE Signal Processing Magazine 2017.

[34] Ahmad BI, Murphy JK, Langdon PM, Godsill SJ. Bayesian intent prediction in object tracking using bridging distributions. IEEE Transactions on Cyber-netics 2017.

Submitted: December 20, 2016. *Revised:* February 11, 2017. *Accepted:* February 15, 2017.

In: Alternative Medicine Research Yearbook 2017
Editor: Joav Merrick
ISBN: 978-1-53613-726-2
© 2018 Nova Science Publishers, Inc.

Chapter 39

THE IMPACT OF THE VISUAL REPRESENTATION OF THE INPUT DEVICE ON DRIVING PERFORMANCE IN A POWER WHEELCHAIR SIMULATOR

Abdulaziz Alshaer[1], MSc, David O'Hare[2], PhD, Simon Hoermann[1,3,4],*, PhD and Holger Regenbrecht[1], DrIng

[1]Department of Information Science, University of Otago, Dunedin, New Zealand
[2]Department of Psychology, University of Otago, Dunedin, New Zealand
[3]Department of Medicine (DSM), University of Otago, Dunedin, New Zealand
[4]School of Electrical and Information Engineering, The University of Sydney, Sydney, Australia

ABSTRACT

Virtual reality-based power wheelchair simulators can help potential users to be assessed and trained in a safe and controlled environment. Although now widely used and researched for several decades, many properties of virtual environments are still not yet fully understood. In this study, we evaluated the effects of the visual representation of the input device in a virtual power wheelchair simulator. We compared the virtual display of a standard gaming joystick with that of a proprietary power wheelchair joystick while

---

* Correspondence: Simon Hoermann, PhD, Research Associate, Positive Computing Laboratory, School of Electrical and Information Engineering, Maze Crescent Bldg J03, The University of Sydney, Sydney, NSW 2006, Australia. E-mail: simon.hoermann@sydney.edu.au.

users used either of the real world counterparts, and measured the effects on driving performance and experience. Four experimental conditions comprising of two visual virtual input modalities and their two real counterparts as independent variables have been studied. The results of the study with 48 participants showed that the best performance was obtained for two of three performance indicators when a virtual representation of the PWC joystick was displayed, regardless of what type of joystick (real PWC or gaming joystick) was actually physically used. Despite not explicitly being made aware of by the experimenter, participants reported noticing the change in the visual representation of the joysticks during the experiment. This supports the theory that the effects of virtual reality representations have a significant impact on the user experience or performance, and visual properties need to be carefully selected. This is specifically important for applications where the transfer effects to real world scenarios is sought and ecological valid simulation is aimed for.

Keywords: power wheelchair, interaction, visualization

INTRODUCTION

Power wheelchairs (PWCs) can improve users' quality of life by enabling them to participate in daily living activities and decrease their dependence on human assistance (1). PWC users have to deal with restricted environments involving limited space to maneuver and are therefore vulnerable to collisions and injuries. Therefore, to use a PWC effectively and safely, individuals have to undertake training and an assessment of their competency. (2) reported that: "the evaluation of user proficiency and the suitability of a given wheelchair is largely guesswork, and user training is limited to practice with a possibly unsuitable wheelchair." This has increased the need for better PWC simulations in order to train users to develop more expertise in driving PWCs and to assess user competency.

This has triggered researchers to investigate systems that could help to overcome the limitations of traditional PWC assessment and training. Already in the 1980s, (3) built a first system to help PWC users to adapt to actual PWCs. They concluded that such a simulation could help with the adaption and/or evaluation of PWC users. Subsequently more studies to evaluate the driving skills of PWC users were conducted. For example (4) measured completion time, number of path boundary violations, and errors between virtual PWC trajectory and desired path and concluded that such data could be useful in assessing and/or training PWC users. Moreover, they noted that a very important aspect of driving a PWC is the input device where the suitability can be objectively assessed through simulation. Previous research shows several advantages of using a PWC simulator: potential utility as an assessment and/or training device, positive skills transfer from VEs to real environments, and objective measures of user performance easily generated by the simulator. These measures can be summarized as number of collisions either with objects or path boundaries, time spent, user trajectories, and combinations of these criteria to formulate a score.

Unfortunately there is a lack of commercially available PWC simulators outside of research that are appropriate for assessment and training (5). Although commercial PWC software (WheelSim) exists, it is deemed unsuitable as a training and assessment system. In a usability inspection, (6) detected severe shortcomings that make it unsuitable for use as a training and/or assessment system. Flaws identified by the authors were: 1) lack of an accurate physical simulation, 2) unknown size and driving speed of the PWC, and 3) inaccurate joystick interaction because the virtual PWC did not move and accelerate accordingly. Furthermore, pure software solutions still require the use of appropriate hardware as input devices which again could cause unwanted results if they are not specific to the software.

Building a realistic and effective virtual-reality-based environment requires the consideration of many factors. Two overview papers by (7, 8) show that movement visualization, feedback and context information can have a significant impact on the user experience as well as on therapy outcomes for patients. This can also apply to virtual-reality-based vehicle simulators such as power wheelchair (PWC) simulators where correct physical simulation, realistic 3D modelling of the environment and the PWC, provision and/or simulation of the physical environment, and an appropriate interaction device may impact user experience and the functionality of the system. An essential hardware component of PWCs is usually a finger-operated joystick. Because actual PWC joysticks are proprietary and expensive, PWC simulators often use commercial gaming joysticks to interact with the simulator (6, 9) or adapted PWC joysticks (10, 11).

Previous research has evaluated different input devices for different applications, either from a usability point of view, or in terms of performance. (12) report that the wrong input device: "can affect performance, increase cognitive workload and increase errors that may lead to the loss of a vehicle." However, none of the previous PWC simulation studies have investigated the impact of using a PWC joystick compared to a gaming joystick. In fact, this also raises the question of the virtual representations of these input devices. According to (13), small changes in the virtual representation of the geometry of objects has an effect on the user experience and affects the perception of spatial location. This was demonstrated in their study where participants were asked to reach and grasp three different shapes in a VE (apple, sphere, and polyhedron) and measured the time participants took to reach the target. They found that users preformed significantly slower to locate and grasp a sphere compared to a polyhedron of the same size. This would indicate that the design of virtual objects, such as PWC components, could have a substantial effect on the performance of users and therefore influence the training and assessment outcomes in PWC simulations.

Our goal in this study is to evaluate the effects of the combination of virtual and real power wheelchair joysticks in the form of a proprietary power wheelchair joystick and a standard gaming joystick. Would one be perceived better than the other and therefore lead to better performance and experience? To our knowledge, this is the first study to investigate the visualization of the input device, in particular, if different input devices are used. In this study, we compared the virtual display of a standard gaming joystick and that of a proprietary power wheelchair joystick in combinations with their real world counterparts. The impact was assessed in the context of driving performance, where users' path and wall collisions, and completion times were recorded as participants drove a simulated PWC. In addition, participants reported on their experience and awareness. This study aims to provide information to help designers/developers to create optimised PWC simulations and extend the knowledge on the effects of visual representation in VE on user performance.

METHODS

The study sample was recruited from people who attended the science festival at Otago University, New Zealand. We performed a statistical power analysis to estimate the required sample size before running the experiment. We used effect size from a similar previous experiment (6) to calculate the required sample size using the power analysis and the required sample size to detect differences was calculated to be 40. We recruited 48 participants (31 males, 17 females). Two participants' data were not analysed, as they were the only two left-handed. The age range of the 48 participants was 18 to 73 years old, with a mean age of 34 (SD = 11.97). Participants were also asked about their joystick experience before the experiment to determine how much information/training participants should receive before conducting the experiment. None of the participants were actual power wheelchair users.

Apparatus

Two aspects of the virtual reality (VR) simulation were considered: (1) the actual joystick, physically operated by the user, and (2) the virtual representation of the joystick within the virtual environment. Two popular joysticks were selected to be evaluated: a standard off-the-shelf gaming joystick (Logitech Attack 3) which is affordable and available in the gaming accessories market, and an expensive, purpose-built PWC joystick (Q-Logic control) which is used on many power wheelchairs and only works with PWC (Figure 1). Due to the specialist design of the PWC joystick, we modified it for use with USB input. To achieve this, an Arduino-based LeoStick (www.freetronics.com/products/leostick) board was electronically connected, programmed, and calibrated to read the PWC joystick outputs. These outputs were then mapped to function in the virtual environment. Hence, both the PWC and the gaming joystick worked the same for the user.

For the virtual joystick representations, realistic 3D designs for both the gaming joystick and the PWC joystick were modelled (Figure 1). In addition, the physical movements of both joysticks were simulated. The 2 degree-of-freedom deflection of the joysticks were mimicked in the virtual representation in the VE. Therefore, pushing the joystick in any direction will immediately be visualized within the VE according to the participant's movements. As with a real PWC, pushing the joystick further in any direction increases the speed of the virtual PWC and rotates the PWC in the direction pushed. None of the joysticks' buttons were used in this experiment. Both joysticks were placed on a wooden frame so that the participant's hand position was similar to that in a PWC (Figure 2). Both joysticks were connected to a laptop via USB. We used a 17" Alienware high-end graphics laptop to run the simulator with a resolution of 1,920 × 1,080 pixels at 120Hz. Google SketchUp was used to design the 3D models, including the indoor environment (house), the virtual mid-wheel PWC, the virtual gaming and PWC joysticks, and the ideal path to be followed by our participants. Unity3D was used as the graphic engine platform for the simulation, which provides also the physics simulation capabilities.

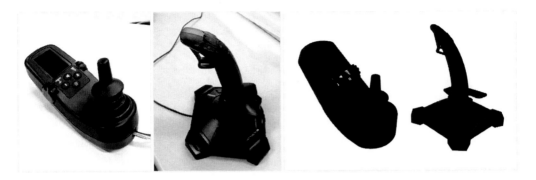

Figure 1. Real PWC and gaming joysticks (left). Virtual PWC and gaming joysticks (right).

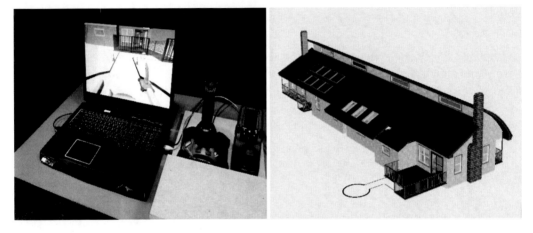

Figure 2. (On the left) experiment setup: Alienware laptop, gaming joystick, and PWC joystick, (on the right) outside view of the house environment used in our simulation.

Environments and driving task

A domestic environment (Figure 2) was used for the simulation. The environment was built to meet the Americans with Disabilities Act (ADA) (14) standards for accessible design. The effective width for internal doors accessed from corridors was 1.2 m and the corridor's minimum width was 1.5 m to facilitate 360° turning (15). The user task was to drive as quickly and accurately as possible through this indoor environment by following an ideal path (driving between two black lines). The path was devised to contain most of the movements a PWC user would make in a domestic environment. These movements were inspired by the wheelchair skills test (WST). The WST is a set of assessment and training protocols developed by Dalhousie University (16). Yellow arrows were placed on the path pointing in the direction of movement. The task (path following) was used in a previous study (6) and yielded a sufficiently variable performance.

Measures

For user performance, the following objective metrics were measured per condition: completion time, path boundary violations (when any of the PWC's wheels went beyond one of the black lines), and wall collisions. The overall performance score was calculated from the number of path boundary violations (pathViolations), the number of wall collisions (wallCollisions) and the total time in seconds (totalTime) required for the completion of the driving route using Eq. (1). The scoring system was used in (6), which was also inspired by (5, 10, 17).

Score = 1000 – (path Violations + 2 x
Wall Collisions + total Time) (1)

To measure user experience and awareness, we developed four questions consisting of seven-point Likert scale items where "-3" means "strongly disagree" and "3" means "strongly agree." The aim of these questions was to obtain participants' experience and therefore were asked once after completion of all conditions. The four questions were as follows: Q1: Overall, I felt as though I was operating the virtual joystick presented on the screen, Q2: Overall, I felt as though I was operating the physical joystick in my hand, Q3: Overall, I was aware of the switching between the virtual joysticks, and Q4: Overall, I was aware of the differences between the joystick on the screen and the one in my hand.

Experiment design

We used a 2 (physical joystick: PWC v Gaming) X 2 (virtual joystick: PWC v Gaming) within-subjects factorial design: the physical joystick handled by the participant (Attack 3 Gaming or Q-Logic Control PWC) and the virtual joystick represented on the screen (Attack 3 Gaming or Q-Logic Control PWC). This yielded four conditions as shown in Table 1.

Table 1. 2×2 factorial design

		Physical Joysticks	
		Gaming	PWC
Virtual Joysticks	Virtual Gaming	G-vG	P-vG
	Virtual PWC	G-vP	P-vP

Counterbalancing

Due to a potential learning effect associated with repeating of the task four times we controlled for ordering effects. First, subjects were randomized in counterbalanced order. Second, although subjects repeated the tasks four times, they were generally unaware of the repetition. The participants followed one layout on a return path, which created a balanced set of comparable paths that the user could traverse without interruption (Figure 3). The users couldn't really predict what was coming next, e.g., it was hard for them to know which direction to travel next as the right turn became left when driving in the reverse direction. In addition, the condition order set was randomized based on Latin Square counterbalancing.

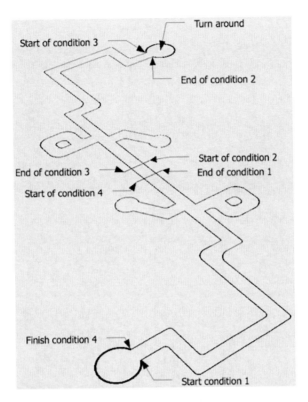

Figure 3. Ideal path through the environment.

Procedure

The experiment was run during a local science exhibition where participants, including school and university students, university staff, and the general public, came to participate in a wide range of scientific activities. All visitors were free to take part in any of the available activities. Upon arrival, participants were welcomed and consent was obtained electronically by clicking 'YES' if they wanted to be part of the experiment.

Participants were informed about the type of the virtual PWC (mid-wheel) and how it moved. They also received instructions on how to use the joystick and were given the opportunity to practice before starting the task. Once participants were ready to start, they were reminded of the task (driving as fast and accurately as possible). They were also told that they would be using two different joysticks and would see virtual counterpart representations in the VE. They were told to follow the ideal path, and stop if they saw a stop sign. Switching between virtual joysticks was done automatically through the simulator depending on the condition order set. When a stop sign appeared on the screen, participants were asked to switch between the physical joysticks. The stop sign appeared according to the condition order as well. At the end, participants were asked to fill in a demographic questionnaire and "overall" perception/awareness questionnaire (four questions).

RESULTS AND DISCUSSION

The means of path boundary violations (driving beyond the black lines), together with standard deviations are reported in Table 2. A two-way, repeated-measures ANOVA was performed. The results showed that neither physical joysticks nor the interaction between physical and virtual joysticks had a significant main effect, but that virtual joysticks had a significant effect where participants had fewer path collisions when the virtual PWC joystick was represented ($F(1, 47) = 4.513$, $p < 0.039$, $\omega^2 = 0.088$).

Table 2. Means and standard deviations for all objective metrics

Path Boundary Violations					Wall Collisions				
		Physical Joystick					Physical Joystick		
		Gaming	PWC				Gaming	PWC	
Virtual Joystick	Gaming	13.27 (9.75)	10.48 (.73)	11.88	Virtual Joystick	Gaming	2.50 (2.24)	1.81 (2.09)	2.15
	PWC	10.71 (7.81)	9.42 (8.43)	10.06		PWC	1.65 (2.22)	1.65 (2.19)	1.65
		11.99	9.94				2.08	1.73	

Completion Time					Overall Driving Performance Score				
		Physical Joystick					Physical Joystick		
		Gaming	PWC				Gaming	PWC	
Virtual Joystick	Gaming	57.35 (12.95)	58.42 (12.49)	57.89	Virtual Joystick	Gaming	924.37 (19.68)	927.46 (18.75)	925.92
	PWC	56.75 (14.18)	58.94 (14.32)	57.84		PWC	929.24 (17.15)	928 (19.65)	928.62
		57.05	58.68				926.81	927.73	

The means of wall collisions, together with standard deviations are reported in Table 2. A two-way, repeated-measures ANOVA was performed. The results indicated that the virtual joystick had a significant effect ($F(1, 47) = 7.009$, $p < 0.011$, $\omega^2 = 0.130$) with participants performing better when the PWC virtual joystick was represented. Neither the physical joystick nor the interaction between the physical and virtual joystick had significant effects on the number of wall collisions.

The means of completion time, together with standard deviations are reported in Table 2. The time spent to complete the task was similar between each condition. Two-way, repeated-measures ANOVA was performed, but neither of the independent variables nor the interaction between them had significant effects on the participants' completion time.

The means of overall driving performance, together with standard deviations are reported in Table 2. The overall performance score was calculated with Equation 1 where a higher score indicated a better performance. A two-way, repeated-measures ANOVA was performed, but neither of the independent variables nor the interaction between them had significant effects on the participants' overall driving performance score.

For the experience and awareness questions (Figure 4), a Wilcoxon signed rank test was performed against the midpoint (0) to see if the participants agreed or disagreed with the statements. Although participant answers to question 1 ("Overall, I felt as though I was operating the virtual joystick presented on the screen") was slightly above the midpoint (M = 0.1, SD = 1.88), the one sample Wilcoxon test did not show a significant difference. On the other hand, the test showed a significant difference on question 2 ("Overall, I felt as though I was operating the physical joystick in my hand," $p < 0.000$, with (M = 2.15, SD = 1.11). A Wilcoxon Signed-Ranks test was performed to compare responses on the two questions. The analysis showed a significant main difference in favour of the physical joystick. Responses to both questions (Q3. "Overall, I was aware of the switching between the virtual joysticks" and Q4. "Overall, I was aware of the differences between the joystick on the screen and the one in my hand") were above midpoint (M = 1.04, SD = 2.0, and M = 0.85, SD = 1.86 respectively). Both questions showed significant effects $p = 0.002$ for Q3, $p = 0.003$ for Q4. A Wilcoxon Signed-Ranks test was performed to compare responses on the two questions. There was no main difference between the two questions.

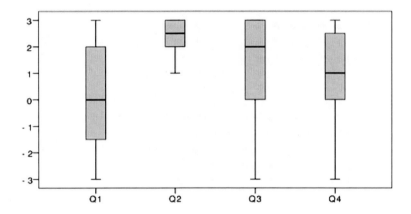

Figure 4. Participants' answers to experience and awareness questions.

CONCLUSION AND FUTURE WORK

In this study, we evaluated the effects of visual representation of input devices in a virtual power wheelchair simulator. We compared the virtual display of a standard gaming joystick to a proprietary power wheelchair joystick while users used either of the real world counterparts. We measured the effects on driving performance and reported experience. Our results showed that for two of three performance metrics driving performance is significantly affected by the form of the virtual joysticks, but not by the type of physical joystick used. This indicates that performance can be influenced by changing visual properties, such as, the type of input device visualised. It also indicates that for the use in a virtual PWC simulator a rather inexpensive gaming joystick might be adequate.

The results of the study suggest that users of the simulator paid attention to the visual representation of the joystick and used it to guide their control of the PWC. We believe that the differences in the driving performance between the two virtual representations of the joystick is due to the level of how participants deduced steering information from the position of virtual joystick's handle. While the PWC joystick is equipped with a straight handle, the gaming joystick has a curved handle pointing forward on the top (Figure 1). This property of the gaming joystick could make it more difficult for participants to notice visual differences between small forward or backward positions of the handle and therefore impede the inclusion of this information in steering decisions; on the other hand, the properly aligned virtual joystick may help to enhance the participants' sense of alignment of the physical joystick. This might have led to better performance, in particular with novice participants. Another explanation could be that the virtual gaming joystick was an out-of-place distraction due to its size in the VE compared to the smaller virtual PWC joystick. Therefore, paying attention to the virtual game joystick degrades performance in a way that the PWC joystick does not.

Future studies may also investigate whether the effects were related to visual dominance theory (18), a felt sense of presence in the environment or both. The visual effect could be investigated more by tracking the user's eyes to determine when and how much time individuals would look directly at the virtual joystick. Moreover, the particular way in which we present the virtual joystick offers a convenient view of the input state near the centre of the display. A larger display could be used so that the physical joystick could be placed and viewed in the same relation to the virtual scene as the virtual joystick. Future studies could also investigate avatar-related conditions where the user's body or body parts are varied in their presence and visualisation characteristics. The participants used in this study were a convenience sample. This enabled us to meet the power requirements for the study. In addition, their unfamiliarity with PWCs and their proprietary joystick controller enhanced the internal validity of the study. The question of external validity or generalizability to the population of wheelchair users remains open for further investigation. Considerable variability in performance was evident between participants, so future studies might consider longer session times or repeated sessions and measures in combination with larger sample sizes.

Our findings suggest that visual properties of input devices represented in the virtual environment need to be carefully selected and chosen specifically for applications where the transfer effects to real world scenarios is sought and ecological valid simulation is aimed for. It also provides guidance on which VR input devices are necessary and appropriate and which virtual device representations can and should be implemented for power wheelchair simulators. In addition, with our simulator we have laid the foundations for a more comprehensive power wheelchair simulation system, including aspects of the use of simulator data to assess individual driving performance, correct physical simulation of power wheelchairs, and to take into account appropriate dimensions of an indoor environment to meet the standards for accessible design. This study provides an interesting test bed for future investigations.

ACKNOWLEDGMENTS

The authors wish to thank all participants and the HCI group. Very special thanks goes to Chris Edwards for his help with the electronic modification of the PWC joystick and to Allied Medical Ltd. for providing the PWC joystick. The first author is sponsored by the Saudi Arabian Ministry of Education.

REFERENCES

[1] Lee S-H. Users' satisfaction with assistive devices in South Korea. J Phys Ther Sci 2014;26(4):509–12.

[2] Swan JE, Stredney D, Carlson W, Blostein B. The determination of wheelchair user proficiency and Environmental Accessibility through virtual simulation. In: Proceedings of the 2nd Annual International Conference: Virtual Reality and Persons with Disabilities. California 1994:156–61.

[3] Pronk CN, de Klerk PC, Schouten A, Grashuis JL, Niesing R, Bangma BD. Electric wheelchair simulator as a man-machine system. Scand J Rehabil Med 1980; 12(3):129–35.

[4] Cooper RA, Ding D, Simpson R, Fitzgerald SG, Spaeth DM, Guo S, et al. Virtual reality and computer-enhanced training applied to wheeled mobility: an overview of work in Pittsburgh. Assist Technol Off J RESNA 2005;17(2):159–70.

[5] Abellard P, Randria I, Abellard A, Ben Khelifa MM, Ramanantsizehe P. Electric wheelchair navigation simulators: why, when, how? In: Di Paola AMD, Cicirelli G, eds. Mechatronic Systems Applications [Internet]. InTech; 2010 [cited 2012 Jun 7]. Available from: http://www.intechopen.com/books/mechatronic-systems-applications/electric-wheelchair-navigation-simulators-why-when-how.

[6] Alshaer A, Hoermann S, Regenbrecht H. Influence of peripheral and stereoscopic vision on driving performance in a power wheelchair simulator system. In: 2013 International Conference on Virtual Rehabil-itation (ICVR). 2013:152–64.

[7] Schuler T, Santos LF dos, Hoermann S. Harnessing the experience of presence for virtual motor rehabilitation: towards a guideline for the development of virtual reality environments. In: Proceedings of the 10th international conference on disability, virtual reality and associated technologies (ICDVRAT): 2–4 September 2014; Gothenburg. Sharkey PM, Pareto L, Broeren J, Rydmark M, eds. Reading: The University of Reading, 2014:373–6.

[8] Schuler T, Santos LF dos, Hoermann S. Designing virtual environments for motor rehabilitation: Towards a framework for the integration of best-practice information. In: 2015 International Conference on Virtual Rehabilitation Proceedings (ICVR), 2015:145–6.

[9] Archambault PS, Tremblay S, Cachecho S, Routhier F, Boissy P. Driving performance in a power wheelchair simulator. Disabil Rehabil Assist Technol 2012;7(3): 226–33.

[10] Hasdai A, Jessel AS, Weiss PL. Use of a computer simulator for training children with disabilities in the operation of a powered wheelchair. Am J Occup Ther 1998;52(3):215–20.

[11] Adelola I, Cox S, Rahman. Adaptable virtual reality interface for powered wheelchair training of disabled children. In: Proceedings of The Fourth International Conference on Disability, Virtual Reality and Associated Technologies. Veszprém, Hungary, 2002: 173–9.

[12] Rupp MA, Oppold P, McConnell DS. Evaluating input device usability as a function of task difficulty in a tracking task. Ergonomics 2015;58(5):722-35.

[13] Powell V, Powell WA. Locating objects in virtual reality – the effect of visual properties on target acquisition in unrestrained reaching, 2014. [cited 2016 Mar 6]. Available from: http://www.academia.edu/21108742/Locating_objects_in_virtual_reality_the_effect_of_visual_properties_on_target_acquisition_in_unrestrained_reaching.

[14] Americans with disabilities act of 1990, as amended [Internet]. [cited 2012 Oct 24]. Available from: http://www.ada.gov/pubs/ada.htm.

[15] Desmyter J, Garvin S, Lefèbvre P, Stirano F, Vaturi A. T1. 4 A review of safety, security accessibility and positive stimulation indicators. In: Seventh Framework Programme, 2010.

[16] Wheelchair Skills Program [Internet]. [cited 2015 Mar 17]. Available from: http://www.wheelchairskillsprogram.ca/eng/.

[17] WheelSim. LifeTool, 2007.

[18] Posner MI, Nissen MJ, Klein RM. Visual dominance: An information-processing account of its origins and significance. Psychol Rev 1976;83(2):157–71.

Submitted: December 15, 2016. *Revised:* February 10, 2017. *Accepted:* February 15, 2017.

In: Alternative Medicine Research Yearbook 2017
Editor: Joav Merrick
ISBN: 978-1-53613-726-2
© 2018 Nova Science Publishers, Inc.

Chapter 40

INFLUENCE OF NAVIGATION INTERACTION TECHNIQUE ON PERCEPTION AND BEHAVIOUR IN MOBILE VIRTUAL REALITY

Wendy A Powell, PhD, BSc(Hons), BA, DC,
Vaughan Powell, PhD, MA, BSc(Hons), Phillip Brown, BSc(Hons),
Marc Cook, BSc(Hons) and Jahangir Uddin, BSc(Hons)*

School of Creative Technologies, University of Portsmouth,
Winston Churchill Avenue, Portsmouth, United Kingdom

ABSTRACT

In recent years the development of affordable virtual reality has opened up enormous possibilities for virtual rehabilitation, and the introduction of ultra-low cost mobile VR such as Google Cardboard has real potential to put virtual rehabilitation right into patient's homes. However, the limited interaction possibilities when a mobile phone is mounted into a headset mean that these devices are generally used for little more than passive viewing. In this paper we present an evaluation of three approaches to supporting navigation in mobile VR, and discuss some of the potential hazards and limitations.

Keywords: mobile virtual reality, navigation, rehabilitation

INTRODUCTION

Until recently, Virtual Reality (VR) has been primarily the domain of experts in specialist laboratories. Whilst it has demonstrated great potential for rehabilitation, the high cost of the technology (1) and technical knowledge required (2) has created a barrier to uptake in many areas. However, in recent years there has been a paradigm shift in the accessibility of VR,

---

* Correspondence: Wendy Powell PhD, Reader in Virtual Reality, School of Creative Technologies, University of Portsmouth, Winston Churchill Avenue, Portsmouth, United Kingdom. E-mail: wendy.powell@port.ac.uk.

with plummeting costs and increasing ease of use driving significant uptake at the consumer level. This opens up unprecedented opportunities for virtual rehabilitation, with the ability to deploy applications not only for use within clinical settings, but also directly into the homes of the patients.

This increased accessibility of VR inevitably presents new challenges for rehabilitation professionals, and in particular for those designing virtual rehabilitation applications. It is well established that interacting with VR can alter behaviour, and indeed, this is the very reason that VR has such potential for rehabilitation. However, it has previously been observed that increased availability of commercial off-the-shelf (COTS) games which involve physical interaction have led to an increase in physical injury amongst users (3), and it has also been demonstrated that there are a wide range of components within VR which may have an (unanticipated) effect on behaviour (4). The rapid proliferation of consumer VR, without a clear understanding of how users will interact with these systems, may not only increase the risk of injury and adverse effects, but also deter future uptake of high quality virtual rehabilitation applications. Indeed, even leading consumer VR hardware suppliers recommend careful design in order to avoid unwanted side effects (5). This will become increasingly important as mobile phone technology improves, and in particular the processing and display of mobile graphics, leading to the emergence of this platform as a base for low cost virtual reality experiences (6).

Background

The introduction in 2014 of the "Google Cardboard" virtual reality headset costing just a few dollars (7), initiated a rapid proliferation of consumer VR applications, with over 1000 applications and 5 million users by January 2016 (8). However, once the phone is mounted in the VR headset, the buttons and screen are generally no longer accessible to provide input to the applications, and control options are very limited. At the present time, they are used primarily for viewing 360 degree photos and videos, or for "passive entertainment" e.g., riding a virtual rollercoaster. The built-in accelerometers or gyroscopes included in most modern mobile phones offer a simple solution to basic tracking of head movement, allowing the user to look around in the virtual space. Active selection of objects can be achieved using head-orientation as a proxy for gaze direction, with extended fixation on an object triggering interaction (9). However, although active exploration is often not an option in mobile VR, the ability to navigate in a virtual environment should be one of the core tasks (10), and for many cognitive and physical rehabilitation applications, the ability to navigate within the virtual space is essential.

Bowman (10) divides navigation tasks into the components of 'way-finding' and 'travel,' and it is this latter component which presents particular challenges for mobile VR. At its core, travel involves the movement of the viewpoint within the virtual environment from one place to another. This movement can be instantaneous or it can involve both temporal and spatial components. The most natural way to travel in VR is to track the actual movements of the body. However, full body motion tracking is challenging (11), and this limits the possibilities for control of travel in low-cost mobile VR platforms.

Designing effective techniques for travel is not a problem unique to VR, and indeed there is a substantial body of Human Computer Interaction (HCI) research exploring navigation in

2D and 3D interfaces. However, the way in which VR is experienced is quite different to traditional interfaces, and we cannot assume that design guidelines from traditional HCI can be applied in the same way to VR (12). VR interaction research is still in fairly early stages, and there is a lack of authoritative guidance regarding many aspects of design (5). Furthermore, different user populations may well have different interaction priorities, particularly where there is already cognitive or motor deficit. Designing VR applications based purely on intuition is driven by highly individual assumptions, and in order to select the most appropriate interaction technique for a specific population, it is important to first understand how it may impact cognitive load and behaviour.

Although in many ways the VR experience is very different from desktop 3D interaction, many of the underlying principles of virtual travel remain the same. An effective travel technique should promote appropriate velocity, spatial awareness, ease of learning, ease of use, a sense of presence in the environment, and the ability to gather information about the environment during travel (13). Which of these elements are most important will depend on both the type of user and the nature of the task, and it could be argued that for physical rehabilitation, the motor response of the user to the interaction is also of key importance.

Travel techniques

In order to create a framework for evaluation of travel techniques in 3D environments, Bowman established a taxonomy to break the techniques into their core components, which he defines as "Direction selection" (specifying direction of travel), "Conditions of input" (requirements for starting or stopping travel), and "Velocity selection" (the ability to accelerate or change/reverse speed) (13). In order to provide these components, it is necessary to mediate interaction between the user and the mobile application. For headset-mounted mobile phones such as Google Cardboard, there are three levels of possible interaction.

Phone-mediated interaction

Most mobile phones already have a number of in-built sensors, and it is possible to leverage these to allow some level of interaction. Accelerometers or gyroscopes are available on most Smartphones, and these can be used to detect movement of the phone, particularly changes in orientation. For mobile VR, head tracking generally relies on motion detected by these sensors, updating tilt and turn, although unable to detect translational movement (14). In practice, this means that rotations of the head can be linked to the viewpoint of the virtual camera, allowing 360 degree viewing from a fixed point, but not directly supporting any movement through the environment. Whilst this is acceptable for experiencing fixed-viewpoint content such as 360° photographs, it is not sufficient for exploration of a virtual environment. A common workaround seen in many applications is to use continuous motion, which is either constrained to a defined path (e.g., a rollercoaster or train ride), or allows free exploration within the bounds of a virtual environment, with travel being limited only by approaching fixed objects, such as walls, within the scene. With the latter technique, head orientation can be used to set the direction, with continuous motion which is effectively in the direction of gaze. This relates to 'Direction selection' in Bowman's taxonomy, and this is the approach selected for the first of our three experimental conditions.

Headset-mediated interaction

Most of the ultra-low-cost VR headsets such as Google Cardboard have a sliding magnet affixed to the side of the headset. Movement of this magnet can be detected by the phone's built-in magnetometer, allowing it to work as a proxy for a switch or button (15). To date, applications using this magnet have focused on its use for selection (e.g., choosing menu items), but it also has the potential to act as a "toggle" for initiating movement. This relates to the 'Conditions of input' in Bowman's taxonomy. Our second experimental condition combines this movement toggle switch technique with the direction selection approach described in 2.1.1.

Externally mediated interaction

The primary appeal of mobile VR is its low-cost and portability. It has no need of any external equipment in order to provide at least an entry level VR experience. However, in order to widen the options for interaction, it may be necessary to add some additional input hardware. As far as possible, this should also meet the criteria of low-cost, portability and ease of use. A number of low-cost headsets come supplied with a small Bluetooth controller, offering the potential for direct control of motion via the mini joystick, and, as the input is analogue rather than digital, it can add an element of velocity control (albeit small due to the small range of input values which can be generated). This relates to the 'Velocity Selection' category in Bowman's taxonomy. For our third experimental condition we used the mini-joystick of the controller to directly control forward and backward motion, whilst retaining head orientation for selection of motion direction. It should be noted that we initially included the ability to strafe (left and right step) in the Bluetooth controls, but preliminary usability testing found that this seemed to trigger a strong feeling of disorientation and nausea. Furthermore, it is generally recommended to minimise the need for strafing within VR design (5), and so it was removed for this study.

Evaluating navigation techniques

Navigation is comprised of 'wayfinding', which is the cognitive process of determining a path, and 'travel', which is the control of the user's viewpoint motion within a Virtual Environment (13). Navigation is not directly dependent on the specific interaction techniques, and thus is not the focus of this current study. Furthermore, the wayfinding component of a navigation task depends on a cognitive process which makes sense of visual cues and other aids within the virtual environment. It requires the acquisition of spatial knowledge, and this causes difficulties for some 20-30% of users (16), and can thus confound the results of an evaluation of travel techniques. Therefore, as far as possible, this confounder has been removed from the study by providing an opportunity to rehearse the navigation task, and by the use of verbal prompts to guide the users between target locations.

Travel is generally not an end in itself, but is necessary in order to move the user to important points within the environment. Moving within a virtual world involves both simple and complex maneuvers, and both should be incorporated into any task designed to evaluate a navigation interface (17). Simple maneuvers should include cornering, 180° rotation, forward movement on a straight line, and reversal of direction. Complex maneuvers include moving around objects or through doorways, and moving towards a specific target location. All of these maneuvers were combined into a structured navigation task.

METHODS

The three techniques to be evaluated were based on Bowman's taxonomy of travel techniques, with increasing levels of control of the movement (see Table 1). Although some authors recommend separating the viewing direction from the travel direction (18), this necessitates an additional input in order to set a travel direction which is independent of the viewpoint orientation. As the goal of this study is to evaluate techniques using restricted input choices, we implemented travel in the direction of head orientation for all three of the travel techniques.

The nature of the study requires a within-subjects repeated measures design. This inevitably introduces two factors which may contribute to an order effect. Firstly, increasing familiarity with the virtual environment may improve task performance and user preferences. The introduction of a rehearsal phase will reduce but not eliminate this effect. Secondly, any travel technique will be evaluated in the context of any previous technique, and with the continuous motion and switch techniques there may also be a learning effect of the travel technique itself. In order to minimise the impact of these order effects on the results, the study was designed as a counterbalanced study, with 6 different sequences of test order. Participants were assigned to the sequences in 3 blocks of 6.

In order to achieve a repeatable task which incorporated the required simple and complex maneuvers, a route was designed around a virtual flat, visiting six locations in sequence (see Figure 1). The travel task involved forward motion, several 90° and 180° turns, reversing direction, maneuvering around objects, passing in and out of two doorways, and planning routes to move towards target objects.

Table 1. The three travel techniques evaluated in the study (counterbalanced order)

Condition	Level of control (Mapping to Bowman's travel taxonomy)
Continuous motion	Can only control the direction ('Direction selection')
Magnetic switch	Travel can be stopped and started using toggle switch ('Input condition')
Bluetooth controller	Direct control of forward and backward travel ('Velocity selection')

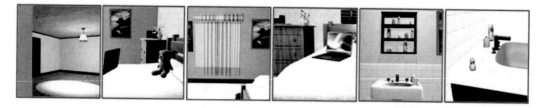

Figure 1. The six target locations visited in the study in sequence from left to right, before returning to the starting location.

Participants

Low-cost VR is designed to appeal to a wide range of the population, and so there was no specific target user group for this evaluation. 18 participants were recruited from academic, support and administrative staff at the University of Portsmouth. There were 12 male and 6 female participants, ranging in age from 22-60 years old, with a mean age of 44, with a mix of background experience from VR enthusiasts to those who had never experienced VR before. Most of the participants were healthy adults, but one had moderate Parkinson's Disease (PD). Each volunteer was given a short introduction to the study and the three techniques to be evaluated, before giving their informed consent to proceed.

Equipment

A virtual flat was built in Autodesk 3D studio max and deployed in the Unity game engine, using the Google Cardboard virtual camera as the viewer. Models and textures were optimised for rendering on an Android phone, running at approximately 30 frames per second (fps). For each technique, the movement was set at the same (steady walking) speed of 1.5m/s. For the Bluetooth controller there was some scope for setting a lower velocity using the analogue joystick. In practice, the small size of the joystick and very small range of motion (+/- 2mm) meant that for all practical purposes it was always used at its maximum input value, equivalent to 1.5 m/s.

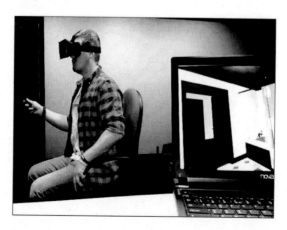

Figure 2. The experimental setup.

The application was deployed as an Android Application Package (apk) file onto a Nexus 6 mobile phone, which was mounted inside a DeFairy VR headset. The controller used was a DeFairy mini Bluetooth controller, mapped to allow only forward and backward movement using the mini joystick. Participants were seated throughout the tasks on a swivel chair with armrests (see Figure 2).

An operator view was mirrored in real-time on a standard PC laptop computer, and this was connected via a local wireless network to the mobile phone. This enabled the observer to track the progress of the participant throughout the task, and provide consistent and timely verbal prompts for each target location.

Procedure

Participants were briefed on the task and the techniques. They were then given an opportunity to rehearse the task and to familiarise themselves with the virtual environment, using keyboard controls and a laptop computer. Following the rehearsal, they completed the navigation task sequence using the VR headset three times, once for each travel technique, and answered a short series of questions after each trial. As the study did not involve memory or cognition testing, each time the participants reached a target location they were given a verbal prompt to direct them to the next location.

Each trial was timed from the start of movement until returning to the hallway at the end of the trial using a digital stopwatch on the operator PC. In order to record natural navigation behaviour, participants were not informed that they were being timed.

RESULTS

The three categories of observations recorded in the study will be discussed in separate sections. Quantitative analysis was carried out using IBM SPSS v22. Qualitative analysis was carried out manually, categorising and coding the free-form text into themes which were then summarised.

Time to complete the navigation task

A repeated measures one-way ANOVA demonstrated a significant effect of travel technique on task completion time ($F2,17$ $F = 10.00$, $p < 0.001$) (see Figure 3). The mean completion time was fastest with the Bluetooth controller (50s), and slowest with the magnetic switch (85s). (Inclusion of the participant with PD disease (number 15) did not impact the results and so was retained in the analysis).

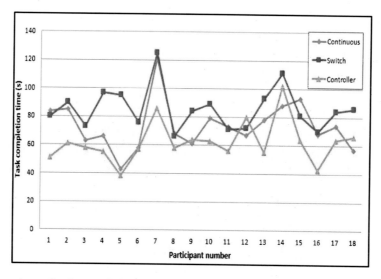

Figure 3. Comparison of task completion times for the three travel techniques.

User experience scores

Participants were asked three questions after each technique (see Table 2). Each question was scored on a Likert scale from 1-5.

A repeated measures one-way ANOVA demonstrated a significant effect of travel technique on the participants perceived ease of use (F2,17 = 8.41, p < 0.01) and on enjoyment of the technique (F2,18 = 4.08, p < 0.05), but there was no significant effect of travel technique on the mini-presence score (F2,17 = 0.90, p = 0.41).

Post-Hoc analysis revealed that the Bluetooth Controller was easier to use than both the continuous motion [t(17) = 3.61, p = 0.00.] and the switch [t(17) = 3.01, p = 0.01.], but there was no significant difference in ease of use between the switch and continuous motion. The controller was liked better than the continuous motion [t(17) = 2.41, p = 0.03.], but comparison with the switch, or between the switch and continuous, showed no significant difference.

There was a strong positive correlation between perceived ease of movement, and enjoyment of the technique (r= 0.78), and a moderate positive correlation between enjoyment and sense of presence (r = 0.38), but no correlation between perceived ease of use, and task completion times (r = -0.19). There was also a weak positive correlation between ease of use and sense of presence (r = 0.24).

Table 2. Mean Likert score for each question (StdDev in brackets)

	Continuous	Switch	Controller
Ease of movement (1 = hard, 5 = easy)	3.3 (1.1)	3.8 (0.7)	4.5 (0.9)
Sense of presence (1 = unreal, 5 = real)	3.4 (0.8)	3.1 (0.7)	3.4 (0.7)
Liked the technique (1 = disliked, 5 = liked)	3.1 (1.1)	3.4 (0.9)	4.1 (1.1)

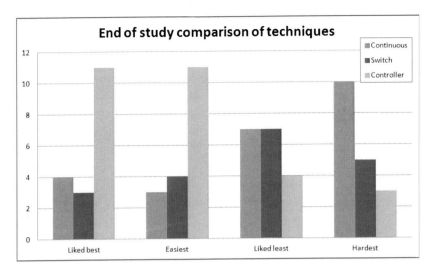

Figure 4. Numbers of participants expressing preferences for each of the three techniques.

At the end of the study, participants were asked to reflect on all three techniques and to compare them. The Bluetooth controller was the preferred travel technique, which was also expressed to be the easiest to use. The continuous motion was both the least liked travel technique, and the one that participants felt was hardest to use (see Figure 4).

Qualitative feedback

After each trial, and at the end of the study, participants were given an opportunity for additional comments on the travel techniques, and these comments were manually coded and categorised to identify common patterns or trends, as well as conflicting opinions. The majority of the responses fell into the broad categories of "control," "discomfort," "ease of use" and "naturalness." Key points for each technique are summarised in individual sections below.

Continuous movement

With regards to control, 61% of participants expressed dissatisfaction with the lack of ability to slow down or stop. 17% stated that they used collision with obstacles in the environment to help them maneuver. In this condition, 39% of participants described some level of disorientation, generally associated with the inability to unlink head motion from the direction of movement, 22% of participants reported some level of dizziness or mild nausea when turning, particularly during sudden or rapid course corrections. For complex movements, 56% of participants highlighted the need to anticipate turns and plan ahead to ovoid overshooting the goals, but nevertheless, 50% of them explicitly reported that this condition was intuitive to use, with low cognitive demands and mapping of movement to head orientation freeing them up to plan the route without explicitly thinking about the controls.

Magnetic switch control

The qualitative feedback from this condition was the least consistent, but key factors emerged primarily around the location and responsiveness of the switch. 33% of participants felt that the switch gave them greater control over their movement, but others noted that on some occasions they either forgot to use it, or made a conscious decision to ignore it. The magnetic switch technique is known to have both false positives and false negatives (15), and together with the small delay between sliding the magnet and the movement response caused 61% of participants to report dissatisfaction with the responsiveness of the control, leading to overshooting of targets and the need for error correction. The inability to control the speed or to reverse or sidestep was reported as a problem for 33% of the participants.

Nearly half of the participants expressed dissatisfaction with the location of the switch, with some feeling the need to hold the headset in place when using the switch, and reports of fatigue and aching in the arm due to prolonged elevation. The switch was felt to be a very unnatural way of controlling movement, with the distinctive sound, and the need to raise the hand to the head to stop or start motion being reported by 50% of participants as factors which diminished their sense of immersion or presence.

Bluetooth controller

The controller received considerable feedback, but much of it was conflicting. The level of control of movement was generally considered to be good, with 72% reporting that the controls were responsive, and that the ability to stop, start and reverse were important features. However, 40% of the participants described some level of mismatch between their expectations of the control and the actual experience. This mostly related either to the lack of strafing (right and left side steps), or to the need to use the head to control direction but the controller for speed. Some participants explicitly described this as making them have to consciously think about how to move around, however overall, 67% expressed satisfaction with the ease of use. 'Naturalness' was quite a polarised category, with positive comments generally relating to prior experience or intuitive use, and negative comments relating to less immersion, and to the mismatch between expectation and experience. Half of the participants felt that this was the least natural and intuitive way of moving around, even if they found it the easiest to use. Interestingly, the participant with Parkinson's Disease particularly liked this technique, and felt that it was less effort and offered "more control than I usually have with tasks."

Additional observations

Whilst there was no explicit remit in this study to record observational data, there were some recurrent behaviours worthy of note.

Movement of the body

There was a distinct difference in the body movements of almost all the participants depending on the technique in use. When using the handheld controller, they generally remained upright and fairly still, using their feet to turn the chair when changing direction, but otherwise showing little movement of the torso. In contrast, when using the other two techniques (and particularly the continuous motion), most participants involved the whole body in the interaction, tilting, turning and twisting the torso and leaning the head in response to anticipated changes in direction.

Frequent stopping

When using either of the controls which had the ability to stop the motion, many participants elected to stop movement for every change of direction, even in places where they had successfully maneuvered in the continuous motion trial.

DISCUSSION

The performance and graphical fidelity of Google Cardboard techniques cannot compete with more expensive VR solutions, but it has the huge advantage of allowing the wider patient population to access truly mobile VR with minimal financial outlay. However, the quality and enjoyment of these first experiences could, for many patients, significantly influence their desire to engage with VR in the future. Furthermore, badly designed interactions may even hinder or undermine rehabilitation goals.

Whilst the findings of this preliminary work are based on a relatively small and heterogeneous group of participants and should be interpreted with caution, they do give some useful insight into the user experience, and offer some guidelines which may be useful to consider when designing mobile applications for virtual rehabilitation.

First and foremost, it is important to remember that we may have little control over the type of headset which is being used. The default position is likely therefore to involve continuous movement, perhaps mediated by head-orientation control or other software-mediated device. In this situation, any requirement to make tight turns or unplanned maneuvers should be avoided, and a suitable collision boundary provided at points where the user may wish to stop. Whilst in ideal circumstances users should be provided with an independent line of sight without changing direction (18, 19), this may prove difficult when input options are limited.

The addition of the switch control to the continuous movement increased the time taken to complete the task without greatly improving the user experience, However, the current magnetic switches are not 100% reliable, and it may be that a more responsive switch might bridge the gap between the immersiveness of continuous movement and the ease of use of the handheld controller. With the recent release of Google's version 2 headset it will be interesting to evaluate whether the new capacitive switch will impact these findings. It was notable that this switch technique was significantly slower than the less controlled continuous motion. Whilst we might have anticipated fewer errors and corrections of direction, this did not seem to be the case, and, furthermore, most users chose to stop and turn at almost every location, even if they had previously navigated them smoothly using continuous motion. However, the unnatural position of the switch on the side of the head, and the implications this has for fatigue and pain, may make this unsuitable for many patient populations. This is of some concern, bearing in mind that a number of VR headsets currently being developed are planned to incorporate headset-mounted controls.

Bluetooth controllers are available at very low cost, and indeed are often included with the purchase of a headset. For many users, particularly gamers, this provides a natural control, but it was reported to create a disconnect between the user and the virtual environment. However, this method was the most efficient for task performance, being nearly 50% faster than the magnetic switch control. This result is likely to vary with different navigation tasks, but is a significant factor, particularly where efficient maneuvering is required in an unfamiliar environment. When combined with head-orientation for direction selection, this technique appeared to have the highest cognitive load, and it may be necessary to use the controller for both direction selection and velocity control in order to lower the cognitive demands of this technique.

In contrast to reported immersion scores, we observed that the physical behaviour of the participants indicated a higher level of immersion when using the continuous controls than with the Bluetooth controller, and this warrants further investigation as it may have implications for certain types of application. Where increase immersion is desirable, for example in exposure therapy, then a hand-held controller may detract from this. However, the increase in movement of the torso and head, may increase the risk of injury or falls, and this is a significant consideration for many patient populations, particularly where there is already compromised balance.

In summary, none of the three techniques evaluated in this study offered an ideal solution for travel within mobile VR, but do point towards some preliminary design guidelines (see Table 3). Further work in clinical population is necessary to establish more robust guidelines. In addition, in this study we only looked at task completion time in our objective measures, but for future work accuracy and error rate will be important additional considerations.

Table 3. Preliminary usage indicators for the travel techniques evaluated in the study. The clinical indicators are tentative, as we have not yet tested directly in these populations

	Continuous movement	Switch on headset	Bluetooth controller
Accurate maneuvering	X	X	✓
Increase immersion	✓[1]	X	✓[1]
Balance impairment	X	X	✓
Parkinson's Disease	✓	X	✓
Cognitive impairment	✓[2]	✓	X
Avoid cyber-sickness	X	X	✓
Efficient travel time	✓	X	X

[1]Depends on individual user; [2]for navigating wide or open areas.

ACKNOWLEDGMENTS

With thanks to Mark Silvester for his contributions to the virtual flat model, and to Dion Willis for assisting with data collection.

REFERENCES

[1] Amer A, Peralez P Affordable altered perspectives: Making augmented and virtual reality technology accessible Paper presented at the Global Humanitarian Technology Conference (GHTC), 2014.
[2] Glegg, SMN, Holsti L, Velikonja D, Ansley B, Brum C, Sartor D. Factors influencing therapists' adoption of virtual reality for brain injury rehabilitation. Cyberpsychol Behav Soc Networking 2013;16(5):385-401.
[3] Bonis J. Acute Wiiitis. N Engl J Med 2007;356(23): 2431-2..
[4] Powell WA, Stevens, B. The influence of virtual reality systems on walking behaviour: A toolset to support application design. Paper presented at the International Conference on Virtual Rehabilitation (ICVR), 2013.
[5] Yao R, Heath T, Davies A, Forsyth T, Mitchell N, Hoberman P. Oculus vr best practices guide. Oculus VR 2014.
[6] Steed A, Julier S. Design and implementation of an immersive virtual reality system based on a smartphone platform. Paper presented at the IEEE Symposium on 3D User Interfaces (3DUI), 2013.
[7] Google. Google Cardboard VR 2014. URL: https:// www.googlecom/.
[8] Google. (Un)folding a virtual journey with Google Cardboard, in Google Official Blog 2016. https:// googleblogblogspotcouk/2016/01/unfolding-virtual-journey-cardboardhtml.
[9] Sibert LE, Jacob RJK. Evaluation of eye gaze interaction. Proceedings of the SIGCHI conference on Human Factors in Computing Systems, 2000.
[10] Bowman DA, Kruijff E, LaViola JJ, Poupyrev I. 3D user interfaces: Theory and practice. Boston, MA: Addison Wesley Longman, 2004.
[11] Slater M. Grand challenges in virtual environments. Front Robotics AI 2014;1:3. doi.org/10.3389/frobt.2014.00003.
[12] Jacob RJK, Girouard A, Hirshfield LM, Horn MS, Shaer O, Solovey ET, Zigelbaum J. Reality-based interaction: a framework for post-WIMP interfaces. Proceedings of the SIGCHI Conference on Human Factors in Computing Systems, 2008.
[13] Bowman DA, Koller D, Hodges LF. Travel in immersive virtual environments: an evaluation of viewpoint motion control techniques. Presented at the Virtual Reality Annual International Symposium, 1997.
[14] Sharma P. Challenges with virtual reality on mobile devices. Paper presented at the ACM SIGGRAPH Talks, 2015.
[15] Smus B, Riederer C. Magnetic input for mobile virtual reality. Proceedings of the 2015 ACM International Symposium on Wearable Computers, 2015.
[16] Sousa Santos B, Dias P, Pimentel A, Baggerman JW, Ferreira C, Silva S, Madeira J. Head-mounted display versus desktop for 3D navigation in virtual reality: a user study. Multimedia Tools and Applications, 2008; 41(1):161-81.
[17] Griffiths G, Sharples S, Wilson JR. Performance of new participants in virtual environments: The Nottingham tool for assessment of interaction in virtual environments. Int J Hum Comput Stud 2006;64(3): 240-50.
[18] Bowman DA, McMahan RP, Ragan ED. Questioning naturalism in 3D user interfaces. Commun ACM 2012; 55(9):78-88.
[19] Sayers H, Wilson S, Myles W, McNeill M. Usable interfaces for virtual environment applications on non-immersive systems. Proceedings of the 18th Annual Eurographics UK Conference, 2000.

Submitted: December 15, 2016. *Revised*: February 10, 2017. *Accepted*: February 15, 2017.

In: Alternative Medicine Research Yearbook 2017
Editor: Joav Merrick
ISBN: 978-1-53613-726-2
© 2018 Nova Science Publishers, Inc.

Chapter 41

EVALUATION OF LEAP MOTION CONTROLLER AND OCULUS RIFT FOR VIRTUAL-REALITY-BASED UPPER LIMB STROKE REHABILITATION

Dominic E Holmes*, BSc,
Darryl K Charles, PGCE, BEng, MSc, PhD,
Philip J Morrow, BSc, MSc, PhD,
Sally McClean, MA, MSc, PhD and Suzanne M McDonough,
BPhysio(Hons), HDip Healthcare, PhD

Computer Science Research Institute and Institute of Nursing and Health Research,
Ulster University, United Kingdom

ABSTRACT

Intensive rehabilitation is important for stroke survivors but difficult to achieve due to limited access to rehabilitation therapy. We present a virtual reality rehabilitation system, Target Acquiring Exercise (TAGER), designed to supplement center-based rehabilitation therapy by providing engaging and personalized exercises. TAGER uses natural user interface devices, namely the Microsoft Kinect, Leap Motion and Myo armband, to track upper arm and body motion. Linear regression was applied to 3D user motion data using four popular forms of Fitts's law and each approach evaluated. While all four forms of Fitt's Law produced similar results and could model users adequately, it may be argued that a 3D tailored form provided the best fit. However, we propose that Fitts's Law may be more suitable as the basis of a more complex model to profile user performance. Evaluated by healthy users TAGER proved robust, with valuable lessons learned to inform future design. The majority of users enjoyed using the Leap Motion controller and VR Headset, the inclusion of visual cues shows a general improvement in target acquiring performance and that Fitts's Law can be used to linearly model user reaching

---

* Correspondence: Mr Dominic Holmes, BSc, Room L037, Computer Science Research Institute, Ulster University Cromore Rd, Coleraine, BT52 1SA, United Kingdom. E-mail: holmes-d2@email.ulster.ac.uk.

and pointing movements in 3D environments. However, in some situations this isn't the case, emphasizing the importance of user profiling to examine the user's kinematic behavior more intricately.

Keywords: virtual reality, leap motion, oculus, stroke, rehabilitation, usability

INTRODUCTION

Upper limb rehabilitation following a brain injury, stroke, or other condition affecting upper limb movement, is carried out by occupational therapists and physiotherapists to recover and adapt the patient's movement and improve activities of daily living (ADL). Research confirms that rehabilitation is capable of improving arm function during both the early and late phases of stroke. However, effective therapy must be intense and requires the repetitive practice of task-related movements and actions (1). Repetitive task training involves intensive repeated practice of appropriate functional tasks and is thought to reduce muscle weakness and form a physiological basis of motor learning (2).

Virtual reality (VR) has significant potential to support self-management of such rehabilitation, in that it allows individuals to interact and train within stimulating, realistic virtual environments. It provides users with the opportunity to practice intensive repetition of meaningful task-related activities necessary for effective rehabilitation (3). A recent Cochrane review of 12 trials involving 397 participants for the upper limb, stated that the use of VR and interactive video gaming might be beneficial in improving upper limb function and ADLs; when used as an adjunct to usual care or when compared with the same dose of conventional therapy (4). This Cochrane review concluded that it is unclear at present which characteristics of VR are most important. However, they emphasized the need for pilot studies assessing usability and validity as part of the development process if designing new VR programs for rehabilitation purposes; these studies may also afford insight on the key VR characteristics for retraining of movement e.g., in reach and pointing tasks.

In this paper we expand on our latest research (5), presenting a multi-sensory VR system, Target Acquiring Exercise (TAGER), and evaluate its usability and performance for upper limb rehabilitation. We evaluate Fitts's law as the basis of an adaptive system to model movement performance for reach and touch tasks in a 3D virtual space. TAGER evolved from previous VR and augmented reality (AR) testbeds developed by our research group (6) and particularly from initial research undertaken with the Leap Motion controller (7). TAGER utilizes several natural user interface (NUI) devices to track the user, namely the Leap Motion, Microsoft Kinect V2, and the Myo armband, and affords the option of wearing a VR headset (in this experiment the Oculus Rift DK1). In the experiment outlined in this paper, the tasks comprise basic 3D reaching and pointing exercises so we can effectively evaluate the system and user model. The experiment reported here focused on testing with healthy users to help us evaluate the user interface ahead of planned experiments with impaired users, and has helped us refine the user profiling system. A participatory approach to system and experimental design was taken; engaging with physiotherapists and occupational therapists in local health trusts, namely the Regional Acquired Brain Injury Unit (Musgrave Hospital, Belfast), the Stroke Unit at the Royal Victoria Hospital (Belfast), and third sector agencies, e.g., Brain Injury Matters (Belfast).

A core interest in VR as a rehabilitation tool is due to its potential to provide an enjoyable experience. However, VR systems are flexible technologies supporting feedback, capability adaptation, high intensity, repetitive, functional exercises to encourage motor control and motor learning. There are an increasing number of studies mainly focused on using commercially available hardware devices to support upper limb rehabilitation (4). Recent cheaper, high-quality commercial technology, such as Leap Motion and the Myo, offer new opportunities for effective, center and home based self-managed rehabilitation. When combined with other existing technology, they have the potential to improve accuracy and reliability of performance monitoring, although research utilising these technologies is still limited. Feedback is of particular importance to patients, and VR systems have the potential to excel in providing rich, informative, personalized, just-in-time responsive feedback. Feedback cues in VR environments, when appropriately designed, can help users improve interaction performance. Rehabilitation systems have implemented multi-modal cues such as visual, tactile and auditory cues. The organization of movement is related to the quality of the viewing environment, particularly visual cues between the user's arm and the objects to improve spatial awareness (8). Tactile cues have also been reported to improve motor performance (9), and are mainly used to help users verify a successful interaction. Positive auditory cues provide user motivation to perform intensified repetitive tasks, represent temporal and spatial information very well and can improve motor learning (10).

Adaptation is an important usability factor within a VR rehabilitation user interface design, to enable a system to adapt both to a diversity of motor control capabilities and as rehabilitation progresses (6). This capability to adapt is important as a user may become frustrated if the tasks are too difficult or bored if tasks are too easy; thus maintaining engagement is vital in rehabilitation. Techniques proposed in the literature for adaptive VR rehabilitation systems include fuzzy logic and Fitts's Law (11). Fitts's Law is well known in the user interface community and has also been applied within the stroke rehabilitation (12) context. Fitts's Law models a user's motor skills by predicting the time to reach and touch a target based on a target's size (W) and the distance (D) from an origin (Eq. 1). The logarithmic element of the equation, known as the "Index of Difficulty" (ID), is used to quantify the difficulty of reaching a particular target. Thus, the movement time (MT) required to acquire a target is linearly dependent on ID, where smaller and further away objects are harder to attain.

$$MT = a + b\log_2\left(2\frac{D}{W}\right) \tag{1}$$

Equation 1 shows Fitts's original equation, but other researchers have devised variations of the equation to provide an improved model in different situations. Two popular adaptations of Fitts's Law are Shannon/McKenzie (eq. 2) and Welford (eq. 3), which were originally tailored to quantifying human movement behavior for 1D and 2D tasks. They have also been applied to 3D environments, but recently new forms of the equation have been devised to represent 3D interactive movements more accurately. Equation 4 (13) adapts Shannon/McKenzie (eq. 2) to include the addition of a movement direction parameter, to account for the consideration that MT is also dependent on the user's angle of motion (θ) on the Y axis from the origin to a target.

$$MT = a + b\log_2\left(\frac{D}{W} + 1\right) \quad (2)$$

$$MT = a + b\log_2\left(\frac{D}{W} + 0.5\right) \quad (3)$$

$$MT = a + b\log_2\left(\frac{D}{W} + 1\right) + \sin\theta \quad (4)$$

METHODS

The research described in this paper has an exploratory emphasis and focuses on investigating VR NUI design, particularly (i) the reliability of tracking systems and the modelling of user motion via Fitts's Law and its variants, (ii) the aesthetic design of multi-modal cues, and (iii) the usability and acceptability of the VR headset. The purpose of conducting this research – and the subsequent follow up with impaired users – is to ensure that the underlying interactive interface and adaptive motion tracking system is as robust as possible before adding further user interface elements, game components, and connected health systems. Ultimately our intention is that the system will be robust enough for unsupervised usage by stroke patients.

Participant recruitment

Healthy participants were enrolled in the experiment from students and staff at Ulster University. Inclusion criteria included that participants should be 18 years old and over, have no vision issues (e.g., blurred vision, color distortion, light sensitivity, depth perception), nor any disability that affected the upper extremity. Participants completed a questionnaire to gather information regarding IT and gaming literacy and to determine inclusion in the experiment.

Target acquiring exercise (TAGER)

TAGER is a custom designed 3D pointing exercise for upper limb rehabilitation, designed based on requirements from research (14) and clinician involvement. TAGER utilizes a number of technologies that work together to monitor and provide feedback to users while completing upper arm rehabilitation tasks. The Leap Motion controller is a small desktop NUI which contains an infrared camera specifically design to track fingers, hands and arms. It tracks up to 20 bones per hand, with 150° field of view and approximately 8ft^3 of 3D interactive space. TAGER uses the Leap Motion as the main interactive device within the virtual world for tracking motion and facilitating target acquisition. Microsoft's Kinect V2 is similar to the Leap Motion, though instead of sensing hands it senses motion of the human skeleton. We collect data of all joints in the upper body in motion with the goal in a future version of providing guidance on suitable functional task movements and other factors. It is natural for a person with an affected limb to move their whole body forward rather than extending their arm, especially if tired. As this would hinder improvement through the rehabilitation process, system feedback and guidance can be crucial. The Oculus Rift DK1 (VR Headset) contains a 7″ screen with a resolution of 1280 × 800 (16:10 aspect ratio) and a 90° field of view and enables head positional and rotational tracking. User head motion controls the viewpoint within a virtual world. The Oculus is investigated in this experiment to determine if it is acceptable for use and could potentially be used to increase spatial awareness. The Myo armband slides onto a forearm, and uses electromyography (EMG) technology with eight medical grade EMG nodes attached, that read electrical signals from the muscles. The Myo armband also includes an accelerometer and gyroscope to track movement and orientation on the forearm. The use of the Myo armband here is to collect data to be stored for future studies helping identify changes in muscles, which could highlight factors such as fatigue and correctness of exercise. The Myo armband also includes tactile feedback capability, for example, vibrations on the skin, which are used to introduce tactile cues into the system.

Experimental setup

The experimental process comprised three stages: (i) a training stage which gives the participant ten minutes to familiarize themselves with the technology and practice interaction. The training tasks are very similar to the real trials. Through system testing and observing users before the actual experiment it was decided that ten minutes training would be sufficient time for the participant to familiarize themselves but not cause fatigue. After training, the patients are given a short two minutes' rest period before the next stage (ii), which is the complete TAGER trial. In stage 3, after each user completes the trial, a short discussion takes place gathering any comments the participant might have and for the investigator to ask questions related to the user's experience of the system. Throughout the experiment, the participant was closely monitored by the investigator who provided assistance if any problems arose. The experiment was strictly controlled; the location of each trial was always the same as was the equipment used. Equipment arrangement was identical for each patient ensuring no other possible variables could affect the collected results. Figure 1 illustrates the layout of the environment.

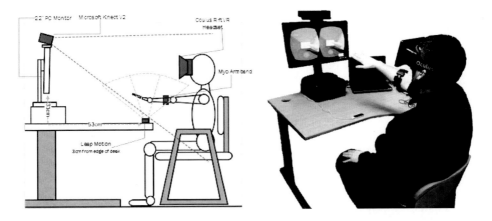

Figure 1. The Experiment setup showing the equipment locations and typically user interactions.

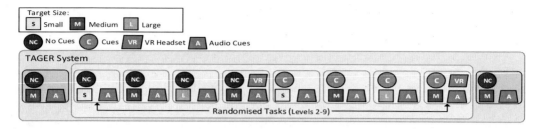

Figure 2. TAGER's level layout and scene attributes.

TAGER's 3D virtual environment is the inside of a basic walled room (no wall at the front) with a large start button on its floor. The user was prompted to push the button with their virtual hand to begin. An icosahedron shape was purposely chosen as the target object for its geometric properties, especially since visual cues are required to enhance spatial awareness. With changes in viewing angles, objects with a greater number of faces and edges such as icosahedrons, provide more clarity of visual cues (15). Each repetition (4 per level) contains 27 icosahedrons to target, all at different locations, a total of 108 per level (4*27). When the start button was pushed a single icosahedron appears randomly at any of the 27 locations. The user moves their virtual hand around the 3D environment touching each icosahedron that appears. When touched, the icosahedron disappeared, and another icosahedron appears on the floor of the room at the location of the start button. We call this object the origin; this approach was used to provide consistent movement trajectories. All objects were intentionally placed at fixed locations and at fixed distances from the user's view to simplify analysis.

The TAGER VR software for this research was constructed with ten levels; the first and last levels were identical enabling us to compare performance over the period of the session – considering learning and fatigue effects. All other levels were unique concerning scene attributes such as target object scale, multi-modal cues and VR headset use; to investigate the impact they had on user movement behavior (see Figure 2). Levels 2-9 were randomized per user to eliminate potential bias in the ordering; a rest period provided between each level and repetition. The unique levels comprise different combinations of scene attributes such as shadowing and proximity color change for visual cueing. Tactile cues were included using the Myo Armband where a vibration was sent to the user's arm upon successful target acquisition. We also changed the scale of the objects; objects were sized accordingly as 2, 3.5 and 5cm. Objects were scaled to discover the impact it has on cues. For example, larger objects were expected to give greater clarity to visual cues and thus quicker arm kinematics. These scene attributes helped build knowledge on the impact they have on arm kinematics, spatial awareness, movement speed and accuracy.

RESULTS

The above experiment was undertaken to investigate core aspects of TAGER. Data was recorded every tenth of a second from all input devices, and *MT* calculated and recorded to file automatically from tasks for analysis of the movement models. Of the 26 participants, three were excluded from data analysis due to missing data or system issues (loss of tracking).

Usability

Of the 26 participants, 77% reported that their experience using the VR headset was enjoyable, no motion sickness or other health-related effects were reported. 43% of people commented that they perceived their performance to have improved while wearing the headset, while 50% said that they needed time to adjust when first wearing the headset. We compared user performance between the VR headset and monitor use, with and without cues. We used a paired t-test to determine significant differences between users' average *MT* and found no significant difference between Cues ($T = 1.681$; $DOF = 21$; $p = 0.053$) or No Cues ($T = 1.591$; $DOF = 21$; $p = 0.063$). Though, there was a consistently slower user response when using the headset (Table 1). In other words, the participant's subjective experience was at odds with the objective measurement. Although this is not a significant issue so long as the effect is consistent among users, it is a consideration for future interaction design. Discussion with health professionals reinforced the importance of aesthetic cues in rehabilitation VR system design. We provided feedback on target proximity and acquisition through lighting and shading, as well as vibration from the Myo armband. Figure 3 shows variation in interaction difficulty with cues (C) or without cues (NC) for different sized objects (large – LRG, medium – MED and small – SML). While results were generally as expected – i.e., cues supported improved efficiency in target acquisition. It was not clear that cues improve performance for MED cue acquisition and more investigation is required. More detail will be covered on the effect of cues in the next sub-section.

Table 1. The mean movement time comparing VR headset and PC monitor: Cues(C), No cues (NC)

Exercise	VR (NC)	Monitor (NC)	VR (C)	Monitor (C)
Mean MT (ms)	1174.2	1107.4	1165.0	1115.4
T-test P = (0.05)	0.063		0.053	

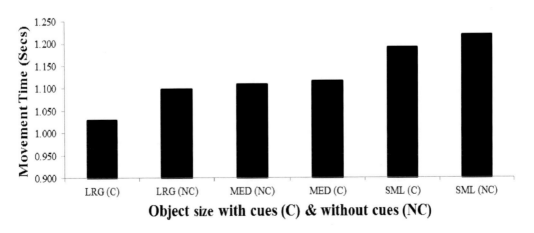

Figure 3. The variation of interaction difficulty arranged by the magnitude of the mean movement time.

An objective way to evaluate system feature effectiveness in TAGER is to record target acquisitions (hits) against movement times. A target has been successfully acquired when the user's hand collides with the surface of the target object without leaving the Leap Motion's detection area. Hits are classified as unsuccessful when the user's hand leaves the boundaries of the Leap Motion's detection area before hitting the target; users were required to return to within the boundaries to hit the target. Users could not progress until they acquired the current target, even after registering an unsuccessful hit. It was found that targets positioned at the center depth (relative to the user) were more successfully acquired – a mean of 29 successful hits per task over all participants (Front = 22, Back = 26). Closer objects appear to have been harder to attain, suggesting we may need to consider moving the minimum distance further away (along the z-axis) or move objects closer to the z-axis along the x and y-axes. The latter suggests a cone area (16) for object placement – with the cone pointing towards the user – rather than a cuboid (which maps well to the Leap Motion's detection area). This approach might account better for arm kinematic differences in attaining targets in close and far locations. Users attained targets in all sectors with reasonable success, though on average there were 31 (28%) unsuccessful acquisitions per level from a total of 108 targets. This may be considered to be quite high for healthy users; if the Leap Motion was mounted on the VR headset, changing position so that the leap camera is pointing forward (user's facing direction) could possibly provide a more natural interactive space, and reduce unsuccessful acquisitions. TAGER's experimental design implemented two identical levels one at the beginning and end of the experiment, enabling investigation of the potential learning effects indicated by improved performance or user fatigue resulting in performance decline. The mean completion times for all users for the start task was 1257.8ms while for end tasks the mean completion time was 1081.4ms suggesting that, despite having 10 minutes training time at the beginning, user performance significantly improved over the experiment (T = 4.60, DOF = 21, p = 7.7E-05). There are also some indications of fatigue (or loss of concentration) among several users. Analysis of experimental data in the next section enabled us to investigate the intricacy of user profiles.

Model effectiveness

As outlined earlier we recorded user motion data in reaching from an origin to touch an object target at various distances. Figure 4 shows the lines fitted to the data through regression for four well-known forms of Fitts's Law.

Table 2. The mean y-intercepts across each TAGER level for all forms of Fitts Law

EQ	SML (NC) (ms)	SML (C)	MED (NC)	MED (C)	LRG (NC)	LRG (C)	VR (NC)	VR (C)	Start	End	Overall Mean
(1)	189.3	77.4	270.7	161.6	392.7	343.4	70.6	-41.6	254.1	356.7	207.5 ± 89.3
(2)	-25.3	-152.2	95.9	-30.8	254.4	209.2	-107.9	-293.5	49.6	213.2	21.3 ± 110.9
(3)	86.4	-37.9	121.5	-7.5	210.2	166.6	-122.8	-250.8	74.7	224.4	46.5 ± 107.0
(4)	319.3	203.3	279.9	243.4	357.7	346.6	203.8	185.0	288.3	374.2	280.2 ± 83.6

Table 3. The mean slopes across each TAGER level for all forms of Fitts Law

EQ	SML (NC) (ms)	SML (C)	MED (NC)	MED (C)	LRG (NC)	LRG (C)	VR (NC)	VR (C)	Start	End	Overall Mean	Bits Per Sec
(1)	339.3	370.1	355.8	406.2	366.9	356.2	463.7	510.8	427.3	308.4	390.5 ± 46.0	2.5
(2)	315.7	343.2	316.6	358.4	311.0	301.9	392.7	454.3	378.1	271.6	344.4 ± 41.1	2.9
(3)	362.8	396.7	396.6	451.2	421.8	409.4	515.8	566.6	475.7	344.6	434.1 ± 51.2	2.3
(4)	247.7	273.1	275.1	290.5	282.1	261.7	318.5	324.1	322.9	236.2	283.2 ± 32.7	3.5

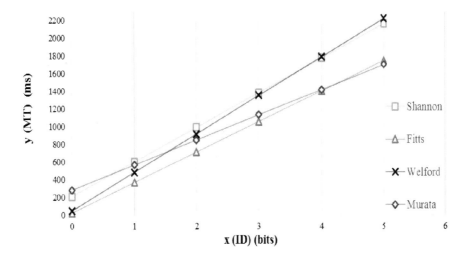

Figure 4. Regression line from our data for the four popular variants of Fitts Law.

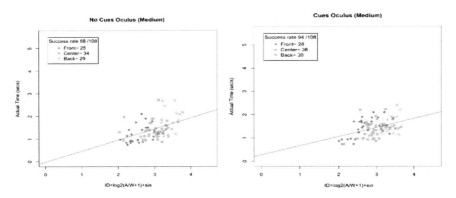

Figure 5. Murata's 3D model of movement for user 1023 while wearing the VR headset, plotting Index of Difficulty against the user's response time to successfully target medium sized objects. Depth (z-axis) is distinguished by 3 locations in the virtual world relative to the user: front (red diamonds), center (green squares), and back (purple crosses).

Tables 2 and 3 show the average regression values of the y-intercept and slope values for all participants. Murata's 3D equation (4) provides y-intercept values ranging from 196 to 363, which are more representative of human movement response (typically 200 to 300 ms); it also provided a more gradual gradient giving a more appropriate model of *MT* against *ID* (17). Thus, while all four equations provided similar results, we focused on Murata for further analysis. Figure 5 shows typical results while wearing the VR Headset with and without cues for medium sized targets and Murata's 3D form of Fitts's law.

Table 4. Participant statistics calculated over time including residual statistics, regression analysis and performance data to define a user performance profile

User	1001	1002	1009	1013	1019	1023	1026
Age : Gender	20 : F	20 : F	42 : M	24 : M	66 : F	54 : F	24 : F
Start (Residual)							
Standard Deviation	0.354	0.461	0.257	0.368	0.313	0.408	0.378
Kurtosis	0.085	-1.141	0.031	-0.238	-0.331	-0.262	0.376
Skewness	0.986	0.394	0.996	0.286	0.394	0.785	0.980
End (Residual)							
Standard Deviation	0.111	0.275	0.194	0.242	0.420	0.285	0.235
Kurtosis	5.852	0.985	2.540	-0.627	1.927	1.197	0.498
Skewness	1.834	1.227	1.515	0.187	0.952	1.143	1.289
Start Regression							
R^2	0.115	0.076	0.228	0.453	0.343	0.112	0.189
P-Value	4.05E-03	9.28E-02	8.60E-07	1.78E-08	1.79E-08	1.17E-03	3.92E-05
Slope	0.268	0.312	0.273	0.602	0.517	0.348	0.388
Intercept	0.352	0.360	0.268	-0.289	-0.212	0.475	-0.121
End Regression							
R^2	0.266	0.024	0.348	0.446	0.224	0.392	0.004
P-Value	3.80E-05	2.54E-01	2.83E-09	7.42E-09	3.18E-06	2.44E-11	5.77E-01
Slope	0.133	-0.109	0.293	0.445	0.481	0.509	0.033
Intercept	0.359	1.220	0.092	-0.070	0.116	-0.216	0.703
Performance							
Targets Hit (1080)	794	554	848	638	828	900	788
Start Hits	70	38	96	55	78	91	83
End Hits	73	57	85	59	88	92	74
% Change Hits	4.29	50.00	-11.46	7.27	12.82	1.10	-10.84
Start Mean Time	1.167	1.292	1.063	1.522	1.391	1.497	1.055
End Mean Time	0.768	0.884	0.952	1.270	1.580	1.262	0.802
% Change Mean Time	-34.19	-31.59	-10.42	-16.54	13.64	-15.66	-23.96

In Figure 5 when cues are included, user 1023 seems to improve her performance shown by a more gradual slope (decrease in value), the y-intercept (reaction time) towards a better representation of the typical human reaction time values and R^2 correlations are very similar. This experiment was fundamentally exploratory in nature. We used Fitts's law and linear regression to develop a user model, which will help us understand how best to create an adaptive system that can personalize interactive tasks. Table 4 provides user profiles from a proposed model comprising parameters such as regression line data, statistics on the residuals of the line fit, task performance and user information. Considering the explicit performance metrics (hits, movement times), target hits provided an informative statistic, and capable users are readily distinguishable from less able. Only one person had a score of less than 500 /1080 with the lowest score 472. The highest score was 900, and the average score was 754.74. Mean successful hits per person rose from 73.91 at the start to 77.22 at the end from a total of 108. The mean percentage improvement in hits over the experiment was 6.92% illustrating diversity of learning and fatigue effects among participants. The mean percentage reduction in MT was 13.79%. The average change in line fit according to R^2 and associated values were not significant (due to the spread of data values there are several valid lines). Change in hits between the start and end tasks in the experiment were potentially revealing of a possible learning effect (improvement) or mental/physical fatigue. A learning effect provided a challenge to adapting task difficulty per user – it is preferable to adapt difficulty based on Fitts's law only after the learning effect stabilizes. Nonetheless, it was helpful to identify that a user remains in a learning phase so that additional support can be provided. However, *MT* and hits should not be considered independently, as some users may slow down deliberately to improve hit performance. The mean slope gradient decreased by 26.85% and the mean intercept decreased by 29.82%. Shallower slopes indicated a more skilled response as there is less difference between acquiring close and far objects, while a rise in the intercept value moves the intercept closer to physiological reflex norms (generally between 200 and 300ms). Additional user profile information can be gained from the residual statistics of regression lines and the changes between start and end tasks. Mean standard deviation dropped by 19.28% and mean variance also fell by 32.49%, suggesting that on average users were becoming more accurate. Range dropped by 10%, supporting this proposal. Kurtosis of residuals increased by over six times the magnitude (positive values) suggesting an increased number of data points with a small deviation from the regression line. On the other hand, skew also increased 44.4% (also positive), which after examining the regression graphs of users we believe was due to users overshooting the target position and having to change direction. From our results, we did not identify a strong relationship between performance and user age or gender.

Data from seven of the twenty-three participants provided a poor fit to the model based on start task motion data. Data after the end session from five participants had a poor regression fit, though two of these participants were different from the seven identified from the start data. These two people may have been overly tired or bored, rather than being less capable, highlighting the need for intricacy and careful analysis of the profiles. To consider this further it was necessary to examine a few representative individual user profiles (Table 4). User 1026 was an informative example, who started well with a strong profile but whose hits and mean MT declined significantly during the end task. Despite having residual statistics during the end task that show less variability (indicating more effective target acquisition for a significant number of targets), hit score actually decreased, while skew and kurtosis both increased (suggesting more overshooting of the target), and R^2 and the associated P-value suggested an unreliable regression fit (possibly due to an increase in outliers). 1026's mean MT dropped by a 23.96%, which suggested, considering the user profile, that during the end task this user may have adopted a high-risk strategy. This is in contrast to 1019, who appeared to have become more conservative, and by moving slower (13.64% increase in mean MT) improved their hit score by 12.82%. This considered approach by user 1019 and other participants seemed to improve the likelihood that the user motion data corresponds to Fitts's law (and variants). User 1002 had the weakest start having the lowest number of hits in the initial task but improved hit performance by 50% and mean MT by 31.59%. However, even by the end task, this user's motion could not be applied to Fitts's law reliably, and they had less than a 50% hit success rate in the final task. User 1023 exhibited arguably the most sustained success, having the highest overall hit success and start and end scores of 90 and 91 respectively and overall an improved profile (based on regression values). As with user 1019, 1023 was not particularly fast but improved speed during the experiment. Three participants got slower over the experiment and all of these achieved higher scores in doing so. Five participants got lower hit scores and all of these, but one had much less adequate regression fit and three of these exhibited faster mean MTs. Further investigation is required to understand whether users with these profiles exhibit a decline of interest – the tasks were repetitive and several of these participants were quite skilled at the tasks – or due to mental/physical fatigue.

DISCUSSION

In this paper, we presented an initial version of the TAGER VR upper arm stroke rehabilitation system, which utilizes several inexpensive, commercially available input devices and a VR headset. We reported on an experiment that focused on the usability of the system and the use of various forms of Fitts's law to linearly model user motion - movement time against an index of difficulty – for reach and touch tasks in a 3D environment using a Leap Motion controller as an input device. Most users enjoyed using the Leap Motion device and perceived tasks to be easier with the VR headset on. No motion sickness or other negative health-related effects were reported. The importance of cues has been reported widely in the literature, and while our results show a general improvement in object acquisition with visual cues, we found the impact on targeting medium sized objects to be unclear. We outlined results from fitting user motion data to four forms of Fitts's law with each of the equations exhibiting a similar success. Examining the statistics of the regression process based on Fitts's law we found that these equations could be used to linearly model user motion with the Leap Motion controller in a range of setups including the utilization of a VR headset. However, the data point variance across the regressed line was quite high, and Fitts's law should not be applied as a simple linear model of user motion equally to all users. We recommend that a form of Fitts's law, for example, Murata's 3D version could be used as part of an intelligent system to profile users. Although the motion of most users could be modelled effectively using Fitts's law, we found a few users who found the NUI so difficult that they could not be modelled linearly. Most of these users required more training than we expected but in some cases, users appeared to become tired or bored. A more complex profiling system will help to identify training requirements and distinguish between loss of interest and mental or physical fatigue. We intend to develop the profiling system with further experiments and subsequently investigate the system with impaired users.

REFERENCES

[1] Kwakkel G, Wagenaar R, Twisk J, Lankhorst G, Koetsier J. Intensity of leg and arm training after primary middle-cerebral-artery stroke: A randomised trial. Lancet 1999;354(9174):191–6.

[2] Bütefisch C, Hummelsheim H, Denzler P. Repetitive training of isolated movements improves the outcome of motor rehabilitation of the centrally paretic hand. J Neurol Sci 1995;130:59–68.

[3] Crosbie J, Lennon S, Basford J, McDonough S. Virtual reality in stroke rehabilitation: Still more virtual than real. Disabil Rehabil 2007;29(14):1139–46.

[4] Laver K, S G, S T, Je D, M C. Virtual reality for stroke rehabilitation. Cochrane Database Syst Rev 2015;2: 8,11,12,13.

[5] Holmes D, Charles D, Morrow P, McClean S, McDonough S. Usability and Performance of Leap Motion and Oculus Rift for Upper Arm Virtual Reality Stroke Rehabilitation. 11th Intl Conf. Disability, Virtual Reality and Associated Technologies, 2016:217–26.

[6] Burke J, McNeill M, Charles D, Morrow P, Crosbie J, McDonough S. Serious Games for Upper Limb Rehabilitation Following Stroke. 2009 Conference in Games and Virtual Worlds for Serious Applications. Ieee, 2009:103–10.

[7] Charles D, Pedlow K, McDonough S, Shek K, Charles T. Close range depth sensing cameras for virtual reality based hand rehabilitation. J Assist Technol 2014;8(3): 138–49.

[8] Levin MF, Weiss PL, Keshner E a. Emergence of virtual reality as a tool for upper limb rehabilitation. Phys Ther 2015;95(3):415–25.

[9] Cameirao M, Bermudez i Badia S, Verschure P. Virtual Reality Based Upper Extremity Rehabilitation Following Stroke: A Review. J CyberTherapy Rehabil 2008;1(1):63–74.

[10] Avanzini F, De Gotzen A, Spagnol S, Roda A. Integrating auditory feedback in motor rehabilitation systems. Proc Int Conf Multimodal Interfaces Ski Transf 2009;232:53–8.

[11] Karime A, Eid M, Alja'am JM, Saddik A El, Gueaieb W. A Fuzzy-Based Adaptive Rehabilitation Framework for Home-Based Wrist Training. IEEE Trans Instrum Meas 2014;63(1):135–44.

[12] Zimmerli L, Krewer C, Gassert R, Müller F, Riener R, Lünenburger L. Validation of a mechanism to balance exercise difficulty in robot-assisted upper-extremity rehabilitation after stroke. J Neuroeng Rehabil 2012; 9(1):6.

[13] Murata A, Iwase H. Extending Fitts' law to a three-dimensional pointing task. Hum Mov Sci 2001;20(6): 791–805.

[14] Hochstenbach-Waelen A, Seelen H a M. Embracing change: practical and theoretical considerations for successful implementation of technology assisting upper limb training in stroke. J Neuroeng Rehabil 2012; 9(1):52.

[15] Powell V, Powell WA. Locating objects in virtual reality – The effect of visual properties on target acquisition in unrestrained reaching. Intl Conf Disabil Virtual Real Assoc Technol 2014;2–4.

[16] Cha Y, Rohae M. Extended Fitts' law for 3D pointing tasks using 3D target arrangements. Int J Ind Ergon 2013;43(4):350–5.

[17] Heiko D. A Lecture on Fitts ' Law [Internet]. 2013:19–25. URL: http://www.cip.ifi.lmu.de/~drewes/science/fitts/A Lecture on Fitts Law.pdf.

Submitted: December 15, 2016. *Revised:* February 10, 2017. *Accepted:* February 15, 2017.

In: Alternative Medicine Research Yearbook 2017
Editor: Joav Merrick

ISBN: 978-1-53613-726-2
© 2018 Nova Science Publishers, Inc.

Chapter 42

STUDY OF STRESSFUL GESTURAL INTERACTIONS: AN APPROACH FOR ASSESSING THEIR NEGATIVE PHYSICAL IMPACTS

Sobhi Ahmed, PhD, Laure Leroy, PhD and Ari Bouaniche, MS*

Paragraphe Laboratory, Université Paris 8, Saint-Denis, France

ABSTRACT

Despite the advantages of gestural interactions, they involve several drawbacks. One major drawback is their negative physical impacts. To reduce them, it is important to go through a process of assessing risk factors to determine the interactions' level of acceptability and comfort so as to make them more ergonomic and less tiring. We propose a method for assessing the risk factors of gestures based on the methods of posture assessment in the workplace and the instructions given by various standards. The goal is to improve interaction in virtual environments and make it less stressful and more effortless.

Keywords: gestural interaction, virtual reality, gestural assessment, human factor

INTRODUCTION

Gestural interactions allow users to manipulate a digital system using gestures, which can be compared to vocabulary for gestural interactions. Saffer 2008 (1) defines a gesture as "any physical movement that a digital system can sense and respond to without the aid of a traditional pointing device such as a mouse or stylus. A wave, a head nod, a touch, a toe tap, and even a raised eyebrow can be a gesture." They differ from 'traditional' interactions

---

* Correspondence: Sobhi Ahmed, PhD instructor and researcher at University Paris 8, Department Hypermedia, 2 Rue de la Liberté, 93200 Saint-Denis, France. E-mail: subhigham@gmail.com.

(mouse or keyboard interactions, for instance) insofar as the latter do not consider the way in which the user performs the action. For example, the way in which the user presses a keyboard button does not matter: the only important thing is the fact that the button has been pressed, not the way of pressing it (2). In addition, more 'traditional' interactions provide a limited set of interactions depending on the structure of the input device (the number of buttons on a mouse, for instance) (3, 4). Gestural interactions, on the other hand, allow users to take advantage of their whole body to interact with systems, therefore providing new interaction modalities and expanding the interaction vocabulary, resulting in a more flexible interface.

One of the purposes of gestural interactions is to facilitate interaction with virtual environments. They aim at being intuitive, easy to use and learn, since lots of them are based on the emulation of natural gestures (5). Some can even fulfill specific needs, such as those of physically disabled people (6). These interactions are supposed to entail less cognitive and physical effort than 'traditional' interactions: for example, the use of a mouse, which demands a physical effort because of its distance from the user, calls for the user's arm to be outstretched while requiring a very accurate gesture when pointing (7). A well-thought gestural interaction could indeed solve those problems.

However, gestural interactions using movements requiring substantial physical effort can be associated with musculoskeletal disorders. What is more, the extended and/or frequent use of such systems can result in an overuse of the muscles in charge of performing expected gestures (8).

There exist stressful, tiring, illogical gestures and some might be impossible to perform for certain people. For instance, interaction with some gestured-controlled TV sets is considered stressful (9) because of the high position of the hand during use. Interaction with touchscreens also affects user comfort negatively because of the need to keep one's arm outstretched (7). The use of big screens is sometimes considered stressful to the neck because of frequent movements of the head and eyes (10).

Few studies have been conducted on how to reduce the physical impact of gestural interactions on the human body and, as a result, non-ergonomic, stressful gestures that are difficult to use are often created, for want of guidelines (11). Interaction using such gestures can lead to various musculoskeletal injuries.

To the goal of analyzing and assessing the health risks associated with gestures, we have studied task assessment methods in the workplace. Just like gestural interactions, those tasks consist of movements repeated frequently. In such assessment methods, physical impact of gestures is affected, for example, by the angle of the joint used in the gesture, the gesture's duration, its repetition, etc. The evaluation of those factors allows the assessment of gesture quality and consequently of their physical impact which, in turn, allows the design and implementation of ergonomic gestures that will cause neither pain nor stress, and which will be easier to use. We aim to implement a gesture assessment method based on certain criteria and factors stated in current studies.

In a first part, we present the medical problems related to gestures used in videogames and the workplace. The second part studies the existing assessment methods of physical movements. In the remaining parts, we propose a synthesis and an analysis of said methods as well as our own approach to assessing gestural interactions.

Potential negative impacts of gestures

As mentioned previously (cf. Introduction), gestural interfaces are used more and more frequently in numerous domains. The use of such interfaces implies the performance of certain types of movements, sometimes repeatedly and/or for a long time, necessitating some effort. The overuse of the muscles in charge of these gestures can cause musculoskeletal disorders (MSDs). "The term MSD groups some fifteen diseases acknowledged as work-related pathologies. These pathologies represent more than 70% of known work-related pathologies" (12). MSDs affect the muscles, tendons and nerves of upper and lower limbs, at the level of wrists, shoulders, elbows or knees.

A lot of MSDs have resulted from the frequent use of gestural interactions, such as those included with the Wii® gaming console (13).

Painful gestures

Painful gestures are often caused by being subjected to an external or internal force and by exceeding the standard angle range at which joints are normally used. Those out-of-range angle values can be occasioned by numerous movements such as extension, flexion, abduction, adduction, pronation, etc. The movement range determines whether the joint is overly used and if the gestures resulting from the movement are potentially painful. Besides, static and dynamic constraints on some parts of the human body impact movement range and interdependence. (14, 15), for example adduction (moving a body part towards the median axis of the body), abduction (moving a body part outwards from the median axis), as well as pronation and supination, which designate limb rotations.

Injuries related to videogames based on gestural interactions

The repeated use of videogames can cause musculoskeletal injuries: for example, the use of the Wii® gaming console has occasioned sore muscles and knee, shoulder and heel injuries (DOMS: Delayed Onset Muscle Soreness) (8). Videogame-related injuries can be classified in four categories:

1. Tendinopathy: tendon injuries.
2. Bursite: swelling and irritation of one or several bursa.
3. Enthesitis: inflammation of the sites where tendons and ligaments are inserted into the bone.
4. Epicondylitis (tennis elbow): painful inflam-mation of the tendon on the outside of the elbow.

The main cause for such injuries and inflammations is the repeated stress undergone by involved muscles. According to the National Electronic Injury Surveillance System (NEISS), a high percentage of MSDs (67%) involve the use of Wii® in playing virtual sports (13).

Work-related injuries

The movements used during gesture interactions are extremely similar to those performed in the completion of some work-related tasks at the level of repetitions, extended time span, involved muscles, postures and the force exerted (8, 16). These movements could occasion injuries called "repetitive strain injuries" (RSIs). Several diseases have been associated with RSIs such as tendinitis, bursite, tenosynovitis, carpal tunnel syndrome, etc. (17). Symptoms such as pain, discomfort, and a sensation of localized fatigue in an overused joint can all point to RSIs.

The risk factors associated with the onset of RSIs and their level of severity depend on time span, frequency and intensity, and have been classified in six categories: awkward postures, force, effort and musculoskeletal load, static muscular work, exposure to certain physical stressors, repetition and the unvarying nature of the work, as well as organi-zational factors.

Effort depends on the joints involved, movement direction, posture and individual characteristics (12).

In gestural interactions, most gestures are deemed natural (natural user interface) (5), and require certain spatial movements, which in turn demand some effort as well as an internal or external force which can over-exert muscles and tendons affected by these activities (8). Moreover, these movements are repetitive, and occur over a long time span (11). It is therefore possible to speculate that videogame- and work-related injuries are similar to those resulting from gestural interactions. It is rather clear that movements with extended arms, device vibrations and activities involving one's arm are very similar.

According to Nielsen (14) the basic principles of gesture ergonomics are: avoiding external positions, avoiding repetition, muscle rest, favoring neutral, relaxed positions, avoiding static positions as well as avoiding internal and external forces on joints and the interruption of the natural flow of bodily fluids.

METHODS

It is crucial to find gesture assessment methods to devise gestures which do not lead to fatigue and health hazards.

Gesture assessment

The reduction of the negative physical impact of gestures requires an assessment procedure. This procedure would allow determining the level of comfort and the stress they cause by measuring risk factors related to said movements. Assessment methods are classified in two categories:

Subjective methods
Most studies on the assessment of the negative impact of gestures and physical movements in general resort to subjective methods (14, 16). Amongst those, one can find:

- The Body Discomfort Diagram method (BDD), which assesses the level of discomfort in different parts of the body using a diagram of the body and an assessment scale. The diagram allows identifying and assessing the places and sources of discomfort by marking the affected areas (18).
- Scoring methods, where a number of points is assigned to each single movement and criterion, resulting in a final score which determines the gesture's level of comfort. Each single score is decided either by the users (14) or by experts (ergonomists, etc.) (19).
- Other methods are used, such as question-naires (20), interviews, open-ended questions (16).

Objective methods and angle measurements

There exist methods and standards which allow the assessment of physical movements in a more objective way:

- Electromyogram. The electromyogram is a tool which measures muscle activity through the detection and recording of electric signals sent by muscle motor cells used during activity. The electric signal is amplified and processed to determine the level of muscle force exerted. (21, 22). This technique is used by (16) to measure muscle activity pertaining to the gestures and effort when interacting with touch-enabled devices.
- RULA (Rapid Upper Limb Assessment). RULA is a risk-factor assessment technique for upper limbs, geared towards individuals subjected to postures, forces and muscle loads potentially leading to MSDs (19). The assessed factors are: number of movements, static work, force, work posture and working time.
- RULA allows the attribution of a final assessment score for each posture ranging from 1 to 7. This score indicates the level of discomfort for the posture: the higher the score, the higher the risk. It follows diagrams specifying the ranges of joint angles for various body parts. In these diagrams, a score is given to each movement depending on its angle (the farther the angle from a neutral position, the higher the score). This numbering system is also used to specify the level of force exerted as well as static and repetitive muscular activity. To calculate the scores, three score charts —defined by ergonomists— are used (19).
- The use of RULA is manual and the assessment is only possible for one side of the body at once (left or right).
- The ISO 11226 standard. The ISO 11226 standard (23) aims at assessing health hazards for workers involved in manual labor. The assessment process involves specifying and classifying posture conditions for each body part as acceptable or not. These conditions comprise joint angle, time-related aspects and movement repetition. The classification is based on experimental studies as well as the current knowledge in ergonomics.
- The assessment procedure is a one- or two-step process. The first step measures joint angles. If said angles do not exceed a given limit, the posture is deemed 'acceptable.' If not, the second step focuses on the time span for which the posture is sustained. Extreme angles are never recommended. There exist several methods to recognize

postures, such as observation, video, etc. Other factors are considered while assessing static postures, such as support (or its absence), sitting or standing position, etc.

- The AFNOR NF EN 1005-4 standard (Safety of machinery – Human physical performance). NF EN 1005-4 is an AFNOR standard (24) aiming to improve machine design in order to decrease health risks by avoiding postures and stressful movements leading to MSDs. This is done through the specification of various recommendations as well as a posture- and movement-related risks assessment method.
- It defines a posture and movement assessment procedure related to working with machinery. The assessment can either be 'acceptable,' 'acceptable under conditions' or 'unacceptable.' The assessed risk factors are: movement angle, gesture time, frequency, etc. In situations determined as 'acceptable under conditions', other risk factors must be considered, such as duration, repetition, period of recovery, the presence of a support to the body, etc.

In addition, some assessment methods for physical movements and some specifications for acceptability status for joint angles ranges were presented by 'Institut National de Recherche et de Sécurité' (INRS, National research and safety institute) (25). Their objective was to better diagnose the work conditions in order to prevent musculoskeletal disorders.

Creating non-stressful gestures

Gesture creation by the user results in gestural interfaces taking user preferences and needs into account. Approaches to creating gestural interfaces are based on the concept of interface adaptability (26). One way is to use predefined (standard) gestures, where standard gestures are conceived from natural human gestures. A set of gesture vocabulary is derived by observing, collecting and assessing natural gestures performed by operators during scenarios (14, 27, 28). The assessment is used to select the final gestures that will be used. Only few studies take physical factors into account during gesture assessment. Another way is to let the user define the gestures he wants to use in a preliminary step before starting to use the system (29). However, the physical impact of the resulting gestures is not assessed.

Designing an assessment method for gestural interactions

We aim to design an assessment method for gestures used during interaction that would minimize their negative physical impacts. A complete gesture consists of a set of single gestures whose assessment results in an overall assessment of the gesture. The assessment of these gestures is done through the assessment of certain conditions and variables of the postures and physical movements effected. These conditions are: joint angles, posture duration, frequency, muscle load and external force.

Variables will be assessed based on specifications for acceptable and unacceptable movements in various studies and standards (24, 23, 25, 19). These specifications assess movement variables, thereby evaluating the quality of the gesture.

Table 1. Recommendations for shoulder joint angles (24, 23, 19)

Movement	Source	Acceptable limit (1)	Acceptable under conditions – Not recommended (2)		Unacceptable limit (3)
Antepulsion (Flexion- front)	AFNOR 1005-4	0° -20°	- 20° - 60° if static: (supported arm) or (short duration + recovery time) - 20° - 60° if frequent. - 20° - 60° if: - frequency < 10 per min - short duration - > 60° if short duration and not frequent		- > 60° if static - > 60° if frequent
	INRS	0° -20°	20°-60°		> 60°
	Tab Reg G				> 60°
	RULA	20° (1 pt)	20° - 45° (2 pts)	45°-90° (3pts)	> 90° (4 pts)
Retropulsion (Extension- back)	AFNOR 1005-4	0°	> 0° if: - not frequent - short duration		> 0° if static > 0° if frequent
	ISO 11226	0°			> 0°
	INRS	0°			> 0°
	RULA	0°-20°(1 pt)	> 20° (2 pts)		
Adduction	AFNOR 1005-4	0°	> 0° if: - not frequent - short duration		> 0° if static > 0° if frequent
	INRS	0°			> 0°
Abduction	AFNOR 1005-4	0° - 20°	- 20°-60° if static: (supported arm) or (short duration + recovery time) - 20° - 60° if not frequent. - 20° - 60° if: - frequency <10 par min - short duration - > 60° if short duration and not frequent		- > 60° if static - > 60° if frequent
	ISO 11226	20°	20°-60° (with support or check max time)		> 60°
	INRS	20°	60°		> 60°
	RULA	stressful (1 pt)			
Elevated shoulder	AFNOR 1005-4		stressful: if not frequent		stressful if frequent
	ISO 11226				stressful
	RULA	stressful (1 pt)			
Hyperadduction of the arm (with shoulder antepulsion)	ISO 11226				stressful
Extreme external rotation					
Arm support	RULA	- 1 pt			
Trunk leaning forward					

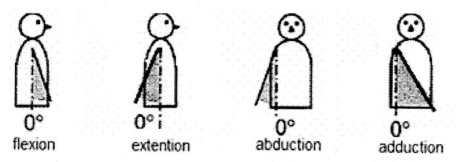

Figure 1. Shoulder movements (25).

The data related to each joint is organized in tables specifying all possible movement types for said joint and giving acceptable or unacceptable values for the various criteria and variables of movement. The angle of movement is a key factor in the assessment process, since it indicates the level of joint stress and, consequently, the potential discomfort to which that stress could lead.

The various levels of acceptability and comfort for shoulder movements (see Figure 1) are shown in Table 1. In this table, the acceptability of postures and gestures is mainly determined with joint angles. What is more, gesture duration, movement frequency and other factors potentially affecting the level of comfort are assessed, such as supports for the body, an even distribution of weight on legs and feet, etc. Joint ranges are classified in 'acceptable,' 'acceptable under conditions' or 'unacceptable' categories. The acceptability of movements is always connected to tasks with enough variation at the mental and physical levels (23). Similar tables for each joint have been compiled and are not printed here for want of space.

The measurement of time is crucial in the assessment of the acceptability of work postures: the longer the gesture and the higher number of repetitions, the more stressful the movement is. The different approaches use various strategies to measure time. Some measure movement frequency (repetition) (24, 19), others measure gesture duration (23), etc.

Table 2. Recommendations for the duration and frequency of movements. The application's inputs are: The physical movements detected by a Kinect device (which will probably be replaced by a more accurate device in the future)

Inputs	Method
ISO11226 (23)	Trunk: for a leaning movement ranging between 20°- 60°, time acceptability is calculated with this equation: $y = -\frac{3}{40}x + \frac{11}{2}$
	Head: For a supported bowing movement ranging between 25°-85°, time acceptability y is: $y = -\frac{7}{60}x + \frac{131}{12}$
	Shoulder: For a supported abduction (elevation) ranging between 20°-60°, time acceptability y is: $y = -\frac{1}{20}x + 4$
RULA (19)	Time is incorporated in the static load (calculate load versus time separately). Scores A or B is increased by 1 point if the posture is static. Scores A or B is increased by 1 point if repeated (more than 4 times per minute).
AFNOR (24)	Movement repetition (if frequency >= twice per minute) Duration (according to ISO 11226).

Table 2 shows ways of assessing time according to various approaches. In ISO 11226, the assessment of gesture duration is necessary when one gets a result that is 'acceptable under conditions'. In that case, time is of the essence in the assessment process. The standard comprises graphs which plot the relationship between joint angle range and the maximum acceptable gesture duration. According to these curves, the movement is deemed acceptable if it does not exceed the maximum time (y) depending on the joint angle (x). The equations in Table 2 are calculated from these graphs (23, 30). Some approaches use a scoring system based on an accumulation of points (19, 14). Besides, other approaches depend on joint angle testing followed by gesture duration to determine its acceptability (23). The information about the levels of acceptability of joint ranges, duration and other risk factors (such as repetition, force, muscle load, etc.) defined in various approaches are collected and organized so as to be used in the assessment process which aims to determine the level of acceptability of the gesture.

SOFTWARE STRUCTURE

Approach

Our goal was to develop a computer application that would allow detecting the conditions and variables of users' freeform empty-handed gestures, assess them, and determine their level of acceptability automatically according to various pre-existing methods and standards. The variables are mainly joint angles, duration, frequency, supports for the body, movement and posture style (weight distribution on both feet, rotation, etc.) This application could be used in the design phase of gestural interactions to decide which gestures are best. What is more, it could be used to assess pre-existing gestural interfaces and find out whether they are stressful.

Input

The application's inputs are:

- The physical movements detected by Kinect (which will probably be replaced by a more accurate device in the future). From the capture, we deduce:
  - angles
  - duration
  - repetition
- The presence of supports for the body and the possible presence of a rotation are manually entered for the time being.
- The tables of acceptable values for the following methods:
  - RULA
  - ISO 11226
  - AFNOR 1005-4
  - INRS

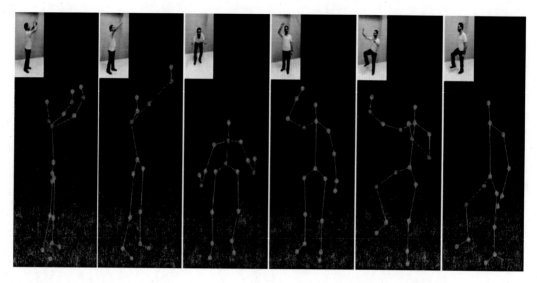

Figure 2. Stressed joints, colored red in the application real-time output (simulated).

Outputs

The application outputs results in a dialog box which includes:

- A binary assessment (acceptable or not) of the evaluated body posture, depending on the analysis through each approach we have implemented (RULA, INRS, ISO, AFNOR). Said assessment will only return 'acceptable' if the collected data is deemed 'acceptable' to each of the aforementioned standards and methods. We have adopted such an approach to ensure a maximum level of safety.
- In the case of a non-acceptable evaluation of the gesture, acceptability results broken down by body part will also be displayed, so as to easily locate the stressful areas which invalidated the assessed gesture.
- On the application interface, stressed joints will be colored in red in real time as shown in Figure 2.

Architecture

The application's design emphasizes clarity, modularity and revisability. It was indeed essential, when envisioning a basis which could be adapted to various uses and custom applications that designers of gestural interactions could modify the software as they see fit without causing the whole program architecture to fall apart. It also makes potential evolution of test methods possible, following progress in the field or, in the case of a custom application, specific constraints or in-house assessment methods. It is thus very easy to modify or add tests to the aforementioned standards and objective methods included in the application. Furthermore, in the perspective of maximum safety, the software was designed to detect the maximum angles reached in the course of a gestural interaction, and it computes its assessments from these maximums, according to the standards and methods stated above.

PERSPECTIVES

The goal of the assessment is to define less stressful standard gestural interactions. We will test a gestural interaction using certain joints (for instance shoulder, elbow, wrist, etc.) to decide on whether it is stressful. If it is, we will be able to point to the problematic joint(s) and the reasons for the stress (extreme angle, repetition, etc.) A subject will perform gestural interactions and the software will assess those gestures and display the assessment result (acceptable / unacceptable). It will also be possible to test several gestures and compare them to find the least stressful. We also collect additional subjective data from users to incorporate them into the assessment process for a better appreciation of user stress.

Validation of the application (Method)

We are aiming at validating our method through performing an experiment where subjects manipulate a gestural interface through performing certain tasks in different conditions. The application then evaluates the physical stress and gives results about the level of fatigue for each gesture and each joint. Furthermore, subjective results are collected from the subjects through a questionnaire about the level of the fatigue they felt in each condition and each joint. The results given by the subjects and those given by the application will be analyzed and compared to find whether they are correlated and by consequence whether the method is valid or not.

- Subjects. 26 potential users of virtual reality systems (students, museum visitors, video-game players, etc.).
- Tasks. We are currently developing several elementary and composite tasks to test our approach. For example, the tasks of selecting and moving an object, exploring a scene, etc. The first one is to arrange items, that is to select an object among several in the stock box, move and drop it in the corresponding box. Each task can be performed in different conditions (box height, number of times, time required, accuracy, etc.) Each subject is asked to arrange objects in various boxes using gestural interaction.
- Physical devices: Microsoft Kinect for Xbox® motion sensor and a computer screen showing the movements and assessment results.

Improving detection accuracy

We are for the moment using the Microsoft Kinect for Xbox® motion sensor to detect the movements. We plan to use more accurate movement detection techniques, such as a multi-Kinect system and/or an ART-Tracking movement detection system. We preferred using the Kinect device for his portability and usage facility (31). We are also thinking of using an EMG to detect the level of physical effort exerted, thereby making the method even more objective.

CONCLUSION AND FUTURE WORK

In spite of the undeniable advantages of gestural interactions, the latter still exhibit several weaknesses, amongst which their negative physical impact on the subject performing them. In order to reduce that impact, it is important to implement a risk-factor assessment procedure to determine the levels of acceptability and comfort of the suggested gestures. This will ensure that the interactions created are more ergonomic and less stressful.

We propose a semi-objective assessment method of the gestures' risk factors based on the assessment of work-related tasks and the specifications found in certain standards.

Our objective is to try to improve interaction in virtual environments and make them easier and less detrimental to subjects. Moreover, our method may be used to assess physical movements in other fields, such as work posture, ergonomics or even physical therapy: the modular nature of our software makes it easily amendable —and, with some little work on the coding side, configurable— by the end-user. It is therefore feasible for a physical therapist in a context of rehabilitation, to change the default joint angle values (as well as other risk factors) provided in the software, taking some trauma into account, and then assess patient movement in real-time while avoiding unnecessary stress on traumatized joints.

REFERENCES

[1] Saffer D. Designing gestural interfaces: Touchscreens and interactive devices. Sebastopol, CA: O'Reilly Media, 2008.

[2] Kurtenbach G, Hulteen EA. Gestures in human-computer communication. In: Laurel B, ed. The art and science ofinterface design. Reading, MA: Addison-Wesley, 1990:309-17.

[3] Baudel T, Beaudouin-Lafon M. Charade: remote control of objects using free-hand gestures. Commun ACM 1993;36(7):28–35.

[4] Isenberg T, Hancock M. Gestures vs. postures: "Gestural" touch interaction in 3D environments. In: Proceedings of the CHI Workshop on "The 3rd Dimension of CHI: Touching and Designing 3D User Interfaces" (3DCHI 2012, May 5, 2012, Austin, TX, USA, 2012:53–61.

[5] Rauterberg M. From gesture to action: natural user interfaces. In: Technical University of Eindhoven. Mens-machine interactie. Diesrede: Technical Univ. of Eindhoven, 1999:15–25.

[6] Jégo J-F. Interaction basée sur des gestes définis par l'utilisateur: Application à la réalité virtuelle. Ecole Nationale Supérieure des Mines de Paris, 2013. [French].

[7] Lalumière A, Collinge C. Revue de littérature et avis d'experts sur les troubles musculo-squelettiques associés à la souris d'ordinateur [Internet]. Montréal : Institut de recherche en santé et en sécurité du travail du Québec, editor. IRSST. Québec: Institut de recherche en santé et en sécurité du travail du Québec, 1999. URL: https://books.google.fr/books?id=ZBrnnQEACAAJ.

[8] Sparks DA, Coughlin LM, Chase DM. Did too much Wii cause your patient's injury? J Fam Pract 2011; 60(7):404–10.

[9] Freeman WT, Weissman C. Television control by hand gestures. In: Proc of Intl Workshop on Automatic Face and Gesture Recognition, 1995:179–83.

[10] Bowman DA, Chen J, Wingrave CA, Lucas JF, Ray A, Polys NF, et al. New directions in 3D user interfaces. IJVR 2006;5(2):3–14.

[11] Yan X, Aimaiti N. Gesture-based interaction implication for the future and. master thesis. Umea: Department Computer Science, Umea University, Sweden, 2011.

[12] Aptel M, Cail F, Aublet-Cuvelier A. Les troubles musculosqueletiques du membre supérieur (TMS-MS)- Guide pour les préventeurs, 2011. URL: http://www. inrs.fr/media.html?refINRS=ED 957.

[13] Jones C, Hammig B. Case report: injuries associated with interactive game consoles: preliminary data. Phys Sportsmed 2009;37(1):138–40.
[14] Nielsen M, Störring M, Moeslund TB, Granum E. A procedure for developing intuitive and ergonomic gesture interfaces for man-machine interaction. In: Proceedings of the 5th International Gesture Workshop, 2003:1–12.
[15] Charles Eaton MD. Electronic textbook on hand surgery, 1997 [Internet]. http://www.eatonhand.com
[16] Muse L, Peres SC. The ergonomic implications of gesturing: Examining single and mixed use with appropriate placement. In: Texas Regional Human Factors and Ergonomics Society Symposium, Texas, 2011.
[17] Simoneau S, St-Vincent M, Chicoine D. Les LATR, mieux les comprendre pour mieux les prévenir. IRSST, editor. Québec: St-Léonard, Québec: Association paritaire pour la santé et la sécurité du travail Secteur Fabrication de produits en métal et de produits électriques, 1996. [French].
[18] Cameron JA. Assessing work-related body-part discomfort: current strategies and a behaviorally oriented assessment tool. Int J Ind Ergon 1996;18(5): 389–98.
[19] McAtamney L, Corlett EN. RULA: A survey method for the investigation of work-related upper limb disorders. Appl Ergon 1993;24(2):91–9.
[20] Ha V, Inkpen KM, Mandryk RL, Whalen T. Direct intentions: the effects of input devices on collaboration around a tabletop display. In: First IEEE International Workshop on Horizontal Interactive Human-Computer Systems (TABLETOP'06), 2006:8.
[21] Long C, Conrad PW, Hall EA, Furler SL. Intrinsic-extrinsic muscle control of the hand in power grip and precision handling. J Bone Jt Surg Am 1970;52(5):853–67.
[22] Freivalds A. Biomechanics of the upper limbs: mechanics, modeling and musculoskeletal injuries. Boca Raton, FL: CRC Press, 2011.
[23] ISO International Organization for Standardization. Ergonomics-evaluation of static working postures. International Organization for Standardization, 2000.
[24] CEN (Comité Européen de Normalisation). Evaluation of working posture in relation to machinery - prEN 1005-4. Saf Mach – Hum Phys Perform – Part 4 Eval Work posture Relat to Mach, 1998;
[25] Aptel M, Gerling A, Cail F. Méthode de prévention des troubles musculosquelettiques du membre supérieur et outils simples [Internet]. Vol. 83, Documents pour le Médecin du Travail. Lorraine; 2000. URL: http://www.inrs.fr/media.html?refINRS=TC 78.
[26] Bobillier-Chaumon M-E, Carvallo S, Tarpin-Bernard F, Vacherand-Revel J. Adapter ou uniformiser les interactions personnes-systèmes? Rev d'Interaction Homme-Machine 2005;6(2):91–129. [French].
[27] Ruiz J, Li Y, Lank E. User-defined motion gestures for mobile interaction. In: Proceedings of the SIGCHI Conference on Human Factors in Computing Systems, 2011:197–206.
[28] Wobbrock JO, Morris MR, Wilson AD. User-defined gestures for surface computing. In: Proceedings of the SIGCHI Conference on Human Factors in Computing Systems, 2009:1083–92.
[29] Jégo J-F, Paljic A, Fuchs P. User-defined gestural interaction: A study on gesture memorization. In: 3D User Interfaces (3DUI), 2013 IEEE Symposium on, 2013:7–10.
[30] ISO International Organization for Standardization. Rectificatif technique 1 à la norme ISO 11226 de décembre 2000 ISO 11226/AC1:2006, 2006.
[31] Zerpa C, Lees C, Patel P, Pryzsucha E, Patel P. The use of microsoft kinect for human movement analysis. Int J Sport Sci 2015;5(4):120–7.

Submitted: December 26, 2016. *Revised:* February 11, 2017. *Accepted:* February 17, 2017.

Chapter 43

BRINGING THE CLIENT AND THERAPIST TOGETHER IN VIRTUAL REALITY TELEPRESENCE EXPOSURE THERAPY

David J Roberts[*], *BSc, PhD, Allen J Fairchild, BSc, PhD, Simon Campion, BSc, PhD and Arturo S Garcia, BSc, PhD*

Department of Psychology, Schools of Health Science University of Salford, Salford, Department of Computer Science, School of Computer Science and Engineering, University of Salford, Salford and THINKLab, School of Built Environment, University of Salford, Salford, United Kingdom

ABSTRACT

We present a technology demonstrator of the potential utility of our telepresence approach to supporting tele-therapy, in which client and remote therapist are immersed together. The aim is to demonstrate an approach in which a wide range of non-verbal communication between client and therapist can be contextualised within a shared simulation, even when the therapist is in the clinic and the client at home. The ultimate goal of the approach is to help the therapist to encourage the client to face a simulated threat while keeping them grounded in the safety of the present. The approach is to allow them to use non-verbal communication grounded in both the experience of the exposure and the current surroundings. While this is not new to exposure therapy, the challenges are: 1) to do this not only when the threat is simulated; and 2) when the client and therapist are apart. The technology approach combines immersive collaborative visualisation with free viewpoint 3D video based telepresence. The potential impact is to reduce dropout rate of exposure therapy for resistant clients.

Keywords: exposure therapy, virtual reality, VRET, telepresence, client therapist relationship, non-verbal communication

---

[*] Correspondence: Professor David Roberts, BSc, PhD, Chair of Telepresence, Psychology, School of Health Science, and Computer Science, Computer Science and Engineering, Alerton Building, Frederick Road Campus, University of Salford, 43 Crescent, Salford, M5 4WT, United Kingdom. E-mail: d.j.roberts @salford.ac.uk.

INTRODUCTION

Exposure therapy is an effective treatment for phobias and post-traumatic stress disorder (PTSD). Yet it suffers high dropout rates, especially in resistant populations. Drop out can come from lack of engagement, symptoms heightening at outset of therapy, or reluctance of clients to travel to the clinic. Virtual Reality Exposure Therapy (VRET) offers potential to address the first two, and its derivative tele-VRET, the latter. We argue that the typical approach of using Head Mounted Displays (HMD) in VRET and desktop displays in tele-VRET focusses attention on threat and blocks or hinders non-verbal communication (NVC).

We present a demonstrator of a new approach to tele-VRET that addresses this. Within this the therapist and client share a virtual space with the simulated threat in such a way likely to both support a wide range of contextualised NVC and promote a feeling of togetherness. In this, the client faces a life sized 3D video of the therapist moving within a virtual environment that contains emotive stimuli. In the current demonstrator the client is captured through 2D video to allow for easy deployment in the home. Both can judge where the other is looking. The therapist can move between the client and the emotive stimuli or stand to one side and gesture toward or away from it, in this way managing their attention. Our approach allows the therapist to determine if the client is looking at them, fixating on or away from the simulated threat, or following instructions to look toward the real world. A limitation of the current demonstrator is that while the therapist can move freely, gaze estimation will be effected if the client moves off the central line of their camera. A symmetrical system that captured 3D video at each side would allow both to move in any direction without fragmenting spatial context. We also demonstrate how video based reconstruction can be used to rapidly create 3D recordings of actors approaching levels of realism that traditionally take much longer capture and rework.

Related work

VRET has been studied across an extensive range of phobias but perhaps most deeply with post-traumatic stress disorder (PTSD). Within PTSD, VRET has demonstrated potential efficacy and appears to be more engaging to resistant groups (1). Yet drop-out rates, at approaching 40%, remain similar to non-technology based exposure therapy (1).

Awareness of both memories and current present-moment experience is seen to facilitate exposure in traumatised individuals (2). Conversely, "immersive virtual environments can break the deep everyday connection between where our senses tell us that we are and where we actually are located and whom we are with" (3). Rothschild explains how the therapist uses non-verbal communication to detect fixation and bring attention back to the present. Yet VRET typically uses Head HMDs (1) that completely block both the present surroundings and therapist from view.

Tele-VRET has been demonstrated but uses desktop interfaces through which avatars representing client and therapist come together in a world, all shrunken to fit within a small monitor. Such systems support little non-verbal communication or feeling of togetherness (4). People seem to react to life-sized virtual humans as if real, following natural patterns that relate gaze and interpersonal distance (5). Subtle changes in gaze and posture of virtual humans alters people's comfort (6). People respond naturally to virtual avatars in distributed immersive collaborative environments (7). We have extended such systems to support mutual eye-gaze (8). However, these avatars still do not look like the person whose movements they copy and do not reproduce faithful facial expressions. We have thus developed 3D video telepresence to communicate both what someone looks like and what they are looking at (4). This technology produces live 3D graphical copies of people, and any items around them, into another space.

Others combined video based reconstruction with an immersive display (9) demonstrating how spatial and visual qualities could be better balanced. However, visual and temporal qualities were still some way behind what could be achieved with motion tracked avatars. Since then, visual qualities of video based reconstruction have significantly improved (10, 11). Recent (12) and current (13, 14) funded EU research focuses on spatial telepresence. The potential utility of our approach in collaborative work has been demonstrated within the realm of space science and exploration (14, 15). This technology could be used to join clinic and home.

Our telepresence system

The ultimate aim of our telepresence system is to situate people from different physical locations into a shared simulated context within which they communicate through a wide range of non-verbal resources. Unlike 2D video based approaches, each can see where the other is looking as they move. This system has been described before (16). Here we summarise what it tries to solve, its approach and current state.

Unlike spoken word, NVC and its use in social interaction is inherently spatial. Just as words link together to provide meaning, so do various non-verbal signals, along with their context. In the natural world, gaze, interpersonal distance and other non-verbal cues of familiarity are linked and used to allow people to manage relationships with each other. Even board room meetings typically start and end with people going up to each other, making eye contact, smiling and sometimes tapping a shoulder or shaking hands. It is these things that grow the trust between people needed for an effective meeting.

Video conferencing supports some of NVC useful in promoting trust and togetherness. Such technology ranges from Skype on a phone to carefully aligned screens and cameras around a table. 2D Video however, loses much of the spatial grounding for NVC. Spatial context can only be accurately determined within the space of the observed, rather than across the spaces of the interactants. While cameras and screens can be aligned to support some approximation of gaze interaction, this only begins to work when people remain in the centre line of the camera. Problems of aligning camera and image of face and the Mona Lisa effect greatly limit this approach and restrict support for relationships between gaze and interpersonal distance. Video conferencing can be said to faithfully communicate visual but not spatial qualities of non-verbal behaviour.

Immersive collaborative virtual environments (ICVE) offer the other extreme, where non-verbal communication between interactants can be situated in a shared virtual context but at the expense of visual faithfulness and many subtleties, such as facial expression. In such a system, people in different displays can move around a shared context together, seeing each other as life sized CGI avatars. We have previously extended ICVE with eye gaze (Roberts

VR'09). Such a system theoretically supports the relationship between personal space and eye gaze although this has not been tested with rigour. ICVEs can be said to faithfully communicate spatial but not visual aspects of non-verbal behaviour.

Numerous video based approaches to reconstructing humans have been applied to telepresence. In theory, these should be able to faithfully communicate both visual and spatial qualities of non-verbal communication. However, balancing the two, especially with temporal qualities remains challenging (16). This is the challenge that our telepresence system is set against. Specifically, we want to faithfully communicate both visual and spatial aspects of non-verbal communication to within the limits of their use in non-touch interaction. This means being able to, for example, look someone in the eye and see if they smile as you enter their personal space, perhaps from the side.

Our approach combines real time free viewpoint video with large projection displays. An end to end description of the system is given in (4). It adopts the video based construction approach of visual hull, using our parallel adaptation (17) of the EPVH algorithm (18). Users stand within an immersive display system and are captured by surrounding cameras, Figure 1. Silhouettes from the images are then used to shape carve a form, onto which the original images are textured. This live textured model can then be sent to another immersive display system to be placed within the spatial context of a shared simulation and another user.

We have built many prototype versions that between them demonstrate that all the fundamental requirements are achievable with our approach. However, we have not yet built a single version that fully meets all. At this point in time, we are able to build demonstrators of principle and undertake perceptual experimentation such as (16). However, we have yet to build complete an end-to-end symmetrical system that would demonstrate a sufficient balance of visual, spatial and temporal interaction to support meaningful behavioural experimentation. This paper presents a novel demonstrator.

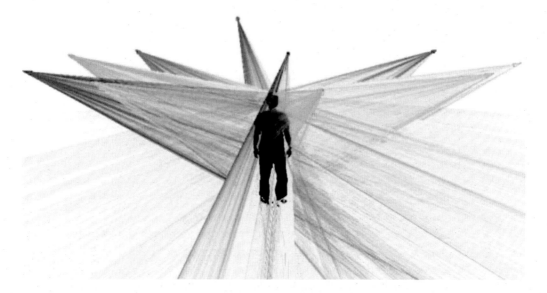

Figure 1. 3D reconstruction of a human in our telepresence system, showing lines from each camera derived from silhouettes.

Demonstration application to virtual reality telepresence exposure therapy

We now describe: the problem we are trying to solve; our general approach; an example scenario; the technology set up; and the limitations.

The problem that we are trying to solve is managing the emotional distance to threat while: 1) the threat is simulated; 2) the client and therapist are in different buildings. The approach we are taking is inspired by Rothschild (2) who attempts to mediate a client's awareness of threat and safety of the present, making use of verbal and non-verbal communication.

Our approach is to share a virtual context through large displays while using video based reconstruction to recreate both the therapist and, in this case, the threat. In another case the threat might be completely virtual. The concept is that the therapist can interpret both attention and emotion of the client through non-verbal signals and use non-verbal communication to direct the client's attention and, by doing so, manage emotion their emotion.

In this scenario, the shared virtual environment represents a non-threatening place. The therapy scenario is one of social anxiety. The people in Figures 2 and 3 are authors playing out parts. The three parts being played are: therapist, client and threatening other. In Figure 1 the "client" looks straight at a threat that has just approach through a door. In Figure 3, the "therapist" steps between them and uses gesture and gaze to direct the client's attention to a neutral object, the sofa.

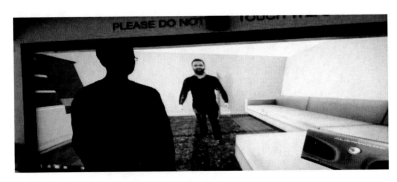

Figure 2. The client in the foreground is approached by a threatening other. The threat is a pre-recorded 3D reconstruction of someone approaching aggressively.

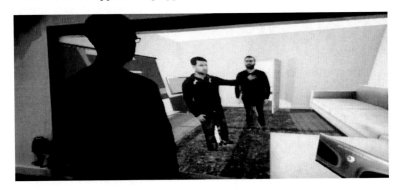

Figure 3. A mock-up of a client fixating on a virtual threat and the therapist stepping in front of it. The therapist (centre) is reconstructed in real time across the telepresence link.

To demonstrate this principle and primary issues we have created an asymmetric system by linking two large displays with two different kinds of mediums (Figures 4 and 5). Asymmetric telepresence systems have been used to demonstrate the impact of differences in VR technology on collaboration (19, 20). Our demonstration does not attempt to address every issue but does attempt to demonstrate the key issues and the fundamental qualities of our approach towards addressing them. The client side uses very simple technology that would be relatively straight forward and inexpensive to replicate in the home. The key components are a large flat screen onto which the shared virtual context is displayed and a camera. The therapist side is more complicated but could still be replicated within a clinic without excessive disruption or expense. The two fundamental differences are the use of two screens and a ring of cameras. The face on view of the "client" is transmitted via skype to a display wall in front of the "therapist." The rear portion of the partially shared virtual environment is displayed behind the therapist. A ring of cameras looks down at the therapist from above the screens. Each is angled so that while capturing the therapist moving within a portion of the space, neither screen is seen. This allows us to use a simpler and faster method of background segmentation that does not need to account for moving images. Between these two displays, the therapist can look ahead to see the client and behind to see the back of the virtual room the client looks into. The "therapist" appears in the foreground of the partially shared virtual space, as seen by the "client."

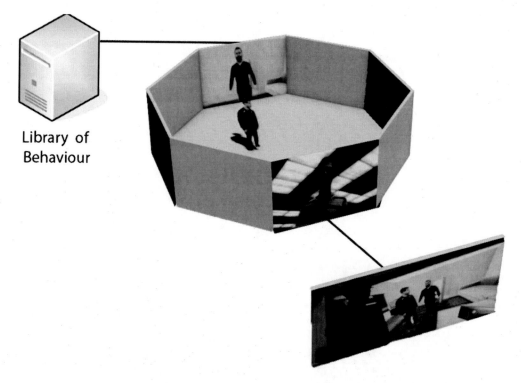

Figure 4. Diagram of the asymmetric telepresence system built for this demonstrator.

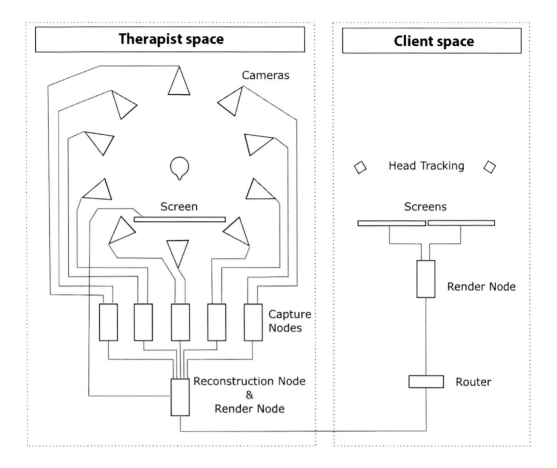

Figure 5. System architecture of this demonstrator.

DISCUSSION

An ideal VRET and teleVRET system would allow client and therapist to be immersed together within the simulation without restricting NVC and its contextualisation in any way. Currently this could nearly be supported for co-located VRET using large immersive display systems. All apart from one potentially significant problem, the need to ware 3D glasses that hide the eyes. TeleVRET is more challenging, not least as it requires easily deployable, unobtrusive, easily maintained, low cost solutions for the home end. We have presented a pragmatic approach to this that uses today's technologies in a novel way. It may be many years before technology is available that allows people in different places to seamlessly share each other's spaces. At present we must make a compromise between freedom of movement across the shared simulation against complexity of system and the issues of each complexity.

The demonstrator we have presented is meant to convey concept, pragmatic approach and issues rather than an ultimate system. It demonstrates a range of technologies put together in a pragmatic way. Both simpler and more advanced approaches could be derived from this. The most advanced would allow a full sharing of virtual context in which client and therapist could move around together. The current and simpler versions provide a partial sharing of context which imposes restrictions on movement within the shared space. However, the demonstrated and simpler approaches are far more deployable, affordable and maintainable given current technology. Our approach could be described as partial as it does not allow both parties to move across the full extent of the shared space. However, we felt it was more important to show a practical solution achievable today within people's homes. Until fully immersive stereo can be achieved without stereo, there has to be a compromise between freedom of movement across shared space and ability to determine eye gaze. We were able to support a "therapist" judging the gaze of a "client" and moving between the client and the "simulated threat" he gazed at, and gesturing to a less threatening part of the simulation.

This is not the first time that immersive projection technology has been used in VRET. However, we are unaware of a publication describing its use to support non-verbal togetherness of client and therapist or communication between them. This is not the first time that immersion and life sized avatars have been used to improve feelings of togetherness or contextualise non-verbal communication. For example, we have previously described our technology approach to faithfully communicating both appearance and attention by combining immersive displays with free viewpoint 3D video based avatars. We have also previously described its application to collaborative working. This is the first time its potential application to exposure therapy has been described.

Conclusion

The primary contribution of this paper is demonstrating how to support the kind of non-verbal communication used between client and therapist in exposure therapy, firstly when the stimuli, and secondly the other, appear through technology. The methodological contribution is using video based reconstruction in tele-therapy for the first time.

We have demonstrated how video-based reconstruction could potentially be used in virtual reality telepresence exposure therapy. This potential utility is in three parts:

- Making the client feel less alone within a threatening simulation. This is because it supports the range of non-verbal resources used to manage social distance and build feelings of trust and rapport.
- Helping the therapist to manage the client's anxiety and attention. Contextualisation of non-verbal communication is necessary for both.
- Potential utility in creation of visually realistic virtual humans, rapid enough to fit within a course of therapy. Conventional approaches take weeks of authoring.

We have sort to demonstrate concept, pragmatic approach and issues:

- The concept is that the therapist and client can be situated together within the simulation, to allow most of the range of non-verbal communication used by many therapists to manage a client's distance to threat.
- The approach is to combine 3D free-viewpoint video based reconstruction with large display systems and simulated environments.
- The issues are around compromise between complexity and deployability of the system.

Rather than demonstrating an approach that maximises the level of sharing of the simulation, we have demonstrated an asymmetric and pragmatic approach that is less complex, cheaper, more deployable and likely to better retain grounding in the real world. This asymmetry also allows us to demonstrate the impact of technology choices.

The potential impact of this approach is in reducing dropout rates of exposure therapy. This is important as dropout rates of 40% are not uncommon in resistant populations. Furthermore, as symptoms typically increase at the beginning of a course of exposure therapy, clients can dropout with negative health impacts. We argue that by allowing clients to both use virtual reality exposure therapy and work with a therapist at home, reduces the risk of non-attendance to therapy sessions. This could impact not only on success rate of treatment but in reducing costs to health providers through reducing missed appointments. We further argue that allowing the therapist and client to see each other and estimate what the other is looking at, would help to manage the grounding of the client in the safety of the present. This again has potential to reduce dropout rates by reducing the risk of retraumatisation and improving the relationship between client and therapist. While remote therapy can be done with conventional video conferencing and CGI avatars, the levels of non-verbal communication used within a clinical therapy session are not supported. Our approach has the fundamental properties to support them much better. Our demonstrator shows both the issues and the principles of the solution.

ACKNOWLEDGMENTS

The authors with to thank Charlie Moritz, Allan Barret from Pennine NHS Care Trust, Warren Mansell from University of Manchester and Linda Durbrow-Marshal from University of Salford for helping us understand the relationship and interaction between client and therapist and what needs to change in VRET to accommodate this. We also wish to thank the technology team at Salford that have helped in the past to develop the telepresence system, including Toby Duckworth, Carl Moore and Rob Aspin and John O'Hare.

REFERENCES

[1] Gonçalves R, Pedrozo AL, Coutinho ESF, Figueira I, Ventura P. Efficacy of virtual reality exposure therapy in the treatment of PTSD: a systematic review. PloS One 2012;7(12):e48469.

[2] Rothschild B. The body remembers casebook: Unifying methods and models in the treatment of trauma and PTSD. New York: WW Norton, 2003.

[3] Sanchez-Vives MV, Slater M. From presence to consciousness through virtual reality. Nature Rev Neurosci 2005;6(4):332-9.

[4] Roberts DJ, Fairchild AJ, Campion SP, O'Hare J, Moore CM, Aspin R, et al. Withyou: An experimental end-to-end telepresence system using video-based reconstruction. Selected topics in signal processing. IEEE J 2015;9(3):562-74.

[5] Bailenson JN, Blascovich J, Beall AC, Loomis JM. Equilibrium theory revisited: Mutual gaze and personal space in virtual environments. Presence 2001;10(6):583-98.

[6] Pertaub D-P, Slater M, Barker C. An experiment on public speaking anxiety in response to three different types of virtual audience. Presence 2002;11(1):68-78.

[7] Steed A, Roberts D, Schroeder R, Heldal I, eds. Interaction between users of immersion projection technology systems. HCI International 2005, 11th International Conference on Human Computer Inter-action, 2005.

[8] Roberts D, Wolff R, Rae J, Steed A, Aspin R, McIntyre M, et al. eds. Communicating eye-gaze across a distance: Comparing an eye-gaze enabled immersive collaborative virtual environment, aligned video confer-encing, and being together. Virtual reality conference, IEEE 2009.

[9] Gross M, Würmlin S, Naef M, Lamboray E, Spagno C, Kunz A, et al. eds. Blue-c: A spatially immersive display and 3D video portal for telepresence. ACM Transactions on Graphics (TOG), ACM 2003.

[10] Grau O, Hilton A, Kilner J, Miller G, Sargeant T, Starck J. A free-viewpoint video system for visualization of sport scenes. Motion Imaging J 2007;116(5-6):213-9.

[11] Waizenegger W, Feldmann I, Schreer O, eds. Real-time patch sweeping for high-quality depth estimation in 3D video conferencing applications. IS&T/SPIE Electronic Imaging, International Society for Optics and Photonics, 2011.

[12] Divorra O, Civit J, Zuo F, Belt H, Feldmann I, Chreer O, et al. Towards 3D-aware telepresence: Working on technologies behind the scene. Proc ACM CSCW: New Frontiers in Telepresence, 2010.

[13] Steed A, Tecchia F, Bergamasco M, Slater M, Steptoe W, Oyekoya W, et al. Beaming: an asymmetric telepresence system. IEEE Comput Graphics Appl 2012;6)10-7.

[14] Garcia A, Roberts D, Fernando T, Bar C, Wolff R, Dodiya J, et al. eds. A collaborative workspace architecture for strengthening collaboration among space scientists. Aerospace 2015: Institute of Electrical and Electronics Engineers, 2015.

[15] Roberts DJ, Garcia AS, Dodiya J, Wolff R, Fairchild AJ, Fernando T, editors. Collaborative telepresence workspaces for space operation and science. Virtual Reality (VR), IEEE 2015.

[16] Roberts DJ, Rae J, Duckworth TW, Moore CM, Aspin R. Estimating the gaze of a virtuality human. Visualization Comput Graphics IEEE Transactions 2013;19(4):681-90.

[17] Duckworth T, Roberts DJ. Parallel processing for real-time 3D reconstruction from video streams. J Real-Time Image Process 2014;9(3):427-45.

[18] Franco J-S, Boyer E, eds. Exact polyhedral visual hulls. British Machine Vision Conference (BMVC'03), 2003.

[19] Slater M, Sadagic A, Usoh M, Schroeder R. Small-group behavior in a virtual and real environment: A comparative study. Presence 2000;9(1):37-51.

[20] Roberts D, Wolff R, Otto O, Steed A. Constructing a Gazebo: Supporting teamwork in a tightly coupled, distributed task in virtual reality. Presence 2003; 12(6): 644-57.

Submitted: January 01, 2017. *Revised:* February 18, 2017. *Accepted:* February 27, 2017.

In: Alternative Medicine Research Yearbook 2017
Editor: Joav Merrick
ISBN: 978-1-53613-726-2
© 2018 Nova Science Publishers, Inc.

Chapter 44

REMOTE COMMUNICATION, EXAMINATION, AND TRAINING IN STROKE, PARKINSON'S, AND COPD CARE: WORK IN PROGRESS TESTING 3D CAMERA AND MOVEMENT RECOGNITION TECHNOLOGIES TOGETHER WITH NEW PATIENT-CENTERED ICT SERVICES

Martin Rydmark, MD, PhD, Jurgen Broeren, PhD, Jonas Jalminger, PhLic, Lars-Åke Johansson*, BSc, Mathias Johanson, PhD and Anna Ridderstolpe, MSc

The Sahlgrenska Academy, University of Gothenburg,
Sweden and Alkit Communications, Mölndal, Sweden

ABSTRACT

This paper describes strategy and work in progress. The combination of patient centered care where many care and nursing units are collaborating with focus on, and in concordance with the patient, the ability to project information focused on the patient's total situation and needs independent where the information was created, the ability to use sensor technology to collect a wide range of aspects of the individual's health situation, the ability to use sensor technology to assess movements both for assessment and intervention purposes, to keep the care and nursing process together through module based information services and a structured care plan containing goals, subgoals, defined activity types and a wide range of health status data involve great opportunities for patients having chronic diseases. This group of patients causes extensive resource consumption for society. Well-structured data and semantic definition of data is a key for the ability to communication between different types of multi-professionals actors with different background. New technology like a wide range of sensor types allows the possibly to catch large amounts of data both for assessment and intervention purposes in

---

* Correspondence: Lars-Åke Johansson, BSc, CEO, Alkit Communications, Sweden. E-mail: johansson@alkit.se.

a continuous way over time. This research group has worked on these issues for several years and some important milestones have been reached. From a chronic point of view three groups of patients are focused: stroke patients, COPD patients and patients with Parkinson's disease. Collaboration approaches, communication technology and adapted information services allow new ways to perform home based care. Integrated monitoring services of planned activities like motion activities using 3D sensors allows professionals and patient to in an exact way follow planned and executed motion activities which is of great importance to many patient needs.

Keywords: serious gaming, rehabilitation, patient centered care process

INTRODUCTION

A stroke or any other neurological disease/damage, like Parkinson's disease, has profound impacts on a person's life. The conditions are often life long and require continuous treatment and rehabilitation, as well as support for the activities of daily life. Communication and the performance of assessment activities as well as intervention activities are tiresome and it is a challenge to create a care situation with continuity for the patient in order to achieve results. Due to the low physical mobility and poor overall condition of these patients, traveling back and forth to doctors, nurses and rehabilitation centres can be exhausting tasks. Communication and interaction with relatives and friends is important but often become cumbersome and may also include long, strenuous trips. More developed forms of home based care, in combination with support from various kinds of professional units, has great potential for innovation, with information technology as an enabler.

Rehabilitation is essential in order to promote and maintain maximal level of recovery by pushing the bounds of physical, emotional and cognitive impairments. It is the foundation to enable full reintegration into the society and pursued occupation. Assessment is a key component in the care of the neurological patient and important for both diagnostic and therapeutic purposes in clinical practice. Patients often perceive their experiences of rehabilitation care as non-connected or non-coherent over time. Continuity and early start for the patient regarding rehabilitation is important to reach constructive results.

For COPD patients the need and importance of performing exercise is similar. Performing exercise can aim at keeping existing capabilities of the individual and to contribute to the avoidance of exacerbation.

For many patients home based care can be an effective way to manage rehabilitation without being required to visit the hospital or other care unit when training has to be performed on a more daily basis. Video mediated remote strategies can be used to support and encourage the individual in being systematic regarding exercises for assessment and intervention purposes. Monitoring can be performed both by observing the individual, using video, but new possibilities are developed by using monitoring services which in detail can monitor how different movements have been performed using worked out representation approaches of sub-movements of each exercise type. Monitoring and storage of detailed results of each exercise instance can be used for feedback, visualization and analysis both for the patient and for the professional.

Stroke, Parkinson's and COPD are examples of diagnoses where movements are of great importance both for assessment and intervention purposes and some exercises can be used for several diagnoses (1, 2), but many types of exercises should be quite different depending on function resources and disabilities of the individual. For example, for stroke patients the rehabilitation service should allow exercises where differences between left and right parts of the body functions are focused.

In earlier work we have documented experiences of developing telemedical tools, tools for support of rehabilitation activities, including, sensor monitoring, 3D visualization and haptics (3-5).

Experiences of this earlier work lead to the insight that:

1. Information services is needed to keep track of the whole set of relevant conditions and goals of the individual to be able to tailor personal plans which can encourage the individual to perform evidence based care activities
2. Be able to perform more of self-managed care activities
3. Make it possible to add new types of sensors and to use the values for them in a structured way so that analysis and conclusions can be drawn related to accepted health condition types and classifications
4. Being able to point out affordable packages of equipment and services which can be affordable to most patients

Games are assumed to stimulate and reward a person, and to make it fun and engaging to perform serious activities. The aim is often and to reach results in terms of keeping up to a structured and individual exercise plan. If exercise activities can be performed through games a lot of encouraging effects can be made. A lot of development work is being performed to create a workable representation structure so that a good representation of exercise types (and its sub-movements) can be associated with one or several game type alternatives. The user can choose between different games for the purpose to perform certain types of evidence based exercises important for the individual.

For Parkinson's disease we are developing tools for remote assessment of motor function. The underlying scientific procedure is called Movement Disorder Society-Sponsored Revision of the Unified Parkinson's Disease Rating Scale (MDS-UPDRS) (6): Process, Format, and Clinometric Testing Plan (7).

Recent work is focusing on monitoring, visualization and assessment of how the planned execution of the exercises really was executed. A specific monitoring part of the services has been developed that monitors and stores how every movement has been performed. This monitoring sub-service used the body representation and body posture to describe how every moment has been performed. Further, we have showed that depth cameras and other types of sensors are useful to follow movements (e.g., prescribed exercises) overtime and can provide a measure of rehabilitation progress in a wide range of remote health monitoring. The objective of this investigation is to develop tools and knowledge to identify if new technology matched with patient oriented services and new care procedures will lead to better rehabilitation in terms of both cost-effectiveness and quality for the individual. The overall goal is a multi-purpose, configurable ICT service platform supporting home based care highlighting the individual patient's specific needs.

Related to monitoring, one type of monitoring can consist of automatic collection of data concerning for example how an exercise has been performed, one other important type of monitoring is self-assessment by the individual him-/herself. For example, to COPD it is of interest to collect data about how tiresome the performance of a particular exercise was experienced by the patient. For this purpose the Borg Scale can be used (8). Borg scale assessments must be linked to the exercise performance and to the elements of the sub-movements.

METHODS

3D sensors like the Kinect and other types of motion sensors like Leap Motion (LM) sensors are markerless motion capture systems which offer an attractive solution for home based rehabilitation (9). Although marker based tracking systems are more accurate, with spatial and temporal correspondence that marker less system lacks, the Kinect and LM devices' precision are sufficient enough for rehabilitation purposes (10, 11). The devices' accessibility and low cost render them an advantageous solution for home based rehabilitation. The video game environment provided by the sensors has the potential to become powerful motivation tools for performing regularly rehabilitation exercises. Data from tracking the execution of the exercises in real time can be used for assessment of patients' physical status, which can trigger the need for interventions. Furthermore, captured data can be utilized to provide guidelines to the user, thereby optimizing the effect of the exercise.

A promising approach, explored in some depth for stroke and COPD patients, is to integrate support for video-mediated communication into the rehabilitation support platform, which includes both LM and Kinect devices. The Kinect device is in this situation used both as a body tracking device and a camera, while the LM device is used for tracking of hand and finger movements. A therapist/doctor can thereby remotely assist or instruct the home cared patient, in cases where direct physical interaction is not needed. Related to patients with Parkinson's disease their motor performance will remotely be registered with the Kinect and LM sensors connected to a laptop or tablet computer. During the fall of 2013 we implemented one of the MDS-UPDRS procedure, namely "alternating movements" and tested it interactively with doctors and patients. Here the patient is instructed to repeatedly approach and remove the thumb and the index finger from each others as much and as fast as possible. For COPD patients there are similar challenges. One of the challenges is the importance of keeping up training and movements and repeatedly meet health care professionals for plan change and updates and also to meet relatives and friends to avoid depressions etc.

For several diagnoses, the risk of falls is significant and structured fall prevention activities are hence important. Many of the tools and technologies explored for Stroke, Parkinson's and COPD patients can also be used for fall prevention. Assessment, risk calculation and intervention activities can be designed to reduce the risk of falls, which can be beneficial for many kinds of home care.

RESULTS

From our previous experiences of stroke rehabilitation, we know that 3D sensor based approaches like Kinect works well in an interactive situation in assessing kinematic information of motor function of the trunk, arm and leg. Now we have developed support for detection of hands and individual fingers. In most cases the interaction/instructions from the examiner can be pre-recorded ´machine´ standards. Our preliminary study of the MDS-UPDRS indicates a drawback, namely that some tests must comprise a physical interaction or/and an, at the actual moment, individualized instructions from the therapist/doctor. In these cases, we have to develop alternative procedures or omit these parts. An added value, as compared to the clinically performed MDS-UPDRS, is that with the ICT tools we can assess kinematic, numerical, values specifying the tested functions. Examples are frequency of tremor, time/velocity/acceleration/precision in movements.

Further findings are that one has to structure the entire set of subservices to really take advantage of the technology potentials which can be used in the home. Development and tests have shown that the following parts are suitable:

- A component that can, in depth, represent a particular exercise type often consisting of a set of sub-movements. This includes variation variables for individual adaptation (see below),
- A component that allows the therapist to define which movement a patient should perform, including definition of regime, intensity, repetition, sets and adapted movements. This is part of the individual-ization and needs and goals for the individual,
- A component that can monitor and store how the patient actually is performing each particular movement at each particular occasion,
- A component that can represent all relevant health condition types and classification related to a set of diagnoses, over all goals, subgoals, goal values of health condition types and relevant relationships to activity types.
- A video-mediated communication tool designed for communication between a professional and a patient where the professionals really can see how different movements are performed in each planned session,
- A component that can describe game types and how they are related to evidence based exercise types.
- A follow-up module where results of each training session are visualized related to goals. This includes more exact monitoring of how each movement is performed by each body part monitored in real time.

To capture, store and analyze large amounts of data about how all exercises have been performed, approached based on Big Data analytics will be used. When monitoring every training instance, e.g., for COPD patients, it can be very fruitful to monitor and store all training instances including sub-movements and also simultaneously monitor medical sensor data such as blood oxygen saturation levels when performing a particular exercise. Based on the collected data, assessments can be performed and conclusions can be drawn about how that patient should perform certain types of exercises, resulting in an updated care plan.

The following plot (Figure 1) shows the distance between the index finger and the thumb on the x-axis with respect to the relative speed between the two fingers on the y-axis. It shows an arc like concentration of dots which is what it typically looks like for a person without any disorder. The more a person is affected the more irregular and flat like are the plotted set of dots. This measure is an indicator of dysdiadochokinesia, the inability to perform rapid alternating movements, a sign of cerebellar and/or frontal cerebral lobe dysfunction. This kind of assessment can be accomplished by having the Leap Motion sensor attached to any home computer and having the patient simply surf to a web URL where the test can be carried out.

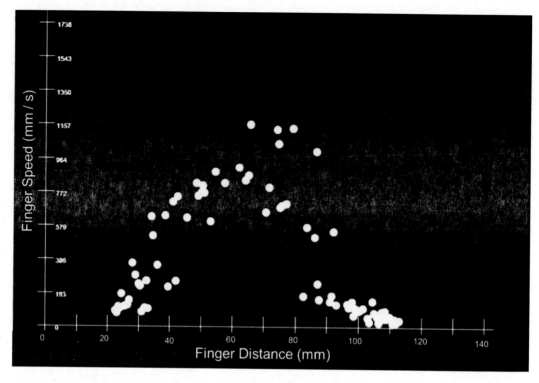

Figure 1. Shows the distance between the index finger and the thumb on the x-axis with respect to the relative speed between the two fingers on the y-axis.

DISCUSSION

The work is in a development and exploration phase but soon more systematic comparative studies will be performed in order to measure effects. Fundamentally, the health cooperation concept is cross organizational process where different care and nursing units and actors can participate. The focus is the patient's overall situation and needs. All actors involved in different types of activities can access selected information in a distributed unit, based on the roles that they have related to the individual. The individual and relatives are heavily involved in the performance of the activities.

The platform architecture has two main parts: the service level and the sensor level. A large number of new sensors have been developed and new sensors will appear. Sensors are typically interpreted in relation to an assessment scale, reflecting a specific health care aspect. The service level is concerned with the logical process oriented interpretation, computation, visualization and storage of data. This architecture will continuously allow new technology to be adapted and integrated. All activities are structured into activity types and activity instances. Some activities are aimed at assessment of conditions and some activities are aimed at interventions related to goals (that change with time). The health plan is an important concept keeping all assessment activities, goals and intervention activities together. The plan can contain prevention as well as assessment and intervention activities.

In this patient/person centric approach, specific e-services, involving sensor technology, can be used for development of other movement oriented health assessment and intervention activities, like prevention of fall injuries and training of motor functions aimed at restoring muscle performance or breathing capacity. The e-services will contain subparts like definition of particular movement oriented activity types, support of how a particular activity instance should be executed, recognition of results of a particular activity instance, reporting of results of an activity instance, video-mediated communication with professional and other actors for support of a particular activity instance. For many activity types, including stroke assessment and rehabilitation, COPD rehabilitation and fall prevention activities, whole body tracking is the most important. For the UPDRS assessment activities, high precision finger tracking is also required.

The tool set outlined here can also contain tool parts supporting powerful assessment scales like the ICF scale. (The International Classification of Functioning, Disability and Health) (WHO) for the purpose of make an extensive analysis and assessment of the situation of the individual. This support can also contain support for setting of goal values related to ICF and the selection of activities for the individual.

CONCLUSION

Sensors, computers, displays and communication technology is getting better and cheaper enabling advanced e-services for home based care, including real time support from remote medical professionals. The developed solutions can be both cost effective and provide high quality for the patients, due to improved continuity of care, less need for travel, and improved motivation to perform physical activities more often. This means that e-health services for home based care, including communication with healthcare professionals, have a great potential to overcome the challenge with increasing demands of care due to an aging population. The services must support both asynchronous communication of patient data, as well as real time interactions for monitoring, assessment, and support. Not only health care personnel, but also relatives and other informal cares need to be included in the communication. By designing an ICT platform supporting both synchronous and asynchronous communication of data from tracking devices and other sensors, including depth cameras and video cameras, a flexible and configurable multi-purpose care solution for home cared patients can be developed. Until such a sophisticated platform is realized, however, experiments with enabling technologies in specific patient groups must be performed, which is the objective of our present study.

ACKNOWLEDGMENTS

This project is partly supported by the Centre for Person-Centered Care at Gothenburg University and by VINNOVA, the Swedish Governmental Agency for Innovation Systems.

REFERENCES

[1] Broeren J, Jalminger J, Johansson L-Å, Rydmark M. A kinematic game for stroke upper arm motor rehabilitation- a person-centred approach. J Access Design All, 2013;4(2):81-93.

[2] Andersson M, Stridsman C, Ronmark E, Lindberg A, Emtner M. Physical activity and fatigue in chronic obstructive pulmonary disease - A population based study. Respir Med 2015;109:1048-57.

[3] Pareto L, Johansson B, Zeller S, Sunnerhagen KS, Rydmark M, Broeren J. VirtualTeleRehab: A case study. Stud Health Technol Inform 2011;169:676-80.

[4] Broeren J, Claesson L, Goude D, Rydmark M, Sunnerhagen KS. Virtualrehabilitation in an activity centre for community-dwelling persons with stroke. The possibilities of 3-dimensional computer games. Cerebrovasc Dis 2008;3(26):289-96.

[5] Goude, D, Björk, S, Rydmark, M. Game design in virtual reality systems for stroke rehabilitation. Stud Health Technol Inform 2007;125:146-8.

[6] Goetz CG, Tilley BC, Shaftman SR, Stebbins GT, Fahn S, Martinez-Martin P, et al. Movement disorder society-sponsored revision of the Unified Parkinson's Disease Rating Scale (MDS-UPDRS): Scale presentation and clinimetric testing results. Movement Disord 2008;23(15):2129-70.

[7] Goetz CG, Leurgans S, Hinson VK, Blasucci LM, Zimmerman J, Fan W, et al. Evaluating Parkinson's disease patients at home: Utility of self-videotaping for objective motor, dyskinesia, and ON–OFF assessments. Movement Disord 2008;23(10):1479-82.

[8] Borg G. Psychophysical bases of perceived exertion. Med Sci Sports Exercise 1982;14(5):377-81.

[9] Goetz CG, Stebbins GT, Wolff D, DeLeeuw W, Bronte-Stewart H, Elble R, et al. Testing objective measures of motor impairment in early Parkinson's disease: Feasibility study of an at-home testing device. Movement Disord 2009;24(4):551-6.

[10] Fernández-Baena A, Susín A, Lligadas X. Bio-mechanical validation of upper-body and lower-body joint movements of kinect motion capture data for rehabilitation treatments. Proc. of 4th International Conference on Intelligent Networking and Collabor-ative Systems (INCoS), 2012:656-61.

[11] Moeslund TB, Hilton A, Krüger V. A survey of advances in vision-based human motion capture and analysis. Comput Vision Image Understand 2006; 104(2-3):90-127.

Submitted: December 20, 2016. *Revised:* February 11, 2017. *Accepted:* February 15, 2017.

Chapter 45

VISUAL IMPAIRMENT SIMULATOR FOR AUDITING AND DESIGN

George W Stewart, BSc
and Rachel J McCrindle*, BSc, MSc, PhD, PGCED

Biomedical Engineering Section, School of Biological Sciences,
University of Reading, Whiteknights, Reading, Berkshire, United Kingdom

ABSTRACT

Individuals within the visually impaired community often have difficulty navigating environments due to the different ways in which they view the world, with even apparently simplistic locations frequently being challenging to traverse. It is therefore important when designing architecture or environments, to consider the differing perspectives of people with visual impairments in order to ensure that design outcomes are inclusive and accessible for all. Although there is documentation regarding guidance and procedures for design of inclusive spaces; architects, designers, and accessibility auditors often find it hard to empathize with visually impaired people. This project aims to make the process of inclusive design easier through the development of a mobile app, VISAD (Visual Impairment Simulator for Auditing and Design), which enables users to capture images or import CAD designs and apply image distortion techniques in order to replicate different visual impairments.

Keywords: visual impairments, inclusive design, mobile application

INTRODUCTION

There are two million people living with some form of visual impairment in the United Kingdom alone including 218,000 people registered with a severe visual impairment or

---

* Correspondence: Professor Rachel McCrindle, BSc, MSc, PhD, PGCED, Professor of Rehabilitation and Assistive Technologies, Biomedical Engineering Section, School of Biological Sciences, University of Reading, Whiteknights, Reading, Berkshire, RG6 6AY, United Kingdom. E-mail: r.j.mccrindle@reading.ac.uk.

blindness (1). The number of people living with a sight threatening eye condition has been predicted to rise over the next decade (2), and it is therefore becoming increasingly important to emphasize inclusive design when producing new products and services, ensuring that they are accessible to, and useable by, as many people as reasonably possible (3).

Architectural design is a key area of interest when it comes to design accessibility. This is especially true for public areas, which often have to abide by various codes of practice, and legislation. There is ample documentation available on the subject of disability access. However, although these documents provide useful information about specific individual architectural aspects, for example, the number of steps in a staircase before a landing, they do not provide the reader with a sense of what it is like to be afflicted with a visual impairment.

Simulating visual impairments is arguably the most effective way to educate uninformed designers about how a person with a visual impairment perceives their environment. Allowing architects to 'see' through the eyes of a visually impaired person makes it much easier for them to empathize with the difficulties individuals might face, and provides them with a greater understanding of the aspects of architecture which can be problematic for people who have visual impairments. Prior research, and subsequent software solutions, related to simulating visual impairments have been predominantly developed on non-mobile PC platforms. This project aims to improve upon, and enhance previous attempts at simulating visual impairments by developing a visual impairment simulator, VISAD, (Visual Impairment Simulator for Auditing and Design) that runs on mobile devices such as smartphones and tablets enabling both in the field simulation as well as the ability to import images at the design stage.

Early research in this field includes that of Fine and Rubin (4) who printed black circles on clear acetate film using an inkjet printer to replicate a scotoma. Test subjects read text through the acetate film, and changes in reading performance were documented. Recent research projects have become increasingly sophisticated with most involving the use of computer graphics and image processing techniques to distort images in various ways to replicate visual impairments. Research by Hogervorst and van Damme (5), involved the production of a software system that allowed the user to import an image and apply simulations of cataract, macular degeneration, glaucoma, retinopathy, myopia, and hyperopia to a 2D image in order to educate and give users an insight into the problems that people with visual impairment conditions faced. Their research provided an in depth perspective on the methods that could be applied to produce visual impairment simulations including a demonstration of how light glare can effect certain impairments. Banks and McCrindle (6) also investigated the use of image processing techniques to replicate the characteristics of common visual impairments in order to provide planners, designers, and architects with visual representations of how people with visual impairments viewed their environment, leading to increased accessibility in the built environment. This research also provided insight into the types of features that could be added to a proposed solution including the ability to import images from CAD files into the system. In addition to 2D image processing solutions, a research project carried out by Lewis, Shires, and Brown (7) involved the application of real time, simulated visual impairments to a virtual 3D environment. This project utilized the Microsoft XNA video game development framework, and allowed the user to walk around a 3D office environment while being afflicted with different visual impairments. This project showed how virtual and real time augmented reality can be used to enhance user experience.

The inclusive design toolkit, developed at Cambridge University, by the Engineering Design Centre (8), features a set of tools that aid creation of products and services that are inclusive or accessible. One such tool is the 'vision simulator' which provides examples of visual impairments applied to a selection of images. The simulator features a variety of impairments that can be applied with different levels of severity. It also includes a section which demonstrates impairments in relation to different objects, including a railway ticket machine and a household toaster. These simulations allow the user to alter certain design aspects of the objects (mainly the colours used) to show how small changes in some of their characteristics can alter their accessibility to someone with a visual impairment. The inclusive design toolkit demonstrates good practices regarding how the user interacts with the system, providing an easy-to-use and intuitive GUI (Graphical User Interface) that incorporates a number of visual impairment presets alongside slider controls for the severity of the impairment. The system also provides users with a short description of the visual impairment being simulated and the demographic of people affected by it.

'Project Rainbow' at the University of Reading (9), investigated the effects that colour and luminance have on the built environment, when viewed by a visually impaired person. The outcome of this project was a set of advisory papers and design guides which provide guidelines and rules to follow when designing the interiors of buildings. The overall aim was to create designs that were accessible to visually impaired people, but also acceptable for 'designers and fully sighted users of the building.'

ViaOpta (10) is one of the first apps to be developed for mobile platforms, however whilst providing a useful tool for simulation of visual impairments in real-time, it falls short with regards to its flexibility to import and export images and simulations.

METHODS

One aspect that many earlier research projects have in common, is that they were designed to run on non-mobile PC platforms. Whilst this approach has benefits such as increased processing power and greater standardization in terms of OS (operating system), mobile device platforms offer greater flexibility of use for architects, designers, and accessibility auditors during the inclusive design, and auditing phases of their projects. Additionally, whilst mobile devices have become incredibly popular over the past decade, for example, by 2013 there were 900 million devices running Google's Android OS (11), PC sales have declined substantially (12), and hence it is timely to develop for the mobile market.

The VISAD application has therefore been developed for use on smartphones or tablets, allowing the user to capture images with the device, and then create instantaneous visual impairment simulations of the images providing users with a better understanding of problems that might occur for people with visual impairments. The app handles all image capturing aspects of the simulation within the app, so that it is convenient to use. The app can produce a series of preset visual impairment simulations as well as allowing for customization of the various image processing effects that are used to take into account severity and layering of conditions. It also provides the user with information regarding specific impairments, including the demographic that is most commonly afflicted. Other key features implemented include the ability for the app to import image files from a range of sources as well as through the integrated camera and the facility to save and export generated image files for external use via their associated Google Drive cloud storage.

Implementation

VISAD has been developed for the android OS platform, implemented in the Java programming language, and created using the android SDK version of the Eclipse IDE (13) and android, version 5.1, API 21 – Lollipop, (14). The app operates with three main classes: the image capturing class; the GUI and user input class; and the graphics rendering class. The overall processing of the app occurs in three stages. First the user captures an image with the devices camera, or imports an existing image. The user then applies a combination of the different image effects, or selects an impairment preset. Finally, the user analyses the resultant image using the comparison tool, or the edge detection tool, and then exports the image by saving it to the devices memory.

Image capture

The image capturing aspect of the app is implemented using the android 'camera' class. This provides access to the device's camera in order to capture images or video, and to retrieve the relevant hardware information. It also provides handlers for setting camera specific features, such as autofocus, capture resolution, and white balance. Image capturing is implemented within the 'CameraPreview' class of the Java project, which provides a custom 'SurfaceView' component that is instantiated within the main class. This ultimately enables the devices camera output to be displayed on the screen.

Image processing

Image processing is used within the app to produce different effects that are then combined to one image to create a visual impairment simulation. This is implemented in the app through a custom 'SurfaceView' component which allows for custom drawing to the screen and to bitmaps. This class defines its own thread which it uses to update the custom drawing every 1/30 of a second. It receives parameters from the GUI thread and produces drawings or image manipulation based on the input. The majority of the work done within this class is produced using the Android 'Canvas' class, which allows for the creation of simple 2D geometry and custom brushes. All of the image processing effects have parameters that can be altered by the user. Each effect has its own menu which contains all of the GUI elements that control the parameters. These menus also include checkboxes which are used to toggle the relevant effect on or off. These parameters are passed to the rendering function and effect what is drawn in the frame. The different effects implemented include:

Brightness

Altering the brightness of the image involves altering the RGB values of the individual pixels in the image. This effect uses the Android Bitmap class to get the pixel value at an x/y coordinate in the image, the pixel's RGB values are then multiplied by a double value, and then set back in the image at the same x/y position. The double value is provided as a parameter and is a value in the range $0 < x < 2$, where any value less than 1 darkens the image, and any value greater than 1 lightens it. This effect, for example, is used in the macular degeneration simulation to increase the brightness of the image replicating the 'washing out' of colours that is commonly associated with this impairment.

Colour filter

The colour filter effect overlays a semi-transparent colour on top of the image. This effect has been implemented using the Android Canvas to draw a rectangle with the same x and y position, and the same width and height of the image. The RGBA values of this effect can be altered to change the colour and opacity of the filter. The colour filter effect is rendered to a separate transparent bitmap, which is then drawn after the image when the rendering loop draws a frame. By implementing this effect in this manner it is easier to implement the option to enable/disable the effect. This effect is implemented in the Cataract preset, where a brownish filter is required to simulate the effect of protein clumps in the lens, which cause cloudy vision.

Warping

The warping effect causes the contents of the objects portrayed in the image to be distorted. Areas of the image are stretched, pinched, and swirled which results in a warped image. This effect uses the JH Labs libraries to perform the warping, and the extent and size of the different kinds of warp can be altered to produce different outputs. There are three types of warping that the system can perform: pinching, twirling, and melting. The pinch warp causes the image to be warped towards the centre of the image; the swirl warp twists the image around its centre; and the melt warp applies random distortions to the image based on a turbulence value. These warping effects are created using forward pixels mapping, where the destination x, y coordinates are mapped using the source v, u coordinates. The warping effects are used during the simulation of Diabetic Retinopathy and Macular Degeneration to replicate the distortions that can occur as a result of these impairments.

Blur

The blur effect applies a Gaussian blur to the image. This effect uses the Android Renderscript API to process the image and produce the resultant blurred image. The Renderscript function for blurring allows parameters to be passed to it which control the extent of the blur. This effect can also produce a blur which fades in from the edges of the screen. A greyscale bitmask is produced that uses a radial gradient that fades from white to black from the centre of the image. This bitmask is then used to alpha composite the original image over the blurred image, leaving the centre more 'in focus' and the edges blurred. This effect can also be inverted, and positioned anywhere on the screen. This means that when inverted, the centre point of the effect is blurred, and it fades out towards the edge. The centre point can be positioned by the user by tapping on the screen, and the centre is set to the point of the tap. These specific aspects of the effect are used for the Myopia (nearsightedness) and Hyperopia (farsightedness) simulations. When selecting these simulations, the user is asked to tap on the screen the most distant point. This effect is used to simulate different aspects of blurred vision that are commonly related to Myopia, Hyperopia and Glaucoma. It can also be combined with the Double Vision effect to produce more severely blurred vision.

Vignette

The vignette effect adds a dark edge to the image which fades out toward the centre. This effect utilizes the Android Radial Gradient shader which allows the creation of a circular gradient which fades between multiple colours that are provided as parameters. In the case of this effect, the colours fade from a user defined colour at the edge (defaulted to black), to a completely transparent colour at the centre. The aperture of the effect is controlled by the radius parameter, which can be adjusted to increase or decrease the size of the vignette. This effect produces an image which has a border with a fading transparent centre. This effect is applied last in terms of layering the effect images onto the canvas and is used in the system to simulate the loss of peripheral vision, which is present in most of the impairments.

Double vision

The double vision effect overlays a semi-transparent copy of the image on top of itself at a slight offset. By using the bitmap variable type that is available in the standard Android API, a copy of the image is made. This copy is then drawn over the original image using the Android Canvas. When drawing the copy, a parameter is passed to the function that draws the bitmap which alters the opacity at which the image is drawn at, and also the x and y position is offset from the original. The image is set to 50% opacity and is offset from the top left corner by a few pixels by default. The results of this effect makes it harder for the viewer to focus on any of the fine detail in the image. This effect is used in the Cataract, Diabetic Retinopathy, and Macular Degeneration presets to replicate some of the blurriness and fuzziness that is associated with these impairments.

Spots

The spots effect draws randomly generated shapes with "fuzzy" edges onto different parts of the image. This effect is produced by initially creating a grid to which a cell is randomly selected, and then adjacent cells are procedurally, randomly selected. This results in a single randomly created shape. The shape is then drawn to fit the canvas using a radial gradient to provide a faded edge. The characteristics of this effect, including: length of shape; size of cells; number of individual shapes; and colour and opacity can all be changed by altering the input parameters. This effect is used mainly in the Diabetic Retinopathy and Macular Degeneration simulations to represent areas where vision is completely lost.

Colour blind

The colourblind effect changes the RGB pixel values of the image in order to simulate colourblindness. This effect can simulate the following types of colourblindness: Protanopia (red blind); Protanomaly (red weak); Deuteranopia (green blind); Deuteranomaly (green weak); Tritanopia (blue blind); Tritanomally (blue weak); Achromatopsia (monochromacy); and Achromatomaly (blue cone). The implementation of this effect is based on research by Wickline (15), which provides the predefined values by which the RGB channels are multiplied by, and then combined to form a pixel. For example, the manipulation values for the Red channel, for the Deuteranopia form of colour blindness are: *(0.625, 0.375, 0)*, which means that the red channel RGB components are calculated using: $R_c = (R_d * 0.625) + (G_d * 0375) + (B_d * 0)$.

Light source

The light source effect is used to simulate the problems that excessive illumination can have on a visually impaired person. This effect creates a pseudo light source and places it on the image. This results in the colours and definition of the image to become 'washed out' due to the increased brightness. The light source effect is produced by creating a radial gradient using the Android RadialGradient class, decreasing the alpha values of the pixels from the centre, and then overlaying a brightened version of the image on top of itself. Essentially it produces a copy of the original image, then increases its brightness and cuts a circular section out of it. The effect then overlays this cut out section on top of the original image in the same location, and fades the edges of the circle to give it a more natural look. This effect has two parameters that can change its properties, the intensity value changes how bright the light source appears to be, and the size which alters the diameter of the effect on the image. The user can add multiple light sources to the same image accessing this feature via the effects menu of the GUI.me.

RESULTS

The effects described above can be applied to the inputted image individually, or the user can choose from a selection of eight preset visual impairments from the presets menu. Each preset simulates a specific visual impairment as defined by the RNIB (16) or the NEI (17) by automatically applying a combination of the individual effects. In addition to this, the user can adjust the severity of the effects using a 'severity slider,' which ranges from mild to severe relating to the selected impairment as shown in Figure 1.

Cataract

Cataracts, defined as the 'clouding' of the lens section of the eye, causing a decrease in the overall quality of vision, are usually identified by the eye turning from its natural colour, to a yellow/brown colour. This yellow/brown colour is the colour of the protein clumps, and the afflicted person's vision is usually 'stained' with this colour as if looking through a coloured filter. The preset for this visual impairment applies a number of different effects to simulate both the clouding of the eye's lens, and also to replicate the loss of peripheral vision. The main effect that is applied is the colour filter effect. A yellow/brown colour filter is placed over the entire image to simulate the lens clouding. To replicate the loss of peripheral vision, a black vignette is placed on the image, and a radial blur is applied to blur the edges of the image in a circular fashion. The brightness of the image is also decreased slightly to account for the lower amount of light able to pass through the lens (Figure 2).

Glaucoma

Glaucoma is a visual impairment that mainly effects the peripheral vision and if left untreated can lead to blindness. The most predominant effect that this preset applies to the image is the vignette effect. This effect is used to create a large black ring around the edges of the image, which is used to replicate a loss of peripheral vision. Also involved in this preset is a slight increase in brightness. This is used in conjunction with a moderate application of blur to simulate the mistiness and 'washed out' colour that are associated with glaucoma symptoms (Figure 3).

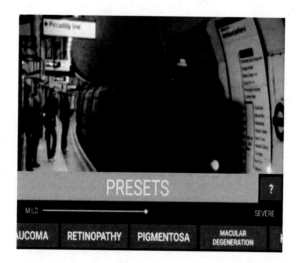

Figure 1. Presets menu.

Retinopathy

Retinopathy affects people who suffer from diabetes. It is caused by microvascular changes in the retina section of the eye, and results in blurred and patchy vision, which ultimately leads to blindness. People who suffer from Retinopathy have areas of their vision which don't function correctly, this causes spots of darkness that are surrounded by blurriness. The preset which is used to simulate Retinopathy makes use of the 'Spots' effect to recreate the patchy areas of vision loss that are associated with this impairment. This is combined with a slight blur and warp effect to simulate the distortion of the vision that occurs around the areas of vision loss. When the severity of this preset is increased to +75%, a vignette is also applied to demonstrate the loss of peripheral vision that occurs in the later stages of this impairments progression (Figure 4).

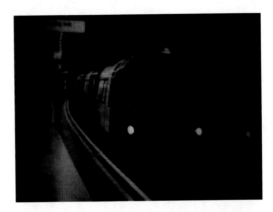

Figure 2. Cataract preset.

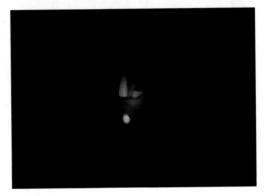

Figure 3. Glaucoma preset.

Pigmentosa

Pigmentosa is an inherited condition which causes severe tunnel vision. It is caused by an inflammation of the retina, and the symptoms can be present from birth. This impairment also causes a decrease in the ability to see in dark conditions, and it is possible for the central vision to also be affected. The preset for this impairment applies similar effects to the Glaucoma preset. The most apparent effect that is used for retinopathy is the vignette effect, which is applied to recreate the tunnel vision symptom that is common with this impairment. A dark grey colour filter is also applied to the image to simulate the decreased vision in low light conditions. The final effect that this preset applies a moderate blur, which is used to replicate the general loss in the quality of vision, which is related to the inflamed retina (see Figure 5).

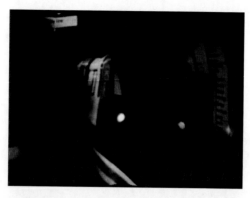

Figure 4. Retinopathy preset.

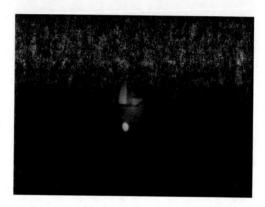

Figure 5. Pigmentosa preset.

Macular degeneration

Macular Degeneration causes issues with the central vision of the eye such that the eye is unable to focus on anything and there is no sharpness or detail in the vision. This impairment is particularly common is older people, and is caused by a build-up of cell debris in the macular section of the retina, which in turn causes scarring and damage. The Macular Degeneration preset applies a special version of the 'Spots' effect to create an irregular, fuzzy, grey coloured circle at the centre of the input image. This is applied to simulate loss of central vision, and the diameter of the circle is increased relative to the severity of the preset. Also applied with this preset, is a blur effect which also increase with the severity, although to a lesser degree of intensity (see Figure 6).

Hyperopia and myopia

Hyperopia and Myopia are both classified as refractive errors of the eye. Hyperopia is commonly known as farsightedness, and myopia is known as nearsightedness. Refractive errors are caused by a combination of factors relating to the size and shape of the various components that make up the eye. The size of the eyeball, deterioration of the lens shape, and alterations of the cornea, can all effect the way that the light that enters they eye can focus on the retina. If the light is incorrectly focused, objects closer or further from the eye appear to be blurry. The preset for hyperopia (see Figure 7) uses the radial blur effect to create an image where object closer to the viewer are out of focus, but ones further away are in focus. This is done by prompting the user to select the point in the image which is of the furthest distance. This is treated as the center point for the radial blur, and the radius of the focused area is adjusted based on the severity of the preset. For the Myopia preset (Figure 8), the same process is used, however the radial blur effect is inverted. This means that the most distant point selected in the image is blurred, and out of focus, and the areas that are closer to the viewer are in focus.

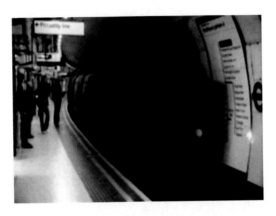

Figure 6. Macular degeneration preset.

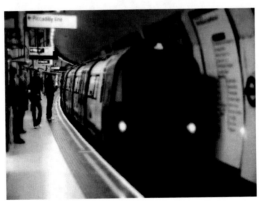

Figure 7. Hyperopia preset.

Colour blindness

Colour blindness, also known as colour vision deficiency, is used to describe the different vision impairments that effect the way in which a person perceives colour. There are eight different types of colourblindness presets that can be simulated by the system, these are: Protanopia (red blind); protanomaly (red weak); deuteranopia (green blind); deuteranomaly (green weak); tritanopia (blue blind); tritanomally (blue weak); achromatopsia (monochromacy); and achromatomaly (blue cone). These are applied with the colour-blindness effect, which works by multiplying the RGB pixels by manipulation values (see Figure 9).

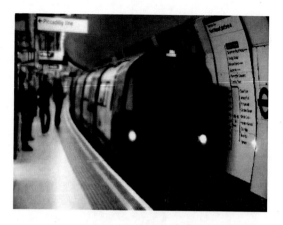

Figure 8. Myopia preset.

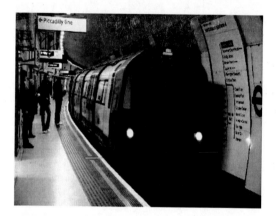

Figure 9. Colour blindness preset.

TOOLS

The analysis components of the app are used to demonstrate the comparisons between the original, unedited image and the newly created image, with the simulation effects applied to it. There are two tools that can be used for analysis: the canny edge detection tool and the side by side comparison tool. These provide the user with an easy way to contrast the differences between how their image appears through the eyes of impaired and unimpaired individuals.

Edge detection

The edge detection tool highlights any perceived edges in the image as green lines (see Figure 10). This can be used to contrast the difference that the visual impairment simulations have on the algorithms ability to detect edges, compared to the original. This feature is implemented using the JHLabs edge detection function which takes in a bitmap image as a parameter, and returns a new image containing the edge detection output. This function applies a 'Canny' edge detection algorithm to the image. The Canny edge detection works in multiple stages, and is fairly complex, however the overall process involves applying a Gaussian blur to the image, then observing the intensity gradients. After this, a non-maximum suppression is applied to reduce the likelihood of false detection, and then a double threshold is applied to examine possible edges. The final step is to suppress the discovered edges that are insignificant, and not connected to the larger edges.

Comparison

The second analysis feature is the comparison tool feature of the app. This provides a side by side comparison of the original image, and the image that has been distorted by the system. This tool places a slider on the screen which overlays the original image on the left side of the slider and the edited version of the image on the right side. The slider can be moved back and forth by the user to display different areas of both the edited, and original images (see Figure 11).

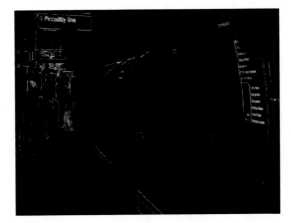

Figure 10. Edge detection tool.

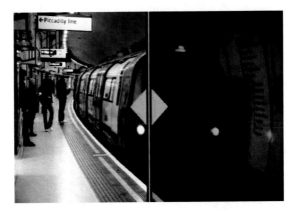

Figure 11. Comparison tool.

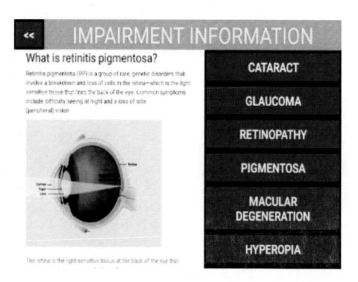

Figure 12. Information tool.

Importing and exporting

The tools section of the app focuses on the more basic aspects of functionality that are expected with any software package including saving and loading options. The user can choose to import an image from the devices file system, instead of capturing their own. The import image tool uses the standard Android 'Image Open Intent', which provides a premade activity that the app can switch to that allows the user to browse images easily. When the user selects an image file, the intent returns the user to the app with the image URI. This URI is then used to copy the image to the image variable used by the app to apply distortions to. Once the user has finished simulating visual impairments with the image, they have the option to export the output as an image file and save it to the device's local storage. Once saved, the images can be used in other applications, or included in documents, or printed. Saving is carried out using the android 'file' object, which works similarly to the standard Java object. The image is saved to a folder within the file system that is created especially for the app which is created when the app is first executed.

Image capturing

While in the "image capture" mode, the app uses the screen to relay the input from the camera, which allows it to be used as a viewfinder. This feature is common among camera applications, and allows the user to capture images more easily. The capture button is placed on the left hand side of the screen, and is used to both capture images, and clear them. When an image has been captured, and the user wants to get rid of it to capture another, they press the capture button again. This deletes the image from memory, and returns the screen to the camera output for capturing.

Information

The app features an information section, which is accessed via the question mark button on the presets menu. This section is dedicated to providing information about the use of the app, and contains specific information about each of the individual impairments that are supported. This information is sourced from the National Eye Institute (17) website, and displays details about the relevant eye disease such as what causes it, and who it affects. This feature is implemented using the android 'WebView' which is a view that displays web pages, and basically allows for a stripped down web browser to be added as a UI element within the app. The information section has a menu of buttons related to the visual impairments that are supported by the app. These buttons are linked to the WebView, and direct it to the relevant web page on the NEI website. This feature was added to allow the user to quickly and easily browse through relevant information about visual impairments without having to leave the app.

DISCUSSION

Evaluations of the effectiveness of the VISAD app, its features and functionality and the accuracy of its simulations was undertaken through comparisons with previous work, a focus group with potential student users, and an interview with a visual impairment expert. With regards to assessing accuracy of the simulated images there is no exact way of knowing whether the actual visual impairment representation is correct, a problem compounded by the visual impairments simulated by the app also have varying degrees of severity. The most plausible way of ensuring the validity of the simulation images, was thus to compare them to other simulations created during past research in this field (8), as well as to the symptom definitions created by official visual impairment organisations, such as the National Eye Institute (17) and the Royal National Institute of Blind People (16). As part of this validation a full comparison of images was undertaken of the VISAD images and those produced by the Cambridge Inclusive Design Toolkit Simulator (8), one example of which is shown in Figure 13. From the images, little difference is evident between the two simulations, both involve rendering a large grey mass in the centre of the image, and include a slight blur to the rest of the image. The only slight difference between the two is that the simulation produced by the VISAD app applies slightly more blurred than the Inclusive Design Toolkit version, from this and the other comparisons we were able to conclude that VISAD simulations were accurate.

During the later stages of the implementation, the app was demonstrated to a focus group of 5 potential student users for testing and feedback purposes. This session involved providing the participants with 'hands on' experience with the app allowing them to test the various features of the app. Afterwards the group was interviewed about their impressions of the app, and what they liked and disliked about it. Overall feedback was very positive with all members of the focus group finding it interesting and easy to use after minimal training on how to use the interface. Some minor errors in the UI were identified, further visual impairment presets were requested and the loading times for some of the more complex effects, such as the edge detection, was considered to be too long.

A meeting and demonstration of the app also took place with Dr. Geoffrey Cook, an expert in the field of accessible design and lighting in regards to the built environment. Overall he was very impressed by the app, and stated that 'he knew of professionals that would be very interested in using the app'. He also expressed interest in the possibility of including further simulated effects of lighting in the app; and how different lighting levels would affect the images.

Overall it can be concluded that this project has created a visual impairment simulator, VISAD (visual impairment simulator for auditing and design), that runs on mobile devices and provides image capture, image processing and image export of visual impairment simulations. Allowing architects, designers, and accessibility auditors to visualize their projects from the perspectives of visually impaired people is essential in providing accessible and inclusive design. The overall benefits of utilizing a mobile platform for visual impairment simulation are that it makes the process more intuitive, more efficient, more educational and more impactful as immediate results can be seen. Using a mobile device allows simulations to be done in situ, with near instant results. This provides a much more fluid and convenient process compared with the previous desktop based systems, which lack integration of image capturing and processing aspects.

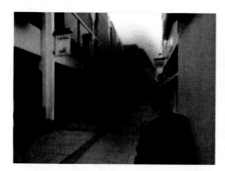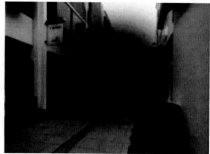

Figure 13. Macular degeneration comparison Cambridge (left) and VISAD (right).

The comparison analysis that was carried out between the simulated images created by the app, and those created in earlier research projects and on visual impairment sites for professional organisations, show that the app can create very similar results. VISAD's simulations for the visual impairment presets were of the same quality, or in some cases better than the ones used for comparison. Discussions with experts and potential users of the app have been highly positive and there is strong interest in using VISAD as part of the University of Reading's Breaking down Barriers project which is embedding inclusive design into teaching and learning in built environment professional education and beyond and in inclusive design workshops run by the Department of Typography and Graphic Communication.

Due to the lower processing power of mobile devices compared to non-mobile devices, optimi-zation is an area of consideration regarding further work on this project. Currently the system is limited to still images due to the processing time of the effects being too long for video, however, real time video processing is an additional feature that will be examined for the future.

An increased focus on the effects of lighting on visual impairments will also be included in future work resulting in increased complexity, sensitivity and accuracy of the 'Light

Source' feature. There is also the potential to incorporate this project into a virtual/augmented reality simulation, which would allow the user to experience the impairments first hand in a more immersive environment. An IOS version of the app is also being considered.

REFERENCES

[1] RNIB, Access Economics. Future sight loss UK (1): The economic impact of partial sight and blindness in the UK adult population, 2009. Accessed 2017 Feb 08. URL: http://www.rnib.org.uk/sites/default/files/FSUK_Report.pdf.

[2] Minassian D, Reidy A. Future sight loss UK (2): An epidemiological and economic model for sight loss in the decade 2010-2020: Executive summary, RNIB Report, 2009. Accessed 2017 Feb 08. URL: https://www.rnib.org.uk/sites/default/files/FSUK_Summary_2.pdf.

[3] Clarkson PJ, Coleman R. History of inclusive design in the UK. Appl Ergonomics 2015;46:235-47.

[4] Fine E, Rubin G. The effect of simulated cataract on reading with normal vision and simulated central Scotoma. Vision Res 1999;39:4274-85.

[5] Hogervorst M, van Damme W. Visualizing visual impairments. Gerontechnol 2006;5(4):208-21.

[6] Banks D, McCrindle RJ. Visual eye disease simulator. Proc. 7th ICDVRAT (International Conference on Disability, Virtual Reality and Associated Technology), Maia, Portugal, 2008:167-74.

[7] Lewis J, Shires L, Brown DJ. Development of a visual impairment simulator using the Microsoft XNA Framework. Proc. 9th ICDVRAT (International Conference on Disability, Virtual Reality and Associated Technology), Laval, France, 2012:167-74.

[8] EDC (Engineering and Design Centre), Inclusive Design Kit, University of Cambridge, 2016. Accessed 2017 Feb 08. URL: http://www.inclusivedesigntoolkit.com/betterdesign2/simsoftware/simsoftware.html.

[9] Cook GK, Bright K. Project Rainbow: a research project to provide colour and contrast design guidance for internal built environments. Occasional Papers, 57. Technical Report. Ascot, UK: Chartered Institute Building, 1999:1-20.

[10] ViaOpta, Visual Impairment Simulator, 2016. Accessed 2017 Feb 08. URL: http://viaopta-apps.com/ViaOpta Simulator.html#.

[11] Business Insider. Google: there are 900 million android devices activated, 2013. Accessed 2017 Feb 08. URL: http://www.businessinsider.com/900-million-android-devices-in-2013-2013-5?IR=T.

[12] Gartner. PC shipments decline globally in Q1. Gartner, 2016. Accessed 2017 Feb 08. URL: http://www.bgr. in/news/pc-shipments-decline-globally-in-q1-2016-gartner/

[13] Google Android. Eclipse Android Development Tools, 2014. Accessed 2017 Feb 08. URL: http://developer. android.com/sdk/installing/installing-adt.html.

[14] Google Android. Android version 5.0 Lollipop, 2014. Accessed 2017 Feb 08. URL: http://www.android.com/versions/lollipop-5-0/.

[15] Wickline M. Colorblind Web Page Filter, 2008. Accessed 2017 Feb 08. URL: http://colorfilter.wickline .org/.

[16] RNIB. Eye Conditions 2017. Accessed on 2017 February 08. URL: https://www.rnib.org.uk/eye-health/ eye-conditions

[17] NEI, National Eye Institute. Eye Condition Topics, 2017. Accessed 2017, Feb 08. URL: https://nei.nih.gov /health.

Submitted: December 22, 2016. *Revised:* February 11, 2017. *Accepted:* February 16, 2017.

In: Alternative Medicine Research Yearbook 2017
Editor: Joav Merrick
ISBN: 978-1-53613-726-2
© 2018 Nova Science Publishers, Inc.

Chapter 46

AUTHENTICATING THE SUBJECTIVE: A NATURALISTIC CASE STUDY OF A HIGH-USABILITY ELECTRONIC HEALTH RECORD FOR VIRTUAL REALITY THERAPEUTICS

Henry J Moller and Lee Saynor*

Knowledge Media Design, Music and Health Research Collaboratory,
Faculties of Medicine, University of Toronto, Toronto,
Digital Futures Initiative, OCAD University,
Toronto and PRAXIS Holistic Health, Toronto, Canada

ABSTRACT

Using data from our established Technology-Enhanced Multimodal Meditation (TEMM) stress-reduction program employing the electronic health record system Wellpad, we illustrate the value of developing a qualitative data-analysis approach to inform clinical practice in the rapidly emerging field of immersive therapeutics. In examining "rich data" of a naturalistic 50-patient TEMM cohort, point out that as with design of VR therapeutics, there is a highly salient role for immersive diagnostics, which ultimately relates to consumer satisfaction, both for patient and health-care practitioner.

Keywords: electronic health records, qualitative research, virtual reality diagnostics

---

* Correspondence: Henry J Moller, Faculties of Medicine, Knowledge Media Design, Music and Health Research Collaboratory, University of Toronto, Toronto, Canada, Digital Futures Initiative, OCAD University Richmond St, Toronto, Canada, PRAXIS Holistic Health, Carlaw Ave, Toronto, Canada. E-mail: drmoller@praxisholistic.ca

INTRODUCTION

Following a rocky era over the past quarter century that industry pioneers might refer to as a multi-industry synergistic vision quest, we are now entering a new era of virtual reality (VR) impact on health and wellness (1). Overlapping with an industrialization of medicine and psychology into models embracing operational protocols, patient management models, and treatment guidelines, a need and opportunity currently exists for setting gold standards to inform clinical practice. In particular for evaluations exploring novel immersive or virtual reality therapy or rehabilitation tools, rather than understanding a patient's experience in terms of rote rating questionnaires, getting at the ultimate experience meaning of wellness and illness is called for at this juncture to optimize care planning.

Information systems are a key success factor for medical research and healthcare. Currently, most of these systems apply heterogeneous and proprietary data models, which impede data exchange and integrated data analysis for scientific purposes (2). In this sense, we note the general problem for reporting of data related to VR mental health treatment and rehabilitation that a *lingua franca* of clinically relevant self-state descriptions and data-capturing that cuts across the wide variety of conditions and circumstances seen and treated in a psychiatry or psychology setting, whether these be anxiety, mood, trauma or organic brain disorders, including often co-occurring complex medical comorbidities such as disturbances of musculoskeletal or sleep health. As we will discuss, this is of essence in being able to inform naturally occurring clinical realities beyond more artificially controlled academic or pre-clinical research studies.

What seems to be important is to arrive at a consensus regarding what "wellness" or "wellbeing" entail on a symptomatic/experiential level in a manner that cuts across rote DSM psychiatric classification categories. This is necessary due to the inherent heterogeneity of patients seeking wellness care. Additionally, finding mechanisms to creatively incentivize patients to offer up rich authentic data, whether though pre- and intra-session data (psychophysiological, gamified self-report, video capture, etc.) makes for a more holistic evaluation potential that should be more fully entertained by clinicians and researchers. There is also the *Zeitgeist* of the "personalized medicine" era to consider. Personalized medicine research ie implies that on a clinical every individual patient is an individual "experiment", with unique circumstances and issues, bearing "rich/thick data", putting the VR industry in pole position to deliver authenticity beyond numbers.

Employing quantitative and qualitative considerations, we now report on our group's experience with ongoing development of Wellpad, an inclusively designed (3, 4) and gamified (5) diagnostic electronic health record (EHR) system intended to optimize the synergistic data flow in a busy operational medical setting.

METHODS

Drawing from a clinical database query of over 450 patients, a sample of 50 patients was identified who had completed between 7 and 15 scheduled TEMM sessions at the PRAXIS Holistic Health and Rosedale Wellness Centre relaxation hubs in Toronto, Canada before

February 14, 2016. These consenting participants resided within the Greater Toronto Area (GTA), the furthest participant being located an hour away from the health centres.

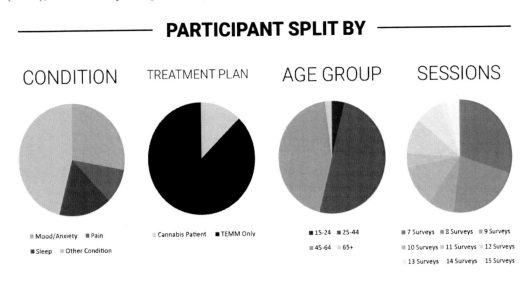

Figure 1. Various proportional classifications of the 50-patient sample.

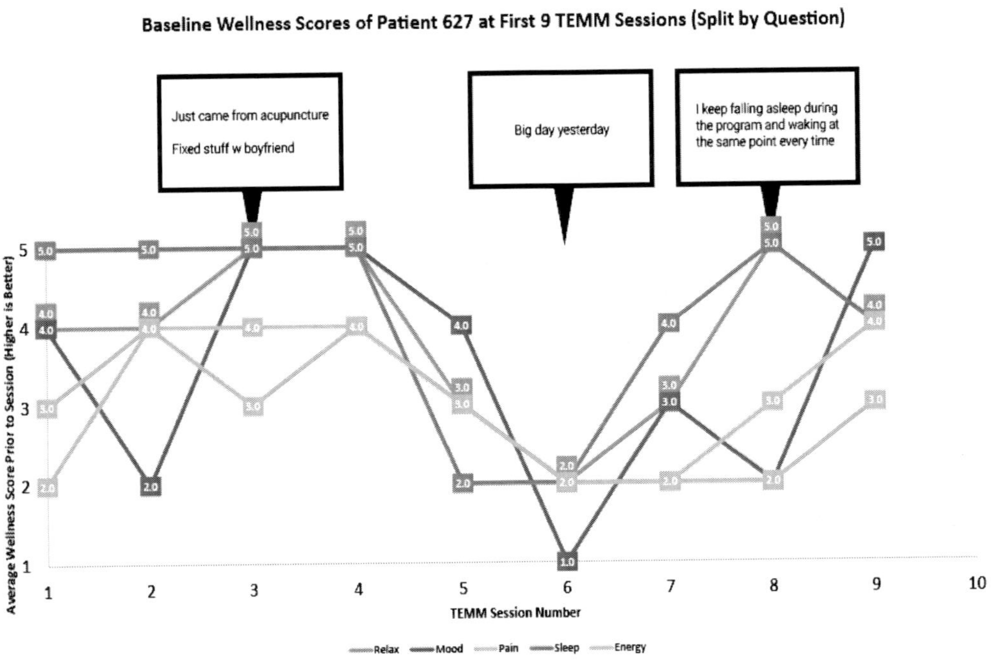

Figure 2. One stress/anxiety patient's wellbeing over time while undergoing TEMM treatment. The plunge before the participant's 6th session suggests the patient may need extra attention.

Easy data collection protocol

Keeping a simple electronic health record of participants, VR practitioners can create personalized wellbeing experiences responsive to the needs and motivations of the modern leisure-seeking consumer. Knowing the balance of demographics like condition, current treatments, age, and length of treatment among a user sample (see Figure 1) is a key driver for praxis by feeding real world results back into the development of more effective new immersive therapeutic programs.

After participant suitability for TEMM is authenticated and she completes a brief intake survey, baseline 1-5 Likert scores for relaxation, pain, sleep quality, and energy in recent times are captured by the inclusively designed iPad-based Wellpad EHR system. Popular medically supervised meditation programs like "Creative problem solving" and "Balancing your moods" are delivered to the patient via non-invasive synthetically packaged leisure-state meditation experiences with relaxing visual, auditory and haptic channels in chair and bed delivery systems (6).

Holistic diagnostic progress tracking

Progress tracking with Wellpad at PRAXIS Holistic Health and Rosedale Wellness Centre currently focuses on a longitudinal visualization of wellbeing captured before each weekly TEMM session. The patient's 1-5 score for each attribute in recent time and potentially significant patient comment/context are plotted visually (see Figure 2) and reviewed with physician during the consultation. The utility of this narrative cue for inclusively exploring the experience user's health over time has been demonstrated before (7, 8) and will be expanded upon by adding followup surveys directly after the treatment session.

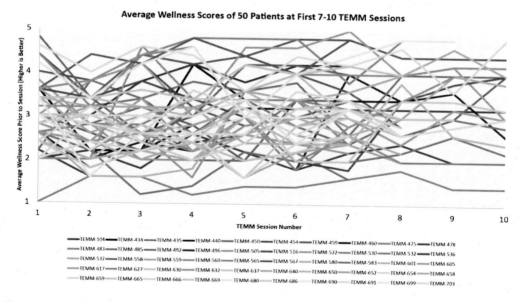

Figure 3. 50-patient spectrum of average patient wellbeing over time may reveal broader trends.

The five attribute scores for each survey submission are averaged into a general Wellness Score, which is readily stacked with peers to identify broader trends. For instance, Figure 3 shows a maximalist 50-patient spectrum of self-reported wellbeing over time, which can also be averaged across the group (see Figure 4) or split by question average (see Figure 5) to check for trends among disparate patients or very specific groups.

Exploring the future potential of rich data

While we believe in evidence-based approaches, evidence does not necessarily consist of structured data points. In VR research, we believe that the life experiences need to be accounted for to derive optimal knowledge. This is particularly true when studying mental health and the complexity of changes in consciousness common in stress and anxiety patients.

This notion feeds into the multimodal nature of the immersive therapies used at our health centre and others endeavouring immersive/VR therapies; we advocate for a further future promotion of multimodal diagnostic data-gathering, which has already been embraced for some time by VR researchers in the form of psychophysiologic (EEG, galvanic skin conductance, EKG heart rate variability, polysomnography etc.) monitoring, eye-movement or blink tracking, motion capture and psychomotor performance tracking inherent to gamified therapeutics. Now that the mobile technology industry is experiencing a commercial proliferation of health and wellness devices and aps (e.g., smart watches, fitness- and brainwave-trackers), we are learning about consumer acceptance, tastes and preferences of what aspects of their daily experiences we can authentically capture to better understand patient wellbeing.

To this end, the actual nascent VR health/wellness therapeutics industry is now at a crossroads of ideally informing the technology market of what is useful and helpful for medical or mental health care, as opposed to the tech sector driving the conversation on a top-down level without the expertise or knowledge of what an individual with an illness or disability actually needs to recover or maintain their wellbeing. The often severe challenges that hospitals, clinics, clinicians and patients have encountered with the vast array of existing EMR's underscores this challenge and opportunity for the VRT community.

How to make an abundance of complex data less overwhelming is a key question in product evaluation for electronic health records. Usability is most certainly one part of the answer, as we have previously argued (7, 8), and here it must be explicitly stated that the "user" is the patient and clinician, and not the "man-behind-the-curtain" digital designer. This means that, as with VR therapeutics, no matter how innovative or aesthetically appealing a VR program may be, without ongoing, often laborious iterative upgrades in arriving at a better and better fit between user needs/preferences and the evaluation tool, it quickly is threatened with obsolescence.

In general, our observation is that patients left with an open invitation to offer up qualitative supplementary data (e.g., unique psychosocial life situations that may significantly affect rote symptom report at the time of therapeutic engagement) will not frequently volunteer this unless specifically monitored or prompted, meaning that much more creativity is needed on behalf of design teams to elicit meaningful qualitative data to inform about user experience.

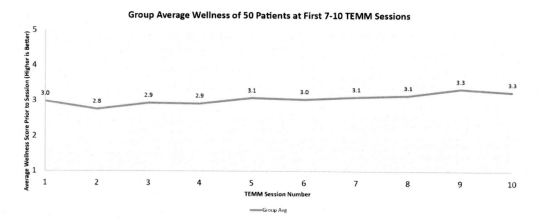

Figure 4. 50-patient trend of average patient wellbeing over time shows a modest net increase.

On a neuroeconomics level, the "low-risk" path of least resistance of putting in minimum effort required to obtain "reward" of completing the therapeutic endeavour likely remains the health-care consumer's most frequent choice on the utility curve (9). For this reason we have previously advocated for inclusive design usability approaches in VR therapeutics that, not just because making things easier to understand or enjoyable for a disabled individual is often the morally right thing to do on a public health level, but also because fun, "easy-to-use" and inherently engaging health-care consumer products are also those with the greatest market potential.

Evidently, most battle-weary clinicians in the mental health or physical medicine rehabilitation trenches would rather look at an easy-to-grasp Gestalt that captures the salient features of clinical progress, compared to "business as usual" standards in paper and/or electronic diagnostics. These currently consist of either manually combing through clinical notes or unorganized spreadsheet of data that is not organized into an experience readily digested by the clinician. In fact, it is puzzling that data visualization optimization has not been a focus of intense research and development by electronic health record vendors (10).

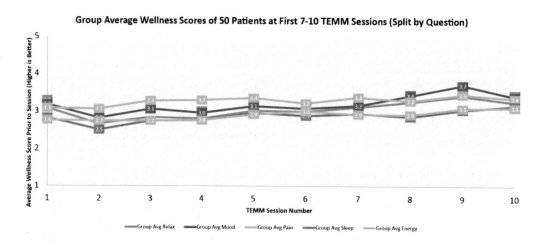

Figure 5. 50-patient wellbeing trend split by question.

RESULTS AND DISCUSSION

In closing, when we introduced the imperative of usability and gold standards in EHR's related to VR/immersive diagnostics based on a generalized health-care culture of managed structural adjustment of patient experiences, we did not intend to imply that there can be no further room for creativity from designer/implementer or clinician.

On a public health level, once patients are assessed on high volume, rapid-fire level in a clinical setting that is more difficult to control than a research environment, the ability to efficiently track salient patient progress patterns is extremely valuable. Rather than viewing clinicians and researchers embracing VR as participating in an increasingly mechanistic or inhumane paradigm, we demonstrate that with the use of inclusive and iterative design processes the entire care flow from demographic data acquisition to symptom elucidation to momentary and longitudinal self-state reports can be optimized and even *authenticated*. With this last term, we refer to the existential Heideggerian notion of *being-in-the-world authenticity* (11) that is also of interest in leisure/recreation experience industries like tourism and hospitality. Here, by accommodating to understandings of consumer tastes, preferences as well as ease of understanding and usability, relevant data can be more readily volunteered in a manner that seems less extractive and more akin to a playful *flow-state,* which we would argue is more akin to our natural state of consciousness (12).

While we do not necessarily suggest that our conceptual digital model of the busy clinician's critical opening line of "how are you doing?" is all-encompassing or negates others, we point to its popularity and acceptance rate in our clinic population amongst frequently quite disabled patients, and our experience in employing it clinically on a routine basis over the past year. Wellpad is driven by a pragmatic need to triage patient care plans (e.g., specialist referrals or medication changes based on specific symptom clusters); alongside this, by a desire to transition the "interview" into a humanized discussion to make the patient/consumer feel understood, while making the experience less burdensome and enjoyable for clinicians.

We continue to support and be engaged in system optimization, including incorporation of real-time data flow, whether physiological or camera-captured. Further research more fully exploring the concept of *Global medical wellbeing* Assessment is also warranted. As a clinical research and development team accustomed to the need for a fluid exchange between theory and praxis, we finally emphasize the importance of iterative design and continuous quality improvements to closer approximate tool optimization, whether therapeutic or diagnostic.

ACKNOWLEDGMENTS

We are grateful to our participants for providing feedback on the Wellpad design and PRAXIS colleagues Kunal Sudan and Robelyn Soriano for collecting data and assisting patient intake.

REFERENCES

[1] Durlach NI, Mavor AS, eds. Virtual reality: Scientific and technological challenges. Washington, DC: National Research Council, National Academies Press, 1995

[2] Dugas M, Neuhaus P, Meidt A, Doods J, Storck M, Bruland P, et al. Portal of medical data models: information infrastructure for medical research and healthcare. Database 2016:pii:bav121. doi: 10.1093/data base/bav121.

[3] Marti P. Enabling through design: Explorations of aesthetic interaction in therapy and care. Eindhoven: Technische Universiteit Eindhoven, 2012.

[4] Nussbaumer LL. Inclusive design: A universal need. New York: Fairchild Books, 2001.

[5] John J. Gamification the name of the game. NZ Business Manage 2015;29(11):42-3.

[6] Moller HJ, Bal H. Technology-enhanced multimodal meditation: Clinical results from an observational case series, Proceed 10th International Conference on Virtual Rehabilitation, Philadelphia, PA 2013 Aug 26-29:1-9.

[7] Moller HJ, Saynor L. Wellpad: An inclusively designed tablet-based digital medical record with optimized efficiency and usability. MobileHCI 2014 Sept 23-26.

[8] Moller HJ, Saynor L, Sudan K, Tabak D. Wellpad: A new standardized assessment and data visualization tool for clinicians and researchers, Proceed IACM 2015 8th Conference on Cannabinoids in Medicine 2015 Sept 17-19, Sestri Levante, Italy

[9] Becker GM, Degroot M, Marschak J. Measuring utility by a single-response sequential method. Syst Res Behav Sci 1964;9(3):226-32. doi: 10.1002/bs.3830090304.

[10] Bach DS, Risko K, Zaran F, Farber M, Polk G. A pharmacy blueprint for electronic medical record implementation success. Hosp Pharm 2015;50(6):484-95. doi: 10.1310/hpj5006-484.

[11] Steiner CJ, Reisinger Y. Understanding existential authenticity. Ann Tourism Res 2006;33(2):299-318.

[12] Csikszentmihalyi M, Kleiber DA. Leisure and self-actualization. In: Driver BL, Brown PJ, Peterson GL, eds. Benefits of leisure. State College, PA: Venture, 1991:91-102.

Submitted: February 10, 2017. *Revised:* March 15, 2017. *Accepted:* March 22, 2017.

SECTION FIVE – ACKNOWLEDGMENTS

In: Alternative Medicine Research Yearbook 2017
Editor: Joav Merrick

ISBN: 978-1-53613-726-2
© 2018 Nova Science Publishers, Inc.

Chapter 47

ABOUT THE EDITOR

Joav Merrick, MD, MMedSci, DMSc, born and educated in Denmark is professor of pediatrics, child health and human development, Division of Pediatrics, Hadassah Hebrew University Medical Center, Mt Scopus Campus, Jerusalem, Israel and Kentucky Children's Hospital, University of Kentucky, Lexington, Kentucky United States and professor of public health at the Center for Healthy Development, School of Public Health, Georgia State University, Atlanta, United States, the medical director of the Health Services, Division for Intellectual and Developmental Disabilities, Ministry of Social Affairs and Social Services, Jerusalem, the founder and director of the National Institute of Child Health and Human Development in Israel. Numerous publications in the field of pediatrics, child health and human development, rehabilitation, intellectual disability, disability, health, welfare, abuse, advocacy, quality of life and prevention. Received the Peter Sabroe Child Award for outstanding work on behalf of Danish Children in 1985 and the International LEGO-Prize ("The Children's Nobel Prize") for an extraordinary contribution towards improvement in child welfare and well-being in 1987. E-mail: jmerrick@zahav.net.il

In: Alternative Medicine Research Yearbook 2017
Editor: Joav Merrick

ISBN: 978-1-53613-726-2
© 2018 Nova Science Publishers, Inc.

Chapter 48

ABOUT THE NATIONAL INSTITUTE OF CHILD HEALTH AND HUMAN DEVELOPMENT IN ISRAEL

The National Institute of Child Health and Human Development (NICHD) in Israel was established in 1998 as a virtual institute under the auspices of the Medical Director, Ministry of Social Affairs and Social Services in order to function as the research arm for the Office of the Medical Director. In 1998 the National Council for Child Health and Pediatrics, Ministry of Health and in 1999 the Director General and Deputy Director General of the Ministry of Health endorsed the establishment of the NICHD.

MISSION

The mission of a National Institute for Child Health and Human Development in Israel is to provide an academic focal point for the scholarly interdisciplinary study of child life, health, public health, welfare, disability, rehabilitation, intellectual disability and related aspects of human development. This mission includes research, teaching, clinical work, information and public service activities in the field of child health and human development.

SERVICE AND ACADEMIC ACTIVITIES

Over the years many activities became focused in the south of Israel due to collaboration with various professionals at the Faculty of Health Sciences (FOHS) at the Ben Gurion University of the Negev (BGU). Since 2000 an affiliation with the Zusman Child Development Center at the Pediatric Division of Soroka University Medical Center has resulted in collaboration around the establishment of the Down Syndrome Clinic at that center. In 2002 a full course on "Disability" was established at the Recanati School for Allied Professions in the Community, FOHS, BGU and in 2005 collaboration was started with the Primary Care Unit of the faculty and disability became part of the master of public health course on "Children and society". In the academic year 2005-2006 a one semester course on "Aging with disability" was started as part of the master of science program in gerontology in our collaboration with the Center for Multidisciplinary Research in Aging. In 2010 collaborations with the Division of Pediatrics, Hadassah Hebrew University Medical Center, Jerusalem, Israel around the National Down Syndrome Center and teaching students and residents about intellectual and developmental disabilities as part of their training at this campus.

RESEARCH ACTIVITIES

The affiliated staff have over the years published work from projects and research activities in this national and international collaboration. In the year 2000 the International Journal of Adolescent Medicine and Health and in 2005 the International Journal on Disability and Human Development of De Gruyter Publishing House (Berlin and New York) were affiliated with the National Institute of Child Health and Human Development. From 2008 also the International Journal of Child Health and Human Development (Nova Science, New York), the International Journal of Child and Adolescent Health (Nova Science) and the Journal of Pain Management (Nova Science) affiliated and from 2009 the International Public Health Journal (Nova Science) and Journal of Alternative Medicine Research (Nova Science). All peer-reviewed international journals.

NATIONAL COLLABORATIONS

Nationally the NICHD works in collaboration with the Faculty of Health Sciences, Ben Gurion University of the Negev; Department of Physical Therapy, Sackler School of Medicine, Tel Aviv University; Autism Center, Assaf HaRofeh Medical Center; National Rett and PKU Centers at Chaim Sheba Medical Center, Tel HaShomer; Department of Physiotherapy, Haifa University; Department of Education, Bar Ilan University, Ramat Gan, Faculty of Social Sciences and Health Sciences; College of Judea and Samaria in Ariel and in 2011 affiliation with Center for Pediatric Chronic Diseases and National Center for Down Syndrome, Department of Pediatrics, Hadassah Hebrew University Medical Center, Mount Scopus Campus, Jerusalem.

INTERNATIONAL COLLABORATIONS

Internationally with the Department of Disability and Human Development, College of Applied Health Sciences, University of Illinois at Chicago; Strong Center for Developmental Disabilities, Golisano Children's Hospital at Strong, University of Rochester School of Medicine and Dentistry, New York; Centre on Intellectual Disabilities, University of Albany, New York; Centre for Chronic Disease Prevention and Control, Health Canada, Ottawa; Chandler Medical Center and Children's Hospital, Kentucky Children's Hospital, Section of Adolescent Medicine, University of Kentucky, Lexington; Chronic Disease Prevention and Control Research Center, Baylor College of Medicine, Houston, Texas; Division of Neuroscience, Department of Psychiatry, Columbia University, New York; Institute for the Study of Disadvantage and Disability, Atlanta; Center for Autism and Related Disorders, Department Psychiatry, Children's Hospital Boston, Boston; Department of Pediatric and

Adolescent Medicine, Western Michigan University Homer Stryker MD School of Medicine, Kalamazoo, Michigan, United States; Department of Paediatrics, Child Health and Adolescent Medicine, Children's Hospital at Westmead, Westmead, Australia; International Centre for the Study of Occupational and Mental Health, Düsseldorf, Germany; Centre for Advanced Studies in Nursing, Department of General Practice and Primary Care, University of Aberdeen, Aberdeen, United Kingdom; Quality of Life Research Center, Copenhagen, Denmark; Nordic School of Public Health, Gottenburg, Sweden, Scandinavian Institute of Quality of Working Life, Oslo, Norway; The Department of Applied Social Sciences (APSS) of The Hong Kong Polytechnic University Hong Kong.

TARGETS

Our focus is on research, international collaborations, clinical work, teaching and policy in health, disability and human development and to establish the NICHD as a permanent institute at one of the residential care centers for persons with intellectual disability in Israel in order to conduct model research and together with the four university schools of public health/medicine in Israel establish a national master and doctoral program in disability and human development at the institute to secure the next generation of professionals working in this often non-prestigious/low-status field of work.

CONTACT

Joav Merrick, MD, MMedSci, DMSc
Professor of Pediatrics, Child Health and Human Development
Medical Director, Health Services, Division for Intellectual and Developmental Disabilities, Ministry of Social Affairs and Social Services, POB 1260, IL-91012 Jerusalem, Israel.
E-mail: jmerrick@zahav.net.il

Chapter 49

ABOUT THE BOOK SERIES "HEALTH AND HUMAN DEVELOPMENT"

Health and human development is a book series with publications from a multidisciplinary group of researchers, practitioners and clinicians for an international professional forum interested in the broad spectrum of health and human development. Books already published:

- Merrick J, Omar HA, eds. *Adolescent behavior research. International perspectives.* New York: Nova Science, 2007.
- Kratky KW. *Complementary medicine systems: Comparison and integration.* New York: Nova Science, 2008.
- Schofield P, Merrick J, eds. *Pain in children and youth.* New York: Nova Science, 2009.
- Greydanus DE, Patel DR, Pratt HD, Calles Jr JL, eds. *Behavioral pediatrics*, 3 ed. New York: Nova Science, 2009.
- Ventegodt S, Merrick J, eds. *Meaningful work: Research in quality of working life.* New York: Nova Science, 2009.
- Omar HA, Greydanus DE, Patel DR, Merrick J, eds. *Obesity and adolescence. A public health concern.* New York: Nova Science, 2009.
- Lieberman A, Merrick J, eds. *Poverty and children. A public health concern.* New York: Nova Science, 2009.
- Goodbread J. *Living on the edge. The mythical, spiritual and philosophical roots of social marginality.* New York: Nova Science, 2009.
- Bennett DL, Towns S, Elliot E, Merrick J, eds. *Challenges in adolescent health: An Australian perspective.* New York: Nova Science, 2009.
- Schofield P, Merrick J, eds. *Children and pain.* New York: Nova Science, 2009.
- Sher L, Kandel I, Merrick J, eds. *Alcohol-related cognitive disorders: Research and clinical perspectives.* New York: Nova Science, 2009.
- Anyanwu EC. *Advances in environmental health effects of toxigenic mold and mycotoxins.* New York: Nova Science, 2009.
- Bell E, Merrick J, eds. *Rural child health. International aspects.* New York: Nova Science, 2009.
- Dubowitz H, Merrick J, eds. *International aspects of child abuse and neglect.* New York: Nova Science, 2010.

- Shahtahmasebi S, Berridge D. *Conceptualizing behavior: A practical guide to data analysis.* New York: Nova Science, 2010.
- Wernik U. *Chance action and therapy. The playful way of changing.* New York: Nova Science, 2010.
- Omar HA, Greydanus DE, Patel DR, Merrick J, eds. *Adolescence and chronic illness. A public health concern.* New York: Nova Science, 2010.
- Patel DR, Greydanus DE, Omar HA, Merrick J, eds. *Adolescence and sports.* New York: Nova Science, 2010.
- Shek DTL, Ma HK, Merrick J, eds. *Positive youth development: Evaluation and future directions in a Chinese context.* New York: Nova Science, 2010.
- Shek DTL, Ma HK, Merrick J, eds. *Positive youth development: Implementation of a youth program in a Chinese context.* New York: Nova Science, 2010.
- Omar HA, Greydanus DE, Tsitsika AK, Patel DR, Merrick J, eds. *Pediatric and adolescent sexuality and gynecology: Principles for the primary care clinician.* New York: Nova Science, 2010.
- Chow E, Merrick J, eds. *Advanced cancer. Pain and quality of life.* New York: Nova Science, 2010.
- Latzer Y, Merrick, J, Stein D, eds. *Understanding eating disorders. Integrating culture, psychology and biology.* New York: Nova Science, 2010.
- Sahgal A, Chow E, Merrick J, eds. *Bone and brain metastases: Advances in research and treatment.* New York: Nova Science, 2010.
- Postolache TT, Merrick J, eds. *Environment, mood disorders and suicide.* New York: Nova Science, 2010.
- Maharajh HD, Merrick J, eds. *Social and cultural psychiatry experience from the Caribbean Region.* New York: Nova Science, 2010.
- Mirsky J. *Narratives and meanings of migration.* New York: Nova Science, 2010.
- Harvey PW. *Self-management and the health care consumer.* New York: Nova Science, 2011.
- Ventegodt S, Merrick J. *Sexology from a holistic point of view.* New York: Nova Science, 2011.
- Ventegodt S, Merrick J. *Principles of holistic psychiatry: A textbook on holistic medicine for mental disorders.* New York: Nova Science, 2011.
- Greydanus DE, Calles Jr JL, Patel DR, Nazeer A, Merrick J, eds. *Clinical aspects of psychopharmacology in childhood and adolescence.* New York: Nova Science, 2011.
- Bell E, Seidel BM, Merrick J, eds. *Climate change and rural child health.* New York: Nova Science, 2011.
- Bell E, Zimitat C, Merrick J, eds. *Rural medical education: Practical strategies.* New York: Nova Science, 2011.
- Latzer Y, Tzischinsky. *The dance of sleeping and eating among adolescents: Normal and pathological perspectives.* New York: Nova Science, 2011.
- Deshmukh VD. *The astonishing brain and holistic consciousness: Neuroscience and Vedanta perspectives.* New York: Nova Science, 2011.
- Bell E, Westert GP, Merrick J, eds. *Translational research for primary healthcare.* New York: Nova Science, 2011.
- Shek DTL, Sun RCF, Merrick J, eds. *Drug abuse in Hong Kong: Development and evaluation of a prevention program.* New York: Nova Science, 2011.
- Ventegodt S, Hermansen TD, Merrick J. *Human Development: Biology from a holistic point of view.* New York: Nova Science, 2011.

- Ventegodt S, Merrick J. *Our search for meaning in life.* New York: Nova Science, 2011.
- Caron RM, Merrick J, eds. *Building community capacity: Minority and immigrant populations.* New York: Nova Science, 2012.
- Klein H, Merrick J, eds. *Human immunodeficiency virus (HIV) research: Social science aspects.* New York: Nova Science, 2012.
- Lutzker JR, Merrick J, eds. *Applied public health: Examining multifaceted Social or ecological problems and child maltreatment.* New York: Nova Science, 2012.
- Chemtob D, Merrick J, eds. *AIDS and tuberculosis: Public health aspects.* New York: Nova Science, 2012.
- Ventegodt S, Merrick J. *Textbook on evidence-based holistic mind-body medicine: Basic principles of healing in traditional Hippocratic medicine.* New York: Nova Science, 2012.
- Ventegodt S, Merrick J. *Textbook on evidence-based holistic mind-body medicine: Holistic practice of traditional Hippocratic medicine.* New York: Nova Science, 2012.
- Ventegodt S, Merrick J. *Textbook on evidence-based holistic mind-body medicine: Healing the mind in traditional Hippocratic medicine.* New York: Nova Science, 2012.
- Ventegodt S, Merrick J. *Textbook on evidence-based holistic mind-body medicine: Sexology and traditional Hippocratic medicine.* New York: Nova Science, 2012.
- Ventegodt S, Merrick J. *Textbook on evidence-based holistic mind-body medicine: Research, philosophy, economy and politics of traditional Hippocratic medicine.* New York: Nova Science, 2012.
- Caron RM, Merrick J, eds. *Building community capacity: Skills and principles.* New York: Nova Science, 2012.
- Lemal M, Merrick J, eds. *Health risk communication.* New York: Nova Science, 2012.
- Ventegodt S, Merrick J. *Textbook on evidence-based holistic mind-body medicine: Basic philosophy and ethics of traditional Hippocratic medicine.* New York: Nova Science, 2013.
- Caron RM, Merrick J, eds. *Building community capacity: Case examples from around the world.* New York: Nova Science, 2013.
- Steele RE. *Managed care in a public setting.* New York: Nova Science, 2013.
- Srabstein JC, Merrick J, eds. *Bullying: A public health concern.* New York: Nova Science, 2013.
- Pulenzas N, Lechner B, Thavarajah N, Chow E, Merrick J, eds. *Advanced cancer: Managing symptoms and quality of life.* New York: Nova Science, 2013.
- Stein D, Latzer Y, eds. *Treatment and recovery of eating disorders.* New York: Nova Science, 2013.
- Sun J, Buys N, Merrick J. *Health promotion: Community singing as a vehicle to promote health.* New York: Nova Science, 2013.
- Pulenzas N, Lechner B, Thavarajah N, Chow E, Merrick J, eds. *Advanced cancer: Managing symptoms and quality of life.* New York: Nova Science, 2013.
- Sun J, Buys N, Merrick J. *Health promotion: Strengthening positive health and preventing disease.* New York: Nova Science, 2013.
- Merrick J, Israeli S, eds. *Food, nutrition and eating behavior.* New York: Nova Science, 2013.
- Shahtahmasebi S, Merrick J. *Suicide from a public health perspective.* New York: Nova Science, 2014.
- Merrick J, Tenenbaum A, eds. *Public health concern: Smoking, alcohol and substance use.* New York: Nova Science, 2014.

- Merrick J, Aspler S, Morad M, eds. *Mental health from an international perspective.* New York: Nova Science, 2014.
- Merrick J, ed. *India: Health and human development aspects.* New York: Nova Science, 2014.
- Caron R, Merrick J, eds. *Public health: Improving health via inter-professional collaborations.* New York: Nova Science, 2014.
- Merrick J, ed. *Pain Mangement Yearbook 2014.* New York: Nova Science, 2015.
- Merrick J, ed. *Public Health Yearbook 2014.* New York: Nova Science, 2015.
- Sher L, Merrick J, eds. *Forensic psychiatry: A public health perspective.* New York: Nova Science, 2015.
- Shek DTL, Wu FKY, Merrick J, eds. *Leadership and service learning education: Holistic development for Chinese university students.* New York: Nova Science, 2015.
- Calles JL, Greydanus DE, Merrick J, eds. *Mental and holistic health: Some international perspectives.* New York: Nova Science, 2015.
- Lechner B, Chow R, Pulenzas N, Popovic M, Zhang N, Zhang X, Chow E, Merrick J, eds. *Cancer: Treatment, decision making and quality of life.* New York: Nova Science, 2016.
- Lechner B, Chow R, Pulenzas N, Popovic M, Zhang N, Zhang X, Chow E, Merrick J, eds. *Cancer: Pain and symptom management.* New York: Nova Science, 2016.
- Lechner B, Chow R, Pulenzas N, Popovic M, Zhang N, Zhang X, Chow E, Merrick J, eds. *Cancer: Bone metastases, CNS metastases and pathological fractures.* New York: Nova Science, 2016.
- Lechner B, Chow R, Pulenzas N, Popovic M, Zhang N, Zhang X, Chow E, Merrick J, eds. *Cancer: Spinal cord, lung, breast, cervical, prostate, head and neck cancer.* New York: Nova Science, 2016.
- Lechner B, Chow R, Pulenzas N, Popovic M, Zhang N, Zhang X, Chow E, Merrick J, eds. *Cancer: Survival, quality of life and ethical implications.* New York: Nova Science, 2016.
- Davidovitch N, Gross Z, Ribakov Y, Slobodianiuk A, eds. *Quality, mobility and globalization in the higher education system: A comparative look at the challenges of academic teaching.* New York: Nova Science, 2016.
- Henry B, Agarwal A, Chow E, Omar HA, Merrick J, eds. *Cannabis: Medical aspects.* New York: Nova Science, 2017.
- Henry B, Agarwal A, Chow E, Merrick J, eds. *Palliative care: Psychosocial and ethical considerations.* New York: Nova Science, 2017.
- Furfari A, Charames GS, McDonald R, Rowbottom L, Azad A, Chan S, Wan BA, Chow R, DeAngelis C, Zaki P, Chow E, Merrick J, eds. *Oncology: The promising future of biomarkers.* New York: Nova Science, 2017.
- O'Hearn S, Blake A, Wan BA, Chan S, Chow E, Merrick J, eds. *Medical cannabis: Clinical practice.* New York: Nova Science, 2017.
- Shek DTL, Leung JTY, Lee TY, Merrick J, eds. *Psychosocial Needs: Success in Life and Career Planning.* New York: Nova Science, 2018.
- Cheuk-Yu Lui L, Wong K-H, Yeung R, Merrick J, eds. *Palliative Care: Oncology Experience from Hong Kong.* New York: Nova Science, 2017.
- Koren N, Moreno M and Merrick J, eds. *Brennan Healing Science: An Integrative Approach to Therapeutic Intervention.* New York: Nova Science, 2017.
- Malek L, Lim F, Angela Wan BA, Diaz PL, Chow E, Merrick J, eds. *Cancer and Exercise.* New York: Nova Science, 2018.

CONTACT

Joav Merrick, MD, MMedSci, DMSc
Medical Director, Health Services
Division for Intellectual and Developmental Disabilities
Ministry of Social Affairs and Social Services
POBox 1260, IL-91012 Jerusalem, Israel
Email: jmerrick@zahav.net.il

SECTION SIX – INDEX

INDEX

A

abuse, viii, ix, xv, xvi, 4, 5, 6, 7, 8, 12, 13, 14, 15, 17, 18, 19, 20, 25, 34, 36, 57, 65, 271, 273, 274, 275, 276, 277, 281, 282, 283, 284, 285, 286, 287, 288, 289, 290, 291, 292, 293, 294, 295, 296, 297, 298, 299, 300, 301, 302, 303, 304, 306, 308, 310, 311, 312, 313, 314, 315, 318, 319, 320, 321, 322, 323, 326, 327, 328, 329, 330, 331, 332, 333, 338, 340, 341, 342, 343, 345, 346, 350, 351, 352, 354, 363, 365, 366, 367, 368, 369, 370, 371, 372, 373, 374, 375, 376, 377, 378, 379, 380, 381, 382, 383, 384, 387, 388, 389, 390, 391, 519
active video games, 193
active wheel device, xv, 263
activity theory, 150
adaptation, 104, 147, 149, 150, 151, 198, 200, 203, 204, 417, 447, 476, 487
adaptations, 153, 154, 157, 447
adaptive functioning, 16
adaptive training, 147
ADHD, 14, 16, 26, 37, 47, 48, 49, 51, 57, 64, 65, 66, 69, 148, 316, 317, 327, 403
adolescent behavior, 377
adolescent boys, 309
adolescents, ix, xiii, 8, 11, 12, 13, 14, 15, 16, 17, 18, 19, 20, 21, 23, 33, 34, 35, 36, 39, 40, 41, 53, 55, 60, 62, 64, 66, 67, 68, 69, 73, 227, 298, 299, 300, 309, 310, 311, 312, 313, 316, 317, 318, 319, 321, 323, 324, 325, 328, 331, 332, 335
adoption incentives, 353
adrenal insufficiency, 340, 342
adrenocorticotropic hormone, 73
adult education, 380
adulthood, 29, 122, 300, 355, 379, 385, 387
adults, xv, 5, 7, 15, 29, 34, 56, 63, 66, 68, 71, 73, 80, 117, 148, 152, 167, 195, 198, 199, 200, 203, 204, 287, 290, 301, 302, 303, 304, 307, 311, 322, 323, 325, 326, 334, 355, 366, 378, 379, 387, 388, 436
advocacy, 117, 118, 157, 166, 292, 319, 329, 334, 344, 361, 377, 519
age, 5, 32, 39, 57, 59, 60, 61, 62, 64, 65, 66, 71, 74, 75, 122, 133, 140, 147, 167, 190, 195, 200, 207, 214, 215, 224, 230, 239, 273, 274, 275, 276, 280, 282, 284, 286, 287, 289, 290, 291, 293, 300, 301, 302, 303, 304, 305, 306, 307, 308, 309, 310, 311, 312,314, 319, 320, 321, 324, 325, 327, 328, 331, 342, 355, 356, 362, 374, 383, 408, 409, 415, 422, 436, 455, 512
ageing population, 205, 210
aggression, 13, 17, 18, 19, 24, 25, 26, 37, 44, 51, 56, 57, 67, 291, 313
aggressive behavior, 29, 33, 301, 310
allocentric reference frame, 205, 210
ambient assisted living, xiv, 139, 140, 144
amputees, xiv, 161, 162, 163, 165, 166
analgesic, 79
anatomy, 294, 298, 342, 380
anger, 18, 29, 33, 34, 37, 51, 326
antibacterial activity, 82, 83, 86, 90
antidepressant medication, 60
antidepressants, 59, 60, 66, 68, 79
antioxidant, xiii, 81, 82, 83, 84, 86, 87, 88, 89, 90, 91, 92
antioxidants activity, 82
antipsychotic, 61, 63, 215
antitumor, 82
anxiety, xiii, 12, 13, 14, 15, 16, 18, 19, 25, 26, 29, 31, 32, 33, 34, 36, 40, 44, 56, 57, 59, 60, 71, 72, 73, 74, 75, 77, 78, 79, 80, 103, 104, 178, 181, 182, 184, 294, 312, 315, 316, 317, 320, 322, 323, 326, 477, 480, 481, 510, 511, 513
anxiety disorder, 13, 15, 16, 19, 26, 33, 34, 36, 56, 57, 59
appointments, 42, 43, 52, 181, 280, 337, 343, 481
arousal, 75, 78, 147, 150, 151, 308, 312

artery, 77, 94, 96, 456
ascorbic acid, 84, 87, 89, 91
assault, 290, 292, 293, 295, 298, 390
assessment, 3, 4, 5, 6, 7, 11, 12, 13, 14, 20, 27, 28, 31, 44, 47, 53, 55, 56, 57, 64, 73, 128, 169, 170, 173, 198, 201, 207, 208, 211, 214, 221, 276, 277, 278, 282, 287, 288, 292, 294, 295, 297, 298, 300, 301, 302, 303, 311, 313, 314, 317, 319, 320, 321, 322, 327, 329, 331, 357, 359, 360, 371, 374, 380, 384, 397, 398, 399, 401, 403, 420, 421, 423, 443, 459, 460, 462, 463, 464, 466, 467, 468, 469, 470, 471, 483, 484, 485, 486, 488, 489, 516
augmented reality, xvi, 110, 115, 140, 145, 211, 253, 395, 446, 492, 507
autism, 12, 13, 15, 16, 27, 56, 61, 67, 131, 132, 135, 137, 299, 300, 317, 329, 331, 332
autism spectrum disorders, 13, 15, 19, 132, 331, 332
avatar, 117, 118, 119, 120, 121, 124, 126, 129, 153, 155, 164, 171, 428
avatar consent, 153

B

Bayesian inference, 406, 412
behavior, v, vi, x, 4, 5, 12, 13, 15, 16, 18, 19, 20, 23, 24, 25, 26, 27, 28, 29, 30, 31, 32, 33, 34, 35, 36, 37, 38, 39, 40, 41, 42, 44, 45, 47, 48, 49, 50, 51, 53, 54, 57, 61, 66, 167, 214, 220, 274, 289, 290, 291, 298, 299, 300, 301, 302, 303, 304, 305, 306, 307, 308, 309, 310, 311, 312, 313, 314, 315, 316, 317, 318, 319, 320, 321, 322, 323, 324, 325, 326, 328, 329, 330, 331, 332, 368, 372, 374, 381, 382, 388, 390, 416, 446, 447, 450, 482
behavior modification, 23, 24, 27, 28, 29, 35, 40
behavior therapy, 20, 23, 24, 27, 35, 37, 38, 39, 40, 54
behavioral assessment, 28
behavioral change, 16, 213
behavioral disorders, 19, 56, 78
behavioral manifestations, 31
behavioral problems, 12, 13, 14, 15, 19, 62, 306
bipolar disorder, 13, 18, 19, 36, 61, 62, 66, 67
birth weight, 275, 277
blame, 43, 100, 101, 103, 276, 327, 379
bleeding, 292, 293
blindness, 229, 230, 232, 234, 235, 236, 238, 239, 243, 268, 492, 497, 498, 501, 502, 507
blood, xiii, 26, 48, 63, 64, 71, 72, 79, 99, 100, 186, 339, 340, 351, 356, 487
blood pressure, xiii, 26, 63, 64, 71, 72, 79, 80
bone, 79, 120, 171, 279, 286, 339, 461
bone growth, 279
bone marrow, 79

borderline personality disorder, 18, 34, 40
braille code, 245, 246
brain, xv, 74, 125, 130, 147, 149, 152, 170, 174, 179, 211, 223, 224, 225, 226, 230, 239, 339, 342, 351, 366, 409, 443, 446, 510
brain activity, xv, 179, 223, 224
brain damage, 351
brain structure, 366
brain-computer interface, 147
brainstem, 74, 339
breast cancer, 95, 96
breathing, 32, 33, 38, 339, 340, 489
breathlessness, 32, 98
brothers, 46, 100, 101, 102
bullying, 57, 308
burn, 276, 280, 281, 282, 283, 284, 285, 288

C

care model, xiii, 41, 42, 43, 44, 336
caregivers, 139, 140, 141, 142, 143, 144, 274, 275, 276, 291, 302, 303, 304, 305, 309, 312, 313, 315, 316, 323, 325, 326, 330, 333, 335, 340, 341, 343, 344, 361, 373, 379
caregiving, 121, 144
carousel maze, 214, 216, 217
case report, xiii, 93, 94, 97, 340, 471
case study, xvii, 111, 135, 332, 490, 509
cerebral palsy, 194, 195, 198, 274, 278, 279, 335, 337, 407, 408, 409, 414
challenges, xvi, 42, 51, 57, 69, 73, 74, 117, 124, 133, 137, 147, 153, 277, 316, 317, 333, 337, 339, 342, 343, 344, 345, 346, 350, 360, 366, 409, 410, 432, 443, 473, 486, 513, 516
child abuse, 4, 5, 6, 7, 8, 274, 275, 276, 283, 286, 287, 288, 289, 303, 314, 319, 320, 331, 333, 334, 340, 341, 342, 343, 345, 346, 352, 363, 365, 366, 370, 371, 373, 374, 375, 376, 377, 378, 382, 383, 384, 387, 388, 389, 391
child development, 300, 301, 302, 322, 370, 371, 372, 383
child labor, 349
child maltreatment, 3, 4, 7, 8, 273, 274, 275, 277, 280, 287, 292, 300, 302, 311, 312, 314, 315, 319, 322, 329, 331, 340, 341, 346, 347, 348, 351, 352, 353, 354, 363, 366, 367, 368, 369, 370, 371, 373, 374, 375, 376, 377, 378, 380, 381, 382, 384, 387, 388, 389, 390, 391
child protection, 7, 329, 343, 347, 351, 352, 353, 354, 355, 356, 357, 358, 359, 360, 362, 375, 390
child protective services, 6, 273, 284, 285, 292, 297, 302, 338, 339, 342, 343, 350, 373, 382, 391

childhood, 13, 29, 44, 51, 54, 56, 62, 274, 275, 277, 284, 287, 291, 300, 301, 302, 303, 305, 306, 307, 308, 319, 322, 329, 330, 346, 366, 373, 377, 378, 380, 382, 384, 385, 387, 388, 389, 391
childhood disorders, 51
childhood sexual abuse, 301
children, x, xiii, xv, xvi, 3, 4, 5, 6, 7, 8, 11, 12, 13, 14, 15, 16, 17, 18, 19, 20, 21, 23, 29, 33, 34, 36, 39, 40, 41, 47, 50, 51, 53, 54, 55, 56, 57, 58, 60, 61, 62, 63, 64, 65, 66, 67, 68, 69, 73, 79, 97, 98, 100, 101, 102, 103, 132, 133, 134, 135, 136, 137, 152, 182, 194, 197, 198, 227, 242, 271, 273, 274, 275, 276, 277, 278, 279, 280, 282, 283, 284, 285, 286, 287, 288, 289, 290, 291, 292, 293, 294, 295, 296, 297, 298, 299, 300, 301, 302, 303, 304, 305, 306, 307, 308, 310, 311, 312, 313, 314, 315, 316, 317, 318, 319, 320, 321, 322, 323, 324, 325, 326, 327, 328, 329, 330, 331, 332, 333, 334, 335, 336, 337, 338, 339, 340, 341, 342, 343, 344, 345, 346, 347, 348, 349, 350, 351, 352, 353, 354, 355, 356, 357, 358, 359, 360, 361, 362, 363, 365, 366, 368, 369, 371, 372, 374, 375, 376, 377, 378, 379, 380, 381, 382, 383, 384, 385, 387, 388, 389, 390, 391, 403, 429, 519, 521, 522
chronic diseases, 99, 275, 483
chronic illness, 24, 36, 98
classroom, 27, 64, 134, 136, 237, 337, 339, 348, 397, 398, 399, 400, 401, 402, 403
classroom environment, 398
client therapist relationship, 473
clinical application, 137
clinical assessment, 398
clinical disorders, 78
clinical judgment, 57
clinical psychology, 211
clinical trials, 60, 61, 67, 115
cognitive behavioural therapy, 132
cognitive deficit, 206, 214, 217, 220, 221, 398
cognitive function, 78, 200, 203, 207, 213, 214, 220, 221
cognitive impairment, 140, 152, 204, 215, 361, 379, 484
cognitive load, 128, 433, 442
cognitive performance, 214, 215
cognitive process, 24, 37, 203, 206, 241, 434
cognitive skills, 73, 149
cognitive tasks, 148, 203
cognitive therapy, 24, 34, 35, 38
cognitive training, xiv, 147, 148, 149, 150, 151
cognitive-behavioral therapy, 24, 68
collaborative virtual environments, 132, 475
collisions, 240, 241, 420, 421, 424, 426
colostomy, 334, 340, 342, 344

colour harmony, 230, 236
colour-check, xv, 229
communication, 6, 15, 30, 43, 46, 73, 117, 118, 119, 131, 132, 135, 140, 143, 157, 181, 184, 247, 254, 276, 293, 297, 325, 328, 329, 336, 372, 402, 473, 474, 475, 476, 477, 480, 481, 483, 486, 487, 489
communication abilities, 73
communication skills, 30, 131, 132, 293, 372
communication technologies, 140
computer, 49, 71, 75, 117, 118, 135, 140, 141, 143, 147, 148, 158, 170, 175, 184, 187, 202, 208, 220, 225, 232, 237, 238, 239, 240, 405, 407, 410, 414, 416, 417, 429, 437, 467, 469, 470, 486, 488, 490, 492
computer models, 237, 238
computer software, 117, 118
computer technology, 240
computer use, 158, 239, 407, 417
computing, 114, 253, 254, 416, 417, 471
conflict, 16, 18, 26, 34, 36, 101, 325, 341
conflict resolution, 16, 18, 36
context information, 123, 126, 127, 129, 421
control condition, 78, 163
control group, 77, 78, 206, 210, 215, 373
cost, xv, 28, 43, 44, 78, 134, 136, 193, 194, 237, 246, 251, 253, 346, 362, 363, 369, 370, 371, 378, 384, 386, 390, 391, 400, 431, 432, 434, 436, 442, 479, 485, 486, 489
counseling, 12, 16, 21, 371, 376, 380, 383
creativity, 113, 345, 369, 513, 515
criminal behavior, 312
criminal justice system, 384
cues, 27, 33, 74, 170, 179, 214, 215, 216, 219, 220, 246, 258, 316, 317, 318, 322, 434, 445, 447, 448, 449, 450, 451, 453, 454, 456, 475
cultural beliefs, 324, 325, 370
cultural conditions, 357
cultural influence, 122, 302, 322
cultural norms, 276, 376
culture, 181, 184, 287, 295, 301, 302, 309, 319, 322, 324, 325, 356, 374, 515
curricula, 328
curriculum, 238, 328, 370
cycling wheelchair, xiv, 185, 186, 192

D

data analysis, 76, 200, 217, 450, 510
data collection, 74, 75, 76, 79, 150, 240, 241, 251, 443, 512
database, 121, 155, 510
deaths, 230, 273, 346, 354, 371

deficit, xv, 15, 49, 56, 57, 59, 64, 148, 210, 213, 214, 217, 219, 316, 339, 433
dementia, 144, 147, 201, 205, 206, 207, 211
depressants, 59
depression, xiii, 13, 14, 15, 16, 17, 18, 19, 25, 34, 35, 36, 40, 56, 60, 63, 66, 68, 71, 72, 73, 74, 75, 77, 80, 97, 99, 103, 104, 178, 291, 320, 338, 366, 383
depressive symptoms, 335
design framework, xiv, 109, 110, 113
development, i, ii, iv, v, vi, viii, ix, xi, xv, xvii, 3, 4, 5, 13, 15, 25, 29, 32, 34, 38, 95, 97, 109, 113, 114, 117, 120, 121, 123, 124, 131, 134, 135, 136, 137, 140, 151, 152, 162, 163, 166, 167, 183, 192, 193, 229, 232, 245, 246, 252, 253, 264, 268, 274, 277, 281, 286, 290, 291, 299, 300, 301, 302, 303, 306, 309, 310, 312, 316, 318, 319, 321, 322, 323, 324, 325, 326, 327, 328, 329, 330, 337, 345, 349, 365, 366, 368, 370, 371, 372, 374, 375, 377, 380, 381, 383, 385, 387, 388, 395, 396, 399, 400, 401, 404, 417, 429, 431, 446, 485, 487, 488, 489, 491, 492, 507, 510, 512, 514, 515, 519, 521, 522, 523
developmental disorder, 16, 300, 316
developmental factors, 27, 311
developmental process, 4, 8
developmental psychopathology, 329
diabetes, 12, 15, 16, 23, 24, 44, 47, 63, 68, 103, 335, 385, 498
diet, 42, 44, 48, 63
disability, xv, 4, 5, 7, 8, 13, 14, 116, 125, 137, 153, 154, 155, 157, 159, 170, 194, 235, 236, 242, 271, 273, 274, 275, 276, 277, 279, 285, 289, 290, 291, 293, 297, 299, 316, 318, 321, 328, 333, 335, 336, 338, 346, 347, 358, 359, 360, 361, 362, 365, 366, 368, 370, 372, 378, 384, 388, 389, 405, 406, 407, 408, 409, 410, 415, 416, 429, 448, 456, 489, 492, 507, 513, 519, 521, 522, 523
disclosure, 154, 277, 291, 292, 293, 294, 295, 296, 297, 313, 379, 390, 391
discomfort, 45, 119, 380, 439, 462, 463, 466, 471
discrimination, 207, 208, 238, 256, 264, 343, 358
diseases, 99, 230, 298, 461, 462
disorder, 13, 14, 15, 24, 32, 49, 50, 56, 57, 58, 59, 60, 61, 62, 63, 64, 66, 67, 104, 137, 148, 185, 220, 299, 300, 312, 316, 322, 323, 329, 332, 335, 338, 339, 340, 366, 487, 490
distress, 29, 32, 34, 38, 79, 326
diversity, 82, 111, 300, 302, 447, 454
doctors, 362, 376, 484, 486
domestic violence, 312, 315, 334, 370, 388
dosage, 59, 67, 370
Down syndrome, 279, 287
drug addict, 37
drug safety, 69

drug testing, 57
drug therapy, 104
drugs, 60, 61, 79, 82, 95, 104, 222, 339, 378
due process, 348, 350, 351
dynamic postural control, xv, 193, 194

E

eating disorders, 13, 15, 17, 18, 19, 20, 59
eating disturbances, 291
education, xiv, 63, 64, 102, 103, 131, 136, 137, 154, 167, 207, 214, 215, 237, 238, 239, 240, 242, 284, 290, 291, 302, 309, 316, 318, 321, 325, 327, 328, 329, 331, 343, 348, 360, 361, 366, 369, 372, 374, 376, 378, 379, 381, 382, 383, 389, 390, 398, 506
educational materials, 359, 389
educational objective, 133
educational programs, 368, 390
educational settings, 132
educational software, 135
educators, 329, 396, 398
egocentric reference frame, 205
elderly, 102, 118, 121, 139, 140, 141, 145, 185, 198, 204, 206, 407, 408, 410, 417
elderly population, 206
e-learning, 161, 162, 163, 164, 165, 166, 404
electronic health records, 509, 513
emotion, 24, 26, 34, 39, 122, 315, 323, 477
emotion regulation, 34, 323
emotional distress, 308, 312, 319
emotional problems, 23
emotional reactions, 16, 303
emotional responses, 24
emotional state, 120, 182
emotional well-being, 73
empathy, 316, 317, 370, 372
empowerment, 371, 390
endophytic fungus, xiii, 81, 82, 83, 84, 86, 87, 90, 91, 92
environment, xiv, 27, 29, 30, 38, 43, 51, 57, 74, 80, 103, 124, 125, 126, 127, 128, 129, 130, 137, 141, 145, 147, 149, 150, 151, 161, 162, 163, 165, 167, 171, 172, 178, 179, 201, 203, 208, 210, 214, 215, 217, 220, 223, 224, 246, 253, 256, 258, 261, 269, 300, 301, 304, 309, 311, 317, 318, 321, 322, 324, 325, 326, 360, 361, 368, 370, 373, 374, 375, 377, 378, 398, 399, 400, 406, 408, 410, 415, 419, 421, 422, 423, 425, 428, 432, 433, 434, 435, 437, 439, 442, 443, 447, 449, 450, 456, 474, 477, 478, 482, 486, 492, 493, 506, 507, 515
environmental change, 322
environmental conditions, 82
environmental factors, 13, 315

environmental influences, 331
environmental stimuli, 74, 220
environmental stress, 315
epilepsy, 338, 339
ethnic background, 120, 275
ethnic diversity, 181
ethnic minority, 302, 343
ethnicity, 75, 309, 324, 378
evaluation, viii, ix, xv, xvi, 4, 5, 6, 13, 57, 64, 65, 68, 104, 113, 116, 122, 132, 135, 151, 152, 162, 167, 174, 178, 186, 189, 190, 191, 195, 201, 205, 206, 210, 273, 276, 277, 281, 282, 283, 286, 288, 289, 291, 292, 293, 294, 297, 298, 315, 321, 329, 331, 344, 352, 359, 360, 361, 371, 375, 377, 389, 399, 416, 420, 431, 433, 434, 436, 443, 445, 460, 468, 471, 510, 513
exploration, 256
exposure, xvi, 14, 24, 32, 33, 35, 68, 77, 94, 119, 180, 222, 242, 292, 300, 301, 306, 309, 311, 314, 315, 318, 319, 320, 322, 325, 326, 378, 382, 383, 388, 442, 462, 473, 474, 477, 480, 481
exposure therapy, xvi, 24, 442, 473, 474, 477, 480, 481
externalizing behavior, 25, 315, 323, 372, 374
externalizing disorders, 15, 16, 19, 37, 57
eye control, 223
eye movement, 170, 173, 223, 224, 226
eye-tracking, 401

F

facial animation, 118
facial expression, 118, 119, 121, 318, 475
fall risk, xv, 199, 200, 202, 204
families, 4, 6, 7, 17, 34, 41, 42, 43, 44, 45, 46, 53, 105, 121, 273, 275, 276, 278, 297, 300, 302, 312, 324, 325, 327, 328, 331, 335, 336, 339, 342, 343, 344, 347, 348, 352, 353, 355, 357, 359, 363, 366, 370, 371, 373, 374, 377, 379, 380, 381, 383, 385, 388, 389
family behavior, 44, 45
family characteristics, 315
family environment, 301, 374
family functioning, 310
family history, 53, 57, 64
family life, 351
family members, 6, 45, 46, 47, 53, 56, 57, 66, 166, 326, 353
family physician, 24
family support, 343, 372, 375, 389
family system, 17, 45
family therapy, xiii, 17, 41, 42, 43, 44, 49, 52, 53, 100, 101, 324

family violence, 287, 291, 306, 311, 315, 383
fear, 30, 31, 32, 34, 37, 43, 45, 200, 291, 327, 380
fear response, 30, 31, 32
feelings, 18, 26, 30, 43, 45, 57, 73, 78, 182, 303, 308, 317, 318, 319, 322, 323, 325, 326, 327, 343, 480
ferrous ion, 81, 85, 87, 91
fidelity, 119, 120, 370, 441
fingerpad, xv, 263, 265, 268
flavonoid, 81, 82, 84, 90, 91, 92
focus groups, xiv, 153, 154, 155, 156, 157, 158, 159, 162, 165, 166, 389
force field analysis, 132
force sensing, 185
freedom, 179, 225, 349, 422, 479, 480

G

games, 49, 52, 109, 110, 115, 116, 159, 211, 215, 225, 229, 231, 234, 235, 306, 308, 329, 399, 404, 432, 457, 485, 490
gamification, xiv, 109, 110, 111, 113, 115, 516
gaze estimation, 169, 474
gender differences, 304, 306
gender role, 306, 307, 308, 309, 320, 326, 376
general practitioner, 97
generalizability, 308, 314, 372, 428
generalized anxiety disorder, 19, 25, 32, 36, 60
genitals, 280, 291, 296, 300, 301, 303, 304, 305, 307, 308, 318, 324, 326
geometry, 140, 141, 421, 494
gestural assessment, 459
gestural interaction, xvi, 459, 460, 461, 462, 464, 467, 468, 469, 470, 471
Google, 401, 402, 404, 422, 431, 432, 433, 434, 436, 441, 443, 493, 494, 507
grief, xiii, 18, 19, 21, 40, 97, 98, 101, 103, 104, 105
guidance, 15, 42, 44, 104, 141, 145, 163, 245, 247, 248, 253, 256, 276, 291, 297, 302, 311, 316, 326, 357, 360, 369, 373, 374, 381, 389, 397, 428, 433, 448, 491, 507
guidelines, 20, 74, 159, 201, 298, 300, 319, 370, 382, 396, 417, 433, 441, 442, 460, 486, 493, 510

H

haptic feedback, xv, 239, 255, 256, 261, 269
hazards, 431, 462, 463
head injuries, 373
head injury, 347, 409
head trauma, 275, 286, 288, 373, 385, 389, 390
headache, 94, 100, 104, 340

healing, 73, 178, 296, 379
health, xiv, xvi, xvii, 7, 8, 11, 12, 16, 19, 20, 37, 41, 42, 43, 44, 45, 46, 47, 49, 52, 53, 63, 74, 97, 98, 99, 100, 101, 105, 116, 118, 121, 137, 140, 153, 154, 155, 156, 157, 159, 161, 162, 163, 166, 167, 177, 178, 179, 181, 183, 203, 206, 211, 274, 275, 277, 279, 280, 290, 293, 294, 295, 296, 297, 298, 300, 310, 322, 330, 333, 334, 335, 336, 337, 338, 339, 340, 342, 343, 344, 345, 346, 347, 349, 353, 354, 356, 358, 360, 365, 366, 368, 369, 370, 371, 373, 375, 376, 377, 378, 380, 381, 382, 384, 385, 386, 388, 390, 391, 399, 405, 406, 408, 410, 411, 414, 415, 446, 448, 451, 456, 460, 462, 463, 464, 481, 483, 485, 486, 487, 488, 489, 507, 509, 510, 511, 512, 513, 514, 515, 519, 521, 523
health care, 7, 8, 11, 12, 17, 20, 37, 41, 42, 43, 44, 45, 46, 49, 52, 63, 97, 98, 118, 140, 153, 154, 159, 162, 167, 177, 178, 179, 211, 274, 278, 279, 280, 294, 295, 297, 298, 300, 333, 334, 335, 336, 337, 338, 339, 340, 341, 342, 343, 344, 345, 346, 347, 353, 358,365, 374, 375, 376, 377, 378, 380, 382, 384, 385, 486, 488, 489, 513
health care costs, 336, 384
health care professionals, 7, 63, 97, 344, 365, 380, 486
health care system, 41, 140, 344, 374, 385
health condition, 277, 335, 336, 345, 346, 399, 485, 487
health effects, 385
health information, 155, 162, 163
health insurance, 356, 377, 378, 385
health problems, 7, 11, 20, 41, 45, 47, 53, 277, 296, 365, 382, 385
health promotion, 183
health risks, 460, 464
health services, 12, 43, 44, 344, 373, 378, 489
health status, 483
healthcare equity, 153
health-induced impairment, 406, 415
hearing impairment, 74, 75
hearing loss, 99, 102
heart attack, 102, 103
heart disease, 102, 385
heart rate, xiii, 26, 30, 31, 64, 71, 72, 79, 80, 182, 513
height, 195, 240, 250, 264, 279, 469, 474, 495
hepatotoxicity, 55, 66
high school, 65, 239, 355, 356, 378
high-risk populations, 378
history, 18, 19, 57, 64, 104, 118, 163, 166, 202, 276, 277, 281, 282, 283, 285, 286, 287, 291, 293, 294, 295, 296, 297, 305, 306, 310, 311, 312, 313, 314, 315, 317, 319, 320, 322, 327, 328, 351, 360, 363, 380
holistic health, 178, 180
home care services, 338
hormones, 72, 73, 79, 94, 316, 366
hospitalization, 17, 18, 221, 336, 372
human, xv, 7, 24, 26, 27, 75, 79, 82, 104, 118, 119, 124, 128, 132, 135, 145, 147, 148, 149, 150, 171, 175, 189, 200, 224, 227, 229, 230, 240, 255, 256, 257, 261, 268, 292, 297, 299, 300, 320, 388, 390, 405, 406, 407, 408, 410, 416, 417, 420, 447, 448, 453, 454, 459, 460, 461, 464, 470, 471, 476, 482, 490, 519, 521, 523
human activity, 150
human body, 82, 460, 461
human brain, 147, 149, 224, 230
human condition, 124
human development, 300, 388, 519, 521, 523
human experience, 24
human factor, 132, 254, 459
human immunodeficiency virus, 292
human machine interaction, 406
hyperactivity, 49, 56, 57, 59, 61, 64, 148, 316
hypothesis, 27, 39, 71, 77, 96, 109, 128, 129, 149, 212

I

immersion, 284, 285, 440, 442, 480, 482
impairments, xvi, 4, 124, 125, 140, 169, 200, 242, 316, 359, 384, 405, 409, 410, 411, 412, 415, 417, 491, 492, 493, 495, 496, 497, 499, 501, 504, 505, 506, 507
inclusive design, xvi, 109, 178, 184, 405, 408, 409, 410, 415, 417, 491, 492, 493, 506, 507, 514, 516
income, 103, 306, 362, 370, 371, 389, 391
individuals, 33, 34, 35, 64, 65, 66, 67, 71, 72, 73, 74, 75, 76, 79, 92, 110, 111, 157, 181, 183, 186, 194, 198, 200, 204, 210, 234, 238, 313, 314, 316, 317, 319, 323, 324, 327, 329, 331, 339, 358, 359, 375, 396, 410, 420, 428, 446, 463, 474, 492, 502
infancy, 299, 303, 368
infants, 5, 276, 286, 287, 368, 371, 373, 388
informed consent, 58, 75, 165, 206, 436
infrastructure, 3, 7, 95, 251, 375, 516
insomnia, 24, 36, 40, 59, 100, 103, 178
integration, 18, 24, 117, 137, 184, 346, 366, 376, 400, 411, 412, 429, 506
intellectual disabilities, 4, 67, 298, 299, 328, 335, 368, 388, 390
intelligence, 145, 149, 331
intelligent agent, 118
intensive care unit, 334, 345

interaction, xvi, 4, 8, 14, 16, 17, 20, 36, 45, 46, 47, 49, 51, 111, 115, 117, 119, 121, 122, 124, 132, 134, 135, 137, 145, 147, 148, 152, 170, 174, 175, 184, 209, 239, 253, 268, 300, 318, 360, 369, 372, 379, 389, 390, 397, 398, 401, 405, 406, 407, 409, 410, 416, 417, 420, 421, 426, 431, 432, 433, 434, 441, 443, 447, 449, 451, 459, 460, 464, 468, 469, 470, 471, 475, 476, 481, 482, 484, 486, 487, 516
interface, xiv, 110, 114, 117, 122, 137, 139, 140, 141, 142, 143, 144, 145, 147, 150, 201, 225, 250, 257, 258, 268, 402, 405, 406, 407, 408, 410, 411, 429, 435, 445, 446, 447, 448, 460, 462, 464, 468, 469, 505
interference, 163, 216, 253, 348, 349, 350
internalizing, 19, 34, 56, 306, 323
intervention, xiv, 12, 13, 14, 17, 18, 21, 26, 34, 37, 44, 47, 49, 52, 53, 57, 72, 73, 78, 79, 97, 101, 104, 128, 133, 135, 137, 141, 161, 162, 163, 165, 166, 167, 220, 229, 278, 303, 312, 313, 319, 322, 324, 341, 366, 368, 370, 371, 372, 373, 374, 375, 379, 380, 388,389, 390, 391, 483, 484, 486, 489
intimacy, 46, 309, 315, 318, 324
investments, 370, 377, 395, 403
irritability, 59, 61, 62, 66, 338
isolation, 13, 51, 83, 90, 92, 118, 327

J

Java, 215, 494, 504
joints, 171, 189, 448, 461, 462, 468, 469, 470
juvenile delinquency, 17, 315, 366, 384
juvenile justice, 296, 311, 322
juvenile sex offender, 332

K

kinect, 144, 193, 194, 195, 196, 197, 198, 406, 445, 446, 448, 466, 467, 469, 471, 486, 490

L

laptop, 403, 422, 423, 437, 486
law enforcement, 6, 292, 338, 343
laws, 6, 276, 292, 349, 352, 356, 358, 369, 373, 378, 389, 390
lawyers, 362
leap motion, 116, 406, 446
learning, iv, 13, 14, 16, 24, 25, 26, 27, 28, 29, 30, 37, 38, 40, 79, 110, 115, 121, 122, 125, 126, 127, 128, 129, 130, 131, 132, 133, 134, 136, 137, 149, 152, 161, 162, 163, 164, 165, 166, 167, 179, 203, 204, 206, 208, 214, 215, 216, 218, 219, 220, 221, 222, 237,238, 239, 241, 242, 274, 289, 290, 291, 296, 309, 310, 329, 358, 361, 375, 377, 388, 396, 398, 409, 417, 424, 433, 435, 446, 447, 450, 452, 454, 506, 513
learning difficulties, 218
learning disabilities, 13, 296
learning environment, 122, 136, 162, 238
learning outcomes, 167
learning process, 24, 237, 238, 241
learning task, 133, 136, 221
legal, xii, xvi, 4, 6, 7, 17, 18, 75, 293, 300, 323, 331, 341, 343, 344, 347, 348, 349, 350, 351, 352, 355, 361, 362, 376
legislation, 347, 348, 352, 354, 357, 373, 385, 492
liver, 66, 85, 286, 334, 337, 338, 345, 366
liver disease, 334, 337, 338, 345, 366
liver failure, 66, 337
living environment, 140, 141
lung disease, 334, 337, 338
lying, 29, 51, 317, 339

M

major depression, 68, 73
major depressive disorder, 60, 63
major issues, 52, 59
maltreatment, xvi, 4, 5, 6, 7, 8, 273, 274, 276, 277, 286, 287, 290, 297, 301, 302, 310, 312, 314, 315, 320, 329, 333, 334, 338, 343, 346, 347, 348, 350, 352, 365, 366, 367, 368, 369, 370, 371, 373, 375, 376, 377, 378, 379, 380, 384, 387, 388, 389, 391
mangrove plants, 82
medical, xvi, 5, 6, 7, 8, 11, 12, 13, 15, 16, 17, 19, 23, 24, 34, 37, 39, 44, 45, 48, 50, 53, 57, 65, 73, 78, 99, 101, 103, 104, 155, 158, 177, 179, 181, 184, 192, 200, 227, 258, 273, 274, 275, 276, 277, 278, 279, 280, 282, 283, 284, 285, 286, 287, 289, 290, 292,293, 294, 295, 296, 297, 298, 312, 316, 320, 333, 334, 335, 336, 337, 338, 339, 340, 341, 342, 343, 344, 345, 346, 349, 352, 353, 359, 360, 362, 371, 373, 374, 377, 378, 380, 381, 384, 385, 386, 387, 391, 449, 460, 487, 489, 510, 513, 515, 516, 519
medical assistance, 377
medical care, 6, 11, 17, 103, 275, 277, 294, 297, 338, 340, 343, 373
medical evaluation, xv, xvi, 5, 273, 276, 283, 287, 289, 292, 293, 294, 295, 296, 297
medical history, 57, 99, 277, 284, 285, 292, 293, 298
medical neglect, 5, 6, 8, 275, 333, 337, 338, 339, 342, 343, 344, 345, 346, 378
medication, 12, 13, 14, 34, 52, 56, 57, 58, 59, 64, 65, 66, 67, 68, 69, 179, 215, 515

medicine, xiii, 9, 73, 79, 510, 514, 523
memory, 73, 99, 117, 140, 141, 145, 148, 152, 204, 206, 207, 211, 214, 215, 216, 220, 221, 222, 321, 409, 437, 494, 504
memory capacity, 148
mental disorder, 20, 104, 300
mental health, 11, 12, 13, 16, 18, 20, 23, 37, 43, 49, 52, 55, 73, 177, 178, 179, 183, 222, 275, 276, 310, 311, 315, 322, 329, 338, 344, 345, 349, 353, 359, 360, 366, 368, 372, 376, 380, 382, 383, 386, 389, 510, 513, 514
mental health professionals, 322, 383
mental illness, 56, 57, 78, 360, 383
mental impairment, 103, 358, 362
methodology, 30, 35, 84, 85, 110, 153, 154, 241
Microsoft, 144, 162, 194, 196, 198, 208, 401, 404, 406, 445, 446, 448, 469, 492, 507
military, 43, 101, 349, 402
mindfulness based stress reduction, 178
misconceptions, 46, 296, 328, 330
mobile application, 433, 441, 491
mobile communication, 409
mobile device, 443, 492, 493, 506
mobile phone, 431, 432, 433, 437
mobile virtual reality, xvi, 431, 443
Morris water maze, 214, 215, 221
motion control, 443, 449
motion sickness, 451, 456
motor actions, 126
motor activity, 223, 227, 401
motor behavior, 50, 416
motor control, 204, 215, 447
motor fiber, 74, 80
motor skills, 125, 128, 284, 447
motor system, 200, 223, 410
movement visualization, 123, 126, 128, 129, 421
multi-user surface, 132
musculoskeletal, 26, 203, 338, 460, 461, 462, 464, 471
musculoskeletal system, 26
music, xiii, 71, 72, 73, 74, 75, 76, 77, 78, 79, 80, 128, 184, 254, 310
music therapy, 73, 74, 79, 80, 184
music-based interventions, 72, 73, 74, 78
myoma, xiii, 93, 94, 95
myopia, 337, 492, 500

N

navigation, xv, xvi, 165, 206, 211, 214, 215, 217, 218, 219, 220, 245, 246, 247, 249, 250, 251, 252, 253, 254, 255, 256, 261, 408, 429, 431, 432, 434, 435, 437, 442, 443

navigation system, xv, 245, 246, 247, 249, 252, 253, 254
navigational assistance, 253
neglect, viii, xv, xvi, 4, 5, 6, 7, 8, 230, 273, 274, 275, 276, 277, 279, 280, 285, 286, 287, 288, 290, 294, 296, 297, 298, 313, 315, 329, 333, 337, 338, 339, 342, 343, 344, 345, 346, 350, 351, 352, 365, 366, 368, 370, 371, 373, 376, 378, 384, 387, 388, 389, 390,391
neural function, 223
neural network, 223, 227
neurological disease, 484
neuropsychological tests, 207, 208, 215
neuropsychology, 152, 211
neurorehabilitation, 198, 208, 223, 224, 227
neuroscience, 55, 105, 211
neurotransmitters, 78
neutral, 30, 181, 462, 463, 477
non-verbal communication, 473, 474, 475, 476, 477, 480, 481
normative behavior, 301, 375
nurses, 12, 17, 371, 484
nursing, 73, 334, 336, 344, 345, 483, 488
nurturance, 48, 311
nurturing parent, 381
nutrient, 83, 279
nutrition, 279, 280, 334, 337, 338, 339, 340, 345
nutritional status, 337

O

obesity, 12, 16, 23, 36, 37, 44, 64, 279, 287
obsessive-compulsive disorder, 13, 60
obstacles, 201, 203, 232, 246, 256, 312, 321, 439
occupational therapy, 125
oculus, xvi, 151, 396, 400, 401, 403, 443, 445, 446, 449, 456
online learning, 396
operating system, 399, 493
organism, 26, 27, 29, 31, 82, 83
outdoor navigation, xv, 245, 246, 250, 253
outpatient, 18, 322, 337, 339, 343
overweight, 279
oxidative stress, 95, 96

P

pain, 7, 29, 33, 64, 72, 73, 79, 100, 163, 182, 276, 277, 284, 285, 287, 291, 292, 303, 338, 365, 366, 442, 460, 462, 512
pain management, 33
panic disorder, 13, 31, 32

parent-child relationship, 322, 374, 385
parenthood, 349
parenting, 3, 7, 13, 15, 17, 19, 29, 45, 306, 311, 322, 350, 351, 358, 368, 370, 371, 372, 374, 375, 376, 377, 378, 380, 383, 389, 390
parents, 4, 7, 8, 11, 14, 16, 17, 23, 29, 31, 35, 36, 43, 45, 46, 47, 48, 49, 50, 52, 58, 59, 65, 66, 100, 101, 102, 121, 134, 273, 275, 276, 290, 295, 300, 301, 302, 304, 306, 308, 309, 313, 315, 317, 318, 320, 325, 326, 327, 328, 330, 333, 334, 340, 341, 348, 349, 350, 351, 353, 354, 355, 356, 357, 358, 359, 360, 361, 362, 363, 368, 369, 371, 372, 373, 374, 375, 376, 377, 378, 379, 380, 382, 383, 389
participant advance preparation, 153
participants, 71, 72, 74, 75, 76, 77, 78, 148, 154, 155, 156, 157, 158, 180, 194, 195, 196, 197, 199, 200, 201, 202, 203, 206, 207, 208, 209, 210, 215, 223, 224, 225, 226, 239, 240, 241, 242, 251, 252, 307, 371, 379, 413, 415, 420, 421, 422, 424, 425, 426, 427, 428, 436, 437, 438, 439, 440, 441, 442, 443, 446, 448, 450, 451, 452, 453, 454, 455, 505, 511, 512, 515
patient centered care process, 484
pediatrician, 41, 42, 43, 44, 49, 52, 278, 279, 280, 286, 287, 380, 387, 389, 391
pediatrics, viii, 3, 8, 41, 53, 69, 276, 278, 287, 288, 297, 298, 330, 345, 346, 365, 366, 374, 381, 387, 388, 389, 390, 391, 519, 521, 522, 523
performance feedback, 123
personal communication, 248
personal views, 304
personality, 19, 118, 119, 121, 129, 311, 315
personality characteristics, 118
personality disorder, 19
personality traits, 129, 311, 315
persons with disabilities, 153, 154, 155, 157
phenolics, 82, 83, 90, 91
physical abuse, 4, 5, 273, 274, 275, 276, 277, 281, 282, 284, 286, 288, 290, 296, 311, 312, 315, 352, 366, 368, 372, 376, 378, 387, 388, 390
physical activity, 17, 42, 63
physical environment, 421
physical health, 42, 73, 104, 294, 366
physical interaction, 326, 432, 486, 487
physical therapy, 165, 204, 279, 470
platform, 208, 211, 214, 396, 398, 399, 400, 406, 410, 422, 432, 443, 485, 486, 488, 489, 494, 506
playing, 48, 49, 52, 198, 225, 284, 301, 308, 461, 477
pneumonia, 83, 86, 87, 280
policy, 183, 206, 242, 294, 328, 334, 352, 366, 369, 376, 377, 378, 381, 382, 385, 523
policy makers, 328, 377

population, 4, 5, 7, 8, 11, 26, 27, 37, 58, 60, 61, 63, 64, 66, 67, 72, 140, 147, 157, 158, 181, 230, 234, 274, 279, 290, 294, 297, 299, 301, 304, 305, 306, 308, 311, 313, 314, 315, 318, 321, 322, 323, 328, 329, 333, 334, 336, 337, 343, 345, 346, 356, 365, 367, 370, 371, 374, 375, 376, 377, 378, 383, 385, 390, 399, 407, 408, 409, 428, 433, 436, 441, 442, 490, 507, 515
population group, 336
positive emotions, 78
posttraumatic stress, 24, 323, 366
post-traumatic stress disorder, 32, 474
postural control, xv, 193, 194, 198, 204
poverty, 275, 312, 337, 343, 344, 369, 376, 377, 378, 380
power wheelchair, xvi, 336, 419, 420, 421, 422, 427, 428, 429
pregnancy, 57, 94, 277, 310, 334, 366, 369, 372
prejudice, 343
prematurity, 275, 334
preparation, xii, 77, 153, 157, 158, 162, 329
prevention, ix, xvi, 3, 4, 7, 8, 12, 14, 16, 32, 33, 38, 63, 65, 80, 235, 275, 277, 287, 289, 298, 332, 338, 344, 346, 352, 365, 366, 367, 368, 369, 373, 374, 375, 376, 377, 378, 379, 380, 381, 382, 383, 384, 385, 386, 387, 388, 389, 390, 391, 486, 489, 519, 522
primary care, xiii, 11, 12, 14, 17, 20, 23, 39, 41, 42, 43, 44, 53, 97, 98, 105, 298, 314, 324, 373, 374, 389
projector camera system, 139, 140
protection, 7, 154, 249, 326, 345, 350, 352, 356, 357, 359, 362, 379, 390
prototype, 134, 139, 143, 144, 152, 242, 245, 253, 263, 268, 476
psychiatric disorder, 55, 56, 68, 73, 201, 311, 313
psychoeducational intervention, 58, 323
psychological assessments, 313
psychological distress, 100
psychological pain, 365
psychological problems, 36
psychological processes, 74
psychological well-being, 74, 80
psychologist, 43, 44, 49, 50, 51, 52
psychopharmacology, ix, xiii, 55, 56, 68, 69
psychosis, 13, 18, 19, 26, 36, 62, 64, 220
psychosomatic, 48, 177, 180
psychotherapy, ii, 11, 14, 15, 16, 17, 18, 20, 21, 23, 26, 34, 40, 100, 104, 105, 344, 358, 390
psychotropic medications, 56, 59, 63
puberty, 303, 308, 309, 316, 317, 318

public health, 3, 7, 8, 65, 105, 178, 289, 297, 369, 375, 376, 377, 381, 382, 390, 514, 515, 519, 521, 523
public investment, 375
public policy, 3, 7, 154, 352, 383

Q

qualitative analysis, 162, 437
qualitative methodology, 153
qualitative research, 509
qualitative study, 245, 249, 250, 253, 390
quality assurance, 249
quality function deployment (QFD), 245, 249, 254
quality improvement, 515
quality of life, 170, 336, 344, 345, 420, 519
quality of service, 375

R

raised-dot, xv, 263, 268, 269
reading, 36, 75, 157, 164, 246, 247, 316, 317, 358, 374, 491, 492, 507
realism, 118, 119, 149, 151, 474
reality, xiv, xv, xvi, xvii, 16, 32, 33, 107, 110, 114, 115, 123, 124, 125, 130, 132, 134, 137, 140, 145, 148, 149, 152, 169, 181, 183, 185, 187, 192, 198, 199, 204, 205, 208, 211, 214, 221, 222, 223, 224, 253, 395, 403, 404, 419, 421, 429, 431, 432, 443, 445, 446, 456, 457, 459, 469, 473, 477, 480, 481, 482, 490, 492, 507, 509, 510, 516
recognition, xvii, 4, 144, 170, 175, 237, 238, 241, 242, 261, 273, 331, 346, 356, 376, 401, 483, 489
recommendations, xii, 12, 115, 131, 132, 135, 161, 162, 319, 322, 325, 363, 366, 464
recovery, xiii, 73, 74, 79, 93, 94, 95, 124, 130, 174, 224, 229, 231, 312, 464, 465, 484
reference frame, xv, 205, 206, 208, 210, 216, 219, 220
rehabilitation, xiv, xv, xvi, 5, 7, 73, 107, 109, 110, 111, 112, 113, 114, 115, 123, 124, 125, 126, 127, 128, 129, 130, 132, 137, 148, 149, 163, 167, 169, 170, 171, 173, 174, 175, 184, 185, 186, 191, 192, 193, 194, 197, 198, 200, 204, 211, 220, 227, 229, 231, 235, 236, 242, 347, 354, 358, 360, 361, 393, 395, 396, 397, 398, 399, 403, 404, 429, 431, 432, 433, 441, 443, 445, 446, 447, 448, 451, 456, 457, 470, 484, 485, 486, 489, 490, 491, 510, 514, 516, 519, 521
rehabilitation game, xv, 109, 110, 111, 112, 229, 235, 236
rehabilitation program, 200

relationship satisfaction, 17
relatives, 98, 99, 101, 484, 486, 488, 489
relaxation, 33, 38, 40, 73, 78, 80, 178, 181, 183, 510, 512
researchers, 32, 43, 73, 75, 76, 110, 111, 114, 132, 137, 166, 194, 227, 239, 241, 299, 304, 306, 308, 320, 324, 328, 377, 395, 396, 398, 420, 447, 510, 513, 515, 516
resources, 5, 11, 14, 20, 42, 45, 53, 58, 101, 103, 134, 238, 297, 323, 329, 338, 343, 362, 366, 374, 380, 381, 382, 383, 384, 409, 475, 480, 485
response, 3, 4, 6, 7, 8, 13, 14, 26, 28, 30, 31, 32, 33, 34, 36, 38, 42, 57, 72, 73, 74, 79, 97, 121, 148, 150, 151, 180, 194, 197, 221, 240, 277, 292, 333, 334, 340, 353, 355, 357, 373, 388, 399, 401, 433, 440, 441, 451, 453, 455, 481, 516
response time, 240, 399, 453
risk factors, 57, 64, 65, 203, 275, 287, 290, 312, 315, 328, 368, 369, 370, 373, 376, 383, 386, 459, 462, 464, 467, 470
risk management, 183
robotics, 110, 120, 175
role playing, 136, 304, 323
rotations, 190, 433, 461
rules, 4, 29, 31, 50, 163, 230, 317, 323, 324, 325, 326, 493

S

safety, 4, 6, 7, 31, 61, 68, 186, 200, 201, 203, 275, 284, 290, 292, 293, 294, 297, 325, 326, 327, 338, 341, 349, 354, 356, 371, 374, 376, 379, 382, 383, 385, 390, 399, 406, 429, 464, 468, 473, 477, 481
schizophrenia, xv, 25, 61, 62, 213, 214, 215, 217, 218, 219, 220, 221, 222
school, 12, 13, 14, 17, 18, 24, 26, 27, 32, 35, 37, 42, 49, 50, 51, 52, 53, 56, 57, 64, 73, 100, 101, 132, 134, 137, 279, 290, 291, 300, 303, 305, 318, 322, 325, 326, 330, 337, 338, 339, 347, 348, 349, 360, 361, 362, 378, 383, 396, 398, 425, 523
school failure, 383
school performance, 49
science, 183, 184, 227, 236, 237, 238, 239, 240, 242, 422, 425, 457, 470, 475, 482, 521
science, technology, engineering and mathematics (STEM), 237, 238, 239
second life, xiv, 153, 154, 155, 156, 157, 158, 159
selective serotonin reuptake inhibitor, 60
self-actualization, 184, 516
self-assessment, 485
self-awareness, 181
self-concept, 16, 18
self-confidence, 326

self-destructive behavior, 34
self-efficacy, 25, 162, 163
self-esteem, 16, 18, 46, 47, 104, 180, 328, 383
self-management, xiv, 161, 162, 163, 166, 167, 446
self-regulation, 315, 324
self-sufficiency, 371
self-worth, 31
senior citizen, 139, 140, 143, 144, 145
sensing, 114, 116, 121, 185, 246, 250, 254, 256, 405, 448, 457
sensitivity, 73, 220, 221, 240, 256, 384, 448, 506
sensor, 139, 141, 143, 144, 192, 196, 202, 404, 408, 409, 412, 469, 483, 485, 486, 487, 488, 489
sensor network, 409
serious gaming, 484
service provider, 4, 117, 121, 344, 358, 369
sex, 36, 101, 214, 215, 296, 297, 298, 302, 303, 304, 306, 308, 309, 311, 313, 315, 316, 318, 319, 321, 323, 326, 327, 328, 329, 330, 331, 334
sex offenders, 311, 323, 330, 331
sexual abuse, xvi, 5, 274, 289, 290, 291, 292, 293, 294, 295, 296, 297, 298, 299, 300, 301, 302, 304, 310, 311, 312, 313, 314, 318, 320, 321, 322, 326, 327, 328, 329, 330, 331, 332, 352, 354, 366, 368, 369, 379, 388, 390, 391
sexual activity, 290, 293, 301, 303, 308, 311, 312, 314, 319
sexual behavior, xvi, 5, 291, 292, 298, 299, 300, 301, 302, 303, 304, 305, 306, 307, 308, 310, 311, 312, 313, 314, 315, 316, 317, 318, 319, 320, 321, 322, 323, 324, 325, 326, 327, 328, 329, 330, 331, 332
sexual development, 5, 299, 301, 302, 309, 316, 324, 325, 326, 327, 328, 329
sexual experiences, 301, 307, 308
sexual feelings, 299, 300, 303, 316, 326, 328
sexual health, 329, 331
sexual identity, 300, 316
sexual intercourse, 94, 309
sexual offending, 315
sexual orientation, 310
sexuality, v, 18, 291, 299, 300, 301, 302, 303, 304, 305, 306, 309, 311, 318, 320, 321, 324, 325, 326, 327, 329, 330, 331, 332, 379, 390
sexually transmitted infections, 292, 294, 295, 379
simulation, 149, 199, 200, 201, 203, 211, 227, 235, 396, 397, 399, 401, 420, 421, 422, 423, 428, 429, 473, 476, 479, 480, 481, 492, 493, 494, 495, 502, 505, 506, 507
situationally-induced impairment, 406
skin, 25, 26, 27, 37, 151, 263, 264, 269, 280, 285, 337, 339, 340, 449, 513
slippage perception, xv, 263, 265
smoking cessation, 375

smooth muscle, 74, 93, 94
social anxiety, 13, 14, 16, 18, 19, 32, 36, 477
social behavior, 307
social cognition, 122, 214
social competence, 132, 137
social environment, 24, 25, 277, 300, 324
social interaction, 74, 137, 328, 475
social learning theory, 37
social norms, 307, 316, 318, 322, 326, 369
social relationships, 372
social situations, 32, 155, 323
social skills, 16, 18, 35, 36, 64, 315, 317, 323
social skills training, 16, 64
social support, 15, 101, 103, 104, 163, 370, 371, 389
social withdrawal, 31, 103
social workers, 12, 338, 344, 352
socialization, 16, 34, 35, 308, 309, 315, 320, 325, 326
societal cost, 384
society, 6, 12, 169, 178, 273, 290, 300, 302, 309, 312, 323, 365, 366, 367, 368, 369, 376, 381, 383, 387, 483, 484, 490, 521
socioeconomic status, 61, 305, 324, 372
software, 110, 113, 115, 120, 121, 131, 132, 134, 135, 136, 137, 157, 162, 163, 165, 171, 196, 208, 215, 226, 231, 232, 235, 241, 258, 395, 396, 397, 399, 403, 420, 441, 450, 468, 469, 470, 492, 504
sonification, 237, 238, 239
spatial navigation, xv, 211, 213, 214, 222
spatial processing, 212
special education, 37, 134, 360, 361, 384
special needs, xiv, 4, 8, 131, 135, 137, 252, 292, 297, 333, 334, 335, 353
speech, 78, 99, 120, 121, 238, 242, 246, 361, 409
spontaneous recovery, 31
state authorities, 349, 350, 351, 352, 354, 355, 357
state intervention, 351
state legislatures, 373
stimulation, 125, 126, 128, 129, 180, 181, 227, 230, 303, 309, 311, 312, 429
stress, 5, 6, 13, 15, 18, 34, 36, 40, 46, 47, 72, 73, 77, 78, 79, 80, 82, 91, 150, 177, 178, 179, 180, 181, 182, 184, 279, 291, 295, 306, 366, 370, 372, 374, 375, 378, 382, 383, 387, 388, 389, 410, 460, 461, 462, 466, 469, 470, 509, 511, 513
stress management, 18, 36
stress response, 34, 72, 73, 79
stressful life events, 315
stressors, 43, 44, 79, 291, 327, 339, 343, 344
stroke, xiv, xv, xvi, xvii, 65, 73, 74, 80, 109, 110, 111, 115, 123, 124, 125, 126, 128, 129, 130, 148, 169, 170, 172, 174, 175, 185, 198, 204, 227, 229,

230, 234, 235, 236, 263, 409, 445, 446, 447, 448, 456, 457, 483, 484, 485, 486, 489, 490
stroke rehabilitation, xvi, 109, 110, 111, 115, 130, 169, 170, 174, 175, 227, 445, 447, 456, 486, 490
substance abuse, 14, 15, 16, 17, 18, 19, 20, 36, 57, 65, 275, 296, 366, 372, 376, 380, 383
substance use, 13, 57, 338, 344
substance use disorders, 13, 344
suicidal behavior, 34, 40
suicidal ideation, 55, 59, 60, 66, 67, 292
suicide, 12, 13, 16, 55, 60, 63, 67, 97, 99, 100, 103
suicide attempts, 13
supervision, 275, 277, 284, 285, 318, 322, 323, 324, 325, 327, 338, 382, 383
survival, 95, 154, 274, 336, 344, 345
survivors, 104, 169, 292, 445
symptoms, 16, 25, 45, 50, 51, 53, 56, 57, 58, 61, 62, 63, 65, 66, 73, 75, 93, 94, 162, 178, 179, 180, 181, 182, 213, 214, 221, 277, 286, 291, 293, 296, 311, 313, 323, 341, 382, 474, 481, 498, 499
syndrome, 8, 15, 18, 19, 37, 50, 57, 68, 186, 222, 279, 331, 334, 338, 339, 340, 346, 352, 363, 376, 378, 389, 409
synthesis, 121, 330, 460

T

teachers, 35, 52, 132, 133, 134, 135, 136, 137, 242, 301, 304, 305, 320, 325, 326, 328, 352, 362
techniques, 12, 18, 25, 26, 27, 29, 31, 33, 34, 35, 36, 38, 39, 53, 78, 110, 113, 117, 119, 136, 140, 162, 177, 246, 297, 324, 331, 383, 407, 410, 432, 433, 434, 435, 436, 437, 438, 439, 441, 442, 443, 491, 492
technology-enhanced multimodal meditation, 178, 179, 184, 516
telepresence, xvi, 473, 475, 476, 477, 478, 480, 481, 482
tension, 31, 33, 78, 181, 182
testing, xvii, 6, 48, 56, 57, 77, 92, 113, 136, 159, 163, 182, 202, 211, 229, 235, 245, 247, 249, 252, 253, 255, 258, 277, 294, 295, 296, 342, 361, 399, 401, 403, 434, 437, 446, 449, 467, 483, 490, 505
theoretical support, 16
therapeutic agents, 82, 91
therapeutic approaches, 15, 24
therapeutic goal, 128
therapeutic interventions, 11, 46
therapeutic process, 15
therapeutic relationship, 15, 35, 73, 74, 342, 374
therapeutics, xvii, 178, 509, 513, 514
therapist, xvi, 17, 35, 36, 38, 43, 44, 45, 46, 47, 48, 49, 53, 399, 402, 473, 474, 477, 478, 479, 480, 481, 486, 487
therapy, xiii, xvi, 6, 14, 15, 17, 18, 20, 23, 24, 25, 26, 27, 30, 35, 36, 37, 38, 39, 40, 41, 42, 44, 53, 60, 63, 73, 79, 80, 104, 105, 110, 111, 123, 125, 127, 128, 130, 132, 137, 169, 170, 172, 174, 178, 179, 180, 181, 183, 184, 211, 220, 224, 227, 323, 372, 390, 404, 421, 442, 445, 446, 473, 474, 477, 480, 481, 510, 516
therapy interventions, 44
thoughts, 8, 24, 26, 31, 32, 38, 39, 60, 300, 302, 312, 317
threats, 312, 313, 338
thuja occidentalis, xiii, 93, 94, 96
toddlers, 275, 287, 389, 390
training programs, 372, 389
trauma, 5, 6, 15, 17, 18, 19, 21, 24, 40, 74, 80, 286, 287, 288, 294, 295, 299, 321, 323, 327, 328, 360, 382, 470, 481, 510
traumatic brain injury, 57, 73, 80
traumatic experiences, 310, 315, 320, 322
treadmill training, 199, 202, 204
treatment, 4, 5, 11, 12, 13, 14, 15, 16, 17, 18, 19, 20, 21, 24, 27, 29, 31, 33, 34, 36, 37, 38, 39, 40, 42, 43, 44, 45, 47, 48, 52, 55, 56, 57, 58, 60, 61, 63, 64, 65, 66, 67, 68, 72, 73, 78, 93, 94, 95, 124, 127, 128, 129, 161, 162, 177, 178, 180, 181, 211, 221, 223, 224, 274, 276, 277, 282, 290, 292, 298, 299, 300, 301, 310, 311, 314, 317, 319, 321, 322, 323, 324, 325, 327, 328, 329, 330, 332, 340, 342, 352, 353, 354, 359, 363, 366, 367, 369, 371, 376, 380, 383, 384, 388, 399, 474, 481, 484, 510, 511, 512
tremor, 409, 410, 415, 487
trial, 52, 60, 68, 78, 79, 105, 115, 151, 162, 163, 166, 208, 209, 210, 215, 217, 218, 219, 258, 259, 260, 350, 351, 371, 372, 373, 375, 388, 389, 403, 415, 437, 439, 441, 449, 456
tricyclic antidepressants, 57, 60
triggers, 31, 32, 34, 320, 322, 361
trustworthiness, 118, 119, 120, 122

U

United Kingdom, 117, 131, 137, 223, 255, 405, 431, 445, 473, 491, 523
United Nations, 4, 8, 376
United States, 3, 4, 11, 23, 30, 72, 153, 161, 230, 273, 289, 290, 299, 307, 333, 337, 343, 345, 347, 348, 350, 351, 352, 356, 365, 366, 380, 384, 391, 519, 523
urban, 72, 74, 158, 245, 246, 253, 391

urban areas, 245, 246
urban population, 391
urinary tract infection, 99
urine, 57, 99, 295, 339
usability, xvii, 113, 137, 162, 175, 184, 236, 245, 249, 250, 251, 252, 253, 254, 406, 408, 410, 416, 417, 421, 429, 434, 446, 447, 448, 451, 456, 509, 513, 514, 515, 516
usability testing, 113, 245, 249, 252, 253, 434
user compliance, 169
uterine fibroid, 93, 94, 95, 96

V

vagina, 296, 304, 320
vagus nerve, 74, 80
velocity, 77, 195, 197, 198, 202, 264, 265, 268, 410, 412, 433, 434, 436, 442, 487
vibro-acoustic therapy, 178
victimization, 5, 8, 273, 290, 313, 316, 323, 328, 330, 379
victims, 6, 235, 256, 274, 276, 286, 290, 291, 292, 295, 297, 298, 315, 366, 368, 384
video games, 159, 193
video-based attention monitoring, 169, 170
videos, 165, 166, 172, 173, 310, 432
violence, 50, 274, 275, 277, 287, 288, 292, 306, 320, 340, 344, 365, 369, 372, 375, 376, 378, 380, 381, 383, 389, 390, 391
virtual characters, xiv, 121, 122, 147
virtual companion, 118
virtual environment therapy, 178
virtual environments, 124, 127, 137, 147, 152, 208, 214, 419, 429, 443, 446, 459, 460, 470, 474, 481
virtual reality, xiv, xv, xvi, xvii, 107, 114, 115, 123, 124, 125, 130, 132, 134, 137, 148, 152, 169, 171, 183, 185, 186, 187, 192, 198, 199, 200, 204, 205, 206, 208, 211, 214, 221, 222, 223, 224, 229, 395, 403, 404, 420, 422, 429, 431, 432, 443, 445, 446, 456, 457, 459,469, 473, 477, 480, 481, 482, 490, 509, 510, 516
virtual reality diagnostics, 509
virtual reality environment, 214, 429
virtual reality exposure therapy (VRET), 473, 474, 479, 480, 481
virtual rehabilitation, xvi, 123, 124, 125, 126, 127, 129, 137, 149, 393, 395, 398, 431, 432, 441
virtual world, xiv, 110, 116, 124, 126, 127, 153, 154, 155, 156, 157, 158, 159, 161, 162, 163, 165, 166, 167, 435, 448, 453

vision, 57, 117, 118, 140, 224, 229, 230, 231, 232, 234, 235, 236, 237, 239, 242, 256, 337, 417, 429, 448, 490, 493, 495, 496, 497, 498, 499, 500, 501, 507, 510
visual acuity, 294, 415
visual impairments, 242, 491, 492, 493, 497, 504, 505, 506, 507
visual modality, 126, 128, 129
visual stimuli, 194, 197, 198, 401
visually impaired, xv, 238, 242, 245, 253, 254, 256, 261, 263, 491, 492, 493, 497, 506
vulnerability, 274, 289, 315, 318

W

walking, 51, 170, 171, 172, 174, 175, 180, 185, 194, 199, 200, 201, 202, 203, 204, 250, 252, 415, 436, 443
water, 83, 84, 85, 182, 194, 195, 197, 198, 214, 215, 221, 222, 240, 284, 285
web, 116, 165, 231, 488, 505
web browser, 505
web pages, 505
websites, 236
weight gain, 63, 64, 279, 337
weight loss, 44, 167, 279, 337, 339
weight management, 279
welfare, xvi, 7, 26, 185, 253, 300, 310, 322, 342, 344, 346, 347, 349, 351, 352, 353, 354, 355, 356, 357, 358, 359, 360, 362, 363, 365, 368, 371, 376, 380, 381, 383, 384, 388, 389, 391, 519, 521
welfare law, 7, 347, 352, 356
welfare system, 7, 358, 360, 380
well-being, 4, 200, 275, 293, 337, 340, 347, 366, 371, 519
wellness, 71, 73, 178, 371, 389, 510, 513
Wii balance board, 193
workflow, 109, 110, 111, 113, 114
working memory, 147, 148, 152, 214, 220, 221
workload, 150, 406, 410, 412, 415, 421
workplace, 78, 80, 178, 183, 459, 460
workplace wellness, 178

Y

young adults, 56, 63, 65, 148, 307
young people, 12, 131, 132, 299, 328